Cardiovascular Diagnosis
The initial examination

Cardiovascular Diagnosis
The initial examination

J. Willis Hurst, M.D., M.A.C.P.
Consultant to the Division of Cardiology
Department of Medicine
(Professor and Chairman, Department of Medicine, 1957-1986)
Emory University School of Medicine
Atlanta, Georgia

with 370 illustrations

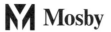 Mosby

St. Louis Baltimore Boston Chicago London Madrid Philadelphia Sydney Toronto

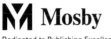 **Mosby**

Dedicated to Publishing Excellence

Executive Editor: Stephanie Manning
Developmental Editor: Laura DeYoung
Project Manager: Gayle May Morris
Production Editor: Judith Bange
Manufacturing Supervisor: Kathy Grone
Designer: Susan Lane
Cover design: GW Graphics

Printed in the United States of America
Composition by Clarinda Company
Printing/binding by Maple-Vail Book Manufacturing Group

Mosby–Year Book, Inc.
11830 Westline Industrial Drive
St. Louis, Missouri 63146

Library of Congress Cataloging in Publication Data

Hurst, J. Willis (John Willis)
    Cardiovascular diagnosis: the initial examination / J. Willis Hurst.
        p.   cm.
    Includes bibliographical references and index.
    ISBN 1-55664-392-6
    1. Cardiovascular system—Examination.   2. Cardiovascular system—
Diseases—Diagnosis.   I. Title.
    [DNLM: 1. Cardiovascular Diseases—diagnosis.
    2. Electrocardiography.   3. Physical Examination.   WG 141 H966
1993]
    RC670.H87   1993
    616.1' 075—dc20
    DNLM/DLC   93-17183
    for Library of Congress   CIP

93 94 95 96 97 / 9 8 7 6 5 4 3 2 1

Because "I am a part of all that I have met,"* this book is dedicated:

To my parents, John Millet Hurst and Verna Bell Hurst, who made many sacrifices for me . . .

To my wife, Nelie, and our sons, John, Steve, and Phil, and their families, who make my life complete . . .

To Harry Harper, V.P. Sydenstricker, William Hamilton, and Perry Volpitto, who were my teachers during the glorious days of medical school and house staff training at the Medical College of Georgia . . .

To Paul Dudley White and his colleagues, who inspired me during my cardiology fellowship at Massachusetts General Hospital . . .

To my many colleagues at Emory University, especially Bruce Logue, Paul Beeson, Robert Grant, James Warren, Robert Schlant, and Wayne Alexander, who have made my professional life exciting and pleasant . . .

To Eugene Stead, Henry Cooper, Proctor Harvey, and Larry Weed, who have profoundly influenced me . . .

To students, house staff, and fellows, who became my second family . . .

To my patients, who became my friends.

*Alfred, Lord Tennyson: "Ulysses," 1842.

Preface

Sir Arthur Conan Doyle created the great detective, Sherlock Holmes. He also created his sidekick, Dr. Watson. It has always bothered me that Doyle, who was a physician, permitted Watson, who was also a physician, to detect the clues but did not program him to appreciate their significance. Doyle allowed Holmes, who was not a physician, to detect the clues *and* appreciate their significance. A physician who engages in diagnostic medicine must be able to detect the diagnostic clues *and* appreciate their significance.

Let us all take a lesson from Helen Keller, who became deaf and blind early in childhood. This brilliant and courageous woman was able to sense many things that were overlooked by others. When a friend communicated that she saw nothing remarkable when she walked through the woods, Helen Keller responded as follows:

> "I wondered how it was possible," Helen said, "to walk for an hour through the woods and see nothing of note. I who cannot see find hundreds of things: the delicate symmetry of a leaf, the smooth skin of a silver birch, the rough, shaggy bark of a pine. I who am blind can give one hint to those who see: use your eyes as if tomorrow you will have been stricken blind.

> "Hear the music of voices, the song of a bird, the mighty strains of an orchestra as if you would be stricken deaf tomorrow.

> "Touch each object as if tomorrow your tactile sense would fail.

> "Smell the perfume of flowers, taste with relish each morsel, as if tomorrow you could never taste or smell again.

> "Make the most of every sense.

> "Glory in all the facets and pleasures and beauty which the world reveals to you."*

This book, *Cardiovascular Diagnosis: The Initial Examination*, highlights the cardiovascular abnormalities that should be seen, heard, or felt during the physician's initial encounter with the patient. This book also emphasizes the significance of the abnormalities. The techniques used in the initial examination are the history, the physical examination, the electrocardiogram, the chest x-ray film, and the "routine"

---

*Reprinted with permission from the American Foundation for the Blind, 15 West 16th Street, New York, N.Y. 10011.

laboratory examination. In today's world these techniques are referred to as being a part of low technology.

The physician-detective who has honed his or her senses of observation, learned to collate the significant information collected by using low-technology techniques, and developed a keen analytic sense should be able to create a specific cardiovascular diagnosis or develop a meaningful differential diagnosis in almost all patients. This approach must be used before high-technology procedures are ordered. This is true because high technology should be used to answer questions raised by the use of low technology. In addition, high technology should not be used unless the anticipated result will enable the physician to improve his or her treatment of the patient. The first four chapters of this book deal with the evolution of our knowledge of the initial cardiovascular examination and the approach to the patient with cardiovascular disease. The next five chapters discuss the information that can be obtained using low technology. The final chapter deals with the indications for, the limitations of, and the cost of high technology.

Every effort has been made to make this book reader-friendly. Accordingly, it is "several books in one," because entire books have been written on most of the chapters included in this book. When the details of the initial examination are discussed in one book, it is more likely that the reader will appreciate the importance of integrating and correlating the results of each technique with the results of the other techniques. A diagnosis can be made, or a differential diagnosis can be created, in almost all patients. Finally, as discussed in Chapter 10, it should be obvious that high technology is used to answer questions raised by the proper use of low technology. When this is not done, high-technology procedures may be used improperly.

Why this book was written

The inital examination is currently being downgraded in training programs and in the practice of medicine. This deficiency should be corrected. The patient with severe chest pain and simultaneous paralysis of the legs does not need a myelogram but does need an esophageal echocardiogram. The diagnosis, based on the symptoms, is dissection of the aorta. The echocardiogram is not needed for diagnostic reasons. It is used to delineate the extent of the aortic dissection and to assist in determining if surgery is needed. This example serves to emphasize that if one is poor at using low-technology procedures, he or she is likely to be disastrous at ordering proper high-technology procedures.

There is evidence that some physicians may go through the motions of performing an initial examination but do not detect or appreciate significant abnormalities that are present. It is a wise physician who extracts all the information that is possible from the history, physical examination, electrocardiogram, chest x-ray film, and "routine" laboratory work. Should physicians "go through the motions" but fail to extract the maximum information that is possible, they are coming dangerously close to performing a deceptious examination. We must remember: the patient believes that the physician is an expert in all aspects of the initial examination that the physician performs.

It is apparent that not all physicians improve the skills they use in performing the initial examination despite ordering a large number of high-technology procedures. The results of properly used high technology should improve the physician's ability to perform an initial examination. For example, the data collected by echocardiography or cardiac catheterization should enable the physician to improve his or her ability to determine the severity of mitral stenosis using the results of the history, physical examination, electrocardiogram, and chest x-ray film.

Many physicians do not know the costs of high-technology procedures. Accordingly, the costs of many diagnostic procedures and tests are listed in Chapter 10. Expensive high technology is needed; no one doubts that. The goal should be to use it wisely. The wise use of high technology depends on the questions raised by low technology. When a question is poorly formulated, the use of high technology will be abused and the cost of medical care will continue to rise.

A final reason for the publication of the book is as follows. I wrote "The Examination of the Heart: The Importance of Initial Screening" for *Disease-A-Month* (1990), a Mosby publication, at the request of Dr. Roger Bone. Because of its warm reception by readers and its success, I was asked to write an expanded version of the booklet. I agreed and proceeded to create this book.

•   •   •

I am indebted to Mary Cotton and Carol Miller, who helped in the preparation of the manuscript. There was much to type and much to "keep straight." They did both beautifully.

I am indebted to Stephanie Manning, Laura DeYoung, and Judi Bange of Mosby. They demonstrated professionalism at its best.

I am deeply indebted to my wife, Nelie. She makes the house we live in a home to enjoy. Although during the creation of this book our home looked like a library, she tolerated the disarray. Even as books, journals, and manuscripts were piled on the tables, floors, and beds of four rooms of our home, she accepted the mess with reasonable equanimity. Truly there could be no book without her help. No Nelie—no book.

J. Willis Hurst

Acknowledgments

This book could not have been written without the help of my predecessors and colleagues. I thank them for passing along to me the diagnostic clues that are discussed in this book.

I thank the publishers and authors for permitting me to use material that has been published elsewhere; the book is testimony to their willingness to share.

Chapter 5

I have written extensively on "the history" in other books and journals and have used the following previously published material as a resource for the creation of this chapter:

- *The Heart* (first 6 editions) by J. Willis Hurst, editor-in-chief; published by McGraw-Hill, Inc., New York, N.Y.
- "The History: Symptoms and Past Events Related to Cardiovascular Disease" by J. Willis Hurst, Douglas C. Morris, I. Sylvia Crawley, and Edward R. Dorney; and "Atherosclerotic Coronary Heart Disease: Historical Benchmarks, Methods of Study and Clinical Features, Differential Diagnosis, and Clinical Spectrum" by J. Willis Hurst. Chapters 9 and 50, respectively, in *The Heart* (seventh edition; 1990) by J. Willis Hurst, editor-in-chief; published by McGraw-Hill, Inc.
- "The History" by J. Willis Hurst. Chapter in *Hurst The Heart* (eighth edition; in press), edited by Robert C. Schlant and R. Wayne Alexander; published by McGraw-Hill, Inc.
- "The Examination of the Heart: The Importance of Initial Screening" by J. Willis Hurst. Article in *Disease-a-Month*, Volume 36, Number 5, May 1990; published by Mosby.
- "Angina Pectoris: Words Patients Use and Overlooked Precipitating Events" by J. Willis Hurst and R. Bruce Logue. Editorial in *Heart Disease and Stroke*, March/April 1993; published by the American Heart Association, Inc., Dallas, Tex.

Chapter 6

Many of the figures in Chapter 6 were originally published in "The Examination of the Heart: The Importance of Initial Screening" by J. Willis Hurst, *Disease-a-Month*, Volume 36, Number 5, May 1990.

I thank Dr. Marilynne McKay, Professor of Dermatology at Emory University, Atlanta, Ga., for her review of the section on skin disorders.

Chapter 7

The chapter on electrocardiography could not have been written without the masterful work of Robert Grant, who created the method of vector electrocardiography. Harvey Estes was at his side, and he should be rewarded for his clear thinking and excellent teaching.

Many of the concepts discussed in this chapter are discussed in greater detail in *Ventricular Electrocardiography* (1991) by J. Willis Hurst; published by Gower Medical Publishing, New York, N.Y.

Most of the electrocardiograms showing cardiac arrhythmias are reproduced from the book *Introduction to Electrocardiography* (1973) by J. Willis Hurst and Robert J Myerburg; published by McGraw-Hill, Inc.

Most of the other electrocardiograms reproduced in this chapter are from the electrocardiographic laboratory at Emory University Hospital and Clinic. They are used through the courtesy of Dr. Wayne Alexander, who is Director of the Division of Cardiology of the Department of Medicine at Emory University School of Medicine, and Dr. Paul Walter, who is Director of the Electrophysiologic Laboratory at the same institution. A few of the electrocardiograms are from other Emory University owned or affiliated facilities, including Crawford Long Hospital, Grady Memorial Hospital, and the Atlanta Veterans Administration Medical Center. They are used through the courtesy of Dr. Douglas Morris, Dr. Robert Schlant, and Dr. David Harrison. I thank my colleagues for permitting me to use electrocardiograms that were recorded on their patients.

Some of the illustrations were recreated from other publications. The sources have been carefully identified in the legends of the figures.

I thank Jan Mulder for her excellent artwork. We worked together for almost 2 years in an effort to create the graphics that would teach the reader. She redrew all of the electrocardiograms in an effort to display clean and clear tracings. She is patient, creative, pleasant, and extraordinarily competent. The computer played an important part in the creation of the artwork, but the computer would just sit there until Jan commanded it to work. We finished the project a short time before the delivery of her baby boy. I recommended the name Vector, because he was exposed to so many vectors prior to birth, but she said she preferred the name Nathan.

Chapter 8

I thank Dr. Wade Shuford, Professor of Radiology at Emory University School of Medicine, for reviewing this chapter and contributing many of the illustrations.

Chapter 9

I thank Dr. Dallas Hall, Professor of Medicine at Emory University School of Medicine, for reviewing this chapter.

Chapter 10

I thank the following experts at Emory University School of Medicine for reviewing the discussions assigned to them. They made useful suggestions for the improvement of the text.

- The sections on ambulatory recording of the electrocardiogram, signal-averaged electrocardiography, and electrophysiologic studies were reviewed by Dr. Sina Zaim, Assistant Professor of Medicine (Cardiology).
- The sections on exercise thallium-201 scan and positron emission tomography (PET) were reviewed by Dr. Randolph Patterson, Professor of Medicine (Cardiology).
- The section on computed tomography was reviewed by Dr. Murray Baron, Professor of Radiology.
- The section on magnetic resonance imaging was reviewed by Dr. Roderic Pettigrew, Associate Professor of Radiology.
- The section on myocardial biopsy was reviewed by Dr. Jerre Lutz, Associate Professor of Medicine (Cardiology).

Finally, I thank Dr. Michael Gravanis, Professor of Pathology, for assisting me in obtaining the costs of the procedures that are performed in the clinical laboratory.

J. Willis Hurst

Contents

Cardiovascular Diagnosis
The initial examination

CHAPTER 1

Evolution of cardiovascular diagnostic thought and methods

I have often wondered whether scientific evolution is subject to the same law that governs the evolution of species: natural selection. Observing the evolution of scientific ideas and concepts, we perceive an everchanging scene that does not seem to differ from the changing panorama of biological evolution. Can the law that governs evolution also determine history of science?

The basis of natural selection is the genetic material with its replications and with the occurrence of mutations, which lead to new variations. It appears to me that the evolution of human thought is also based on the genetic material, because mind is the distillation of soma and thus is determined by natural selection. The thoughts and ideas of a genius represent mutations. They are newly created concepts. In the creation of both species and ideas, natural selection blindly wields its unrelenting scythe. But while natural selection of the species is blind and random, science does have a definite goal, that of finding solutions. In medicine, moreover, applicability and usefulness play an important role. Natural selection of ideas occurs from within: the individual personality, the intellectual capacity, or the innovations of a genius. Natural selection is also influenced from without: the tenure and temper of time and foremost their applicability, in medicine their usefulness. This confers on the history of science and of medicine a personal and often heroic aspect. It is this human element that links science to art.

RICHARD J. BING 1990[1]*

The survival of diagnostic thought and methods depends on their usefulness in day-to-day work. The purpose of this chapter is to trace the evolution of cardiovascular diagnostic thought and methods to the present. Although the same approach could be used to trace therapeutic thought and action, this discussion is limited to the diagnostic portion of the physician's work.

History teaches us that at any point in time diagnostic methods can be divided into (1) the method used in the initial examination and (2) other methods that are used to answer questions not fully answered by analyzing the results of the initial examination. Invariably, the diagnostic methods that have survived over time are those that permit the physician to make diagnoses using the results of the initial ex-

---

amination and those that answer questions raised by the initial, routine examination. In addition, new diagnostic procedures that survive but are not used initially, may yield information that improves the diagnostic skills used in the initial examination. In other words, a feedback loop is commonly created that improves the physician's skills. The feedback loop will not be completed, however, without the conscious effort of the physician.

This chapter highlights the evolution of diagnostic thought and methods currently used to examine the cardiovascular system. Subsequent chapters deal with the information and skills required to perform the initial cardiovascular examination. Indications for the use of diagnostic procedures that are not used initially are discussed in Chapter 10.

The reader should remember that this text does not deal with the evolution of all of our knowledge concerning the heart and circulation but relates exclusively to the evolution of diagnostic thought and methods required to examine the cardiovascular system.

DIAGNOSTIC THOUGHT AND METHODS BEFORE THE MID-TWENTIETH CENTURY

In the past, physicians used the symptoms expressed by patients to identify the presence of heart disease. Many excellent observers contributed to this type of examination, and William Heberden's description[2] of angina pectoris in 1768 is representative of the type of observations that were made by perceptive physicians in England, Germany, France, Italy, and other countries throughout the world. Heberden did not know what caused the angina pectoris he described. However, he posed the question regarding its cause, and Edward Jenner, who performed autopsies on patients who died with prolonged angina, answered it in 1799[3]; angina, he determined, was caused by atherosclerosis of the coronary arteries. These events indicate how physicians learned during that period; inquisitive physicians correlated the patient's symptoms with the information they discovered at autopsy. Accordingly, because they were correlators, their skill in the analysis of symptoms improved.

Although many physicians contributed to the method of physical examination, the work of René T.H. Laennec[4] particularly illustrates the contribution of physical examination to the examination of the heart. Laennec invented the stethoscope and reported on its use in 1819. Prior to his invention physicians had to apply their naked ear to the chest and precordium in order to examine the heart and lungs. Initially there was considerable resistance to the use of Laennec's stethoscope, but it was finally accepted as an instrument to be used routinely on every patient. Laennec and others began to correlate the sounds and noises they heard by using the stethoscope with the abnormalities they discovered at autopsy, and they thereby improved their auscultation skills.

The next instrument to be developed was the mercury sphygmomanometer by Scipione Riva-Rocci[5] in 1896. Initially only the systolic pressure could be measured; then in 1905 Nicolai S. Korotkoff[6] devised the current method of auscultation and sphygmomanometry so that the diastolic pressure could be measured. Prior to the development of the sphygmomanometer, physicians tried to estimate the patient's arterial blood pressure by palpating the arterial pulse. However, by correlating their estimate of the blood pressure with the actual blood pressure obtained by using the new device, they soon learned that they could not estimate the arterial blood pressure accurately. Accordingly, the effort to estimate blood pressure by palpating the arterial pulse was discontinued, and the device was used routinely to measure the arterial blood pressure in all patients. This example is an illustration of a new and better method of examination replacing an old and inaccurate method.

Sir James Mackenzie[7] investigated the pulsations of the neck veins in subjects with normal hearts and in patients with heart disease, and invented the polygraph in 1902. Never used routinely as part of the initial examination of the cardiovascular system, the polygraph was used to learn more about the cardiac physiology responsible for normal and abnormal pulsations of the neck veins. Physicians then correlated their observations of the pulsations of the patient's neck veins with the patient's symptoms, other abnormalities found on physical examination, and the findings at autopsy. Accordingly, their diagnostic and clinical skills improved. The development of the polygraph illustrates how, at times, the information supplied by the use of a new instrument, even when the instrument is later discarded, is used to encourage physicians to observe normal and abnormal phenomena more carefully.

Augustus D. Waller,[8] using a mercury capillary manometer, recorded the first human electrocardiogram in 1887. In 1901 Willem Einthoven[9] improved the galvanometer, which was then used to record the electrocardiogram in selected patients. Sir Thomas Lewis[10] used the instrument before 1913 to study and diagnose cardiac arrhythmias. Although his ability to recognize cardiac arrhythmias was improved by correlating the electrocardiographic abnormalities with his clinical observations, he also identified arrhythmias in the electrocardiogram that could not be identified by physical examination. Frank N. Wilson and many others studied the ventricular electrocardiogram and correlated their findings with the patient's symptoms, the results of physical examination, and the abnormalities found at autopsy.[11] They soon learned that the ventricular electrocardiogram revealed useful information that could often be correlated with the abnormalities found at autopsy. They also discovered that abnormalities could be observed in the electrocardiogram that could not be explained by the findings of the usual routine autopsy of the heart. In addition, they learned that the electrocardiogram could remain normal even though the history, physical examination, and findings at autopsy indicated the presence of serious cardiac disease. As time passed and instrumentation improved, the electrocardiogram was used routinely as a method of examining the heart.

Wilhelm C. Roentgen's discovery of x-rays[12] in 1895 led eventually to the development of the chest x-ray film, which provided physicians with a new method of identifying heart and lung disease. As this method of examination became available to the general population of patients, it replaced certain methods of examining the lungs. Physicians soon learned that physical examination did not permit the diagnosis of small lesions in the lungs and that an x-ray film of the chest was superior to physical examination of the lungs. However, they also learned that physical examination of the lungs was occasionally superior to x-ray examination of the chest. For example, the wheezing of bronchial asthma is detected by physical examination rather than by roentgenography of the chest. Again, however, physicians learned more as they correlated the patient's complaints, findings on physical examination, and findings on the chest x-ray film with the abnormalities found at autopsy.

The x-ray film of the chest also revealed signs of heart disease. The size of the heart and its individual chambers could be determined more accurately by examination of the chest x-ray film than by physical examination. This was determined by correlating the abnormalities found at autopsy with the abnormalities found by physical examination and those found on the chest x-ray film. The posteroanterior x-ray film of the chest soon gained its place in the routine examination of the heart and lungs, and the technique of percussion of the chest to determine the size of the heart and individual cardiac chamber enlargement was discontinued. Physicians then learned that palpation of the precordium and auscultation of the heart revealed abnormalities of the heart that could not be detected on the chest x-ray film.

Angiocardiography, which was simultaneously developed by Augustin Castellanos et al.[13] and by George P. Robb and Isreal Steinberg[14] in the late 1930s, provided anatomic information of the heart that was not previously available. As discussed later, the technique has been improved to the point where it is commonly used, but it is not part of the initial examination of the heart. The information it yields, however, has improved the skill of physicians who wish to improve their ability to perform an initial examination of the heart. Diagnostic skill is improved when the patient's symptoms, abnormal physical signs, abnormalities detected on the chest x-ray film, abnormalities found in the electrocardiogram, and abnormalities found at autopsy are correlated with the abnormalities found by angiocardiography.

The phonocardiogram was used extensively during the late 1930s and 1940s in an effort to understand heart sounds and murmurs. Never performed as a routine initial procedure, it was used to elucidate the physiologic mechanisms responsible for heart sounds and murmurs. Today it is rarely used, but the information gained by correlators such as Samual A. Levine and W. Proctor Harvey,[15] as well as Aubrey Leatham,[16] should be used each time the stethoscope is placed on the precordium.

Just before and around the time of the mid–twentieth century, the kinetocardiogram, ballistocardiogram, and vectorcardiogram were used extensively. However, they were never performed routinely and did not withstand the test of time. The information these procedures yielded was either not unique or sufficiently useful to justify their continued use. Accordingly, other techniques replaced them.

Before the mid–twentieth century, examination of the urine consisted of determination of the specific gravity, identification of white and red blood cells and casts, and identification of albuminuria and glycosuria. Examination of the blood consisted of measurement of the hemoglobin, red and white blood cell counts, the differential white blood cell count, measurement of nonprotein nitrogen, and a fasting blood glucose determination. Although these measurements were of value in screening the patient for anemia, infection, renal disease, and diabetes, however, they did not provide diagnostic clues to the presence of cardiovascular disease. Obviously, these tests did reveal evidence of renal disease that might be related to the hypertension; red blood cells in the urine that occasionally provided a clue to the presence of infective endocarditis; and glucose in the urine or an abnormally elevated fasting blood glucose level that identified the patient with diabetes mellitus, who might also have coronary atherosclerosis.

As time passed, physicians continued to correlate the complaints of patients, the results of physical examination, the observations made by electrocardiography, the findings on the chest x-ray film, and the abnormalities discovered by routine examination of the blood and urine with the abnormalities found at autopsy. During this period clinical pathologists were making great advances, and their insights were being incorporated into the thought processes of practicing clinicians. In addition, cardiac physiologists were explaining how the heart worked in health and in disease, and this information was also correlated with data collected through an analysis of symptoms, the results of physical examination, data obtained by electrocardiography and the interpretation of the x-ray film of the chest, the findings of the routine laboratory examination, and the findings at autopsy.

Thus by the mid–twentieth century the initial cardiovascular examination consisted of the history, including the analysis of symptoms and other subjective information; the physical examination; the interpretation of the electrocardiogram; the interpretation of the chest x-ray film; and the routine laboratory examination (which yielded few diagnostic clues to the presence of cardiovascular disease).

DIAGNOSTIC THOUGHT AND METHODS AFTER THE MID–TWENTIETH CENTURY

The turning point in the development of cardiovascular medicine came when cardiac catheterization became commonplace. Although a "catheter" was used by Stephen Hales[17] in 1796 to record the blood pressure in a mare and "catheters" were inserted into the hearts of animals by Auguste Chauveau and Ettienne J. Marey[18] in 1861, it was the brilliant Claude Bernard[19] who in 1879 published a diagram showing how he performed cardiac catheterization in animals. Werner Forssmann[20] performed the first human cardiac catheterization on himself in 1929 but was not allowed to continue his work. O. Klein[21] used the procedure on 18 patients in 1930. André Cournand and H.A. Ranges (1941),[22] John McMichael and E.P. Sharpey-Shafer (1944),[23] and Richard J. Bing et al. (1947)[24] used cardiac catheterization in humans to study cardiac physiology.

In 1945 E.S. Brannon et al.[25] at Emory University were the first to report the use of the technique for diagnostic purposes when they catheterized a patient with an atrial septal defect. Eugene A. Stead, Jr.,[26] and others at Emory studied patients with heart failure. E. de F. Baldwin et al.[27] reported the diagnosis of ventricular septal defect in 1946. L. Dexter et al.[28,29] contributed significantly to the use of the technique in the late 1940s. Henry Zimmerman performed cardiac catheterization of the left side of the heart soon after he developed his catheterization laboratory in 1947.[30]

Mason Sones was the first to perform selective coronary arteriography in a human in 1958.[31] This procedure has influenced the practice of cardiology more than any other single procedure; it led the way for improved diagnostic and therapeutic advances, including coronary bypass surgery. Coronary angioplasty, as developed by Andreas R. Gruentzig,[32] could not have been developed without the development of coronary arteriography.

Cardiac catheterization and visualization of the chambers of the heart and coronary arteries are not used routinely, so why are they mentioned in a book that deals primarily with the initial examination of the heart? It is because the results of these procedures have taught clinicians to become better observers. Accordingly, history taking, physical examination, interpretation of the electrocardiogram, and interpretation of the x-ray film of the chest improved when clinicians began correlating the data collected from these methods of examination with the data collected from cardiac catheterization and cardiovascular angiography. A trainee in cardiology who spends a year working in a cardiac catheterization laboratory and does not correlate the data collected through the use of these procedures with the data collected using the routine skills of examination might, at the end of the year, know little more about the initial examination of the heart than he or she did before the year of training. I once asked a third-year cardiac fellow to discuss the x-ray film of a patient with a secundum atrial septal defect with a group of medical residents and cardiac fellows; I was chagrined to discover that despite his spending almost a year in one of our cardiac catheterization laboratories, he could not comply with my request. He was embarrassed, and I was embarrassed for him. He later asked me for special sessions in the interpretation of chest x-ray films.

Having the results of cardiac catheterization and cardiovascular angiography, including coronary arteriography, not only improves the skill of physicians in performing the initial examination of the patient but also encourages clinicians to think physiologically. This improvement, however, cannot occur unless physicians are obsessed with the correlation of medical data; the feedback loop must be completed!

Although Arthur M. Masters and H.L. Jaffee[33] reported the use of the exercise electrocardiogram in 1941, this procedure was not used extensively until after about 1960, when it became possible to correlate the patient's symptoms and the results of coronary arteriography with the abnormalities found in the exercise electrocardiogram. The test is not part of the initial examination. However, as discussed later, the need for and safety of the test are determined by the results of the initial examination.

Working at Emory University, Robert P. Grant created the vector method of interpreting the electrocardiogram in 1947.[34] New information regarding the depolarization sequence of the heart and the conduction system was added by D. Durrer[35] and Mauricio B. Rosenbaum et al.,[36] respectively. This new information was then added to the knowledge base used in routine electrocardiography. In addition, it has become possible to perform electrophysiologic studies on patients with certain troublesome arrhythmias. Obviously, electrophysiologic procedures are not used routinely; their use is determined by questions raised by the initial, routine examination.

Body surface mapping of the electrical potential has improved our understanding of the standard electrocardiogram, but it is not, as yet, used routinely as part of the initial examination.[37]

Echocardiography was introduced to diagnostic cardiology by Inge Edler and C.H. Hertz[38] in 1953. Harvey Feigenbaum[39] was one of the major leaders in its clinical development and usage. Three-dimensional echo-Doppler and transesophageal echocardiography are now used commonly. The size of the cardiac chambers, the contractility of the ventricles, the ejection fraction, the structural appearance of heart valves, the magnitude of the aortic valve pressure gradient and pulmonary artery pressure, intracardiac shunts, the presence of calcification, and cardiac masses and vegetations on the heart valves can be identified by using this technique. These procedures are not used in the initial examination, but some type of echocardiography may be used routinely in the future. The progress made in this field has been achieved by correlating the patient's symptoms, the results of the physical examination, the results of the interpretation of the electrocardiogram, the results of the interpretation of the chest x-ray film, the results of cardiac catheterization and cardiovascular angiography (including coronary arteriography), and the findings at autopsy with the abnormalities found with the echo-Doppler technique. A trainee working in the echocardiographic laboratory should become highly skilled in auscultation of the heart. However, such trainees may not improve their auscultatory skill unless they make a conscious effort to correlate their auscultatory findings with the echocardiogram.

As radioisotopes became available, it was predictable that they would be used to study the heart. Herman L. Blumgart and Somma Weiss[40] used a radium C salt to measure the circulation time in 1927, and Myron Prinzmetal et al.[41] used a radioisotope to create a radiocardiogram in 1948. By 1980 radioactive technetium and thallium were used to identify the contractile ability of the ventricles and myocardial perfusion deficits, respectively. At the time of this writing the positron emission tomography (PET) scan is being touted by some as being superior to the thallium scan as a method of identifying myocardial ischemia.[42] Here again, the clinician must learn to correlate the results of these tests with the patient's symptoms, the results of the physical examination, the interpretation of the electrocardiogram, the interpretation of the chest x-ray film, the results of cardiac catheterization and coronary arteriography, the results of echo-Doppler studies of the heart, and the abnormalities found at autopsy. Tests using radioisotopes are not used in the initial examination of the heart, but the results of the initial examination are used to determine if important remaining questions can be answered by nuclear testing.

The computed tomography (CT) scan[43] and magnetic resonance imaging (MRI)[44,45] are remarkable techniques. Although they are not part of the initial examination of the heart, the results of these techniques should be correlated with the data collected through the analysis of the patient's symptoms, the results of the physical examination, the results of the interpretation of the electrocardiogram, the results of the interpretation of the chest x-ray film, the results of echo-Doppler technique, the results of cardiac catheterization and cardiovascular angiography (including coronary arteriography), the results of nuclear studies, and the abnormalities found at autopsy. When this type of correlation is performed, the skill of the clinician improves.

After the midpoint of the twentieth century routine laboratory work increased a great deal for three reasons: the discovery that diseases and conditions could be identified by testing the blood and urine, because in some instances the abnormalities were present in the blood or urine long before other abnormalities could be identified; the development of an automated system of chemical analysis that permitted the measurement of many items quickly and relatively inexpensively (the SMA); and the ability to order a liver profile, complete lipid profile, clotting profile, etc., with the stroke of a pen. Some of these tests are not ordered routinely, and information is needed from other sources to justify the testing. For example, the measurement of the level of the cardiac enzymes (serum glutamic-oxaloacetic transaminase [SGOT], lactic dehydrogenase [LDH], and creatine kinase) is a great advance, but these tests are not done routinely; they are usually ordered in an effort to diagnose the cause of chest pain.

The diagnostic clues to the recognition of cardiovascular disease through the identification of abnormalities in the routine blood and urine examination remain the same as they were before the midpoint of the twentieth century with a few exceptions. Now the blood lipids, including total serum cholesterol, low-density lipoproteins, high-density lipoproteins, and triglycerides, should be measured routinely and then, if they are in the desirable range, not be measured again for several years.[46] If these values are abnormal, appropriate action should be taken. The serum electrolyte values are abnormal sufficiently often to be measured on the routine SMA panel of tests. A low level of serum potassium may suggest hyperaldosteronism but is more commonly due to diuretic therapy. The liver tests, which are also included on the modern routine SMA panel of tests, may also become abnormal when certain drugs are used by the patient.

The last 50 years have been filled with new and effective surgical procedures, including cardiac transplantation. Although these advances are therapeutic rather than diagnostic procedures, the cardiac surgeons have stimulated all of us to improve our diagnostic skills.

Except for the routine measurement of serum lipids and triglycerides, the measurement of the level of serum electrolytes, and tests for liver dysfunction, the diagnostic laboratory procedures that have been developed during the last 40 to 50 years are not used in the initial, routine examination of the cardiovascular system. These include cardiac catheterization and cardiovascular angiography, including coronary arteriography; exercise electrocardiography, Holter monitoring, total body mapping, and electrophysiologic studies; echo-Doppler techniques; nuclear techniques; and the CT scan and MRI. Why, then, are they mentioned in this book, which deals with the initial, routine examination of the cardiovascular system? These techniques are important advances in the field of diagnostic cardiovascular medicine for two reasons:

- They are used to answer questions generated by the physician who performs a careful initial examination. The physician should not use these techniques unless he or she believes the answers provided by them will benefit the patient. Obviously, the more skilled the physician is in performing the initial examination, the clearer his or her questions will be. This in turn leads the clinician to use the new procedures wisely.
- The results of the techniques that are not used routinely should, when they are used, be correlated with the patient's symptoms, the data collected from the physical examination, the data collected by interpreting the electrocardiogram, and the data collected by interpreting the chest x-ray film. When this is done, the skill of the physician in performing the initial examination of the cardiovascular system improves. In addition, in many instances the physician is able to understand the pathophysiology responsible for the abnormalities he or she discovers.

LOW TECHNOLOGY VERSUS HIGH TECHNOLOGY

Eugene A. Stead, Jr.,[47] emphasized that if one wished to make a point during the process of teaching, he or she should make the point several times but should say it differently each time. Accordingly, I wish to make the points discussed up to now by saying them a different way.

We hear a great deal about high technology. The use of the word *high* implies that there is a *low* technology. If so, what is low technology? One can assign the term *low diagnostic technology* to the analysis of symptoms, the performance of a physical examination, the interpretation of the resting electrocardiogram, the interpretation of the chest x-ray film, and the interpretation of the routine laboratory data. The label *high diagnostic technology* can be applied to exercise electrocardiology and Holter monitoring, body surface mapping, and electrophysiologic studies; cardiac catheterization and cardiovascular angiography, including coronary arteriography; echo-Doppler techniques; nuclear studies; and CT scans and MRI.

Low diagnostic technology can be viewed as the first step, and high diagnostic technology can be considered the second step. Obviously, if a physician plans to take a diagnostic walk, it is wise to take a well-placed first step before attempting a second step. However, this simple fact seems difficult for some trainees to understand. One student told me that it was so difficult to obtain a history that it seemed easier to have coronary arteriograms performed on all patients with chest pain. He could then have someone else interpret the coronary arteriogram, and the patient's problem would be solved. I pointed out that coronary arteriography cannot be done without risk, that it costs a great deal, that there are many patients with obstructive coronary artery disease whose chest pain is actually due to another cause, and that many patients have several different types of chest pain due to several different causes. The student replied, "It's hard, isn't it?" I responded, "Yes, like being a professional violinist or any professional person." Learning to use low technology properly is a professional approach to the problem; in addition, it places one in the position of using high technology wisely.

APPROACH OF MODERN CLINICIANS

For many years clinicians made excellent observations but did not catalogue them so that they could be subjected to statistical analysis. Despite this, many superb clinicians became experts in determining the diagnostic value of the presence or absence of abnormalities determined from the initial examination of the heart.

Today the diagnostic value of the presence or absence of diagnostic clues is viewed in the light of Bayes' rule, the sensitivity of the clue, the specificity of the clue, and the predictive *value* of the clue.

Bayes' rule is as follows: the predictive value of a test result (or diagnostic clue) for a particular disease is predetermined by the prevalence of the disease in the population of people being studied. Stated another way, according to Bayes' rule, the probability that the presence or absence of an abnormality indicates the presence or absence of a certain condition depends on the prevalence of the condition in the population of people being tested. In other words, a positive test for pregnancy in a 25-year-old man is a false positive test; it cannot be a true positive test, because pregnancy does not occur in a population of males. An electrocardiogram that reveals no abnormalities (a normal electrocardiogram) made at rest in a 60-year-old man with what is believed to be angina pectoris does not indicate the absence of coronary artery disease, because the resting electrocardiogram is known to be normal in about 80% of a population of 65-year-old men with angina pectoris in whom obstructive coronary disease has been proved to be present by coronary arteriography.

Whereas many clinicians have understood the value of determining the predictive value of abnormalities of laboratory data, few clinicians have understood that the concept is also applicable to the response to a question posed in the history; to the presence or absence of physical abnormalities; and to the presence or absence of abnormalities found in the electrocardiogram, chest x-ray film, and routine laboratory data.

Clinical investigators use the following formula to determine the *predictive value* of a test result (or diagnostic clue)[48]:

$$\text{True positive} = \frac{\text{True positives}}{\text{False positives} + \text{True positives}}$$

$$\text{True negative} = \frac{\text{True negatives}}{\text{False negatives} + \text{True negatives}}$$

The predictive value of a test indicates the likelihood (probability) that a condition is present when the test result (or diagnostic clue) is positive (or present) or the likelihood (probability) that a condition is absent when the test result (or diagnostic clue) is negative (or not present).

Clinical investigators use the following formula to determine the *sensitivity* of a test result (or diagnostic clue)[48]:

$$\text{Sensitivity} = \frac{\text{True positives}}{\text{True positives} + \text{False negatives}}$$

The sensitivity of a test indicates the percentage of times the disease, or condition being sought, is actually present when the test result is positive (or the diagnostic clue is present).

Clinical investigators use the following formula to determine the *specificity* of a test result (or diagnostic clue):

$$\text{Specificity} = \frac{\text{True negatives}}{\text{True negatives} + \text{False positives}}$$

The specificity of a test indicates the percentage of times the disease, or condition being sought, is actually absent when the test result is negative (or the diagnostic clue is absent).[48]

In years past there was little effort to weigh the value of diagnostic clues. For example, when one clue supported the presence of a certain condition and another clue supported the absence of the condition, the inexperienced or disinterested physician was confused. Now an effort is made to know the predictive value of each of the test results (or clues). By assigning a mathematical value to each test result, it becomes obvious which test result has the greatest diagnostic value. A problem remains, however, because predictive values have not as yet been assigned to all test results (or diagnostic clues). The lack of information of this type highlights areas of clinical work that should be subjected to clinical research.

In day-to-day clinical work I tend to use the concept of predictive value of test results (or diagnostic clues) more than I use the concepts of sensitivity and specificity.

Finally, it is useful to recognize that the concept of predictive value should not be applied solely to a single test result (or single diagnostic clue). Clinicians often work with clusters of clues. When several abnormalities are present, all indicating that a certain condition is present, the consortium of clues may have a powerful predictive value for a specific disease. This is true even when the predictive value of individual clues making up the cluster is not great. I often use the comments of the cartoonist Charles Schultz to emphasize this point. To paraphrase: Lucy, speaking with anger to Charlie Brown, says, "See this hand. The individual fingers mean nothing, but when I use them to make a fist, it makes a weapon that is a terror to behold."

Modern clinicians use the diagnostic value found in the initial examination to estimate the pretest probability that a disease process or condition is present. The pretest probability is then used to determine the need for a specific type of high-technology procedure.

Key Points

- The routine initial examination of the cardiovascular system evolved over a period of centuries.
- The initial examination of the cardiovascular system consists of the analysis of symptoms, the results of the physical examination, the interpretation of the electrocardiogram, the interpretation of the chest x-ray film, and the interpretation of the routine laboratory data.
- Before 1940 to 1950 physicians improved their skills of history taking; physical examination; and interpretation of the electrocardiogram, chest x-ray film, and routine laboratory data by correlating the information obtained through these methods with the abnormalities found at autopsy and identified in the polygram and phonocardiogram, which, of course, were not used routinely.
- None of the diagnostic procedures that have been added since about 1940 is used in the initial examination of the cardiovascular system. An exception to this statement is the routine measurement of blood lipids and serum electrolytes.

The new diagnostic procedures are used to clarify problems — to answer questions — identified by analyzing the results of the initial examination. Clinicians must extract all of the diagnostic information they can from the initial examination in order to pose the proper questions that may be answered by procedures that are not used routinely. The clinician who correlates all of the diagnostic data that is collected should be able to improve his or her skills in the use of the initial examination.

- Low diagnostic technology includes the history; the physical examination; and the interpretation of the electrocardiogram, chest x-ray film, and routine laboratory data. High diagnostic technology includes the exercise electrocardiogram; Holter monitoring; electrophysiologic testing; body surface mapping; cardiac catheterization and angiocardiography, including coronary arteriography; echo-Doppler studies; nuclear testing; and the use of CT scans and MRI.

- Clinicians who use low diagnostic technology with great skill are more likely to use high diagnostic technology properly. Clinicians who use low diagnostic technology poorly are likely to use high diagnostic technology poorly.

- Modern clinicians must understand Bayes' rule, predictive value, sensitivity, and specificity of diagnostic clues. Modern clinicians must also develop the ability to determine the pretest probability that a disease process is present, because this probability determines the need for a high-technology procedure. These concepts should be applied to individual clues, as well as to clusters of clues.

REFERENCES

1. Bing RJ: Evolution of cardiology: triumph and defeat, *Perspect Biol Med* 34(1):1, 1990.
2. Heberden W: Some account of a disorder of the breast, *Med Trans* (published by the College of Physicians in London) 2:59, 1772.
3. Baron J: *The life of Edward Jenner, M.D.*, London, 1838, Henry Coburn, p 39 (letter to Dr. William Heberden, dated 1786).
4. Laennec RTH: *Traite' de L'auscultation mediate*, ed 2, Paris, 1826, Brosson et Chaude.
5. Riva-Rocci S: Un nuovo sfigmomanometro, *Gazz Med Torino* 47:981, 1896.
6. Korotkoff NS: On method of studying blood pressure, *Izv Voennomed Akad* 11:365, 1905.
7. Mackenzie J: *Principles of diagnosis and treatment in heart affections*, London, 1916, Oxford Medical Publications, p 48.
8. Waller AD: Demonstration on man of the electromotive changes accompanying the heart's beat, *J Physiol* 8:229, 1887.
9. Einthoven W: Un nouveau galvanomètre, *Arch Néerl Sci*, ser 2, 6:625, 1901.
10. Lewis T: *Clinical electrocardiography*, London, 1913, Shaw & Sons.
11. Johnston FD, Lepeschkin E, editors: *Selected papers of Dr. Frank N. Wilson*, Ann Arbor, Mich, 1954, Edwards Brothers.
12. Roentgen WC: Ueber eine neue Art von Strahlen, *Sitzung Physikal-Medicin Gesellschaft* 137:132, 1895. (English translation: *Science* 3:227, 1896.)
13. Castellanos A, Pereira R, Garcia L: L'angiocardiographie chez l' enfant, *Presse Med* 46:1474, 1938.
14. Robb GP, Steinberg I: Visualization of chambers of the heart, the pulmonary circulation, and the great blood vessels in man: a practical method, *AJR* 41:1, 1939.
15. Levine SA, Harvey WP: *Clinical auscultation of the heart*, ed 2, Philadelphia, 1959, WB Saunders.
16. LeathamA: Phonocardiography, *Br Med Bull* 8:333, 1952.
17. Hales S: *Statical essays: haemastaticks*, vol 2, London, 1733, Innys & Manby, p 361.
18. Chauveau A, Marey J: Determination graphique des rapports du choc du coeur avec les mouvements des oreillet-

tes et des ventricles; experience faite a l'aide d'un appareil enregistreur (sphygmographe), *C R Acad Sci* 53:622, 1861.

19. Bernard C: *Lecons de physiologie operatoire*, Paris, 1879, JB Baillière et Fils, p 278.
20. Forssmann W: Die Sondierung des rechten Herzens, *Klin Wochenschr* 8:2085, 1929.
21. Klein O: Zur Bestimmung des zirkulatorischen Minutenvolumers beim Menschen nach dem Fickschen Prinzip (Gewinnung des gemischten venosen Blutes mittels Herzsondierung), *Munch Med Wochenschr* 77:1311, 1930.
22. Cournand A, Ranges HA: Catheterization of the right auricle in man, *Proc Soc Exp Biol Med* 46:462, 1941.
23. McMichael J, Sharpey-Schafer EP: Cardiac output in man by direct Fick method: effects of posture, venous pressure change, atropine, and adrenaline, *Br Heart J* 6:33, 1944.
24. Bing RJ, Vandam LD, Gray FD Jr: Physiological studies in congenital heart disease. I. Procedures, *Bull Johns Hopkins Hosp* 80:107, 1947.
25. Brannon ES, Weens HS, Warren JV: Atrial septal defect: study of hemodynamics by the technique of right heart catheterization, *Am J Med Sci* 210:480, 1945.
26. Stead EA Jr: The role of the cardiac output in the mechanisms of congestive heart failure, *Am J Med* 6:232, 1949.
27. Baldwin E de F, Moore LV, Noble RP: The demonstration of ventricular septal defect by means of right heart catheterization, *Am Heart J* 32:152, 1946.
28. Dexter L, Haynes FW, Burwell CS et al: Studies of congenital heart disease. I. Technique of venous catheterization as a diagnostic procedure, *J Clin Invest* 26:547, 1947.
29. Dexter L, Haynes FW, Burwell CS et al: Studies of congenital heart disease. III. Venous catheterization as a diagnostic aid in patent ductus arteriosus, tetralogy of Fallot, ventricular septal defect, and auricular septal defect, *J Clin Invest* 26:561, 1947.
30. Hurst JW: History of cardiac catheterization. In King SB III, Douglas JS Jr, editors: *Coronary arteriography and angioplasty*, New York, 1985, McGraw-Hill, p 4.
31. Ibid, p 5.
32. Gruentzig AR: Transluminal dilatation of coronary artery stenosis, *Lancet* 1:263, 1978.
33. Masters AM, Jaffee HL: Electrocardiographic changes after exercise in angina pectoris, *J Mt Sinai Hosp* 7:629, 1941.
34. Grant RP, Estes EH: *Spatial vector electrocardiography*, Philadelphia, 1952, Blakiston.
35. Durrer D: Electrical aspects of human cardiac activity: a clinical physiological approach to excitation and stimulation, *Cardiovasc Res* 2:1, 1968.
36. Rosenbaum MB, Elizari MV, Lazzari JO et al: The differential electrocardiographic manifestations of hemiblocks, bilateral bundle branch block, and trifascicular blocks. In Schlant RC, Hurst JW, editors: *Advances in electrocardiography*, vol 1, New York, Grune & Stratton, p 145, 1972.
37. Mirvis DM: Current status of body surface electrocardiographic mapping, *Circulation* 75:684, 1987 (editorial).
38. Edler I, Hertz CH: The diagnostic use of ultrasound in heart disease, *Acta Med Scand* 208:32, 1955.
39. Feigenbaum H: *Echocardiography*, ed 2, Philadelphia, 1976, Lea & Febiger.
40. Blumgart HL, Weiss S: Studies on the velocity of blood flow. II. The velocity of blood flow in normal resting individuals, and a critique of the method used, *J Clin Invest* 4:14, 1927.
41. Prinzmetal M, Corday E, Bergman HC et al: Radiocardiography: a new method for studying the blood flow through the chambers of the heart in human beings, *Science* 108:340, 1948.
42. Schelbert HR, Mody FV: Positron emission tomography. In Pohost GM, O'Rourke RA, editors: *Principles and practices of cardiovascular imaging*, Boston, 1991, Little, Brown, p 293.
43. Bateman TM: X-ray computed tomography. In Pohost GM, O'Rourke RA, editors: *Principles and practices of cardiovascular imaging*, Boston, 1991, Little, Brown, p 423.
44. Bloch F: Nuclear induction, *Phys Rev* 70:460, 1946.
45. Doyle M, Cranney GB, Pohost GM: Basic principles of magnetic resonance. In Pohost GM, O'Rourke RA, editors: *Principles and practices of cardiovascular imaging*, Boston, 1991, Little, Brown, p 455.
46. Brown WV: Lipoproteins: what, when, and how often to measure, *Heart Dis Stroke* 1(1):20, 1992.
47. Stead EA Jr: *What this patient needs is a doctor*, Durham, NC, 1978, Carolina Academic Press (edited by GS Wagner, B Cebe, and MP Rozear,) p 111.
48. Leaverton PE: *A review of biostatistics: a program for self-instruction*, ed 2, Boston, 1978, Little, Brown, p 95.

CHAPTER 2

Goals of the initial examination

If the confidence of the patient is secured at the start and he is put at once at his ease, the results for both patient and doctor may mean the difference between success and failure in the proper handling of the case, which is more than simply the establishment of the correct diagnosis and the outline of the special cardiovascular treatment. Sometimes trivial remarks, actions, or occurrences may destroy the confidence or ease of the patient and so prevent the successful evolution of the case. It is at the very outset that the physician must use the greatest care.

PAUL DUDLEY WHITE 1931[1]*

Practicing physicians, medical students, house officers, and fellows examine patients. At the same time that they are being examined, patients are examining the practicing physician, medical student, house officer, or fellow. Patients try to determine if the individual who is examining them is kind, thoughtful, gentle, patient, and trustworthy. Simply stated, patients try to decide if they like the examiner. If they do, they may draw the conclusion that the examiner is competent. If they do not like the examiner, they may draw the conclusion that the examiner is not competent. During the examination practicing physicians, medical students, house officers, and fellows must collect useful scientific data and, equally important, must establish an appropriate personal relationship with the patient. As discussed later, it is during the history-taking period that both of these goals can and should be achieved.

Practicing physicians almost invariably believe they have an excellent relationship with their patients. They probably do, because in the long term, dissatisfied patients seek their medical care elsewhere. Accordingly, established members of the practicing physician's clientele generally like the physician and have a good relationship with him or her. The initial encounter is a different matter, however, and practicing physicians, medical students, house officers, and fellows must develop the sensitivity to determine whether they are, at that moment, establishing an excellent doctor-patient relationship. This is a great challenge, because patients come from different worlds—a farmer's world is different from that of a lawyer whose world is different from that of a statesman, whose world is different from that of an 80-year-

---

*Reprinted with the permission of Macmillan Publishing Company from *Heart Disease* by Dr. Paul Dudley White, p 9. Copyright 1931 Macmillan Publishing Company; copyright renewed © 1959 Paul Dudley White.

old woman. Somehow, though, even beginners must learn to slip into the world of each of the patients they see—and be accepted.

The methods used in the initial examination of the cardiovascular system include eliciting the patient's history and other subjective data, the physical examination, interpretation of the electrocardiogram, interpretation of the chest x-ray film, and interpretation of certain routine laboratory data.

CREATION OF A TRUSTFUL RELATIONSHIP

The proper doctor-patient relationship is usually established during the history-taking period, when the examiner asks questions and the patient gives answers. The skilled examiner learns to listen to the patient, and it is during this exchange that the patient draws his or her conclusions regarding the trustworthiness and competence of the physician. Because the examiner usually continues to converse with the patient during the time that the physical examination is being performed, the effort to establish a trustful relationship should continue during that part of the examination. Finally, when the examination is completed, the relationship between the physician and the patient becomes firmly established when the physician summarizes his or her medical findings and treatment plans with the patient and family. Simply stated, the proper doctor-patient relationship is created by talking and listening. Although there are many opportunities to establish a trustful relationship with a patient, the initial encounter between the examiner and the patient is of primary importance. If the initial encounter is poorly managed, it is unlikely that a good doctor-patient relationship will be attained.

We sometimes hear that physicians today have poorer relationships with patients than they did formerly. Furthermore, the problem is often blamed on the excessive use of high technology. However, high-technology machines neither interfere with nor encourage a relationship between the physician and the patient. If the accusation of poorer doctor-patient relationships is true, it is because physicians are not talking with or listening to their patients; or when they do talk with their patients, they do not talk with them properly. Talking improperly with a patient can cause far more harm than a silent high-technology machine.

COLLECTION OF SCIENTIFIC INFORMATION

The examiner obtains scientific information from the history, the physical examination, the interpretation of the electrocardiogram, the interpretation of the chest x-ray film, and the interpretation of certain laboratory data. The data per se should be interpreted as scientifically as possible.

To summarize, taking the history has a dual purpose. The history-taking exercise must be used by the practicing physician, medical student, house officer, or fellow to establish the proper relationship with the patient and to elicit excellent scientific data from the patient. Each of the methods of examination may yield scientific information, but a trustful relationship between the examiner and the patient is established for the most part during the history-taking period.

INITIAL CARDIOVASCULAR EXAMINATION IN CONTEXT

The initial examination of the cardiovascular system must never be implemented as an isolated event for obvious reasons: it is not possible to formulate a diagnosis or to create diagnostic and therapeutic plans about one body system without knowing the medical problems of all of the body systems. The value of this admonition is explained best with an example:

A 65-year-old man has advanced cancer of the lung, insulin-dependent diabetes, and stable angina pectoris (Class 2). The detection of stable angina pectoris (Class 2) would usually prompt one to order a coronary arteriogram, but cancer of the lung, discovered on the chest x-ray film, determines the approach to the patient. This is because the survival curve for cancer of the lung is worse than the survival curve for stable angina pectoris (Class 2). A judgment is made by the physician that it would not be wise to pursue any further definition of the heart disease, because a serious disease has been found in another body system.

Accordingly, an important goal for the physician is that he or she must collect scientific data about all of the body systems in order to make a judgment regarding the need to pursue conditions involving the cardiovascular system (see Chapter 4).

Key Points

- The purpose of the history (and the collection of all subjective data), the physical examination, the interpretation of the electrocardiogram, the interpretation of the chest x-ray film, and the interpretation of certain routine laboratory data is to collect information that is analyzed in a scientific manner.
- The history-taking exercise, more than any of the other techniques of examination, has a dual purpose. In addition to collecting the scientific information revealed by the history, it is equally important for the physician to use the history-taking period—the interview—to establish a trustful relationship with the patient.
- The physician must collect sufficient data about all of the body systems so that diagnostic and therapeutic judgment can be made about the conditions found in the cardiovascular system. Cardiovascular conditions must never be viewed in isolation; they must be viewed in the context of all of the patient's illnesses.

REFERENCE

1. White PD: *Heart disease*, New York, 1931, Macmillan, p 9.

CHAPTER 3

A disciplined approach, thoroughness, good judgment, communication, and records

System, or as I shall term it, the virtue of method, is the harness without which only the horses of genius travel.

SIR WILLIAM OSLER[1]

I have worked with practicing physicians, medical students, house officers, and cardiology fellows for 40 years. As medicine has become more complex, it has become increasingly evident that all of us need a map and a compass in order to achieve our goals in the care of patients. The map, designed to create order and to simplify, must be teachable. The compass must always point toward the goal. Together the map and the compass should create a linkage between medical knowledge and the actions used to care for the patient. Larry Weed[2] drew the best map and designed the best compass.

DISCIPLINED APPROACH

Modern medicine demands a disciplined approach. Without a system, a physician may lose his or her way. That is, intellectual goals may not be clearly defined, and patient care objectives may be poorly formulated. As stated in the preceding paragraph, Weed[2] created the best system. His approach is referred to as the problem-oriented system and is discussed later in this chapter.

THOROUGHNESS[2]

The word *thoroughness* sounds good, but without a definition it cannot be implemented. In an effort to satisfy an open-ended definition of thoroughness, a physician could spend all day taking a patient's history and more than an hour performing the neurologic examination, as well as require the patient to spend several days in a clinical laboratory. This extreme example is mentioned in order to emphasize that in the practical world efficiency demands that the data required to screen the patient for illness be collected in a reasonable time period and cost as little as possible. Furthermore, the practice of good medicine requires that we collect only the scientific data needed. It is not proper to collect data just because the information is interesting; it must be useful in the care of the patient. With these constraints being placed on us, it is necessary to define the data to be collected during the initial examination of the patient (see Chapters 5 through 9).

The constraints imposed by the rules of a basketball game, or any other game, can be used as a metaphor for the limitations placed on the examiner during the initial examination. The rules of the basketball game are clearly stated: the game is to last a specified period of time; the players must handle the ball in an agreed-on manner, as well as follow other rules regarding their behavior; and the playing court is a certain size. The objective of the game is clear—to place the ball through a hoop that is located at a specific height—and the score must be kept according to specified guidelines. The initial examination also involved certain rules: the information to be collected must be defined in advance of the examination; the skill required to collect the data must be perfected; the data must be collected in a reasonable amount of time; and the data collected must be recorded and displayed in such a way that the information can be readily understood by associates and other health workers.

Thoroughness, then, should be defined in terms of the type and amount of data to be collected within a reasonable and specified amount of time. To make this point, let us assume that there are 100 items to be sought in the initial examination and that an examiner identifies only 50 of them; one could conclude that the examiner is only 50% thorough. The importance of each omission is a separate issue; the data to be collected must be of significant value and, if collected every time a patient is examined, should be useful in establishing the illnesses that affect the patient.

GOOD JUDGMENT[3]

Good judgment is as difficult to define as wisdom. Good judgment implies that assessments and decisions have been made and that these assessments and decisions are accurate. The following are two examples of good judgment:
- When a physician senses that he or she has embarrassed a patient by discussing a sensitive subject, the physician should direct the questioning to more pleasant subjects. To delay the questioning shows good judgment, because if the answers to the embarrassing questions are important, they can be probed again later—after a trustful relationship with the patient has been established.
- Suppose a physician realizes that two treatment options—medical and surgical—are available for the treatment of a specified disease. The physician must compare the operative risk and morbidity with the survival curve and complication rate of medical treatment alone. When the track record of the physician

reveals that he or she usually makes the correct choice, we state that the physician has good judgment.

Some people maintain that good judgment cannot be learned or taught and that a physician either has it or does not have it. I do not agree with this view. I believe that good judgment is difficult to learn and to teach but that with effort it can be learned and taught.

The following points are relevant to the development of good judgment:

- The physician must realize that there are more diagnostic and therapeutic options in modern medicine than there were in years past. Accordingly, during the initial examination it is necessary to collect the appropriate data that will permit the physician to formulate the questions clearly, determine if the questions should be answered, choose the proper diagnostic option(s), and finally choose the proper therapeutic action.
- The creation of a problem list that displays all of the patient's problems is essential (see later discussion). This list should be studied with the following specific question in mind: what diagnostic or therapeutic plan should be implemented for any one of the problems when it is viewed in the light of the other problems?
- The physician must know the predictive value of individual diagnostic clues and clusters of clues.
- The physician must be sensitive to the feelings the patient has regarding his or her illness. This statement does not imply that the physician allows the patient to decide which diagnostic or therapeutic approach he or she should accept; it is the physician's responsibility to make medical decisions. The physician should, however, know the patient's reactions and emotional makeup well enough that the physician can present the decision in such a way that it is acceptable to the patient. When the decision is not acceptable to the patient, the relationship with the physician should be such that an excellent doctor-patient relationship continues.
- The physician must know the indications, risks, and contraindications for the diagnostic and therapeutic procedures he or she recommends. It is not sufficient to use the medical literature as the only source of this information; the physician must use data collected from his or her own institution.
- Physicians struggling to have good judgment know the medical literature relative to the problem being solved. The literature reporting clinical trials is of great value but should not be viewed as gospel. A major drawback of clinical trials is that the patients selected to enter them have usually been chosen according to the results of the initial examination, which may have been inadequately performed. If the initial examination was faulty, the entire trial will be faulty. Despite this limitation, performing an analysis of clinical trials improves the judgmental ability of an experienced physician.

- A physician's judgment improves when he or she analyzes his or her own track record of decision making. Such analysis is not possible without appropriate records.
- Perhaps the most important aspect of good judgment is that physicians must recognize that there is such a thing and be sufficiently mature to focus their efforts on making proper choices when several options are available.

COMMUNICATION

Communication implies that the individual who is talking or writing is able to convey his or her thoughts to the individual who is listening or reading. Communication requires the use of language that is understood by the sender and receiver. It also implies that the talker or writer has the ability to sense if his or her message is actually understood by the listener or reader. Communication in medicine is more important today because medicine is more complex than it was a few decades ago. Accordingly, the proper use of words is more important than it was some years ago. For example, many diseases have been divided into subsets of illness that must be carefully defined, because the diagnostic procedure and therapy used for one subset may be different from the diagnostic procedure and treatment used for another subset of the same medical condition. For example, stable angina pectoris and unstable angina pectoris are subsets of angina pectoris, but the molecular biology and pathophysiology responsible for each type of angina are different, the procedures used to study each type of angina are different, and the treatment for each type of angina is different. The physician of today must use words and terms with great care.

PROBLEM-ORIENTED MEDICAL RECORD

Weed's perception of the medical record[2] is that of a document that leads and guides the examiner to elicit the right items (data base), analyze data properly, create a numbered problem list, formulate plans for each problem, and describe the patient's response to the plans in a follow-up note.

When implemented properly by the physician, the problem-oriented medical record encourages the self-discipline that is necessary to work through the complex medical problems that confront the modern clinician, and it becomes a document that communicates to associates, nurses, and other health care personnel. These benefits of the problem-oriented record can be recognized immediately. Other benefits will accrue for the examiner who takes the problem-solving approach seriously. This approach (which educators claim is lacking in American education) leads one to think in terms of things that really matter. In addition, the problem-oriented record is helpful to medical teachers.[4] When used properly, the problem-oriented record displays the facts that have been collected by the examiner, the analysis of the facts and the formulation of a set of problems based on the facts, the action taken for each problem, and the follow-up of each problem. Teachers should review and discuss each of these steps with medical students, house officers, and fellows rather than lecture (announce facts) and give exams to determine if facts alone are being transiently memorized.[4] The problem-oriented record also provides a map for the seasoned physician to follow so that he or she does not omit important items but does become increasingly skilled at transferring medical knowledge to the care of the patient.

The problem-oriented record, as described by Weed,[2] consists of four parts: the defined data base, the problem list, initial plans, and follow-up progress notes.

Defined data base

As indicated earlier, it is necessary to define in advance the medical information that should be collected from the patient in order to identify diseases or abnormalities. The goal of the endeavor must be kept clearly in mind, because an ophthalmologist, for example, does not need to collect the same data from the patient that a primary care physician should collect. Also, the examiner must possess the skill and time to collect the information from the patient.

This book deals with the initial examination of the cardiovascular system. Accordingly, Chapters 5 through 9 deal with the data that should be collected from the patient in order to identify abnormalities of the cardiovascular system. The techniques used to collect information about the cardiovascular system are history taking, the physical examination, electrocardiography, chest roentgenography, and the performance of a few laboratory tests.

As emphasized throughout this book, abnormalities of the cardiovascular system and cardiovascular disease processes should not be viewed as isolated conditions; they must always be viewed in the context of all of the patient's disease processes. This is especially true when the treatment of cardiovascular disease is being considered. For example, should coronary bypass surgery be offered to a 75-year-old man with mild, stable angina pectoris whose memory is failing and who, in addition, has a bronchogenic carcinoma of the lung? It is not wise to treat an organ, such as the heart, with disregard for the diseases that are present in other organs. It is wise to collect information from the patient that will screen each organ for disease processes and abnormalities. In other words, it is wise to treat the patient as a whole; it is erroneous to consider an organ a separate and unrelated part of the person. One does not admit coronary arteries to a coronary care unit; coronary arteries are attached to people, who have their own unique personalities and commonly have other, noncardiac diseases that may influence the investigation and treatment of a coronary artery event. Thus data must be collected during the initial examination that will enable the examiner to identify any abnormalities or disease processes in any of the body systems. The reader is referred to other books for discussion of the type of data to be collected during the initial examination of organs other than the heart.

Problem list

Let us assume that the items in the defined data base have been collected (see Chapters 5 through 9). The examiner must then determine which items are normal and which items are abnormal. The examiner must survey the data and, when he or she is able to do so, create clusters of abnormalities that seem to identify a new perception—a new understanding of the patient's illness. For example, suppose a patient with severe essential hypertension exhibits a large heart due to left ventricular enlargement, dyspnea on exertion, and a left ventricular gallop sound. The physician deduces that the patient has hypertensive heart disease and heart failure. This perception should be placed on the problem list, and a complete diagnosis can be made (see Chapter 4 for a discussion of the creation of a complete cardiovascular diagnosis). On the other hand, suppose a patient has a temperature elevation of 2 degrees and no other abnormalities are detected. The problem—elevation of temperature—should be placed on the problem list, but a complete diagnosis cannot be made. The former example represents the problem statement for a diagnosis, and the later example represents the problem statement for an abnormality that must be investigated. All abnormalities identified in the data base must be accounted for in the problem list, either as attributes of diagnoses or as separate problems.

The problems should be numbered and titled on a specially designated sheet of paper that is placed at the front of the medical record.

Obviously, different physicians may create different problem lists for the same patient, because the problem list depends on the data collected, which in turn depends on the skill of the examiner. In addition, one examiner may have a different knowledge base and may be more experienced than another in interpreting abnormalities and analyzing data. The problem list is a table of contents of the patient's conditions as viewed by the examiner. The beginner should be making an effort to improve his or her data collection skills and should look up every abnormality he or she finds; as times passes, the examiner will be able to fit the abnormalities he or she finds into more highly refined problem statements. More experienced physicians must not forget this discipline, because they will continue to discover abnormalities that they do not understand, and when this occurs, they must look them up.

The creation of an excellent problem list is an intellectual accomplishment. It requires a knowledge of the information needed to make a diagnosis. Accordingly, all diagnoses listed must be defensible in terms of modern medical thinking. On the other hand, as the examiner looks up abnormalities he or she has listed on the problem list, he or she may reconstruct the problem list and pull the abnormalities together into a diagnosis. This is accomplished by marking through (but not erasing) several problems and listing the new perceived diagnosis as a separate numbered problem. An arrow should be placed after each abnormality as a signal that it is being pursued. Also, as new data become available, the problems should be updated to a higher level of understanding. The date of the progress note that explains how the problem was updated should be placed above the arrow, and the new perception should be placed after the arrow.

Teachers of medicine should check the data bases and problem lists created by all students, house officers, and fellows.[4] A skilled teacher should determine if the data are correct and, by studying the problem list, determine if the data were used correctly to formulate the problem statements.

Initial plans

Initial plans should be written for each problem in which a judgment has been made that plans are needed. The problem number and title should be restated in the record, and three types of plans should be written: diagnostic plans, therapeutic plans, and educational plans.

There are two types of *diagnostic plans*. When the cause of the problem is not understood—such as chest pain—a differential diagnosis should be developed. It is useful to write down the diagnostic tests that will be done to identify the conditions listed in the differential diagnosis. Furthermore, it is wise to establish the priority of the workup. Diagnostic plans are also written when the complete diagnosis is known but further diagnostic work is needed in order to implement a specific treatment. For example, when unstable angina pectoris due to coronary atherosclerosis has been diagnosed from data in the defined data base, it is proper to write that a coronary arteriogram is needed to delineate the anatomy of the coronary arteries. An order for the coronary arteriogram should be written on the order sheet of the hospitalized patient with the order numbered and titled exactly as it is numbered and titled on the problem list. It is important that the numbers and titles of the orders match the numbers and titles on the problem list so that a colleague, nurse, or other health care worker can determine at a glance why a procedure is being ordered.

Therapeutic plans are stated in writing for each problem. The plans may be to use drugs, surgery, or some other type of treatment. The order written on the order sheet of a hospitalized patient must be numbered and titled to match the number and title of the problem as it is listed on the problem list; communication breaks down if this is not done.

Educational plans are written for each problem. It is here that the responsible physician recounts what he or she has told the patient. Such items as the side effects of drugs, the operative risks compared with the outcome without surgery, the risks of procedures, and anything else that the patient needs to know to be a knowledgeable partner in his or her diagnostic workup and treatment should be included. The educational plan is important in that it documents the discussion the physician has with the patient and notifies all others who participate in the care of the patient what the patient has been told. This note is usually brief, but in some situations it may be the longest note in the record.

To repeat, plans are written for a problem when a decision is made by the physician that a plan is needed for the problem. The plans are numbered and titled to match the numbers and titles of the problems that are stated on the problem list. Diagnostic, therapeutic, and educational plans should be written for each problem. All orders are numbered and titled to match the numbers and titles of the problems.

Follow-up progress notes

The results of the diagnostic plans for each problem must be sought and recorded. Obviously, the physician must have the medical knowledge to make the appropriate diagnostic observations that are needed to determine if the treatment is succeeding or failing. When the cause of a poorly understood problem is being investigated, the physician incorporates the results of the diagnostic procedures into his or her thought processes.

The progress note is numbered and titled to match the problem list. The physician's observations and new data are organized under four headings: new *S*ubjective data, new *O*bjective data, *A*ssessment of the data, and new *P*lans (SOAP). New plans should always be subdivided into diagnostic, therapeutic, and educational aspects, just as they were subdivided when the initial plans were developed.

The follow-up progress note just described is called a narrative progress note. A flow sheet is also a progress note and should be used when it is useful to correlate several different variables over a period of time. For example, it is easier to correlate the blood glucose level, urine glucose and acetone levels, state of coma, and insulin dosage in a patient with diabetic coma when the appropriate data are plotted on a flow sheet.

Key Points

- Weed's problem-oriented medical record[2] enables the physician to translate medical knowledge into medical care. The medical record that is so brief that it reveals nothing is of no value. Even worse is the long medical record that rambles on endlessly in a completely disorganized manner. The problem-oriented record demands that the one who writes it address the items required for the care of the patient. It forces the physician to focus his or her efforts and to communicate the proper elements of the patient's care to others who are involved in the patient's care.

- The record is created during the examiner's initial encounter and subsequent encounters. This book deals exclusively with steps one and two of the four-step system—the defined data base and the problem list; it does not deal with plans or follow-up. An excellent problem list depends on the ability of the examiner to collect the appropriate data and to synthesize the data into new perceptions. If one cannot collect the proper data and cannot synthesize the data into new perceptions, then the plans will be incorrect and the follow-up will be misdirected.

REFERENCES

1. *Osler aphorisms*, New York, 1950, Henry Schuman (collected by RB Bean; edited by WB Bean), p 72.
2. Weed LL: *Medical records, medical education, and patient care*, Chicago, 1971, The Press of Case Western Reserve University.
3. Feinstein AR: *Clinical judgment*, Baltimore, 1967, Williams & Wilkins.
4. Hurst JW: *The bench and me*, New York, 1992, Igaku-Shoin.

CHAPTER 4

Cardiac appraisal

The adoption during the last few years of a simple and clear-cut classification of heart disease has been of such service to us in the cardiac clinic at the Massachusetts General Hospital and to practicing physicians with whom we have discussed it that a brief paper outlining it has seemed desirable. We have assembled this classification in its present, fairly stable form from our experience in the cardiac clinic in particular, and from the writings of Mackenzie, Lewis and Cabot.

. . . There are three main headings, under each of which every patient with cardiac symptoms or signs should be classified. They are, first, etiology; second, structural change; and third, functional condition. . . . One of the most important reasons for insisting on the etiologic diagnosis, besides allowing much greater accuracy in prognosis, is to forward the prevention of heart disease, about which the medical world is beginning to take more action than in the past.

PAUL DUDLEY WHITE and MERRILL M. MYERS 1921[1]*

1921

Paul Dudley White and Merrill M. Myers[1] wrote a two-page article in 1921 that revolutionized the way physicians thought about, talked about, and wrote about heart disease. The quotation that introduces this chapter is from their article.

White developed a defined data base that was printed on thick, durable paper that folded on itself so that there were six writing surfaces. On this "case record" card, which measured 6 by 4 inches, he recorded the results of his examination of the patient in a meticulous fashion and stated his appraisal of the patient in terms of the etiology, structural change, and functional condition on the front of the record (Box 4-1). These standardized records were later used by White as background information for his first book, *Heart Disease,*[3] which established him as the father of American cardiology.

White and Meyers[1] indicated in their 1921 article that an "additional functional grouping such as that suggested by the New York Association of Cardiac Clinics is also very useful."

---

*Reproduced with permission from White PD, Myers MM: The classification of cardiac diagnosis, *JAMA* 17(18):1414-1415. Copyright 1921, American Medical Association. White,[2] who wrote many scientific articles and shaped American cardiology, believed that this brief communication was one of the most important articles he wrote during the 1920s.

Box 4-1 Case record*

Name _____ Serial No. _____ Date _____

Address _____ Tel. _____

Age _____ M S W D   Occupation _____ 1 2 3 4 5

Seen in office, at home, hospital _____ * _____

Referred by _____ Dec. _____

Address _____ Nec. _____

Cardiac diagnosis

Etiological
Structural
Functional
How much is normal activity limited by cardiac condition?

Other diagnoses

Chief complaint (duration) _____

PI, onset _____

_____

_____

_____

_____

Reprinted with the permission of Macmillan Publishing Company from *Heart Disease* by Dr. Paul Dudley White, p 5. Copyright 1931 Macmillan Publishing Company; Copyright renewed © 1959 Paul Dudley White.

*This box shows the "front card," or first page, of White's "case record" card. Abbreviations and special designations are as follows: *Tel.*, telephone number; *M*, married; *S*, single; *W*, widowed; *D*, divorced; *1* to *5* refer to grades of financial status of the patient from *1*, of very limited means, to *5*, wealthy; *, for special study; *Dec.*, date of death (deceased); *Nec.*, postmortem examination (necropsy); *PI*, present illness.

1928 TO 1973

The New York Heart Association expanded the concept of classifying heart disease in 1928 in a publication titled *Criteria for the Classification and Diagnosis of Heart Disease.*[4] The New York Heart Association has subsequently created eight editions of this book, which I consider a conceptual breakthrough in medicine and one of the most important contributions to cardiology. Every physician who examines the heart should understand the concepts set forth in this book.

These concepts continued unchanged through six editions of the book (until 1973). The committee responsible for the book insisted that a *complete cardiac diagnosis* should include the etiologic diagnosis, the anatomic diagnosis, the physiologic diagnosis, and the physical capacity of the patient (functional diagnosis) (Box 4-2). The implication was that the examining physician could not understand the patient's cardiac condition unless these elements of the complete diagnosis were identified. As new knowledge about the heart and circulation was developed, the etiologic, anatomic, and physiologic components of the complete cardiac diagnosis could be stated more accurately than was possible when White first published his views on the subject. The functional condition of the patient continued to be listed as a separate cat-

---

Box 4-2 New York Heart Association's classification of a complete diagnosis of cardiovascular disease*

Old (prior to 1973)[4]	New (1973)[5]
Etiology	Etiology
Anatomy	Anatomy
Physiology	Physiology
Functional capacity	Cardiac status and prognosis
Therapeutic	Specific recommendations

*See Box 4-3. The category Functional Capacity has been abandoned and replaced by Cardiac Status and Prognosis. The old category, Functional Capacity, was determined by the amount of effort required to produce symptoms in a patient. The new category, Cardiac Status and Prognosis, is determined by integrating all of the data (natural history, anatomy, physiology, laboratory data, and symptoms) into the category. Cardiac status is then classified as (1) uncompromised, (2) slightly compromised, (3) moderately compromised, or (4) severely compromised. Prognosis is designated as (1) good, (2) good with therapy, (3) fair with therapy, or (4) guarded with therapy. Additional diagnostic work, medical and surgical treatment, and the amount of exercise permitted are designated under Specific Recommendations.

The New York Heart Association's functional classification for heart failure is still used, but it should be listed under Physiology. The Canadian Cardiovascular Society's classification of angina has replaced the New York Heart Association's classification and should be listed under Physiology.

Box 4-3   Functional classification*

Class I. Patients with cardiac disease but without resulting limitations of physical activity. Ordinary physical activity does not cause undue fatigue, palpitation, dyspnea, or anginal pain.

Class II. Patients with cardiac disease resulting in slight limitation of physical activity. They are comfortable at rest. Less than ordinary physical activity causes fatigue, palpitation, dyspnea, or anginal pain.

Class III. Patients with cardiac disease resulting in marked limitation of physical activity. They are comfortable at rest. Less than ordinary physical activity causes fatigue, palpitation, dyspnea, or anginal pain.

Class IV. Patients with cardiac disease resulting in inability to carry on any physical activity without discomfort. Symptoms of cardiac insufficiency or of the anginal syndrome may be present even at rest. If any physical activity is undertaken, discomfort is increased.

Reprinted with permission from the Criteria Committee of the New York Heart Association: *Diseases of the heart and blood vessels: nomenclature and criteria for diagnosis*, ed 6, Boston, 1964, Little, Brown and Company, pp 112-113.

*This classification is now used to categorize the patient's symptoms of heart failure; angina pectoris is classified and categorized according to the guidelines created by the Canadian Cardiovascular Society.

---

egory. Accordingly, angina pectoris and the dyspnea of heart failure were classified into four groups (Box 4-3).

This classification of the functional capacity of a patient was used until 1973.[5] However, although the functional classification served a useful purpose for almost half a century, it was misused by some physicians, who erroneously believed that a patient with no symptoms always had a good prognosis, that patients with mild symptoms always had a fairly good prognosis, and that all patients with severe symptoms had a poor prognosis. This misconception created problems in relation to work, retirement, and insurability. Still, the intention of this discussion is not to fault a system that classified patients according to symptoms because there was inadequate information available to do otherwise. In fact, as discussed subsequently, such a system is still extremely valuable; however, it must be viewed in a different way than it was formerly.

AFTER 1973

The Criteria Committee of the New York Heart Association made a bold and proper move in the seventh edition of their book, which was published in 1973.[5] They recognized the contribution of modern diagnostic technology to our understanding of asymptomatic, but serious, heart disease that could be treated successfully; mildly symptomatic, but serious, heart disease that could be treated successfully; severely symptomatic heart disease that could be treated successfully; and the natural history of the various subsets of a specific type of heart disease. The committee recognized the therapeutic advances that were being made in surgery, pharmacology, and preventive cardiology, which, of course, altered the prognosis of any given patient. Thus in the seventh edition of the book, which was titled *Nomenclature and Criteria for Diagnosis of Diseases of the Heart and Great Vessels,* and which was published in 1973, the committee made a change in the classification (see Box 4-2).[5] A portion of the preface is presented here:

> The most radical change from previous editions is the abandonment of the Functional and Therapeutic Classification. A new classification of the patient's overall cardiac status and prognosis seemed indicated by the greater precision of modern diagnostic techniques and the improvements in specific surgical and medical therapies.
>
> The Functional and Therapeutic Classification of previous editions required that the physician classify the patient's cardiac status on the basis of symptoms alone, without regard to the etiologic, anatomic, or physiologic diagnoses. Although a consideration of symptomatology is essential for a correct physiologic diagnosis, it is now recognized that a classification of cardiac status based on symptoms alone may be misleading. Symptoms may be absent in the presence of serious anatomic and physiologic abnormalities, and the necessity for medical or surgical intervention may not be appreciated. In addition, symptoms may appear only after serious changes have taken place in the heart and lungs, which can prevent an effective attack upon the underlying defect. Further, some therapies may alter the symptoms and the course of the disease only briefly, whereas others may fundamentally change the course of the disease. Recommendations for therapy can rarely be based on a single diagnostic category; the implications of the other two categories also must be considered.
>
> With these considerations in mind, a new classification, Cardiac Status and Prognosis, is presented. This classification should reflect an accurate assessment of each patient based on the etiologic, anatomic, and physiologic diagnoses and on an understanding of the benefits of present therapies.*

The eighth edition of the book was published in 1979.[6] A portion of that preface is presented also:

> The classification of the patient's overall Cardiac Status and Prognosis (which, in the seventh edition, replaced the old Functional and Therapeutic Classification) continues to be indicated in view of modern diagnostic techniques that have been capable of enlarging the concepts of a single diagnostic statement to include the stage of a disease as well as its name. Furthermore the interplay of the more specific medical and surgical ther-

---

*Reprinted with permission from the Criteria Committee of the New York Heart Association: *Nomenclature and criteria for diagnosis of diseases of the heart and great vessels,* ed 7, Boston, 1973, Little, Brown and Company, pp vii-viii.

apies and their effects upon the basic disease picture must be part of modern cardiac appraisal. The use of this classification also recognizes the changing picture that may characterize the cardiac subject's performance and thus be a more practical and meaningful evaluation. Although it is difficult at times to relinquish an old and well-used method, a more vital and functional one, when it exists, is to be preferred.*

The functional classification of the dyspnea of heart failure has not changed (see Box 4-3). The classification of angina pectoris has changed; the New York Heart Association's classification has been abandoned in favor of the Canadian Cardiovascular Society's classification (Box 4-4). The classification of heart failure and angina should be recorded under the physiology portion of the complete diagnosis.

The reader may ask why so much of this text is devoted to the problem of classifying heart disease. The following encounter explains why this chapter has been included in this book. I recently reviewed the problem list of a patient created by a second-year medical resident in medicine. The list included:

Problem 1. Atrial fibrillation

Problem 2. Congestive heart failure

That this could occur in the last decade of the twentieth century was astounding. I explained, "Heart failure occurs in patients with heart disease—it is a measure of

---

*Reprinted with permission from the Criteria Committee of the New York Heart Association: *Nomenclature and criteria for diagnosis of diseases of the heart and great vessels*, ed 8, Boston, 1979, Little, Brown and Company, p vii.

Box 4-4   Canadian Cardiovascular Society's classification of angina pectoris*

1. Ordinary physical activity does not cause . . . angina, such as walking and climbing stairs. Angina with strenuous or rapid or prolonged exertion at work or recreation.
2. Slight limitations of ordinary activity. Walking or climbing stairs rapidly, walking uphill, walking or stair climbing after meals, or in cold, or in wind, or under emotional stress, or only during the few hours after awakening. Walking more than two blocks on the level and climbing more than one flight of ordinary stairs at a normal pace and in normal conditions.
3. Marked limitation of ordinary physical activity. Walking one to two blocks on the level and climbing one flight of stairs in normal conditions and at normal pace.
4. Inability to carry on any physical activity without discomfort—anginal syndrome may be present at rest.

From Campeau L: Letter to the editor, *Circulation* 54:522, 1976. Reproduced by permission of the American Heart Association, Inc.
*This classification of angina pectoris has replaced the New York Heart Association's classification, which was abandoned in 1973.[5]

the severity of the heart disease. Although heart failure may be treated as an independent problem, the long-range treatment is also determined by the etiology of the heart disease."

The point is, if we fail to emphasize the five components of a complete cardiac diagnosis, it is highly likely that we will slip into a superficial approach to the patient's problem and might not develop the skills needed to examine the heart and circulation. One final point: the classification of heart disease as proposed by the New York Heart Association should serve as a paradigm—a model—because the concept can be applied to lung disease, kidney disease, liver disease, neurologic disease, etc. The self-discipline this approach engenders is priceless. Such an approach also highlights the areas of ignorance that should be eliminated by further research.

The following example illustrates the change in approach to a patient with chest pain that has occurred during the last 100 years. The patient, a 64-year-old man who has retrosternal chest discomfort, first experienced the discomfort 2 days before his visit to the physician. The discomfort is produced by walking up a hill and lasts for 3 minutes after the patient stops walking. The discomfort is not severe and radiates into the left arm. The physical examination is normal.

1779   If the patient visited Dr. William Heberden, the physician would diagnose angina pectoris. Another physician would diagnose "indigestion."

1810   If the patient visited Dr. Edward Jenner, the physician would diagnose angina pectoris due to coronary atherosclerosis. Another physician might diagnose "indigestion."

1912   If the patient visited Dr. James Herrick, the physician would diagnose angina pectoris due to coronary atherosclerosis and would admonish those who said it was "indigestion."

1921   If the patient consulted Dr. Paul White, the physician would perform a resting electrocardiogram and would find it to be normal. He would diagnose:
    Heart disease
    Etiology: *Coronary arterosclerosis with angina pectoris*
    Structure: *Normal heart size; obstruction in coronary arteries*
    Function: *Angina produced by climbing a hill*
    Some physicians were still diagnosing patients as having "indigestion."

1950   The diagnosis would be viewed as follows:
    Heart disease
    Etiology: *Coronary atherosclerotic heart disease*
    Anatomy: *Normal heart size; coronary atherosclerosis*
    Physiology: *Normal rhythm, no heart failure, angina pectoris*
    Function: *Angina Class 2 to 3 (New York Heart Association classification)*
    Some physicians were still diagnosing such a patient as having "indigestion."

1980   The diagnosis would be viewed as follows:
    Heart disease
    Etiology: *Coronary atherosclerotic heart disease*

Anatomy: *Normal heart size; coronary atherosclerosis*

Physiology: *No heart failure, normal rhythm, unstable angina pectoris Class 2 (Canadian Cardiovascular Society Classification)*

Cardiac status: *Undetermined*

Prognosis: *Undetermined*

Some physicians were still diagnosing such a patient as having "indigestion."

By 1980 many physicians recognized that the predictive value of the history of chest discomfort as described in this 64-year-old man indicated obstructive coronary atherosclerosis 90% of the time. Furthermore, they realized, because the chest discomfort had been present for only 2 days, that the patient had unstable angina pectoris. This indicated progression of the obstruction in the coronary artery, which caused a decrease in oxygen supply to the myocardium, rather than angina due to an increase in myocardial oxygen demand. By 1980 it was also appreciated that unstable angina is inherently serious regardless of its severity. Physicians also realized that a resting electrocardiogram was usually normal in such patients and that the performance of an exercise stress electrocardiogram was usually contraindicated. By 1980 it was clear that the proper assessment of the patient could not be made without a coronary arteriogram. So the knowledgeable physician obtained a coronary arteriogram. Let us suppose that it revealed an ejection fraction of 40%, as well as 90% obstruction of the left main coronary artery and 75% obstruction of the midportion of the right coronary artery. With this new information the patient could be more accurately classified. The classification after coronary arteriography would be:

Heart disease

Etiology: *Coronary atherosclerotic heart disease*

Anatomy: *Normal heart size; 90% obstruction of the left main coronary artery and 75% obstruction of the mid–right coronary artery*

Physiology: *Normal sinus rhythm, no heart failure; unstable angina pectoris Class 2 (Canadian Cardiovascular Society classification); ejection fraction 40%*

Cardiac status: *Class 4; severely compromised*

Prognosis: *Class 2; good with coronary bypass surgery*

Unfortunately, some patients and physicians still interpret these symptoms as being due to "indigestion" and do not pursue the diagnosis with appropriate diagnostic procedures. Even when the condition is perceived as angina pectoris, they may not perceive the seriousness of unstable angina and the need for a coronary arteriogram. The example given shows how the cardiac appraisal changes as appropriate data are collected.

CARDIAC PROBLEMS VIEWED IN CONTEXT

It is essential for the physician to view cardiac problems in the context of the patient's other medical problems. Good medical judgment cannot be exercised without this approach. The same cardiac problem may be managed differently in different patients depending on noncardiac problems the patients have. For example, a beta-blocker may be indicated in a patient with angina pectoris who has no other medical problems, but the drug is not indicated in a patient with the same class of angina if the patient has chronic obstructive lung disease and bronchospasm. A 70-year-old man with Class 3 angina (Canadian Cardiovascular Society classification) may be a candidate for coronary bypass surgery if no other illnesses are present, but such an operation would not be indicated if the patient exhibited definite signs of Alzheimer disease.

Key Points

- White and Myers[1] pointed out that it is necessary to classify heart disease according to its etiology, structural change, and functional capacity.

- Before 1973 the New York Heart Association emphasized that a complete cardiac diagnosis consisted of identifying the etiology, altered anatomy, altered physiology, and functional capacity of the heart disease. The functional capacity was determined by the amount of activity required to produce dyspnea or angina.

- In 1973 the New York Heart Association abandoned the functional classification and substituted cardiac status in its place.[5] Cardiac status is determined by analyzing all of the data rather than symptoms alone. This change represents a benchmark in medicine, because by 1973 the increase in knowledge generated by modern technology plus an improved knowledge of the natural history of the subsets of cardiac disease had improved our ability to judge the seriousness of heart disease as compared with making a judgment on the basis of symptoms alone.[5] Accordingly, now we use all data, including symptoms, to determine the seriousness of heart disease in an individual patient.

- It is not wise to diagnose and treat heart disease in isolation. The physician must always view a patient's heart disease in the context of all of the patient's problems.

REFERENCES

1. White PD, Myers MM: The classification of cardiac diagnosis, *JAMA* 17(18):1414, 1921.
2. White PD: *My life and medicine*, Boston, 1971, Gambit, p 46.
3. White PD: *Heart disease*, New York, 1931, Macmillan, pp 1-931.
4. Criteria Committee of the New York Heart Association: *Criteria for the classification and diagnosis of heart disease*, ed 1, Boston, 1928, Little, Brown.
5. Criteria Committee of the New York Heart Association: *Nomenclature and criteria for diagnosis of diseases of the heart and great vessels*, ed 7, Boston, 1973, Little, Brown, pp vii-347.
6. Criteria Committee of the New York Heart Association: *Nomenclature and criteria for diagnosis of diseases of the heart and great vessels*, ed 8, Boston, 1979, Little, Brown, pp vii-349.

CHAPTER 5

The history

To take an accurate and relevant history is one of the most difficult and important arts in medicine. Sometimes, a complete diagnosis can be made from the history alone, and not infrequently the possibilities can be whittled down to two or three. A good history should at least indicate the system involved, or it should point unerringly to some group or groups of diseases. A common mistake is the failure to analyse any given symptom sufficiently; in cardiovascular work this applies especially to pain, breathlessness, palpitations, and syncope. The student is usually taught to encourage the patient to tell his story in his own words, and to record them more or less verbatim. Yet such an account may be verbose, irrelevant, inaccurate, and misleading. It is an axiom that the leading question must be avoided at all cost; yet again, an experienced physician must know that the ability to put the appropriate leading question at the right moment, and the intelligent interpretation of its reply, are invaluable. It is not pretended that leading questions may not lead to false information, if the power of their suggestion is not appreciated by the questioner; and it is agreed that much may be lost by failure to allow the patient freedom and time to express his complaints in his own way; but the average patient will not mention half the available information until he is pressed, and the data freely given must be checked as at the bar. For example, in the differential diagnosis between a neural and non-neural somatic lesion, an accurate description of the quality of the pain may determine the issue immediately; yet the majority of patients will volunteer no information concerning the quality of pain, and if asked to describe it will do so inadequately. They may say it is aching or sharp, but fail to enlarge on this, even when urged to do so. In answer to the leading question, "Does it tingle?", however, they may reply at once in the affirmative. It is essential to realise that the matter does not end there: that such a positive reply to a leading question demands the most penetrating cross-examination, until the questioner is satisfied that the pain really does tingle, and that the patient is not merely saying so because it seems the easier answer. It is scarcely too much to say that the best history-taker is he who can best interpret the answer to a leading question. Appropriate leading questions can only be asked, however, when the proffered history has provided sufficient data upon which to work, and if the physician has sufficient knowledge of the possibilities that entailed. It is this latter factor which makes it easier for the expert than the student.

PAUL WOOD 1956[1]*

When physicians "take the history of the patient," they elicit the patient's symptoms, past medical events, and family illnesses that might have an important bearing on the patient's current or future health.[1-4]

History taking is the most difficult skill that the physician must try to master. Make no mistake about the following point—the history must be taken by the physician; it cannot be taken by someone else who relates it to the physician, because much is lost in the transfer of the information. The purpose of history taking is to achieve two goals: the physician must obtain useful, accurate, scientific information and, equally important, must establish a trustful relationship with the patient.

The physician will not be viewed by the patient with kindness if the physician performs a courtroomlike interrogation without concern for the patient's feelings. Should this occur, the physician will not obtain an accurate history and the patient will view the physician as being automated, rushed, inhumane, and noncaring. The physician must remember that each patient is an individual and that each reacts differently to questions asked by the physician.

The history-taking period is when the skilled physician "fits" his or her personality with the personality of the patient, who may be a laborer, teacher, secretary, physician, lawyer, farmer, homeless person, political figure, etc. The skilled physician uses the history-taking period to get to know the patient as a person and to establish a bond between them. The sensitive physician can detect when he or she is not achieving these goals and immediately and imperceptibly alter his or her approach. It is not always necessary to obtain a complete history at the first encounter. The physician identifies the emotionally sensitive points in the history and, unless the information is essential for immediate action, will wait until he or she knows the patient better to continue the questioning. The physician must remember that more harm is done when the history-taking process is "cold" and inhumane than is done by the "coldness" of the modern machines that are inert until someone presses a button (unless, of course, the technician upsets the patient by talking inappropriately).

The patient must be made to feel emotionally and physically comfortable in the examining room. When first meeting a new patient, I have found it useful to initially ask about the patient's referring physician or to ask about other people who live in the patient's home town. Somehow, the fact that I know and respect the people that they know seems to "break the ice" of the interview.

In summary, the history-taking session serves two purposes: the physician collects scientific data from the patient, and the physician makes friends with the patient. When it is over, the patient should view the physician as a kind, thorough, caring person who will be his or her advocate.

Although the discussion in this book is confined to the cardiovascular system, it should be emphasized that a physician should never examine only one organ system of the body and disregard the other organ systems; the data gathered from one organ system may influence the decision-making process regarding another organ system. Accordingly, a defined history must be obtained for each organ system. The data to be collected from the patient regarding the cardiovascular system include information about symptoms such as chest pain or discomfort, breathlessness, palpitation, syncope, intermittent claudication, stroke, and less common complaints; past cardiovascular events; and any family history of conditions that might increase the likelihood of current or future cardiovascular events in the patient.

CURRENT HISTORY (THE PRESENT ILLNESS)

Chest pain or discomfort caused by myocardial ischemia

The most common cause of myocardial ischemia is coronary atherosclerosis that has progressed to the stage where there is obstruction to coronary blood flow. Other causes of myocardial ischemia are coronary artery spasm, anomalous origin of the coronary arteries, coronary artery thrombosis, coronary artery embolism, aortic dissection or coronary artery dissection, coronary ostial disease due to syphilis or previous cannulation of the coronary ostia, Fabry disease, Kawasaki disease, syndrome X, aortic valve stenosis, aortic valve regurgitation, left ventricular hypertrophy due to hypertension, right ventricular hypertrophy due to pulmonary hypertension or severe pulmonary valve stenosis, and hypertrophic or dilated cardiomyopathy.

Clinical characteristics[5]

Description of the discomfort. At the outset it must be emphasized that patients may not refer to the discomfort of myocardial ischemia as "pain." William Heberden assigned the term *angina pectoris*, which means "strangling in the chest," to the discomfort. Heberden[6] wrote:

> But there is a disorder of the breast marked with strong and peculiar symptoms, considerable for the kind of danger belonging to it, and not extremely rare, which deserves to be mentioned more at length. The seat of it, and sense of strangling and anxiety with which it is attended, may make it not improperly be called angina pectoris.
>
> With respect to the treatment of this complaint I have little or nothing to advance; nor indeed, is it to be expected we should have made much progress in the cure of a disease which has hitherto hardly had a place or a name in medical books. Quiet, and warmth, and spiritous liquors help to restore patients who are nearly exhausted and to dispel the effects of a fit when it does not soon go off. Opium taken at bed-time will prevent the attacks at night.

If the physician asks only about chest pain, he or she will fail to identify angina pectoris in a significant number of patients. The patient may describe the chest discomfort as tightness, indigestion, pressure, a weight on the chest, ache, or constriction. Every physician collects a number of unusual terms patients use to describe the sensation caused by myocardial ischemia. One of my patients described his angina pectoris as feeling like a "shoe box in my chest." Another patient called the sensation a "wad." One patient described two types of discomfort; he said the severe attack felt like a "hook was caught beneath my jaw and was pulling upward" and the less severe attack felt like a "needle and thread were being pulled through the space between my two lower front teeth." A medical school dean felt a "flame in my hard palate." The patient may simply refer to the discomfort as "it." Some patients use their hands to communicate the way the sensation feels. Samuel Levine described the clinched fist sign, in which the patient clinches his or her fist in front of the sternum. One of my patients indicated that when he was walking up a hill, someone seemed to "grab and squeeze my throat from behind." Another patient, whose angina pectoris had been overlooked for several months, described his sensation as a "sternal whisper," which teaches us that angina pectoris is not always intensely uncomfortable for the patient. This same patient suggested that I teach medical students to take any patient seriously who relates to them that there is simply a new feeling in the chest that is produced by walking and that was not there previously.

It is important to understand that myocardial ischemia can occur and that the patient may experience no discomfort. This is especially likely to occur in patients with diabetes mellitus and in the elderly.

Location, size of the area, and duration. The discomfort associated with myocardial ischemia is usually located in the midretrosternal area. It may be felt in the neck, lower jaw, hard palate, lower teeth, left or right shoulder, left or right upper arm, left or right elbow, left or right wrist, little finger, upper back, epigastric area, or left precordial area. The common location is the retrosternal area with radiation to the neck and some portion of the left arm.

The area of retrosternal discomfort due to myocardial ischemia is usually about the size of a clinched fist. It is useful to have the patient circumscribe the area of discomfort with a single finger. An area of discomfort located in the left precordium that is no larger than a fingertip is rarely due to myocardial ischemia.

Angina pectoris due to myocardial ischemia usually lasts 1 to 3 minutes if the precipitating cause is discontinued. For example, when the patient develops angina pectoris while walking up an incline, the discomfort will subside within a few minutes if the individual discontinues the effort. Angina pectoris precipitated by anger or some other emotion may last longer than angina precipitated by effort, because it is not as easy to decrease the level of serum catecholamines associated with emotional stress as it is to discontinue walking up an incline.

When the discomfort that is characteristic of myocardial ischemia lasts 10 to 20 minutes or longer, it should not be referred to as angina pectoris. Angina pectoris is brief in duration, and the heart returns to its previous condition after the episode is over. When the discomfort of myocardial ischemia lasts longer than 10 to 20 minutes, it is a serious sign that the heart may not return to its previous state when the discomfort subsides. This condition can be called prolonged angina if the physician and patient realize that it may represent a more serious condition than ordinary transient angina (see later discussion). I prefer to use the term prolonged chest discomfort due to myocardial ischemia with or without signs of myocardial infarction.

A series of sensations, each of which lasts no longer than it takes to "snap your fingers," is not characteristic of myocardial ischemia. This common complaint is often referred to by the patient as "sticks or stabs."

Precipitating causes. Angina pectoris may be precipitated by several events, or it may occur spontaneously. Angina pectoris is commonly precipitated by effort, such as walking up a slight incline, rushing to catch a plane, or climbing stairs. It is useful to ask the patient to "live through a day" in a historical sense: the patient describes his or her usual day, including walking to and from the mailbox, and the exact activity expended at work. The physician should be able to envision the terrain, the buildings, and every aspect of the patient's environment, including the physical and emotional experiences of the day. It is useful to use the Samuel Levine approach and ask a carefully crafted leading question, such as "Walking downhill brings on the discomfort, doesn't it?" If the patient corrects the physician and states, "No, indeed; it only bothers me when I walk up the hill," the act of correcting the physician indicates that the patient has studied the discomfort and is clear on the fact that the discomfort is produced by the effort of going uphill. This type of observation by the patient is likely to be reliable and aids enormously in the identification of angina pectoris.

Emotional stress, such as anger or fright, may also precipitate angina pectoris. These are rather obvious types of emotional behavior. More subtle emotions, such as winning or losing a hand at poker, being startled by the rush of a covey of birds, or hearing a beautiful song that brings back significant memories, may also precipitate angina pectoris. A physician cannot always determine the emotions that will produce stress in a patient. For example, a professional Santa Claus told me that he developed angina each time he observed another Santa Claus "handle the children improperly." Thus it is important to know the patient as a person. Everard Home,[7] John Hunter's son-in-law, described Hunter's angina pectoris as follows:

Although evidently relieved from the violent attacks of spasm by the gout in his feet, yet he was far from being free from the disease, for he was still subject to the spasms, upon exercise or agitation of mind; the exercise that generally brought it on was walking, especially on an ascent, either of stairs or rising ground, but never on going down either the one or the other; the affections of the mind that brought it on were principally anxiety or anger: it was not the cause of the anxiety, but the quantity that most affected him; the anxiety about the hiving of a swarm of bees brought it on; the anxiety lest an animal should make its escape before he could get a gun to shoot it brought it on; even the hearing of a story in which the mind became so much engaged as to be interested in the event, although the particulars were of no consequence to him, would bring it on; anger brought on the same complaint and he could conceive it possible for that passion to be carried so far as to totally deprive him of life; but what was very extraordinary, the more tender passions of the mind did not produce it; he could relate a story which called up all the finer feelings, as compassion, admiration for the actions of gratitude in others, so as to make him shed tears, yet the spasm was not excited; it is extraordinary that he ate and slept as well as ever, and his mind was in degree depressed; the want of exercise made him grow unusually fat.

In the autumn 1790, and in the spring and autumn 1791, he had more severe attacks than during the other periods of the year, but of not more than a few hours duration; in the beginning of October, 1792, one, at which I was present, was so violent that I thought he would have died. On October the 16th, 1793, when in his mind, and not being perfectly master of the circumstances, he withheld his sentiments, in which state of restraint he went into the next room, and turning around to Dr. Robertson, one of the physicians of the hospital, he gave a deep groan, and dropt down dead.

Angina pectoris may also be precipitated by exposure to cold wind (especially on the face); walking in cold weather; drinking ice water; using the arms above the head, such as struggling to raise a window (see later discussion); sexual intercourse; eating a large meal; walking after a large meal; smoking tobacco; or walking and smoking after a large meal.

Angina pectoris may be precipitated when the patient gets up to go to the bathroom at 3:00 AM. Myocardial ischemia and myocardial infarction are more likely to occur in the first few hours after getting up in the morning because of the biologic changes that are related to circadian rhythm and because of the act of changing from the recumbent, sleeping state to the upright, nonsleeping state. These changes include an increase in thrombotic tendency, hypotension, and an increase in serum catecholamines.

Early-morning angina may occur as the patient takes a bath or shower, or when he or she is toweling afterward. Such patients may not have angina pectoris the remainder of the day, even with moderate effort, which often leads the physician to doubt the diagnosis of angina pectoris.

Angina pectoris may be precipitated by using the arms above the head, whereas walking does not produce it. Isometric exercise, such as raising a window, produces an elevation of blood pressure. The heart rate–pressure product increases significantly, so that heart work is abruptly increased.

Walk-through angina pectoris is always surprising. The patient develops angina pectoris while walking and, rather than stopping, continues to walk. Despite the continued effort, the angina pectoris vanishes.

Angina pectoris may occur while the patient is smoking a cigarette. This occurs because nicotine is a potent stimulus for the release of catecholamines.

Angina pectoris may also occur when the patient is resting in a chair or in bed. As discussed earlier, when the discomfort lasts longer than a few minutes, it should not be viewed as angina pectoris but should be perceived as more prolonged myocardial ischemia in which objective signs of infarction may or may not appear. Angina pectoris occurring at rest and chest discomfort due to prolonged myocardial ischemia are caused by different pathophysiologic mechanisms than are responsible for long-standing angina pectoris produced by effort or emotional stress (see later discussion).

Patients who have disturbing dreams or "nightmares" may wake up with angina pectoris. The heart rate is usually rapid, suggesting an excess of catecholamines. For example, a patient dreamed that he was walking in a tunnel but could not see the end of the tunnel. He walked faster but still could not see the end of the tunnel. He then began to run, felt frightened, and woke up with angina pectoris.

Actions taken by the patient. Patients who have had angina pectoris produced by effort for some time learn to walk slower, avoid stair climbing, and refrain from walking while carrying a suitcase or some other heavy object. This emphasizes a point in history taking: it is important for the physician to determine if the patient's angina pectoris is occurring less because the patient does less or because of some therapy that has been prescribed.

At times, when walking with a friend, the patient may pause periodically to talk and make a point because walking and talking at the same time may precipitate angina whereas doing either alone may not. A patient who is walking alone may stop and pretend to examine a building when he or she develops angina pectoris.

Angina pectoris that is induced by assuming the recumbent position and relieved by sitting up may lead the physician to believe that such discomfort is due to esophageal reflux.

Unlike the patient with stable angina pectoris produced by effort, the patient with prolonged chest discomfort due to myocardial ischemia may walk the floor, searching for relief.

Patients who have had episodes of angina pectoris for many weeks may learn to discontinue the effort that produced it and perform a Valsalva maneuver. The angina pectoris subsides when the heart rate slows.*

The discomfort of myocardial ischemia is not aggravated by deep inspiration, whereas the pain of pericarditis is. One must recall, however, that myocardial infarction may be responsible for pericarditis. On rare occasion a patient may have a painless myocardial infarction with a presenting complaint of chest pain due to the pericarditis of infarction.

Characteristics of chest discomfort that strongly suggest myocardial ischemia. Chest discomfort that is clearly related to effort is more likely to be caused by myocardial ischemia than is discomfort that is not related to effort. The relationship to effort is more important than the location of the discomfort in determining if the discomfort is due to myocardial ischemia. In addition, radiation of the discomfort to the mandible, shoulder, or arm is more suggestive of myocardial ischemia than is discomfort that is limited to the chest. However, although these points are true, their

---

*Dr. William Dock taught me this technique. He appeared to use the maneuver to relieve his own angina pectoris.

negative predictive value is inadequate to exclude myocardial ischemia. That is, their absence will not exclude myocardial ischemia in a patient with chest discomfort.

Two overlooked clues to the recognition of myocardial ischemia should be stressed:

- The reproducibility of the discomfort is a powerful clue. When the patient observes that the discomfort occurs each time he or she walks up an incline, the physician has reliable information to diagnose angina pectoris due to myocardial ischemia. When the patient has chest discomfort but cannot identify the precipitating factors, because the episodes have occurred only two or three times or because he or she has not studied that aspect of the problem or is a sedentary person, the physician has inadequate data to make a definite diagnosis of myocardial ischemia. Chest discomfort occurring at rest may be due to myocardial ischemia, but the likelihood is less than when the discomfort is produced by effort. Angina at rest, however, represents one of the more serious types of myocardial ischemia.
- The recognition that different grades of effort are associated with angina pectoris has considerable diagnostic value. For example, if the patient has observed that walking rapidly produces chest discomfort and walking slowly does not produce the discomfort, the discomfort is likely to be due to angina pectoris. Discomfort that is due to musculoskeletal causes is likely to occur with either slow or rapid walking, whereas discomfort that occurs only with rapid walking is commonly due to angina pectoris. My best example of this was provided by an unschooled but highly intelligent farmer who made the following observation. He noted that when he walked down the hill to his barn, he had no chest discomfort, but when he expended more effort by walking up the hill, he experienced retrosternal pressure. By trial and error he discovered that when he walked up the hill in a zigzag manner, even though the distance was greater, he had no chest discomfort.

Physical examination during an episode of angina pectoris. It is unavoidable— the physician performs part of the physical examination during the history-taking period. Accordingly, there are times when the physician has an opportunity to observe a patient experiencing an episode of angina during the interview session. The patient may develop circumoral palor, perspire, and appear anxious. The male patient with angina pectoris is commonly 40 years of age or older, and the female patient is commonly 50 years of age or older. Angina pectoris can, however, occur at an earlier age, even in children, and the etiology may be a condition other than coronary atherosclerosis. The physician should listen to the heart during the episode of chest discomfort; he or she may hear an atrial or ventricular gallop sound that vanishes as the chest discomfort subsides.

Predictive value of the history. The predictive value of a history of chest discomfort is an important concept that has not achieved the diagnostic status it deserves.

It is important because it determines the type of procedure the physician orders after the discomfort has been analyzed. The concept begins by accepting that different histories have different diagnostic values depending on the age and gender of the patient and the type of discomfort. There is no history of chest discomfort that always indicates myocardial ischemia, and there is no history of chest pain that always excludes myocardial ischemia as its cause.

At the time of this writing, the following approach can be defended:

- Suppose a man who is beyond the age of 40 years has retrosternal discomfort that lasts 1 to 5 minutes. The discomfort is produced by effort and relieved by rest. He indicates that he has had the discomfort for several weeks. He expresses his symptoms in a clear manner. The predictive value of this history indicating myocardial ischemia of some cause is about 90%.

- Suppose a man who is beyond the age of 40 years has chest discomfort but has difficulty stating whether it is located in the retrosternal area, to the left of the sternum, or at the cardiac apex. Furthermore, the patient has trouble stating how long the discomfort lasts but states that it "does not last too long." He is not certain what precipitates the discomfort but states, "I think it comes on with effort—but I also have it when I'm sitting down, looking at television." The patient thinks he has had the discomfort for a few weeks but adds, "I really don't know exactly when it started." The predictive value of this history indicating myocardial ischemia is much less than it is in the first example. In this case the likelihood that the discomfort is due to myocardial ischemia is 50% to 75%.

- Suppose the patient is a 50-year-old woman who has retrosternal chest discomfort that lasts 1 to 5 minutes and is precipitated by effort. The symptoms have been present for several weeks and are related to effort. The predictive value of this history indicating myocardial ischemia is about 75%.

- Suppose the same history is obtained from a woman who is under the age of 50. The predictive value of this history indicating myocardial ischemia is about 50%. One reason for this low predictive value is that the prevalence of coronary atherosclerosis in women who are less than 50 years of age is less than it is in men of similar age. However, this prevalence may be changing, because there is evidence that coronary atherosclerosis is increasing in women who are 30 to 50 years of age.

Classification of myocardial ischemia. Herrick[8] pointed out in 1912 that there were different types of myocardial ischemia. He wrote:

All attempts at devising these clinical manifestations into groups must be artificial and more or less imperfect. Yet such an attempt is not without value, as it enables one to better understand the gravity of an obstructive accident, to differentiate it from other conditions presenting somewhat similar symptoms, and to employ a more rational therapy that may, to a slight extent at least, be more efficient.

Box 5-1   Classification of myocardial ischemia

Transient myocardial ischemia
    Stable (chronic) angina
    Unstable angina
    Prinzmetal (variant) angina´
    Angina pectoris following myocardial infarction
    Angina equivalents
    Symptomless myocardial ischemia
Prolonged myocardial ischemia
    Prolonged myocardial ischemia without objective evidence of myocardial infarction
    Prolonged myocardial ischemia with objective evidence of myocardial infarction
        Evolving myocardial infarction
        Completed myocardial infarction
        Symptomless myocardial infarction
Sudden death
Syncope
Cardiac arrhythmias
Positive exercise electrocardiogram response
Positive thallium scan

I recommend the classification shown in Box 5-1. It meets the criteria for a meaningful classification in that it is possible to link the clinical features of the subset to the pathophysiology responsible for the subset and to link both to the diagnostic and therapeutic approach to the subset. Thus when the physician analyzes symptoms produced by myocardial ischemia, he or she should be thinking in terms of the pathophysiology responsible for them. This approach makes it possible to determine the appropriate diagnostic and therapeutic approach to the patient's problem. Accordingly, the clinical features of the various subsets that are assigned specific names must be carefully defined (see following sections).

Transient myocardial ischemia

Stable angina pectoris. Stable angina pectoris is said to be present when the chest discomfort, which usually lasts 1 to 3 minutes, has not changed in frequency, duration, or precipitating causes for 60 days.

Stable angina pectoris occurs when there is an increase in cardiac work; it is usually caused by effort. An electrocardiogram made when the patient is resting and having no chest pain is usually normal. An electrocardiogram made during an episode of angina may show the ST segment displacement of subendocardial injury. The working myocytes need more oxygen-laden blood during the period of increased work, but the obstructed coronary arteries cannot deliver it. When angina is due to aortic valve stenosis, the coronary arteries may be normal or exhibit atherosclerosis. In either case the obstructed left ventricular outflow tract prevents the increase in myocardial perfusion of blood that is needed to prevent the occurrence of ischemia of the heart muscle during the increased cardiac work associated with exercise. In fact, regardless of the etiology of stable angina pectoris, it is caused by an increase in myocardial oxygen *demand* rather than an alteration in the *supply* end of the myocardial oxygen supply-demand system.

For years now, physicians have estimated the amount of effort required to precipitate angina pectoris in their patients. At an earlier time physicians assumed that patients who had to perform a great deal of effort to produce angina had only mild coronary artery disease, whereas patients who developed angina with little effort had severe coronary artery disease. Although this may be true as a general rule, there are many exceptions. The same is true for the severity of each episode of angina. A severe episode of angina does not always signify terrible coronary artery disease, and a mild episode does not guarantee that the coronary lesions are benign. We now know that the severity of coronary artery disease and its prognosis are determined by the findings at coronary arteriography, left ventriculography, and exercise testing (if not contraindicated), as well as by the amount of effort required to cause angina pectoris. Also, many other factors may conspire to produce myocardial ischemia, including thrombosis and spasm in patients with mild coronary atherosclerosis.

It is important, however, to determine the exercise tolerance of patients with angina pectoris, because the information is used to determine the degree of disability the disease is imposing on the patient. This in turn is one of the variables used to determine the need for angioplasty or coronary artery bypass surgery. Still, it is important to remember that some patients with serious, triple-vessel coronary atherosclerosis have no angina, or only mild angina after moderate effort.

The current system of classification of angina pectoris was created by the Canadian Cardiovascular Society. Most randomized trials dealing with therapeutic approaches to coronary atherosclerosis and angina pectoris use this classification (see Box 4-4).

All classifications have limitations, and the Canadian Cardiovascular Society's classification is no exception. I believe that the Canadian Cardiovascular Society's classification applies, for the most part, to patients with stable angina pectoris rather than patients with unstable angina pectoris. Patients with unstable angina pectoris may not have had time to determine the reproducibility of their angina. For example, many patients with unstable angina are seen by the physician the first day the patients have chest discomfort. Also, unstable angina is serious even when the symptoms are mild, because other coronary events are likely to occur hours, days, or weeks later.

Unstable angina pectoris. The label *unstable* should be applied to angina pectoris that occurs for the first time; to angina pectoris that has made its appearance during the last 60 days; and to angina pectoris that has been present for weeks or months but is now increasing in severity, duration, or frequency or is precipitated with less effort or emotional stress than formerly. The chest discomfort usually lasts 1 to 3 minutes. It often occurs when the patient is at rest. An electrocardiogram made during an attack of angina may show an ST segment displacement that is characteristic of subendocardial injury.

Unstable angina pectoris is usually due to coronary atherosclerosis and occurs because of a crack in an atheromatous plaque, which leads to coronary thrombosis and coronary spasm. Accordingly, the ischemic episode is caused by an alteration in the *supply side* of the myocardial oxygen supply-demand system.

There is undoubtedly a difference in the patient with unstable angina who developed the symptoms a month earlier as compared with the patient who has an episode of angina for the first time. Obviously, a more aggressive diagnostic and therapeutic strategy is needed for the latter case. The pathophysiology is probably the same but is more severe or accelerated in the second patient.

Prinzmetal angina. The angina pectoris occurs at rest and lasts 1 to 20 minutes. The angina often occurs at about the same time each day. It may be precipitated by smoking tobacco. An electrocardiogram made during an episode of angina reveals transient ST segment displacement. A mean vector representing the ST segment is directed toward a segment of epicardial injury. The electrocardiogram may occasionally reveal transient abnormal Q waves and atrioventricular block.

Prinzmetal angina pectoris is usually due to obstructive coronary atherosclerosis plus coronary artery spasm or, on occasion, may be due to coronary artery spasm alone.

Angina pectoris following myocardial infarction. There are two subsets of postinfarction angina pectoris. One is characterized by angina pectoris occurring during the first few hours or days following myocardial infarction. Dead myocardial cells do not produce discomfort. Therefore the occurrence of angina implies that other myocytes are ischemic. The pathophysiology responsible for the angina is the same as the pathophysiology that caused the infarction. Infarction is usually caused by coronary thrombosis and coronary spasm superimposed on obstructive atherosclerotic coronary disease.

The other subset of postinfarction angina pectoris is characterized by angina occurring several weeks after myocardial infarction. The ischemic episodes occur about the time the patient becomes more active, and although some cases may be caused by an alteration in the *supply side* of the oxygen supply-demand system, many of these patients have angina because of an increase in the *demand side* of the oxygen supply-demand system.

Angina equivalents. Patients with angina equivalents do not have chest discomfort but must be included in this classification. These patients have dyspnea, fatigue, or both, which can be caused by many other diseases. Accordingly, the predictive value of these complaints signifying myocardial ischemia is much less than it is with chest discomfort.

The *dyspnea* may be noted on effort. When this occurs in a patient without pulmonary disease, or any other condition, such as anemia or thyrotoxicosis, it must be considered an angina equivalent until it has been proved otherwise. The patient may complain of experiencing the unpleasant symptom, produced by effort, for weeks or of experiencing abrupt, but transient, dyspnea in the middle of the night. When the symptom has been present for more than 60 days, it falls into the stable category. When it is of recent onset and occurs at rest, it is considered part of the unstable syndrome. The stable syndrome is caused by an increase in myocardial *demand* for oxygen, and the unstable syndrome is caused by an alteration in the *supply side* of the oxygen supply-demand system. In either case the dyspnea is due to left ventricular diastolic dysfunction and an elevation of left ventricular diastolic pressure due to myocardial ischemia.

The *fatigue* may be chronic, or exhaustion may be produced by effort. For example, an executive complained of exhaustion each morning after he walked from the door of his house to his car. He would lean against the steering wheel of the car, too exhausted to start the motor, and wait for the extreme exhaustion to subside. Fatigue and exhaustion occur because myocardial ischemia produces left ventricular myocardial dysfunction, which results in a decrease in cardiac output. When this occurs, the blood supply to the skeletal muscles is decreased, and this decreased blood supply produces the symptoms.

Symptomless myocardial ischemia. This subset of myocardial ischemia is usually referred to as silent ischemia. The condition is usually recognized because of an abnormal response in the patient's electrocardiogram that is made during exercise. Although this text is primarily concerned with the initial examination of the patient, symptomless myocardial ischemia is included here in the classification of myocardial ischemia because it is important and common.

Symptomless myocardial ischemia is usually caused by coronary atherosclerotic heart disease. It occurs in patients who have angina pectoris, as well as in patients who do not. Patients who have diabetes mellitus are more likely to have symptomless myocardial ischemia than are patients without diabetes.

Prolonged myocardial ischemia. Patients who experience the characteristic chest discomfort of myocardial ischemia that persists longer than angina pectoris are believed to have prolonged myocardial ischemia, which is usually caused by coronary atherosclerosis. The episode commonly occurs in the early-morning hours—usually before noon—because of the influence of circadian rhythm, a more active clotting mechanism, and the physiologic adjustments that must be made after several hours of sleep. The condition may, however, also be caused by effort. Obviously, an absolute number of minutes cannot be assigned to the duration of the chest discomfort in order to distinguish it from angina pectoris. However, angina pectoris is transient and usually lasts 1 to 3 minutes if the patient discontinues the effort that produced it. Chest discomfort suggesting myocardial ischemia that lasts longer than 20 minutes should not be considered the same transient, reversible myocardial ischemia that is characteristic of angina. Myocardial ischemia lasting 20 minutes or longer is likely to produce dead myocytes, whereas transient angina pectoris usually does not.

The subset of prolonged chest discomfort due to myocardial ischemia may be divided into two additional subsets: prolonged chest discomfort due to myocardial ischemia without objective signs of myocardial infarction and prolonged chest discomfort due to myocardial ischemia with objective signs of infarction.

Prolonged discomfort without objective signs of infarction. This subset of myocardial ischemia should be identified when the chest discomfort is characteristic of myocardial ischemia and lasts longer than angina pectoris, transient ST segment and T wave changes may or may not develop in the electrocardiogram, and the level of serum cardiac enzymes remains normal. This syndrome may overlap the syndrome of unstable angina pectoris and Prinzmetal angina. Prolonged chest discomfort due to myocardial ischemia without objective signs of myocardial infarction is a serious condition. There is an alteration in the *supply side* of the myocardial oxygen supply-demand system caused by a crack in an atherosclerotic plaque, thrombosis, and coronary artery spasm. Patients with this syndrome are likely to have additional ischemic cardiac events during the subsequent days, weeks, or months.

Prolonged discomfort with objective signs of infarction. This subset of myocardial ischemia can be divided into two additional subsets: non–Q wave infarction and Q wave infarction.

Non–Q wave infarction is said to be present when persistent ST segment and T wave abnormalities develop in the electrocardiogram of the patient who has chest discomfort that is characteristic of prolonged myocardial ischemia. The ST segment and T wave abnormalities are characteristic of epicardial injury and ischemia (see Chapter 7). No abnormal Q waves develop in the electrocardiogram. The level of serum cardiac enzymes is usually elevated. A few years ago some clinicians labeled this syndrome a subendocardial infarction. Others referred to the condition as a nontransmural infarction. These designations are no longer used, because many of these patients actually have a transmural infarction. The syndrome is caused by a crack in an atheromatous plaque, thrombosis, and coronary artery spasm, resulting in an alteration in the *supply side* of the myocardial oxygen supply-demand system.

Q wave infarction is said to be present when abnormal Q waves, along with ST segment and T wave abnormalities, develop in the electrocardiogram of the patient who has chest discomfort that is characteristic of prolonged myocardial ischemia (see Chapter 7). The level of serum cardiac enzymes is usually elevated. A few years ago clinicians referred to these abnormalities as being caused by a transmural infarction. This label is no longer used, because these electrocardiographic abnormalities can occur with nontransmural infarction. The syndrome is caused by a crack in an atheromatous plaque, thrombosis, and coronary artery spasm, resulting in an alteration in the *supply side* of the myocardial oxygen supply-demand system.

It is important to determine the interval of time that elapses between the onset of chest discomfort and the time the patient is seen by the physician. Suppose the patient's chest discomfort lasted an hour but he or she was not seen until 5 or 6 hours later; this patient has a *completed* infarction. Suppose, however, the patient is seen an hour after the discomfort started; this patient has an *evolving* infarction; that is, salvable myocardium is still present. The longer the delay in following the onset of chest discomfort due to myocardial ischemia, the less myocardium can be salvaged by thrombolytic therapy.

Subendocardial infarction does occur, although it is uncommon. It occurs in the clinical setting that includes left ventricular hypertrophy from aortic valve stenosis or hypertension, coronary atherosclerosis, and hypotension from some other condition such as trauma or hemorrhage. Laplace's law dictates that there will be more ischemia of the subendocardial region of the left ventricle than elsewhere. Accordingly, the entire left ventricular endocardial area may become infarcted. The chest discomfort due to myocardial ischemia may be prolonged, or the patient may have no chest discomfort. The electrocardiogram shows an ST segment vector directed away from the cardiac apex (see Chapter 7). When this vector persists for hours and the level of cardiac enzymes is elevated, a subendocardial infarction can be diagnosed. The electrocardiogram may then change to show the abnormal Q waves and ST-T changes of epicardial injury and ischemia.

Symptomless myocardial infarction. Symptomless myocardial infarction is not rare. It is usually discovered by abnormalities noted in the resting electrocardiogram or may be identified by left ventriculography and coronary arteriography performed for angina pectoris. Silent infarction is common in patients with diabetes mellitus and in the elderly.

Chest pain or discomfort from other cardiovascular causes

Pericarditis.[9] The pain of pericarditis is located in the precordial area and may be felt at the top of the shoulders. The pain is aggravated when the patient takes a deep breath and is relieved somewhat when the patient sits and leans forward. The patient will often admit that he or she breathes in a shallow fashion in order to avoid breathing deeply. The pericarditis of myocardial infarction usually occurs several days after the infarction. The pain of viral or bacterial pericarditis is commonly associated with a temperature elevation. Uremic pericarditis may not produce pain or be associated with a temperature elevation. A pericardial friction rub may or may not be present in patients with pericarditis (see Chapter 6).

Pericarditis may be caused by infection, collagen disease, neoplastic disease, myocardial infarction (including Dressler syndrome), cardiac surgery, uremia, or trauma, or it may follow the use of procainamide.

Dissection of the aorta.[10] Dissection of the aorta is usually caused by medial cystic necrosis of the media of the aorta. The vasa vasora may rupture and hemorrhage into the loose media. This produces a poorly supported area of the intima and permits the development of an entry site through which blood enters the media of the aorta.

The pain, which is severe in 90% of patients, is located in the anterior portion of the chest but is commonly felt more severely in the back of the thorax. It usually lasts until an injection of an opiate is given to the patient. The pain reaches its maximum almost immediately, which is somewhat different from the pain of myocardial infarction, which reaches its maximum a bit more gradually.

The abnormalities that may occur on physical examination are discussed in Chapter 6. The peripheral arteries may become occluded, a neurologic deficit may occur simultaneously with the chest pain, and the blood pressure usually remains elevated. The coronary ostia may become involved and produce a myocardial infarction.

Pulmonary artery hypertension.[11] Some years ago the chest discomfort associated with pulmonary artery hypertension was thought to be caused by abrupt distention of the pulmonary artery. The relationship of the discomfort to effort was explained by the abnormal rise in pulmonary artery pressure that occurs in patients with pulmonary artery hypertension during exercise. The chest discomfort is similar to angina pectoris. Patients with mitral stenosis, Eisenmenger physiology, or primary pulmonary hypertension are likely to have chest discomfort associated with pulmonary hypertension.

The current view is that the discomfort is actually due to right ventricular angina, because myocardial perfusion via the coronary arteries may be diminished when there is an elevation of systolic and diastolic pressure in the right ventricle, poor cardiac output, and right ventricular hypertrophy. This pathophysiology is reminiscent of the mechanism responsible for angina in patients with severe aortic valve stenosis.

Cardiac arrhythmias.[12] Patients with rapid heart action, such as paroxysmal supraventricular tachycardia, paroxysmal atrial fibrillation, or ventricular tachycardia, may complain of an uncomfortable feeling in the center of the chest. Some patients with premature atrial or ventricular contractions may complain of a "sucking feeling" in the chest. Generally, however, the patient with an arrhythmia can distinguish the tumultuous sensation associated with it from angina pectoris. Patients with chest discomfort associated with rapid heart action may have no intrinsic coronary artery disease, but rapid heart action can and often does precipitate angina in a patient with obstructive coronary artery disease. Accordingly, great care must be exercised to avoid making a diagnostic error in a 50-year-old man or woman who may have coronary atherosclerosis.

Chest pain or discomfort caused by skin disease[13]

Herpes zoster. Herpes zoster is the only skin disease I have encountered that may be confused with myocardial infarction. The chest pain may be in the precordial area, and the skin itself is extremely sensitive to the touch. Vesicles may appear a day later, confirming the diagnosis.

Mondor disease. This unusual condition is due to phlebitis of the veins located in the region of the left breast. The patient complains of discomfort in the area, and the skin is sensitive. The condition can be diagnosed when the veins can be palpated as tender cords just beneath the skin's surface.

Chest pain or discomfort caused by neuromusculoskeletal disease[13]

Tietze syndrome. Tietze syndrome is characterized by pain, swelling, and tenderness in the costochondral, chondrosternal, or xiphisternal joints. There are no systemic symptoms. The swelling and tenderness, usually located in the second costochondral junction, may persist for weeks but eventually disappear. This condition is occasionally confused with myocardial ischemia, although there are few signs to suggest it.

Chest wall pain. Chest wall pain is common, and the exact cause is rarely discovered. The discomfort may be located anywhere in the chest wall; there may be tenderness on pressure, or pain may occur as a result of twisting or turning the trunk.

Chest wall pain is common after cardiac surgery. The pain is usually located in the area where the incision was made or where tubes were inserted, but the pain may also be located in intercostal spaces where intercostal muscles were stretched when the rib cage was spread apart as a necessary part of the surgery.

This type of pain may occasionally simulate myocardial ischemia but is usually identified correctly because of the location and tenderness of the painful area.

Thoracic outlet syndrome.[13] Thoracic outlet syndrome is due to compression of the arteries and nerves as they pass over the upper border of the thorax and into the left or right arm. It is a marvel that this disorder does not occur more commonly, because the tissues are quite crowded in these areas. There are many subsets of this condition, because different structures may be compressed. The discomfort is due to nerve or arterial compression and may be felt in the left or right arm. The pain commonly follows the distribution of the ulnar nerve, is usually located in either hand or arm, and may be felt in the shoulder, neck, and left or right anterior portion of the chest wall. The patient may indicate that certain body positions, such as sleeping with the arms above the head or reaching above the head, may trigger the onset of the discomfort. The condition must be differentiated from carpal tunnel syndrome, cervical disc syndrome, and cervical arthritis.

When the patient's symptoms suggest a type of thoracic outlet syndrome, the physician should perform certain physical maneuvers in order to diagnose the condition (see Chapter 6).

Chest pain or discomfort caused by pulmonary disease

Pulmonary embolism and infarction.[14] Pulmonary embolism, along with subsequent infarction, is a common cause of chest pain. Pulmonary embolism is especially likely to occur in patients with congestive heart failure and in patients who are confined to bed. The postoperative patient is perhaps the most vunerable. Patients who have had hip or knee replacement or prostate surgery are particularly at risk for having pulmonary emboli, which is due to thrombosis in the leg veins. There may or may not be signs of phlebitis.

The patient may experience acute dyspnea and a feeling of tightness in the chest. Acute pleuritic chest pain develops either acutely or subsequently, depending on the size of the embolus and the presence or absence of pulmonary congestion.

Other data, including information derived from the electrocardiogram (see Chapter 7), serum cardiac enzyme determinations, blood gas determination, and chest radiography (including radionuclear scanning), are often needed to identify pulmonary embolism and infarction, rather than myocardial infarction, as the cause of chest pain. Pulmonary embolism may precipitate myocardial ischemia in patients with coronary atherosclerosis. When this occurs, there may be clues pointing toward both pulmonary infarction and myocardial infarction.

Pleurisy. Pleurisy is usually caused by pulmonary infection or pulmonary infarction. The pain, which is usually located in the lower lateral portion of the thoracic cage, is commonly severe and may be described as "cutting." It is aggravated by inspiration.

Postmyocardial infarction syndrome (Dressler syndrome) consists of pleurisy, pericarditis, and the accumulation of pleural fluid. This condition may occur days to weeks after myocardial infarction. A similar condition may occur days to weeks following cardiac surgery.

The physical signs of pleurisy are described in Chapter 6.

Spontaneous pneumothorax. Spontaneous pneumothorax is usually caused by rupture of a pulmonary bleb. It is associated with acute dyspnea and pain, which is located in the lateral portion of the chest. This condition is often missed on physical examination and may be overlooked on the x-ray film. The electrocardiogram may become abnormal (see Chapter 7).

Mediastinal emphysema.[15] Hamman disease, or mediastinal emphysema, occurs when the pulmonary alveoli rupture into the tissue space surrounding the smaller pulmonary arterioles, so that air dissects its way into the mediastinal area. The condition may occur spontaneously or be caused by pulmonary infection or trauma. The patient experiences acute chest pain and dyspnea. At times the patient hears a peculiar noise that emanates from the inside of the chest. On rare occasions the patient notices subcutaneous emphysema and crepitation in the neck and chest wall. The telltale auscultatory signs are discussed in Chapter 6.

Chest pain or discomfort caused by gastrointestinal disease[16]

Esophageal reflux. Esophageal reflux produces lower retrosternal discomfort that may simulate angina pectoris or more prolonged myocardial ischemia. The patient may refer to the discomfort as "indigestion" or "heartburn," but the patient may also label angina pectoris with the same names. Usually precipitated by the ingestion of spicy food or liquid containing citric acid, the discomfort of esophageal reflux may occur when the patient assumes the recumbent position; it is not precipitated by effort. At times the condition is associated with esophageal spasm that may be relieved by nitroglycerin; this response further confuses the clinical picture, because it may be interpreted as further evidence of angina pectoris due to coronary atherosclerosis.

The condition is caused by an incompetent lower esophageal sphincter. An incompetent lower esophageal sphincter is commonly associated with a hiatal hernia, but a hiatal hernia alone does not usually produce retrosternal discomfort.

It is important to remember that angina pectoris or more prolonged chest discomfort due to myocardial ischemia can also be precipitated by a heavy meal, and one must resist diagnosing esophageal reflux simply because the discomfort followed the consumption of a large meal that perhaps was too "spicy." The physician must also realize that both angina pectoris (or more prolonged discomfort due to myocardial ischemia) and esophageal reflux may occur in the same patient. In fact, some patients who have both conditions may complain more of the discomfort due to esophageal reflux than of that due to angina pectoris.

To restate, when the chest discomfort is produced by effort, it is more likely to be due to angina pectoris. Additional studies are commonly required to separate the discomfort of esophageal reflux from that of angina pectoris due to coronary atherosclerosis.

Esophageal spasm. Esophageal spasm may cause retrosternal discomfort that mimics angina pectoris or prolonged chest pain due to myocardial ischemia. The discomfort may or may not be precipitated by the ingestion of food. Esophageal spasm is not precipitated by effort. Nitroglycerin is commonly used to relieve angina pectoris. The discomfort due to esophageal spasm may also be relieved by nitroglycerin. Accordingly, such relief cannot be used as proof that the discomfort is due to angina. Patients with esophageal reflux may also have esophageal spasm, and both may occur in a patient who also has angina pectoris.

When the chest discomfort is caused by effort, it is more likely to be due to angina pectoris. Additional studies are commonly needed to diagnose esophageal spasm and esophageal reflux and to distinguish the discomfort caused by them from that of angina pectoris.

Acute esophageal impaction. The discomfort of esophageal impaction may simulate the discomfort of myocardial infarction. The sequence of events may be as follows. The patient eats some solid food, such as meat, and develops severe pain in the retrosternal area. He or she senses that the discomfort is related to the food that has just been swallowed and drinks a glass of water. The water, however, will not "go down." The patient has no trouble talking. This scenario is diagnostic of esophageal impaction and is in sharp contrast to the problem associated with a "cafe coronary," in which the meat becomes impacted in the larynx or trachea and the patient cannot talk or breathe.

Esophageal impaction may occur in a patient with an esophageal stricture or Schatzki ring.

Esophageal rupture. Perforation of the esophagus may be produced by forceful retching and vomiting. The pain may be severe and is located in the center of the chest and back. Mediastinal emphysema commonly develops. The physician should be alerted to this condition by the clinical setting in which it occurs.

Gallstone colic. Patients with colic due to gallstones usually experience pain in the right upper quadrant of the abdomen. The pain may be felt in the right scapular area. It usually lasts for 30 minutes to an hour and may be confused with prolonged myocardial ischemia due to coronary atherosclerosis. This confusion is especially likely when the pain is felt in the lower retrosternal area and the right lower portion of the chest. The pain is not produced by effort, and there may or may not be tenderness in the gallbladder area.

Patients with gallstones commonly have coronary atherosclerosis, and some clinicians believe that gallbladder colic can precipitate coronary artery spasm. Thus, once again, the possibility exists that two diseases—gallstones and coronary atherosclerotic heart disease—may be present in the same patient. Additional studies are commonly needed to diagnose gallstone colic and to identify associated coronary artery disease.

Peptic ulcer disease. The discomfort of peptic ulcer disease is usually located in the epigastric area. On occasion the discomfort is located a little higher than the usual area and may be confused with angina pectoris at rest or prolonged myocardial ischemia. There is, of course, no relationship to effort, and the discomfort is relieved by food. Additional studies are usually needed to diagnose peptic ulcer disease.

Chest pain or discomfort from emotional, psychologic, or mental causes

There are no perfect labels for the syndromes that are usually characterized as being behavioral problems without identifiable heart disease. They are, however, usually discussed under the following headings.

Depression.[17] Depression is common, although it is uncommonly diagnosed. Both men and women are affected. After a superficial interview the patient may be misdiagnosed as having anxiety. The patient may complain of insomnia, fatigue, and lack of interest in events and people and may feel that every day is a "bad day." Such patients have many other complaints, including chest discomfort, that may simulate some of the features of angina pectoris or prolonged myocardial ischemia. The cause of the chest pain in depressed patients is not known.

At times it is not possible to differentiate the chest pain of myocardial ischemia from the chest discomfort associated with depression. The location of the discomfort may be similar in the two conditions, and although the discomfort associated with depression is not as clearly related to effort, unstable angina and prolonged myocardial ischemia may also occur at rest. Accordingly, these subsets of myocardial ischemia are difficult to differentiate from the chest discomfort associated with depression.

Coronary artery disease and depression are common. Therefore both conditions may occur in the same patient. Additional studies are often needed to determine if the depressed patient has or does not have coronary artery disease.

Neurocirculatory asthenia.[18] Neurocirculatory asthenia (NCA) is rarely diagnosed today, whereas it was commonly diagnosed 40 years ago. It is not that the syndrome itself has vanished but that its cumbersome name has disappeared and new names have been created to label certain parts of the syndrome. For example, a part of the syndrome is currently called a *panic attack* (to be discussed later), and some people attribute some of the attributes of NCA to *mitral valve prolapse, vasoregulatory asthenia, hyperdynamic syndrome,* and *syndrome X*. Stated simply, if NCA appears to have "disappeared," it is because physicians call it, or parts of it, by different names.

During the American Civil War DeCosta described a syndrome in soldiers that had some of the clinical features of what was later called NCA. During World War I the cluster of symptoms appearing in soldiers was called NCA. Many distinguished physicians, including Sir Thomas Lewis, Paul Dudley White, and Samuel Levine, described the syndrome, and it remained an accepted diagnosis until the midpoint of this century. The best description of NCA was by Mandel Cohen and White,[18] who emphasized that the condition was composed of many symptoms—not simply chest discomfort.

During the period of World War II, NCA occurred predominantly in young men. When peace came, the syndrome was seen more commonly in women. The age range was about 20 to 60 years, although it was also seen in children whose mothers or fathers had NCA.

The chest pain that is part of NCA may be of two types. The patient may complain of a *dull ache* near the cardiac apex. The area of discomfort is about the size of the hand, and the discomfort lasts continuously for hours to days. The pain is not directly related to effort, because some degree of discomfort is always present. The other type of chest discomfort is opposite the one just described: the patient may experience short *sticks and stabs* of chest pain near the cardiac apex. This pain lasts no longer than it takes to snap the fingers and is also not related to effort. In fact, it commonly occurs when the patient is sitting and relaxed.

There may be periods of time when the chest pain, be it the continuous ache or the sticks and stabs, may, for unexplained reasons, disappear only to return days or weeks later.

Patients with NCA have two types of dyspnea. One type, *sighing respiration*, is common. The definition of sighing respiration is that the patient feels that normal respiration is not adequate—it is not satisfying. The patient, who may complain that the "air does no good," takes a deep breath in an effort to get a "satisfying breath."

Normal individuals exhibit sighing occasionally, but patients with NCA do so frequently. The patient with NCA is usually unaware of the sometimes noisy, sighing respiration. As stated before, children may imitate their sighing parents.

In the second type of dyspnea patients have episodes of overt *hyperventilation*. Feeling "short of breath," the patient may breathe more deeply and more rapidly and may begin to note "an unreal feeling" and numbness around the mouth and in the hands. In severe episodes tetany of the hands may develop. At times the episode is so terrifying to the patient that he or she may not be aware of or complain of dyspnea but may complain of a feeling that he or she is dying. At times only a few deep breaths will precipitate the uncomfortable feeling. These patients may have chronic hyperventilation that is unrecognized by them or their physicians[19] and, accordingly, may develop the symptoms that are usually associated with advanced hyperventilation after only a few deep inhalations and exhalations.

The physiologic reason for the patient's symptoms during hyperventilation are well known: the patient's P_{CO_2} declines, and ionizable calcium decreases. The episodes themselves may be precipitated by an apparently stressful situation or may occur "out of the blue." Part of the "new" *panic attack syndrome* is the "old" hyperventilation syndrome.

Patients with NCA may complain of fatigue, which is present continuously and is not diminished by sleep or rest. They may also complain of claustrophobia. They do not like crowded places, such as a room full of people or a crowded elevator, and they may prefer the end seat of a row in a crowded theater. These patients may also have other simple phobias.

Patients with NCA may complain of palpitation. Definite episodes of supraventricular tachycardia or ventricular tachycardia are rarely documented, however; the patient is simply conscious of the normal heartbeat or ectopic beats.

In addition, patients with NCA have multiple unexplained complaints that may involve any of the body systems.

Today it is popular to blame the complaints mentioned above on mitral valve prolapse. I do not believe that the complaints are all due to mitral valve prolapse for the following reasons:

- Expert cardiologists such as White and Levine did not detect a midsystolic click at the cardiac apex. One can say that they did not detect the midsystolic click because no one was aware of its significance at the time they observed patients with NCA; however, they also did not observe mitral regurgitation in their patients with NCA, and they were very good at hearing the systolic murmur of mitral regurgitation. It would be unusual, indeed, for patients with a midsystolic click (which was overlooked) due to mitral valve prolapse to have symptoms and for patients with mitral regurgitation (which was not overlooked) due to mitral valve prolapse to be asymptomatic.

- Many patients with mitral valve prolapse have no symptoms whatsoever. Some patients become symptomatic after they are told they have mitral valve prolapse.

Two other syndromes are confused with NCA: hyperdynamic syndrome and vasoregulatory asthenia.

Hyperdynamic syndrome, originally discussed by Gorlin,[20] is characterized by hyderdynamic activity of the heart. The patient complains of the increased force of cardiac activity and carotid artery pulsation. The condition is caused by the action of an overactive sympathetic nervous system on the heart.

Vasoregulatory asthenia is caused by the action of an overactive sympathetic nervous system on the peripheral arteries.[21] Blood is shunted away from the skeletal muscles, and the patient complains of fatigue, left-sided chest discomfort, and decreased ability to exercise. The heart rate is faster than normal at rest and when standing. Although a planned exercise program may alleviate the symptoms and signs to some degree, the symptoms and signs return promptly after the program is discontinued. It may be the cause of an abnormal ST segment displacement in the exercise electrocardiogram. The abnormal response is prevented by a beta-blocking drug.

Two or more of these syndromes are occasionally intertwined in the same patient, and the physician's challenge is to distinguish between them.

Although some patients with mitral valve prolapse may have palpitation, a hyperdynamic circulation, and precordial discomfort, many patients with mitral valve prolapse have superimposed symptoms of NCA.

Recently a new name has appeared. The label *dysautonomia* is now used by some physicians to describe the dysfunction of the autonomic nervous system. Such a label is not needed, and the word frightens anxious patients.

Chest discomfort and self-gain.[17] Some patients may fake the symptoms of myocardial ischemia for self-gain. For example, a patient known to have angina pectoris may "develop" angina in order to create sympathy and win an argument. The narcotic addict may "experience chest pain" in order to obtain a narcotic, or a patient may claim disabling angina in order to receive disability insurance payments.

Some of these patients are so knowledgeable of the symptoms of angina pectoris that it is impossible for the physician to exclude its presence. At times it is virtually impossible to make an accurate appraisal of the complaints of such patients when they have coronary arteriographic evidence of coronary artery disease.

Cardiac psychosis.[17] Patients with cardiac psychosis may believe that their heart is severely damaged when it is not. Some will state that their heart has deteriorated— that it is "rotten." They are obsessed with their belief that their heart is so diseased that it will not function when in reality there is no heart disease. A middle-aged man once called me on the telephone and stated that his heart had stopped beating. He said he was lying on the floor and was administering cardiac resuscitation to himself!

Dyspnea[22]

Dyspnea is defined as the uncomfortable feeling of "shortness of breath."[23] The physician determines that heart failure is the cause of the dyspnea on effort by identifying the presence of heart disease and other signs of heart failure through physical examination and chest x-ray examination (see Chapters 6 and 8).

Dyspnea related to heart disease

Dyspnea at rest. Patients with chronic congestive heart failure may complain of dyspnea at rest or on very little effort.[23] An observer may see little change in respiratory rate when the patient complains of "shortness of breath."

The patient with heart failure may have *orthopnea*. He or she discovers that lying flat in bed produces dyspnea and learns to elevate the trunk with pillows to avoid the unpleasant feeling. In addition, the patient with heart failure may go to sleep at night and awaken a few hours later with profound dyspnea. The patient will usually sit on the side of the bed until the "shortness of breath" subsides and then return to the recumbent position without difficulty. This type of dyspnea is labeled *paroxysmal nocturnal dyspnea* and is almost diagnostic of congestive heart failure caused by disease of the left ventricle.

The patient may have dyspnea due to *acute pulmonary edema*. He or she may develop abrupt, severe dyspnea and wheezing. In severe cases the patient coughs up frothy, blood-streaked material. This life-threatening event is caused by acute dysfunction of the left ventricle, as with myocardial infarction; an arrhythmia, such as uncontrolled atrial fibrillation in a patient with coronary artery disease, cardiomyopathy, or aortic or mitral valve disease; or rupture of the papillary muscle or chordae tendineae of the mitral valve. Papillary muscle rupture is usually due to myocardial infarction, and rupture of the chordae tendineae is caused by endocarditis or myxomatous degeneration of the chords and mitral valve leaflets. The pulmonary edema may subside spontaneously when it is due to a subset of coronary artery disease in which there is transient ischemia of the left ventricle. This event may occur, and the patient may not experience angina pectoris, leaving the physician bewildered as to the cause of the frightening event.

Another cause of acute pulmonary edema is uncontrolled atrial fibrillation or sinus tachycardia in a patient with mitral stenosis. In these patients the left ventricle functions normally but left atrial pressure rises abruptly because the time for diastolic filling of the left ventricle is curtailed significantly by the tachycardia.

Cheyne-Stokes respiration is characterized by periods of hyperpnea alternating with periods of apnea.[23] The patient may become agitated during the hyperpneic phases of the abnormal respiratory cycle, and cardiac arrhythmia may occur. Patients who exhibit Cheyne-Stokes respiration commonly have heart failure and cerebral vascular disease.

Dyspnea on effort.[23] The patient with heart failure may note that he or she cannot walk fast, climb stairs, or walk up a slight incline without experiencing "shortness of breath," whereas these activities did not previously produce any difficulty. Other causes of dyspnea produced by effort are lung disease and obesity, as well as effort in a patient who is usually sedentary.

The patient with coronary artery disease may experience dyspnea on effort; it is labeled as an angina equivalent and is actually caused by a transient rise in left ventricular diastolic pressure and poor myocardial contractibility. This, of course, is transient heart failure due to transient myocardial ischemia.

Patients with *hypoxia due to congenital heart disease* who have a right-to-left shunt experience dyspnea on effort related to increased activity.[24]

Patients with an *acute pulmonary embolism* may experience abrupt dyspnea,[14] because hypoxia may develop acutely and respiration is altered by pleuritis.

Patients who have pain due to *pericarditis* or *pleuritis* due to pulmonary infarction may alter their breathing pattern to avoid pain,[9] and this change in breathing pattern may produce dyspnea. Patients with *constrictive pericarditis* have dyspnea on effort as a result of diastolic dysfunction and pulmonary congestion.

Patients with primary pulmonary hypertension or Eisenmenger physiology may have an increase in hypoxia and dyspnea on effort.[11,24] A right-to-left shunt through the foramen ovale develops in patients with primary pulmonary hypertension; patients with Eisenmenger physiology have pulmonary hypertension and reverse the shunt through a ventricular septal defect, patent ductus arteriosus, or atrial septal defect.

Patients with *cor pulmonale* have dyspnea on effort because of the associated lung disease due to emphysema, pneumoconiosis, or neoplastic disease.[25]

Noncardiac causes of dyspnea

Anxiety. Patients with anxiety, with or without the full-blown picture of NCA, have two types of breathing difficulty.[4,18] They may complain of feeling that the air they inhale "does not satisfy" them. Accordingly, they take deep breaths—they sigh frequently. These patients do not complain of dyspnea on effort. When a patient complains of dyspnea at rest but denies dyspnea on effort, is is highly likely that the patient does not have heart or lung disease.

Patients with anxiety may also have episodes of *hyperventilation* in which they develop numbness, especially around the mouth and in the hands, tetany, and an "unreal" sensation.[19] The symptoms usually disappear when the physician indicates that the patient can stop the hyperventilation. The current term for this condition is "panic attack." When this syndrome occurs at night, it may be difficult to distinguish it from paroxysmal nocturnal dyspnea due to heart failure. There are differences in the two conditions, but the patient cannot always describe them to the physician. For example, the patient with a panic attack may not feel better when he or she sits up in bed. The panic attack lasts longer, and the patient may not return to the recumbent position.

Lung disease. Patients with chronic lung disease of any kind without heart disease may experience dyspnea on effort. A pneumothorax or mediastinal empyema[4,15] may produce acute dyspnea, and patients with pneumonia may develop dyspnea when the pneumonic process involves a significant portion of the lungs.

Patients with asthma often notice wheezing at rest. Wheezing may also be produced by effort, especially in cold weather. Patients with heart failure may wheeze and are labeled as having cardiac asthma. Commonly the patient has obvious heart disease and other signs of heart failure, but at times the cause of the asthma may not be readily apparent. The diagnosis may be difficult when there is a long-standing history of asthma (wheezing) and the patient also has heart disease. The diagnosis is difficult, because patients who have a long-standing history of wheezing are likely to wheeze more when they develop heart failure.

Anemia, thyrotoxicosis. Patients who are severely anemic may complain of dyspnea on effort, as may patients with thyrotoxicosis.[4]

Hyperpnea. Women who are in the last few months of pregnancy may develop hyperpnea on effort. They are not alarmed by the obvious respiratory movements and are detached from the hyperpnea; they are not truly dyspneic, because the hyperpnea does not alarm them.[4]

Patients with diabetic ketoacidosis have hyperpnea due to low serum pH, but they do not complain of shortness of breath.[4]

Caveat. Although there are many causes of dyspnea, only a few types of dyspnea are relatively specific for heart disease and heart failure. Newly developed orthopnea and paroxysmal nocturnal dyspnea are perhaps the most specific signs of heart failure. Newly developed dyspnea on effort in the absence of lung disease is likely to be caused by heart failure. The physician must seek other clues indicating heart disease and must rule out noncardiac causes of dyspnea in order to diagnose the condition correctly.

Palpitation

Palpitation is defined as an awareness of the heartbeat.[4] The patient may notice the normally beating heart, a single atrial or ventricular beat, supraventricular or ventricular ectopic tachycardia, or an extremely slow beat due to any of several mechanisms. The patient may detect a periodic fullness in the neck veins when the atrium contracts against a closed tricuspid valve, as well as precordial discomfort due to the tumultuous action of the heart. The patient may or may not notice whether the onset and offset of the rapid heart action is sudden or gradual. A gradual onset and offset of a rapid heartbeat suggests sinus tachycardia, whereas an abrupt onset and offset of a rapid heartbeat suggests supraventricular or ventricular tachycardia. An abrupt return to normal rhythm produced by certain actions, such as a Valsalva maneuver, suggests supraventricular tachycardia. A rapid but irregular heart rhythm suggests atrial fibrillation or atrial flutter with varying degrees of atrioventricular block.

The fact that some patients feel every benign ectopic heartbeat whereas others may not detect treacherous ventricular tachycardia serves to emphasize that the patient cannot separate benign arrhythmias from malignant ones.

Patients with heart disease may develop heart failure as a result of tachycardia. For example, a patient with mitral stenosis may develop dyspnea, even acute pulmonary edema, when uncontrolled atrial fibrillation or sinus tachycardia occurs. A patient with symptomatic or asymptomatic coronary heart disease may develop the chest discomfort of myocardial ischemia when an abnormal, rapid heart rhythm occurs.

Syncope[26]

Syncope is usually serious; the mechanisms responsible for syncope are the same mechanisms that cause death. Syncope may be viewed as temporary death, or death may be viewed as permanent syncope.

Syncope is defined as the transient loss of consciousness. Having said that, it is necessary to define transient and loss of consciousness. Transient is defined as a few seconds, and loss of consciousness implies that the patient's mental status is normal before the event and returns to normal a few seconds after the event. The patient has no warning that he or she is about to faint. Also, the patient may have no memory of syncope. There may, however, be signs of injury that suggest that the patient has fallen. Near syncope is defined as a transient loss of postural tone. The patient feels as though he or she is about to faint but does not do so.

Cardiac syncope is caused by an abrupt decrease in cerebral blood flow resulting from a sudden decrease in cardiac output.

Decrease in cardiac output due to cardiac arrhythmia.[26] Certain cardiac arrhythmias—including episodes of complete heart block due to coronary artery disease, Lenegre disease, Lev disease, sick sinus syndrome (bradycardia-tachycardia syndrome), ventricular tachycardia, and ventricular fibrillation—may produce cardiac syncope. These arrhythmias may produce syncope when there are no obstructive lesions in the heart. Atrial fibrillation may produce syncope in association with preexcitation of the ventricles, because the ventricular rate may be 300 depolarizations of the ventricles per minute. Atrial fibrillation, or supraventricular tachycardia, may precipitate syncope when there is obstructive heart disease, such as aortic valve stenosis, obstructive cardiomyopathy, or mitral stenosis. Syncope can also occur when rapid tachycardia occurs in a patient with a decreased ejection fraction from any cause.

A young patient with a *long QT interval* in the electrocardiogram may have ventricular arrhythmias, which may cause syncope (see Chapter 7).

Carotid sinus syncope is due to profound bradycardia or asystole. The diagnostic problem is to determine whether the carotid sinus is hypersensitive or whether the atrioventricular node is hypersensitive (see later discussion).

Decrease in cardiac output due to obstructive cardiovascular disease.[26] Patients with *severe aortic valve stenosis* may have syncope even when there is no evidence of cardiac arrhythmia.

Patients with *idiopathic hypertrophic subaortic stenosis (IHSS)* may have episodes of syncope. Endogenous and exogenous catecholamines may precipitate syncope in such patients. For example, one of my patients fainted in bed when he used a nasal decongestant for coryza. Patients with IHSS may also faint when they develop atrial fibrillation or ventricular arrhythmia.

Patients with primary pulmonary hypertension or Eisenmenger physiology may also be included in this group of patients, because they have *obstructive pulmonary arteriolar disease.*

Acute *pulmonary embolism* may produce syncope, in part because of abrupt pulmonary artery obstruction; however, a cardiac arrhythmia may also contribute to the event.

Patients with a *decrease in blood flow to the lungs*, a right-to-left shunt, and arterial oxygen unsaturation, such as occurs with tetralogy of Fallot, may have episodes of syncope as a result of the obstruction to pulmonary blood flow plus severe hypoxia. To avoid syncope, the small child with tetralogy of Fallot learns to squat, which increases the peripheral resistance and decreases the right-to-left shunt. The parent of an infant with tetralogy of Fallot learns to detect a "hypoxic spell" by observing an increase in cyanosis. The parent simulates the child's squatting by holding the infant and pulling the infant's legs upward to abort the episode.

Decrease in effective blood volume and/or peripheral arterial resistance.[26] *Postural hypotension* may produce syncope. It is diagnosed by identifying a fall of 10 mm Hg or more in the systolic blood pressure when the patient assumes the upright position.

The patient with *blood loss* may have syncope when he or she assumes the erect position, because the effective blood volume decreases to a critical amount when the patient stands; this is due to further pooling of the blood in the veins of the legs.

The patient who has been *bedridden for several weeks* may faint when he or she stands, because the normal increase in peripheral arterial resistance does not occur as promptly following a period of inactivity.

Patients with *heart failure who have been diuresed* may develop postural hypotension and syncope because the effective blood volume is inadequate.

Postural hypotension and syncope may be caused by *autonomic dysfunction*, such as occurs in patients with diabetes mellitus. These individuals are unable to increase their peripheral resistance when they stand up. They do not sweat normally, and their heart rate does not increase when their systemic blood pressure declines.

Other causes/types of syncope[26]

Common faint. The common faint (vasodepressor syncope) occurs when susceptible persons find themselves in a situation from which they would prefer to run but are prevented from doing so by the rules of maturity and society. For example, a strong-appearing man may faint when he views a venipuncture being performed on another person; I was present when several healthy young football players fainted at the funeral of a friend. The patient feels slightly nauseated, salivates slightly, and if he or she is standing or sitting, loses consciousness. The pulse is slow, and the blood pressure is low. The skin is pale, and the patient has a deathlike appearance. The sympathetic and parasympathetic systems are in bitter conflict. The peripheral arterial resistance is decreased, and the heart rate is slow. These two abnormalities conspire to produce the decrease in cardiac output that causes the syncope.

Vagovagal syncope. Vagovagal syncope is caused by stimulation of the afferent end of the vagus nerve. Pleural shock, which occasionally occurs with needle aspiration for hydrothorax, is an example of this type of syncope.

Cough-and-sneeze syncope. Although cough-and-sneeze syncope can occur in anyone, it is most often observed in men with chronic bronchitis. An abrupt increase in intrathoracic pressure occurs during the cough or sneeze, leading to a marked decrease in stroke output, an increase in cerebrospinal fluid pressure, and compression of arteries and veins in the brain. These events may be accompanied by bradycardia, atrioventricular block, and sinus arrest.

Micturition syncope. Syncope may occur during or following the act of urination. It is usually seen in men who have nocturia, and the cause is multifactorial. Bradycardia seems to occur at a time when there is a decrease in peripheral resistance. This suggests parasympathetic stimulation similar to that which occurs when pleural or ascitic fluid is removed. The reflex caused by performing a Valsalva maneuver during the time the man is standing may also be a factor.

Defecation syncope. Syncope may occur during the act of defecation. The same mechanism that causes micturition syncope may be responsible for defecation syncope.

Conditions that simulate syncope. It is not always possible to separate syncope from other conditions that alter the mental status. Petit mal epilepsy may mimic syncope, and an electroencephalogram and Holter monitoring may be needed to determine the cause of the episode. A grand mal seizure, on the other hand, is associated with characteristic muscular movement that starts on one side and moves to the other, and the patient may detect an aura prior to the seizure. A hypoglycemic episode is characterized by excessive sweating. A transient ischemic attack is recognized by its accompanying transient neurologic deficit; the patient rarely faints.

Caveat. Patients with syncope should be asked if they are taking medication such as a beta-blocking drug, calcium antagonist, any antiarrhythmia drug, digitalis, or diuretic, because the action of these drugs may be responsible for, or contribute to, the development of syncope.

The patient with syncope may not be diagnosed accurately by the history alone. In addition, the physical examination may not reveal a cause for the syncope. The purpose of this discussion has been to emphasize the importance of asking every patient if he or she had ever fainted or felt like he or she was about to faint. The spouse of the patient with syncope should also be asked if the patient has ever fainted, because the patient may not recall the episode. Commonly other procedures are necessary to determine the exact cause of the syncope. For example, Holter monitoring and electrophysiologic testing may be needed (see Chapter 10).

Intermittent claudication

The pain of intermittent claudication of the skeletal muscle is due to temporary ischemia that is usually (but not always) caused by atherosclerosis of the artery or arteries that supply a particular anatomic part of the body.[27] Intermittent claudication is produced by effort and relieved by discontinuing the effort. In that respect it is similar to angina. However, it is never related to emotional distress, as is angina. The arterial obstruction is located proximal to the location of the intermittent claudication. Intermittent claudication of the toes or arches of the feet is produced by arterial obstruction in the small arteries of the feet and in the posterior tibial arteries. Intermittent claudication of the calves, the most common site, is due to obstructive disease of the popliteal and femoral arteries. Intermittent claudication of the thighs and buttocks is caused by obstructive disease of the iliac arteries or terminal aorta (Leriche syndrome).[27] Intermittent claudication of the hands or forearms indicates obstruction of the radial, ulnar, or brachial arteries. Intermittent claudication of the masseter muscles suggests Takayasu disease rather than atherosclerosis.

Acute, persistent pain in the calf, thigh, or other muscle groups suggests an embolus to the artery or acute thrombosis of an obstructive lesion.[27] This occurs at rest and may lead to gangrene of the toes or lower leg. From a pathophysiologic standpoint this condition is similar to myocardial infarction. The "blue toe" syndrome is caused by cholesterol emboli to the toes from proximal atherosclerotic lesions of the arteries proximal to the feet.

Raynaud phenomenon

The patient with Raynaud phenomenon complains of pain in the fingers that is usually precipitated by exposure of the whole body to cold or exposure of the hands to cold objects such as ice.[27] The fingers become white (ischemic), then blue, and finally red (reactive hyperemia).

Raynaud disease occurs in patients with no other disease. Raynaud phenomenon occurs in patients with progressive systemic sclerosis (scleroderma) or some other collagen disease.

Symptoms due to emboli

Patients with the following conditions may have embolic episodes: atrial fibrillation by itself; atrial fibrillation with mitral stenosis; mitral stenosis and normal rhythm; myocardial infarction with a left ventricular mural thrombus; a large, dilated heart with a mural thrombus; endocarditis of diseased native or prosthetic aortic, mitral, or, rarely, tricuspid valves; marantic endocarditis; thrombosed prosthetic aortic or mitral valves; mitral valve prolapse; myxoma of the left atrium; carotid atherosclerosis; aortic atherosclerosis; and a "crossed embolus" that travels from the leg veins through a foramen ovale to the systemic arterial circulation.[28] Such patients may have transient cerebral ischemic attacks or, when the embolus is large, a completed stroke; acute pain and weakness of the leg or arm; pain in the flank from renal infarction; or abdominal pain. It is likely that some of the unexplained episodes of abdominal pain in elderly individuals are caused by an embolus to the mesenteric arteries.

A stroke occurring in a patient who is under 50 years of age with no other disease is likely to be due to a *crossed embolus*. That is, a silent thrombus within the veins of the leg may break off and pass through a foramen ovale, resulting in the stroke.[28]

The newly delineated syndrome of multiple emboli to the brain, to abnormal viscera, or to the arteries of the lower extremities is sometimes related to a *shaggy thoracic aorta*.[29] The shagginess is due to numerous small, villouslike lesions composed of platelets and cholesterol. The lumen of the aorta, when viewed by transesophageal echocardiography, is filled with wheat field–like projections.

Fatigue

Fatigue has many causes.[4] Fatigue related to heart disease occurs in patients with heart failure from any cause, with excessive diuresis, or with angina equivalent, which is caused by transient myocardial ischemia (see earlier discussion). Fatigue may also be caused by hypokalemia and thyrotoxicosis, both of which may be related to heart disease.

Hemoptysis

Hemoptysis is the act of coughing up blood.[4] The frothy fluid coughed up by patients with pulmonary edema is often blood tinged, but this is not hemoptysis. Patients with pulmonary infarction, mitral stenosis, or Eisenmenger syndrome may cough up blood.

Hoarseness

The patient with mitral stenosis may become hoarse, because the large left pulmonary artery may compress the left recurrent laryngeal nerve.[4] The voice may be low pitched in patients with myxedema.

Nausea

Heart disease rarely produces nausea. Occasionally it may occur in a patient with myocardial infarction or be related to medication such as an opiate or digitalis.

Chills and fever

Fever is almost a constant feature of bacterial endocarditis; chills may also occur. Rheumatic fever is almost always accompanied by fever, but chills do not occur unless aspirin has been given. Patients with pulmonary infarction may have a low-grade fever, and fever may occur following myocardial infarction. Fever may also occur in pericarditis and myocarditis.

Edema

The patient with heart failure may give a history of edema of both lower extremities; it subsides at night, when the patient is recumbent, and returns during the day, when the patient is upright. Edema is, however, a late sign of heart failure and can be caused by many other conditions. The most common cause of lower-extremity edema in relatively active people is venous disease of the lower extremities. Lower-extremity edema occurs in healthy people after long periods of sitting, such as occurs with long trips in an airplane or automobile. Elderly patients who sit in wheelchairs all day in nursing homes develop stasis edema, which is commonly mistaken as being due to heart failure.

Nocturia and polyuria

Patients with congestive heart failure may have nocturia, because the cardiac output and renal blood flow is greater during recumbency than during the activity of the day. Patients with supraventricular tachycardia may have an increase in urine production, because the abnormal rhythm causes a decrease in atrial antinatriuretic hormones.[30]

Noises heard by the patient

Patients may hear the following murmurs: the murmur caused by mitral regurgitation secondary to a ruptured chordae tendineae of the mitral valve; acute aortic regurgitation due to a retroverted aortic valve cusp or rupture of a porcine prosthetic valve; and the loud murmur of aortic valve stenosis or interventricular septal defect.

Weight gain or loss[23]

A patient may gain weight as a result of chronic heart failure. In fact, several pounds of fluid can be retained without edema formation. Weight loss may occur when the patient has severe chronic heart failure. Cardiac cachexia occurs because of poor food intake and poor assimilation.

Hiccups

Patients with myocardial infarction may develop hiccups.[5] In fact, on rare occasions hiccups may be an early sign of myocardial infarction. Hiccups may also occur following cardiac surgery.

PAST HISTORY

It is always important to ask the patient, "When were you last perfectly well?"[31] Each of the patient's complaints should then be explored from its onset.

The physician should inquire if the patient had rheumatic fever as a child. However, a negative past history for rheumatic fever does not exclude the presence of rheumatic heart disease. Today we demand that the modified Jones criteria be fulfilled to diagnose rheumatic fever but tend to accept a vague history of rheumatic fever occurring in the distant past. Accordingly, the acceptance of a vague past history of rheumatic fever may be misleading.

The patient should be asked when a heart murmur was first detected. A murmur heard early in life is a clue to the diagnosis of congenital heart disease. It is, however, essential to ascertain if the patient was actually examined early in life.

How long has the patient had hypertension? Hypertension discovered early in life suggests coarctation of the aorta, congenital renovascular disease, or renal disease. Hypertension first discovered in the sixth decade of life suggests acquired renovascular disease. Essential hypertension usually develops in the third or fourth decade of life.

The febrile patient with a heart murmur who had dental work a few days or weeks before examination is considered to have infective endocarditis until it has been proved otherwise.

Has the patient been in an accident that could have produced injury to the heart and aorta? Has the patient had radiation of the chest that could have caused constrictive pericarditis, coronary artery disease, or heart valve disease?

The lifestyle of the patient is very important. The physician must inquire about the use of alcohol, tobacco, or addicting drugs; the amount of exercise; and the diet. If the blood lipid levels have been measured in the past, does the patient remember their values?

It is important to note all of the drugs the patient is taking, or has taken, and to be familiar with their side effects.

FAMILY HISTORY

It is important to ask if any member of the patient's family has hypertension. It is likely that a hypertensive patient has essential hypertension if several members of the family, including the parents, have, or had, hypertension.

It is also valuable to determine if other members of the family have, or had, atherosclerotic coronary heart disease. The patient is more likely to have, or to develop, atherosclerotic coronary heart disease if other members of the family who are under 50 years of age have been diagnosed as having it.

A subset of hypertrophic cardiomyopathy is genetically determined. Thus a history of death at an early age that was attributed to heart disease may have been due to hypertrophic cardiomyopathy.

Diabetes mellitus is also genetically determined, and because of its role in producing coronary artery disease, the family history should include an inquiry as to its occurrence.

The age and cause of death of the parents, brothers, and sisters should be recorded. Paul Dudley White believed strongly that the longevity of a patient was predetermined by the life span of the patient's parents.[31] If the patient's mother and father lived to be 90 years of age, he viewed this as evidence that the patient's outlook was good—even if the patient had heart disease.

Key Points

- The medical history yields many diagnostic clues, and it takes a physician a lifetime to fully learn the art of history taking.

- There are two objectives to history taking: to obtain scientific data and to establish a trustful relationship with the patient. The scientific data include the identification and analysis of symptoms, past medical conditions (including the patient's lifestyle), and the medical conditions in family members. The development of a trustful relationship depends on the skill of the physician and his or her ability to place the patient at ease, to listen to the patient, and to be sensitive to the patient's feelings.

- Each organ of the body has its own language. The patient translates the body's language into symptoms, and the physician must then translate the patient's symptoms into diagnostic clues. In many ways it is like learning a foreign language, with all of the dialects associated with it.

- The past medical history (including determining the lifestyle of the patient and environmental factors) and the family history are also important and commonly supply the most powerful diagnostic clues.

- Patients with no symptoms may have serious disease that can be discovered by techniques other than history taking, and patients with numerous severe symptoms may have a good prognosis depending on the cause of the symptoms. Obviously, in day-to-day work, the physician must correlate the data found by history taking with the data found by physical examination, the results of the interpretation of the electrocardiogram, the results of the interpretation of the chest x-ray film, and the results of the routine laboratory tests.

REFERENCES

1. Wood P: *Diseases of the heart and circulation*, Philadelphia, 1956, JP Lippincott, p 1.
2. Fuster V: The clinical history. In Brandenburg RO, Fuster V, Giuliani ER, McGoon DC, editors: *Cardiology: fundamentals and practice*, St Louis, 1987, Mosby, p 185.
3. Braunwald E: The history. In Braunwald E, editor: *Heart disease*, Philadelphia, 1980, WB Saunders, pp 3-12.
4. Hurst JW: The history and physical examination. In Hurst JW, editor-in-chief: *The heart*, ed 7, New York, 1990, McGraw-Hill, pp 122-134.
5. Hurst JW: Atherosclerotic coronary heart disease: historical benchmarks, methods of study and clinical features, differential diagnosis, and clinical spectrum. In Hurst JW, editor-in-chief: *The heart*, ed 7, New York, 1990, McGraw-Hill, pp 965-967.
6. Heberden W: Some account of a disorder of the breast, *Med Trans* 2:59, 1772 (published by the College of Physicians in London).

7. Home E: *A treatise on the blood, inflammation, and gun shot wounds by the late John Hunter*, Philadelphia, 1796, Thomas Bradford (earlier edition published in England in 1794).

8. Herrick JB: Clinical features of sudden obstruction of the coronary arteries, *JAMA* 59:2015, 1912.

9. Hurst JW: Atherosclerotic coronary heart disease: historical benchmarks, methods of study and clinical features, differential diagnosis, and clinical spectrum. In Hurst JW, editor-in-chief: *The heart*, ed 7, New York, 1990, McGraw-Hill, pp 984-985.

10. Lindsay J Jr, Beall AC Jr, DeBakey ME: Diseases of the aorta. In Hurst JW, editor-in-chief: *The heart*, ed 7, New York, 1990, McGraw-Hill, p 1408.

11. Kuida H: Primary and secondary pulmonary hypertension: pathophysiology, recognition, and treatment. In Hurst JW, editor-in-chief: *The heart*, ed 7, New York, 1990, McGraw-Hill, p 1191.

12. Hurst JW: Atherosclerotic coronary heart disease: historical benchmarks, methods of study and clinical features, differential diagnosis, and clinical spectrum. In Hurst JW, editor-in-chief: *The heart*, ed 7, New York, 1990, McGraw-Hill, p 984.

13. Ibid, pp 993-994.

14. Dalen JE, Alpert JS: Pulmonary embolism. In Hurst JW, editor-in-chief: *The heart*, ed 7, New York, 1990, McGraw-Hill, p 1207.

15. Talley JD: Pneumomediastinum. In Hurst JW, editor-in-chief: *Medicine for the practicing physician*, Boston, 1992, Butterworth, pp 921-922.

16. Hersh T: Gastrointestinal causes of chest discomfort. In Hurst JW, editor-in-chief: *The heart*, ed 7, New York, 1990, McGraw-Hill, pp 987-991.

17. Hurst JW: Atherosclerotic coronary heart disease: historical benchmarks, methods of study and clinical features, differential diagnosis, and clinical spectrum. In Hurst JW, editor-in-chief: *The heart*, ed 7, New York, 1990, McGraw-Hill, pp 982-984.

18. Cohen ME, White PD: Life situations, emotions, and neurocirculatory asthenia (anxiety neurosis, neurasthenia, effort syndrome), *Psychol Med* 13(6):335, 1951.

19. Okel BB, Hurst JW: Prolonged hyperventilation in man, *Arch Intern Med* 108:757, 1961.

20. Gorlin R: The hyperkinetic heart syndrome, *JAMA* 182:823, 1962.

21. Holmfewn A: Vasoregulatory asthenia, *Can Med Assoc J* 196:904, 1967.

22. Hurst JW, Morris DC, Crawley IS, Dorney ER: The history: symptoms and past events related to cardiovascular disease. In Hurst JW, editor-in-chief: *The heart*, ed 7, New York, 1990, McGraw-Hill, pp 127-129.

23. Spann JF Jr, Hurst JW: The recognition and management of heart failure. In Hurst JW, editor-in-chief: *The heart*, ed 7, New York, 1990, McGraw-Hill, pp 421-423.

24. Nugent EW, Plauth WH Jr, Edwards JE, Williams WH: The pathology, abnormal physiology, clinical recognition, and medical and surgical treatment of congenital heart disease. In Hurst JW, editor-in-chief: *The heart*, ed 7, New York, 1990, McGraw-Hill, p 664.

25. Newman JH, Ross JC: Chronic cor pulmonale. In Hurst JW, editor-in-chief: *The heart*, ed 7, New York, 1990, McGraw-Hill, pp 1220-1229.

26. Weissler AM, Boudoulas H, Lewis RP, Warren JV: Syncope: pathophysiology, recognition, and treatment. In Hurst JW, editor-in-chief: *The heart*, ed 7, New York, 1990, McGraw-Hill, pp 581-603.

27. Smith RB III, Perdue GD: Diseases of the peripheral arteries and veins. In Hurst JW, editor-in-chief: *The heart*, ed 7, New York, 1990, McGraw-Hill, pp 1424-1425.

28. Lechat P, Mas JL, Lascault G, et al: Prevalence of patent foramen ovale in patients with stroke, *N Engl J Med* 318(18):1148, 1988.

29. Hollier LH, Kazmier FJ, Ochsner J, et al: "Shaggy" aorta syndrome with atheromatous embolization to visceral vessels, *Ann Vasc Surg* 5(5):439, 1991.

30. Hartle DK, Hill RD, Talley JD: Atrin—a cardiac hormone: diagnostic and therapeutic possibilities, *Emory Univ J Med* 1(1):66-75, 1987.

31. White PD: Personal communication, circa 1950.

CHAPTER 6

Physical examination

At the outset I wish to emphasize the importance of the very first impression that the patient makes on the physician as he enters the consulting room, or as he looks up from bed or chair of sick room or hospital ward. This first general impression may be more valuable than any other finding of the examination, and this is one reason why the physician can handle a case which he himself sees better than one described to him by spoken or written word. Details of attitude, mental and physical, and data of history and of examination, be they ever so thorough, are really incomplete without the actual sight and contact of the patient. A passing look, a slight gesture, a chance remark may give valuable hints as to the proper handling of the case. For example, a strained look with wide open eyes seen from across the room may lose itself on closer scrutiny and yet it may be one of the most important clews for the search and discovery of thyrotoxicosis when there is little or no definite exophthalmos or thyroid gland enlargement.

Is the patient timid or courageous, gloomy or cheerful, excited or at ease, worried or placid, suspicious or trustful, reserved or frank, silent or loquacious? Is his memory good or bad? Is he old or young for his years? Is he heavy or light for his height? Is he strong or weak? Has he obviously lost weight recently? Has he any deformities, scars, paralyses, tics, or defects of sight or hearing to worry or to hamper him? Is he breathing normally? Is he hoarse? Does he stammer? Is he alone or are friends or relatives with him and what are their attitudes towards each other? All these points come to notice during the first few minutes of observation and scrutiny and during the history telling. They are frequently of considerable value and yet most of them are not recorded except more or less unconsciously in the mind of the physician; it is well to enter definitely in the written record at least those that are striking or that seem significant.

PAUL DUDLEY WHITE 1931[1]*

The questions asked during the history-taking interview are usually organized along the lines of body systems. That is, inquiries are made regarding the circulatory system, the digestive system, the endocrine system, the neurologic system, etc. The physical examination, however, is usually performed by beginning at the top of the head and progressing toward the feet. This is more convenient than completing the physical examination on one body system before proceeding to examine another body

---

*Reprinted with the permission of Macmillan Publishing Company from *Heart Disease* by Dr. Paul Dudley White, p 38. Copyright 1931 Macmillan Publishing Company; copyright renewed © 1959 Paul Dudley White.

system, but there is a disadvantage to performing the physical examination in this manner: it breaks the continuity of the physician's thought process. It would seem to make more sense to perform the physical examination on the entire cardiovascular system than to begin the examination by checking the blood pressure, which is an attribute of the arteries, and then examine the head and neck rather than completing the examination of the arteries. Still, it would be cumbersome, indeed, to examine the circulatory system as a unit rather than examining from "head to foot," as is customarily done. Accordingly, when the physical examination is completed, the physician would do well to arrange the data that have been collected so that the data collected on the cardiovascular system are viewed as a unit and the data collected from the endocrine system are viewed as another unit, etc.

The examination of the cardiovascular unit includes general inspection, examination of the eyes, examination of the arteries, examination of the veins, examination of precordial pulsations, and auscultation of the heart. However, the remainder of the physical examination is also extremely important, since the abnormalities found in any body system may influence the physician's view about another body system. My failure to discuss the examination of other systems must not be construed as suggesting that it is less important than the examination of the cardiovascular system. It only indicates that this book is about the cardiovascular system.

As emphasized by Paul Dudley White,[1] the physical examination begins during the history-taking interview. The first glance the physician has of the patient may yield information that is gained in no other way. For example, the stare associated with thyrotoxicosis is usually noted initially, or it is overlooked. The blue sclerae associated with osteogenesis imperfecta may be noted instantly, suggesting the possibility of aortic or mitral valve regurgitation. Xanthelasma of the eyelids should lead the physician to think of hyperlipidemia and coronary atherosclerosis, and abnormalities of the eyes, such as those occurring in patients with Down syndrome, may be an indication of congenital heart disease such as an ostium primum type of atrial septal defect. As the interview proceeds, the perceptive physician notes the sighing respiration of anxiety and the despondency of depression. The signs of discomfort or respiratory difficulty are obvious during the interview. The hoarse voice of myxedema is usually detected during the history-taking period, as are abnormalities of communication, such as aphasia. A limp, weak arm or aphasia may be due to a previous stroke, which should stimulate the physician to wonder about the presence of hypertension or a cardiovascular source of cerebral emboli. Deafness in a child should lead the physician to think of osteogenesis imperfecta, along with its cardiac abnormalities, or Jervell and Lange-Nielsen syndrome, which consists of a long QT interval, arrhythmias, and sudden death.[2] Cyanosis of the lips and clubbing of the fingers may be noted during the interview and should lead the physician to consider the possibility of congenital heart disease with a right-to-left shunt.[3] Diseases of the skin, arthritis, ankylosing spondylitis, other skeletal abnormalities, and an abnormal appearance of the face are clues alerting the physician to the possibility of heart disease.

These, as well as other conditions, are often detected during the interview and are discussed in detail in the following sections of this chapter.

ABNORMALITIES FOUND ON GENERAL EXAMINATION AND THEIR CARDIOVASCULAR IMPLICATIONS

Abnormalities of height and weight

The height and weight of the patient must be measured and recorded.

Exceedingly tall patients may have Marfan syndrome, with its associated abnormalities of the aorta, aortic regurgitation, mitral regurgitation, and cardiomyopathy.[4] One must remember, however, that not all patients with Marfan syndrome are tall and that not every tall person has Marfan syndrome.

Obesity may aggravate congestive heart failure, angina pectoris, and hypertension and may, when it is extreme, produce heart failure in the absence of other heart disease.[5] Coronary atherosclerosis and diabetes, with its renal and vascular complications, are more common in obese patients, as is sleep apnea syndrome.

Excessive thinness may be due to anorexia nervosa in young girls, and this condition may be associated with myocardial disease.[6] Cachexia may be related to neoplastic disease, and such patients may have pericarditis and/or myocardial disease, as well as nonbacterial thrombotic endocarditis.

Fever

Temperature elevation may occur in patients with heart disease in the following situations. Bacterial endocarditis is almost always associated with an elevation of temperature.[7] Fever is also commonly associated with rheumatic fever, myocarditis, and pericarditis. Fever may accompany septic arthritis and the arthritis of sickle cell anemia, both of which may be associated with heart disease. Endocarditis may accompany septic arthritis, and myocardial disease, mitral regurgitation, and heart failure may accompany the arthritis of sickle cell anemia. The temperature may be elevated a degree or two in patients with large myocardial infarctions, and patients with thrombophlebitis or pulmonary infarction may have an elevation of temperature. In addition, patients with systemic diseases that may involve the heart, including neoplastic and collagen diseases, may have elevations of temperature.

Hypothermia

Hypothermia may produce atrial fibrillation, a QRS conduction defect, and an Osborne wave in the electrocardiogram.[8]

Abnormalities of the voice

A patient with a low-pitched voice who talks slowly may have myxedema, which may be associated with pericardial effusion, low QRS voltage in the electrocardiogram, cardiomyopathy, and bradycardia.

Aphasia may be apparent and, in conjunction with any clue gained from observing the gait or use of the arms, plus facial signs of a former stroke, should alert the physician that the patient may have hypertension or a cardiovascular cause of cerebral emboli.

EXAMINATION OF THE EARS

Deafness

The deaf child with blue sclerae who breaks his or her bones easily in addition to being deaf has osteogenesis imperfecta.[9] The physician should listen for aortic or mitral valve regurgitation in such patients.

The deaf child who has cardiac arrhythmias and syncope may have the Jervell and Lange-Nielsen syndrome, which is indicated by a long QT interval in the electrocardiogram.[2] Unfortunately, sudden death is also part of this syndrome.

The adult may gradually detect a hearing loss as part of the aging process. Diuresis from the drug furosemide (Lasix) may, however, be the cause of deafness in a small percentage of patients who take it.[10] Paget's disease may also produce a hearing defect, and this disease can cause high-output cardiac failure[11,12] (see later discussion).

Elliot[13] believes that earlobe creases are a marker for coronary atherosclerosis. However, they are so common in older patients that they have little diagnostic value.

EXAMINATION OF THE EYES

Inspection of the eyelids and external structures of the eyes

Inspection of the eyes may provide many clues to diseases that may affect the cardiovascular system. Thyrotoxicosis, which may occur at any age, is an example of such a disease. The patient may have a stare, exophthalmos (Fig. 6-1), and a lid lag. (In the elderly, thyrotoxicosis may not produce exophthalmos.) The patient's eyes may fail to converge—signifying weakness of the extraocular muscles—when the examiner asks the patient to follow the examiner's fingertip as it moves toward the eyes. Thyrotoxicosis may produce atrial fibrillation with a ventricular rate of 170 to 180 beats per minute whereas the euthyroid patient with untreated atrial fibrillation (and no other problem) will usually exhibit a resting ventricular rate of 140 to 160 beats per minute. In some cases atrial fibrillation may be the only clinical indication of thyrotoxicosis. Thyrotoxicosis may augment and accelerate angina pectoris or heart failure from any cause and on rare occasion may be the only recognizable cause of heart failure. The condition may produce a systolic murmur and "scratch" in the second left intercostal space near the sternum and a venous hum in the neck. The former is due to an increase in blood flow in the pulmonary artery, and the latter is due to a series of contact sounds due to distention of the pulmonary artery.

Abnormalities of the eyelids. The shape of the eyelids may be characteristic of Down syndrome (Fig. 6-2).[14] Patients with Down syndrome may have congenital heart disease with an ostium primum type of atrial septal defect.

External ophthalmoplegia and ptosis of an eyelid may be associated with cardiomyopathy. Ptosis may also be secondary to a stroke, which is often associated with an embolus from the cardiovascular system.

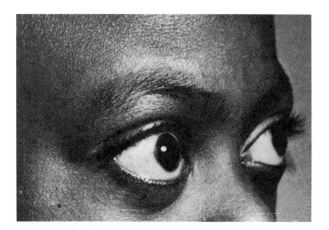

Fig. 6-1. Thyrotoxicosis with typical exophthalmos in a young boy.

Reproduced with permission from Logue RB, Hurst JW: General inspection of the patient with cardiovascular disease. In Hurst JW, Logue RB, editors: *The heart,* ed 1, New York, 1960, McGraw-Hill, p 60.

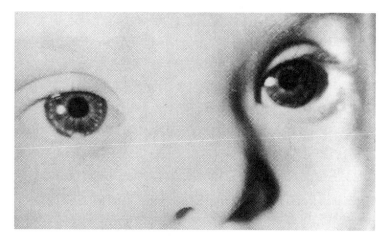

Fig. 6-2. Down syndrome. Note Brushfield spots in the iris of each eye. Epicanthal folds are apparent.

Reproduced with permission from Logue RB, Hurst JW: General inspection of the patient with cardiovascular disease. In Hurst JW, Logue RB, editors: *The heart,* ed 1, New York, 1966, McGraw-Hill, p 57.

Xanthelasma may be noted on the eyelids. This skin lesion suggests the possibility of hyperlipidemia and coronary atherosclerosis[15] (see later discussion).

Petechial hemorrhages may be seen on the inner surface of the lower and upper eyelids, suggesting the possibility of infective endocarditis (Fig. 6-3, A).[7]

Pupillary abnormalities. The pupils of patients with syphilis may be unequal and irregular in shape and fail to constrict when exposed to light. Patients with syphilis may have aortic regurgitation, an aortic aneurysm, or coronary ostial disease.

Blue sclera. Blue sclera indicates osteogenesis imperfecta, which may be accompanied by aortic or mitral regurgitation.[9]

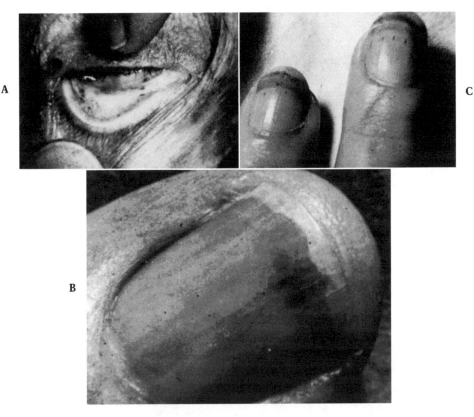

Fig. 6-3. Bacterial endocarditis. **A,** Petechial hemorrhages of the lower eyelid of a patient with infective endocarditis. **B,** Splinter hemorrhages beneath the nails may occur in patients with bacterial endocarditis. Splinter hemorrhages may also be due to other conditions. The splinter hemorrhages shown here occurred in a normal, healthy individual (they were probably due to trauma). **C,** The splinter hemorrhages shown here were due to trichinosis.

Reproduced with permission from Logue RB, Hurst JW: General inspection of the patient with cardiovascular disease. In Hurst JW, Logue RB, editors: *The heart,* ed 1, New York, 1966, McGraw-Hill, p 62.

Corneal arcus. The white ring around the cornea is a marker for abnormal blood lipids and atherosclerosis (especially in young men). The sign is uncommonly present, however, in patients with coronary or peripheral atherosclerosis.

Corneal microdeposits. Patients who are treated with amiodarone for cardiac arrhythmias may develop microdeposits of the cornea.

Cataracts. Cataracts may be seen in young children with rubella syndrome (Fig. 6-4).[16] This syndrome occurs in the children of mothers who had rubella during the first few months of pregnancy, is associated with eighth cranial nerve deafness, patent ductus arteriosus, aortic septal defect, pulmonary valve stenosis, and coarctation of the pulmonary arteries. Cataracts may also occur in patients with myotonia dystrophica, who often have cardiomyopathy.[17]

Dislocation of the lens. Dislocation of the lens of the eye may occur in patients with Marfan syndrome (Fig. 6-5, *C*). Such patients may have an aneurysm of the proximal portion of the aorta, annuloaortic ectasia, mitral valve prolapse and mitral regurgitation, or possibly myocardial disease.

Abnormalities of the iris. The iris may tremble when the head is moved[18]; this abnormality also suggests Marfan syndrome, which may be associated with aortic and cardiac abnormalities, as indicated in the preceding paragraph.

The iris may exhibit spots arranged in an incomplete circle. These spots, known as Brushfield lines, occur in patients with Down syndrome (see Fig. 6-2). Such patients may have an ostium primum type of atrial septal defect or some other abnormality of the endocardial cushions.

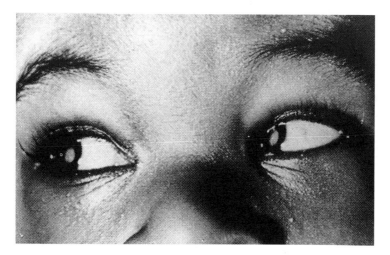

Fig. 6-4. Rubella syndrome. Note the cataracts in each of the eyes.
Reproduced with permission from Logue RB, Hurst JW: General inspection of the patient with cardiovascular disease. In Hurst JW, Logue RB, editors: *The heart,* ed 1, New York, 1966, McGraw-Hill, p 57.

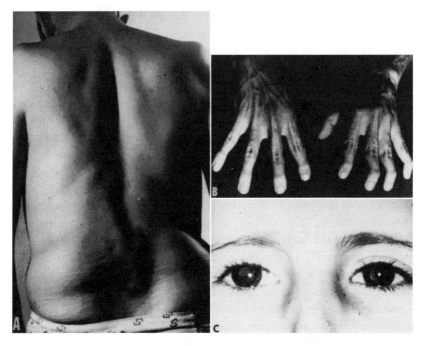

Fig. 6-5. Marfan syndrome. This patient experienced painless dissection of the aorta with aortic regurgitation following a vigorous game of basketball. **A,** Note the scoliosis. Not all patients with this syndrome are asthenic; note the muscular build of this patient. **B,** Long, tapering fingers (arachnodactyly) of the same patient). **C,** Dislocation of the lens in the eyes of another patient with Marfan syndrome.

Reproduced with permission from Logue RB, Hurst JW: General inspection of the patient with cardiovascular disease. In Hurst JW, Logue RB, editors: *The heart,* ed 1, New York, 1966, McGraw-Hill, p 56.

Examination of the ocular fundi*

Atherosclerosis. Atherosclerosis does not affect the arterioles. Accordingly, the retinal arterioles are spared from this disease. However, three signs of atherosclerosis can occasionally be seen in the retina:

- A Hollenhorst plaque (embolus) may be noted in one of the retinal arterioles. It appears as a small white spot in an arteriole and, with the passage of time, moves more distally in the arteriole. This unique embolus usually originates in an atherosclerotic plaque in the carotid artery or aorta. It is composed of platelets, white blood cells, and thrombi.   Coronary atherosclerosis is likely to be present, or to develop, in such a patient.

---

*Modified with permission from Wilber JA: Examination of the retinal fundi. In Hurst JW, Logue RB, editors: *The heart,* ed 1, New York, 1966, McGraw-Hill, p 126.

- Atherosclerosis may occur in the central retinal artery. Obstruction of this artery produces abrupt blindness and pallor of the entire retina. The macula may exhibit an isolated red spot.   Coronary atherosclerosis is likely to be present, or to develop, in such a patient.
- Occlusion of the central retinal vein, or occlusions in the veins near the optic disk, may be due to atherosclerosis. The mechanism for this development is as follows. The arterioles and venules share the same adventitia in areas where the arterioles cross the venules. The atherosclerotic lesions responsible for obstruction of the central retinal vein, or venules near the optic disk, are actually located in the adjacent central retinal artery. This situation does not occur in the more distal arterioles of the retinas.   The vision of the affected eye is lost suddenly when the central retinal vein becomes occluded. The retina appears edematous with sheets of hemorrhages, and papilledema develops.

Coronary atherosclerosis is likely to be present, or to develop, in such a patient.

Arteriolosclerosis. The major cause of retinal arteriolosclerosis is hypertension. The cause of the hypertension cannot, however, be determined from the appearance of the arterioles. The intima of the arteriolar wall becomes hyalinized, and medial hypertrophy develops, along with adventitial fibrosis. This change in the histologic makeup of the arterioles is responsible for the change in their appearance. The color of the arterioles may initially change from red to a copper color; then, as the walls of the arterioles become thicker, they become silver colored. Arteriolovenous nicking is produced when the rigid arterioles cross the venules. This phenomenon is augmented because, as discussed above, the arterioles and venules share the same adventitia at the point where the arterioles cross the venules. There is also generalized arteriolar spasm, but this is not always easy to detect.

Retinal exudates. Although there are other causes of retinal exudates, the most common cause is hypertension. Exudates are caused by leaking arterioles. "Cotton-wool" exudates have fuzzy borders. "Hard" exudates are whitish yellow in color and shine more than cotton-wool exudates. A "macular star" is created when hard exudates are clustered around the macula.

Retinal hemorrhages. Hemorrhages in the retina occur in patients with hypertension. They also occur in patients with anemia, leukemia, diabetes mellitus, macroglobulinemia, subarachnoid hemorrhage, or collagen disease, and they may be the result of emboli. The shape of the hemorrhage is determined by the layer of the retina that is involved.

Roth spots. Roth spots are retinal hemorrhages with a white center. They may occur in patients with infective endocarditis, leukemia, or severe anemia.

Papilledema. Papilledema is recognized when the physiologic cupping of the disk is no longer evident. It is noted in both eyes, and vision is not affected during the early stages of the condition. Later the disk margins become indistinct, the retinal veins become prominent, and retinal hemorrhages and exudates may develop near the optic disks.

Accelerated hypertension is a common cause of papilledema. Papilledema may also be secondary to an increase in intracranial pressure from any cause. Brain tumors, as well as other cerebral lesions, can cause papilledema. In such cases arteriosclerosis does not occur, as it does when the papilledema is caused by hypertension. Papilledema may also be caused by severe pulmonary disease with respiratory acidosis.

Papillitis, which must be differentiated from papilledema, occurs in one eye, and vision is not impaired during the early stage of the disease. The retinal veins may become swollen. The cause of papillitis is usually not identified; it may occur with encephalitis or multiple sclerosis.

Capillary aneurysms. Capillary aneurysms, which are usually located between the optic disk and the macula, produce small red dots in the retina. Capillary aneurysms occur in patients with diabetes mellitus, and the cardiovascular implications are obvious: arterial disease, including coronary atherosclerosis, is common in diabetic patients.

Angioid streaks. Angioid streaks appear as cracks in the retina that extend from the optic disk toward the periphery of the retina. The color of the streak is produced

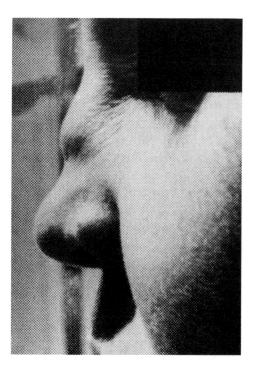

Fig. 6-6. Relapsing polychondritis. Note the collapse of the bridge of the nose. This patient developed aortic regurgitation.
Courtesy Dr. Warren Sarrell, Anniston, Ala. Reproduced with permission from Logue RB, Hurst JW: General inspection of the patient with cardiovascular disease. In Hurst JW, Logue RB, editors: *The heart*, ed 1, New York, 1966, McGraw-Hill, p 58.

by the choroid layer of the eye. Angioid streaks occur in patients with pseudoxanthoma elasticum, Paget disease, or sickle cell disease, each of which has cardiovascular implications.

Caveat

Clinical signs and symptoms are valuable diagnostic clues when they are present. There are, however, many diseases in which the absence of certain signs and symptoms does not eliminate the possibility that the disease is present. All of the diseases discussed in this chapter may occur in the absence of abnormalities of the eye. For example, patients with coronary atherosclerotic heart disease rarely have abnormalities of the eyes due to atherosclerosis.

EXAMINATION OF THE NOSE

Physical examination of the nose offers few clues to the presence of heart disease. The saddle nose of syphilis, along with its associated heart and aortic disease, was seen many years ago but is not seen today. An abnormality of the nose with related cardiovascular implications can be seen in the rare patient with necrotizing chondritis in which aortic regurgitation may be observed (Fig. 6-6).

EXAMINATION OF THE MOUTH AND TONGUE

The tongue may be large (macroglossia) in patients with acromegaly[19] or amyloidosis.[20] When the base of the tongue is infiltrated with amyloid, the tongue may depress the submaxillary glands, which may also be involved with amyloid, so that they become visible (Fig. 6-7). The hard palate may be "arched" more than usual in patients with Marfan syndrome, and petechial hemorrhages may be seen in the mucous membranes of the mouth in patients with infective endocarditis.

EXAMINATION OF THE SKIN*

Abnormalities of skin temperature and texture

The skin may be warm and moist in patients with thyrotoxicosis and dry and thick in patients with myxedema. These abnormalities can sometimes be detected at the time of the introductory handshake. The skin of the lower extremities may be thick and indurated in patients who have had recurrent edema due to heart failure.

---

*Most of this section is abstracted from Goldfarb MS, Gaspari AA, Sturm RL: The skin and the heart. In Hurst JW, editor: *Clinical essays on the heart*, vol 5, New York, 1985, McGraw-Hill, p 197. The copyright has been transferred by the publisher to me. Dr. Mark Goldfarb, the lead author of the original text, has given me permission to abstract the material.

Fig. 6-7. Amyloidosis. Macroglossia may
be due to amyloid infiltration of the
tongue. This young woman had amyloid
deposits in the base of the tongue and
amyloid involvement of the submaxillary
glands.

Reproduced with permission from Logue RB,
Hurst JW: General inspection of the patient
with cardiovascular disease. In Hurst JW,
Logue RB, editors: *The heart,* ed 1, New York,
1966, McGraw-Hill, p 64.

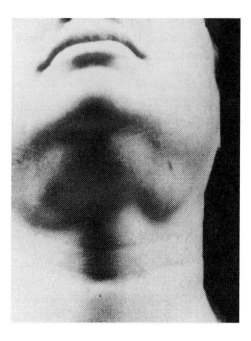

Abnormalities of skin color

Cyanosis (bluish color). It is difficult for the physician to detect minor degrees
of cyanosis. Accordingly, inspection of the patient for cyanosis is a poor method of
assessing arterial hypoxemia unless the cyanosis is definite. Also, when the patient is
anemic, it may not be possible for the patient to develop cyanosis, because the development of "blueness" depends on the presence of at least 5 g of reduced hemoglobin per deciliter of blood. When cyanosis is definitely noted, it is necessary to
determine if it is central or peripheral.

Persistent *central cyanosis* implies that the tongue and mucous membranes of the
mouth are reddish blue. This color is caused by erythrocytosis and a decrease in arterial oxygen saturation, both of which occur in right-to-left shunts associated with
congenital heart disease, such as tetralogy of Fallot, transposition of the great arteries, tricuspid atresia, truncus arteriosus, and rarer forms of defects.

Persistent *peripheral cyanosis* may also be due to congenital heart disease with a
right-to-left shunt. In such cases the fingers and toes are cyanotic; central cyanosis is
also present, and clubbing of the fingers and toes may be obvious. When there is
cyanosis and clubbing of the toes, fingertips of the left hand, and tongue, and no
cyanosis or clubbing of the fingertips of the right hand, the patient has Eisenmenger
physiology with pulmonary hypertension and reversed blood flow in a patent ductus
arteriosus.[21]

Peripheral cyanosis, however, may also be caused by local factors, such as exposure to cold. Central cyanosis does not occur with exposure to cold, because the tongue and mucous membranes of the mouth are usually warmer than the lips, fingertips, or tips of the toes. A young child who remains in a cold swimming pool too long will exhibit blue lips, fingers, and toes. This is due to peripheral arteriolar constriction and an increased extraction of oxygen from blood that enters the capillary bed. Some patients without heart disease have cold feet and cyanosis of the toes without cyanosis of the fingers or tongue; this does not necessarily indicate a decrease in arterial oxygen saturation.

Jaundice (yellow color). Jaundice due to heart disease is rare. When it does occur, it is noted in the sclerae and on the dorsal surface of the hands. Jaundice may be observed when there is severe liver congestion due to heart failure or constrictive pericarditis. The serum bilirubin level is almost never above 2 mg/dl in patients with heart failure and liver congestion. A large pulmonary infarction in a patient with severe heart failure may cause slight icterus.

The patient with myxedema may exhibit a yellow color of the skin, because the liver cannot convert carotene into vitamin A. Myxedema may be the cause of pericardial effusion, myocardial disease, and low voltage in the electrocardiogram.[22]

Patients with long-standing renal failure may develop a dirty yellow color to the skin, often referred to as sallow, because the kidney is retaining urochromes and carotene.[23] The patient is often anemic. Signs of scratching (excoriations) may be evident, since many uremic patients have severe itching of the skin. Such patients may have hypertension, left ventricular hypertrophy, and heart failure.

Green color. Slight cyanosis and slight icterus may occur in a patient with far-advanced heart failure and severe tricuspid valve regurgitation or stenosis. This combination may produce a faint green color to the face and neck.[24]

Bronze color. Hemochromatosis may produce a bronze color to the skin.[25] The discoloration is generalized. Hemochromatosis is seen in patients with diabetes who have evidence of cirrhosis of the liver. Such patients may have cardiomyopathy. Early diagnosis is important, because early recognition can lead to appropriate treatment, which can prevent the cardiomyopathy.

Slatelike color. Argyria is rarely seen today, because nose drops containing silver have been discontinued. Occasionally, however, a patient with recurrent aphthous ulcers may overuse silver nitrate sticks to treat the lesions, and the absorption of silver can be significant; such patients may acquire a silver-slate color.[26] Although argyria is not associated with heart disease, the condition may be confused with cyanosis.

Formerly seen more often than it is today, methemoglobinemia was caused by drugs such as sulfanilamide. The condition may be caused by nitrates given to patients with coronary artery disease.[27] It causes a dusky, slatelike color to the skin of the entire body. Methemoglobinemia may be confused with cyanosis.

Amiodarone toxicity is not rare.[28] This drug, usually given in an effort to prevent serious ventricular arrhythmias or atrial fibrillation that is not controlled by usual medications, may produce a slatelike color to the skin of the ears, nose, and dorsal surface of the hands. These patients may also develop liver, lung, or thyroid disease as a result of amiodarone toxicity.

Ochronosis may produce a slatelike color to the cartilage of the ears and sclera (see later discussion).[29]

Red flush. The most common cause of a transient red flush to the skin is the common, emotionally provoked, blush. The "hot flush" associated with the estrogen deprivation of the menopause is also considered a normal phenomenon. When, however, a red flush develops in a man, or in a woman who is not undergoing the menopause, it may be due to a carcinoid tumor with metastases to the liver.[30] When the tumor is isolated to the small intestine, where it usually originates, the liver destroys the substances that produce the flush. When the carcinoid tumor metastasizes to the liver, the toxic substances are not detoxified; the toxic substances are delivered into the venous system, which enters the right side of the heart. The patient with a carcinoid tumor of the ovary may, however, have episodes of flushing without liver metastasis, because the venous drainage of the ovary enters the superior vena cava and the right side of the heart without passing through the liver.[30]

My experience with patients with carcinoid tumors has been that the red flush is more intense in the face and upper trunk. The red flush may last for several minutes, and it is unpleasant to the patient. It is precipitated by unusual pressure on the liver or abdomen, emotional stimuli, a small amount of alcohol, and certain salad dressings.

The numerous toxic substances produced by carcinoid tumors enter the venous system and the chambers on the right side of the heart and produce carcinoid plaques in the right ventricular endocardium, pulmonary valve stenosis, tricuspid valve regurgitation and stenosis, and conduction defects in the electrocardiogram.[30]

A persistent red flush of the skin, especially of the face and neck, may be due to polycythemia.[31] This is called plethora and may be associated with chronic lung disease or may be idiopathic. Excoriations may be evident on the skin, because the skin may itch, especially after a hot bath. Patients with polycythemia may develop coronary thrombosis more readily than patients without polycythemia. Cerebrovascular events are also more common in these patients.

White discoloration (pallor). Vasodepressor syncope (the common faint) is recognized by the clinical setting, intense pallor to the face, moist palms, and bradycardia. The face has the appearance of death.

Chronic pallor of the lips, face, and fingertips may be present when there is persistent anemia. Anemia may aggravate heart failure or angina pectoris.

Facial pallor may also appear during an episode of angina pectoris.

Sequential white, blue, and red discoloration of the fingers. Patients with Raynaud disease or Raynaud phenomenon have a special type of discoloration of the fingers[32] that occurs when the body is exposed to a cold environment or the hands are used to grasp cold objects. The skin of the fingers becomes pale and numb, and a bluish discoloration follows. These characteristics are due to arteriolar constriction and constriction of the venous end of the capillaries of the fingers. The skin of the fingers then becomes red as a result of reactive hyperemia.

Raynaud disease implies that the condition is not an attribute of another disease. Raynaud disease can only be diagnosed as an isolated entity after several years of observation, because the signs of collagen disease, such as progressive systemic sclerosis (scleroderma) or lupus erythematosus, may not become obvious until this amount of time has passed. *Raynaud phenomenon* is said to be present when the condition occurs as an attribute of another disease.

Lacy brown discoloration of the shins. The reticulate brown pigmentation that is typical of erythema ab igne is located on the shins. It is rarely seen today except in impoverished patients with edema due to severe chronic heart failure, or in patients with edema of the legs from any cause, who sit near an open fire for long periods of time. The heat is not felt because of the edema, and infrared radiation stimulates the melanophores of the skin. This condition should not be mistaken for diabetic dermopathy, a scarring process occurring on the shins of patients with diabetes. The latter is due to microinfarcts, not pigment (see later discussion).

Abnormalities of the skin due to specific diseases

Myxedema. The skin is dry and puffy, especially around the eyes (Fig. 6-8).

Petechiae. Petechiae may be seen in the skin in patients with infective endocarditis.[7] Petechial hemorrhages may also be seen in patients with fat emboli (Fig. 6-9).[33] The petechial hemorrhages are seen in the skin of the upper portion of the body and may be associated with cerebral and pulmonary insufficiency.

Amyloidosis.[34] Patients with *primary amyloidosis* have no other diseases that account for the condition. Such patients may exhibit recurrent *purpura,* or the purpura occurs in response to minimal trauma to the skin,[35] such as a gentle pinch. This occurs because vascular walls are fragile. Purpuric lesions are usually located around the mouth, nose, and neck. *Yellow or reddish brown papules* may develop in the same areas of the body, and these lesions become hemorrhagic when episodes of purpura occur.

Involvement of large areas of the skin may *simulate scleroderma* of the face and extremities; the fingers may be painful, swollen, and red. Rarely, patients with generalized amyloidosis may exhibit signs *suggesting myxedema,* with swelling and puffiness of the face.

Patients are said to have *secondary amyloidosis* when the condition occurs in con-

Fig. 6-8. Typical facies of myxedema in a patient in near-coma.

Reproduced with permission from Logue RB, Hurst JW: General inspection of the patient with cardiovascular disease. In Hurst JW, Logue RB, editors: *The heart*, ed 1, New York, 1966, McGraw-Hill, p 61.

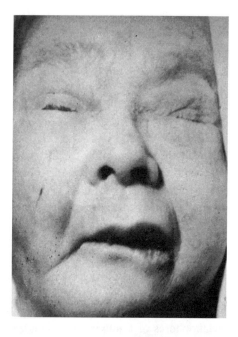

Fig. 6-9. Characteristic axillary petechiae in fat embolism syndrome.

Reproduced with permission from Peltier L: The diagnosis and treatment of fat embolism, *J Trauma* 11:661, © by Williams & Wilkins, 1971.

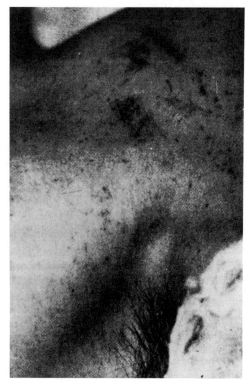

junction with rheumatoid arthritis, bronchiectasis, Crohn disease, or chronic infection. The skin is rarely involved with amyloid in such patients, although internal organs are commonly affected.

Cutaneous amyloidosis may occur in patients with multiple myeloma. Although the amyloidosis is classified as the secondary type, it has some features of primary amyloidosis.

Patients with amyloidosis may have restrictive cardiomyopathy. The heart may not be greatly enlarged, but heart failure is progressive once it begins. Postural hypotension may develop. The electrocardiogram may exhibit conduction defects of the QRS complexes, and abnormal Q waves may develop, suggesting myocardial infarction. The QRS voltage is almost always low.

Neurofibromatosis. Patients with neurofibromatosis may have café au lait spots. Such patients may have hypertension secondary to a pheochromocytoma.[36]

Sarcoidosis. Sarcoidosis may involve the nervous system, lungs, lymph nodes, eyes, skin, and heart (Fig. 6-10). It is a granulomatous disease of unknown cause. Because skin lesions due to sarcoid may simulate other diseases and vice versa, the diagnosis is often established through histologic examination of a biopsy specimen of a lesion. Red, painful, tender nodules, which are characteristic of erythema nodosum, may occur on the anterior portion of the lower extremity. Sarcoidal papules with

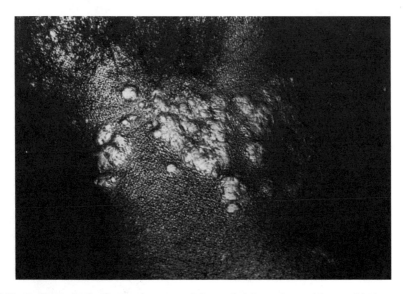

Fig. 6-10. Infiltrated papules on the nape of the neck in a patient with sarcoidosis.
Courtesy Marilynne McKay, M.D., Department of Dermatology, Emory University School of Medicine, Atlanta, Ga. From Goldfarb MS, Gaspari AA, Sturm RL: The skin and the heart. In Hurst JW, editor: *Clinical essays on the heart*, vol 5, New York, 1985, McGraw-Hill, p 201. The copyright has been transferred from the publisher to me.

atrophic centers may develop around the nose and mouth. Sarcoidal skin lesions may be diffuse, with serpiginous borders; in some cases plaques may form and simulate psoriasis. *Lupus pernio* may be suspected when the plaques involve the ears, nose, toes, and fingers.

Most patients with systemic sarcoidosis do not have cardiovascular symptoms; there seems to be no direct correlation between the skin lesions and systemic involvement. However, the myocardium may become involved with the lesions of sarcoid, and heart failure and arrhythmias may develop. Atrioventricular block may occur, as may QRS conduction disturbances. The electrocardiogram may show Q wave abnormalities suggesting myocardial infarction.

Rheumatic fever.[37] *Subcutaneous nodules* may occur on the elbows, the forehead, some other bony prominences, or the tendons (Fig. 6-11). These nodules are nontender and movable. *Erythema marginatum* is a pink plaque with a clear center and occurs on the abdomen, trunk, and proximal portions of the legs and arms. Neither of these lesions is specific for rheumatic fever; nodules can also be seen in patients with lupus erythematosus or rheumatoid arthritis, and annular erythema may occur in patients with acute glomerulonephritis, drug toxicity, or sepsis.

The cardiovascular manifestations of acute rheumatic fever include pericarditis,

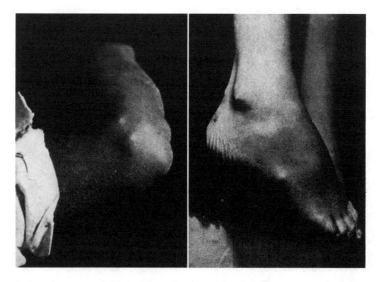

Fig. 6-11. Subcutaneous nodules on the elbow, ankle, Achilles tendon, and foot in a child with acute rheumatic fever.

Courtesy Cardiac Clinic, Children's Hospital, Boston, Mass. Reprinted with the permission of Macmillan Publishing Company from *Heart Disease* by Dr. Paul Dudley White, p 60. Copyright 1931 Macmillan Publishing Company; copyright renewed © 1959 Paul Dudley White.

myocarditis, acute mitral regurgitation, and, rarely, acute aortic regurgitation. The electrocardiogram may show a long PR interval, but complete heart block is rare.

Hyperthyroidism. The skin is warm and smooth. The palms are pink and moist, and the nails may show onycholysis.[38] Hair loss may occur. Dermatographism and lower-extremity edema may occur. Pretibial myxedema may appear as flesh-colored plaques in a small percentage of patients (Fig. 6-12).

Atrial fibrillation is common in patients with hyperthyroidism. The hypermetabolic state will aggravate heart failure and angina pectoris. Patients with thyrotoxicosis may rarely develop high-output cardiac failure when no other cause of heart disease is apparent.[39]

Myxedema. The skin becomes puffy, dry, and swollen but does not pit with pressure (see Fig. 6-8).[40] There may be a slightly yellow color to the skin, because carotene is metabolized poorly by the liver in such patients. The outer portion of the eyebrows may disappear, and the scalp hair may become brittle. The axillary hair and pubic hair become sparse.

Patients with myxedema may develop bradycardia, pericardial effusion, low volt-

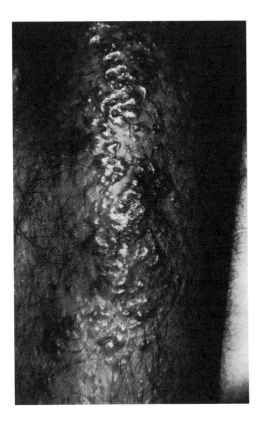

Fig. 6-12. Pretibial myxedema. Flesh-colored papules have coalesced to form a plaque on the anterior shin of this patient with Graves disease.

Courtesy Hiram M. Sturm, M.D., Clinical Professor of Dermatology, Emory University School of Medicine, Atlanta, Ga. From Goldfarb MS, Gaspari AA, Sturm RL: The skin and the heart. In Hurst JW, editor: *Clinical essays on the heart,* vol 5, New York, 1985, McGraw-Hill, p 213. The copyright has been transferred from the publisher to me.

age of the QRS complexes in the electrocardiogram, myocardial disease, and coronary atherosclerosis.[41,42]

Kidney failure. Sallow skin may be due to the combination of anemia, which produces pallor, with carotene and urochrome, which produce a yellow color.[23] Petechial hemorrhages and purpura may occur in the skin, which may become hyperpigmented when exposed to the sun. Scratch marks may be evident, because pruritus is common. Splinter hemorrhages may occur in the nail beds, and white transverse bands may develop in the nails.[43,44] The white band may make up as much as one half of the nail.[45] Hyperkeratotic pruritic papules may also occur in the skin of patients with renal failure, and this characteristic is known as Kyrle disease (Fig. 6-13).

Patients with uremia may develop pericarditis, and patients receiving renal dialysis may develop infective endocarditis.[46] Hyperkalemia is common with renal failure, and the electrocardiogram may show sinus arrest, QRS conduction abnormalities, and abnormal T waves (see Chapter 7). The serum triglyceride level may be elevated in uremic patients, and there is an increased risk that patients will develop atherosclerotic coronary heart disease, especially during dialysis. The hypercalcemia

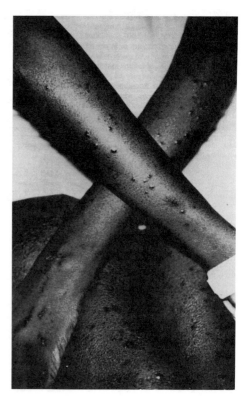

Fig. 6-13. Kyrle disease. Widespread keratotic, pruritic papules in a patient with renal failure undergoing dialysis.

Courtesy Marilynne McKay, M.D., Department of Dermatology, Emory University School of Medicine, Atlanta, Ga. From Goldfarb MS, Gaspari AA, Sturm RL: The skin and the heart. In Hurst JW, editor: *Clinical essays on the heart,* vol 5, New York, 1985, McGraw-Hill, p 216. The copyright has been transferred from the publisher to me.

associated with end-stage renal disease may produce a short QT interval in the electrocardiogram, and calcification of the conduction system, heart valves, and arteries may occur.[47] Although myocardial function may deteriorate in the uremic patient, no single factor can be held responsible.[48]

Systemic lupus erythematosus. An increase in sensitivity of the skin to sunlight is common in systemic lupus erythematosus, but such sensitivity also occurs with other skin diseases. Exposure to the sun may produce a persistent flush, urticaria, or discoid lesions.[49] The damage is primarily produced by ultraviolent light in the B wavelength range. The dorsum of the hands, the face, and the neck are typical areas where the skin lesions develop. The discoid lesions are characterized as scaly, reddish areas with follicular plugging. Ulceration of the lesions may occur. The classic malar rash is usually a reddish macular eruption but may be urticarial. It is often

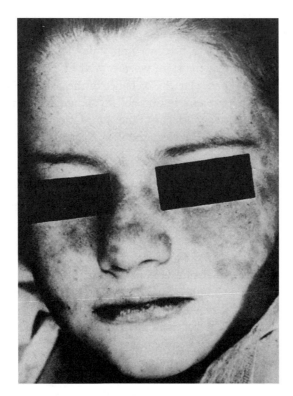

Fig. 6-14. Young girl with lupus erythematosus showing the typical "butterfly" rash of the face. The rash may not be so obvious and may not be present at all.

Reproduced with permission from Logue RB, Hurst JW: General inspection of the patient with cardiovascular disease. In Hurst JW, Logue RB, editor: *The heart*, ed 1, New York, 1966, McGraw-Hill, p 61.

found over the nose and cheeks, giving the appearance of butterfly or bat wings (Fig. 6-14). Telangiectasis may develop. Finally, patients with lupus may have Raynaud phenomenon, purpura, subcutaneous nodules, and areas of panniculitis.

The patient with systemic lupus erythematosus may have pericarditis.[50] Libman-Sacks disease, which is characterized by fibrous, or warty, lesions on the heart valves, may also occur.[51] The most common sites are the undersurface of the mitral valve, chordae tendineae, and papillary muscles. Emboli may produce a stroke or arterial obstruction of other peripheral arteries. Patients with lupus may develop mitral and aortic valve regurgitation, and lupus arteritis may involve the coronary arteries.[52] In fact, myocardial infarction is a common cause of death in such patients. However, significant myocarditis is uncommon.

Scleroderma (progressive systemic sclerosis). This connective tissue disease is characterized by tight, thick skin and vasculitis. Patients with progressive systemic sclerosis often have Raynaud phenomenon.[53] In severe cases the pulp of the distal digits of the fingers may show ulcerations or scars. The nails may become abnormal in these patients, and calcium may escape from some of the lesions. The skin of the face also becomes involved in the sclerotic process. The face becomes expressionless, and the tissue around the mouth becomes immobile. The skin is tightly bound to the bony prominences, so that the skin, when moved by the examiner's hand, does not slide over the frontal bone, clavicle, or bones of the hands (Fig. 6-15). Telangiectasia occurs, as does hyperpigmentation and hypopigmentation. Four of the five features of CREST syndrome are lesions of the skin: Calcinosis cutis, Raynaud phenomenon, Sclerodactyly, and Telangiectasia. The E stands for esophageal dysfunction.[54]

The heart involvement in this condition includes myocardial fibrosis and abnormalities of the conduction system.[55] Although coronary arteritis may be present, coronary artery spasm may also be a cause of the myocardial damage seen in such patients. This characteristic has been likened to Raynaud phenomenon in the coronary arteries. Some patients have angina, myocardial infarction, or cardiac arrhythmia. Pericarditis may occur, but in my experience it is less likely to occur in patients with progressive systemic sclerosis than it is in patients with lupus.

Pulmonary hypertension is apparently being identified more commonly in patients with progressive systemic sclerosis than it was previously. It is common in CREST syndrome.[54] This condition, which may produce severe right ventricular hypertrophy and heart failure, may be caused by pulmonary disease associated with progressive systemic sclerosis, but more commonly it is due to necrotizing arteritis, medial and intimal hyperplasia, or spasm of the pulmonary arterioles.

It is possible, indeed likely, that some patients with primary pulmonary hypertension are victims of progressive systemic sclerosis in whom the skin and renal lesions have not yet appeared. Accordingly, patients with what appears to be primary pulmonary hypertension should be followed carefully for the skin and renal lesions that accompany progressive systemic sclerosis.

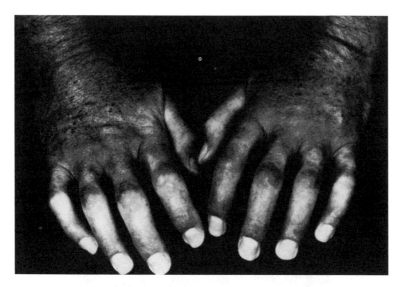

Fig. 6-15. Sclerodactyly occurring in a patient with scleroderma. The sclerosis starts distally and extends proximally. The fingers are cold, and the skin is sclerotic and bound down.

Courtesy Lynn A. Drake, M.D., Department of Dermatology, Emory University School of Medicine, Atlanta, Ga. From Goldfarb MS, Gaspari AA, Sturm RL: The skin and the heart. In Hurst JW, editor: *Clinical essays on the heart,* vol 5, New York, 1985, McGraw-Hill, p 233. The copyright has been transferred from the publisher to me.

Dermatomyositis. Dermatomyositis is believed to be a connective tissue disorder that involves both the skin and the skeletal muscles, whereas polymyositis involves only the muscles. The myositis of dermatomyositis commonly produces muscle weakness before skin lesions become apparent. The skin lesions include violaceous macules on the face, trunk, and extremities.[56] Typically, they involve the eyelids or periorbital tissues, where telangiectasias may develop. Scaly reddish lesions may appear on the joints. Many of these skin lesions are transient during the initial stages of the disease, but they later become persistent, resembling the lesions of lupus. Raynaud phenomenon and urticaria may occur.

When the lesions become permanent, certain specific abnormalities are noted. Gottron papules occur only in dermatomyositis (Fig. 6-16).[57] These small, flat, violaceous plaques overlie the interphalangeal joints of the hands, as well as other joints. The nail folds become red and glistening. Small areas of pigmentation and depigmentation, similar to the lesions seen in progressive systemic sclerosis, may occur. Subcutaneous calcium deposits may occasionally cause the skin to break down, and calcium may be extruded from the lesions, leading to cutaneous ulcers.[58] The skin may become thick, and vesicles and bullae may develop.

Cardiac lesions are less likely to occur in patients with dermatomyositis than in

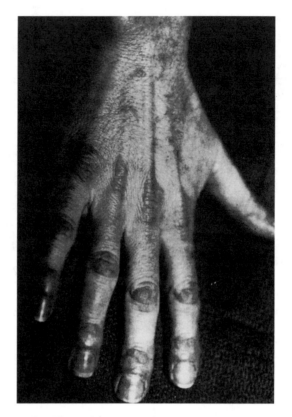

Fig. 6-16. Gottron papules. These violaceous scaly papules on the knuckles are pathognomonic of dermatomyositis.

Courtesy Marilynne McKay, M.D., Department of Dermatology, Emory University School of Medicine, Atlanta, Ga. From Goldfarb MS, Gaspari AA, Sturm RL: The skin and the heart. In Hurst JW, editor: *Clinical essays on the heart*, vol 5, New York, 1985, McGraw-Hill, p 232. The copyright has been transferred from the publisher to me.

patients with lupus or progressive systemic sclerosis. Cardiac arrhythmias, conduction abnormalities, and complete heart block have been reported.[59]

Mixed connective tissue disease. Patients with mixed connective tissue disease exhibit signs of lupus, progressive systemic sclerosis, and dermatomyositis. This condition has been called undifferentiated or incomplete connective tissue disease by Braverman.[60]

Patients with mixed connective tissue disease may have pericarditis, myocardial disease, cardiac arrhythmias, and QRS complex conduction abnormalities.

Rheumatoid arthritis. Rheumatoid arthritis is a systemic disease involving the joints, arterioles, lungs, heart, skin, and nervous system. It is considered an autoimmune disease involving connective tissue and collagen.

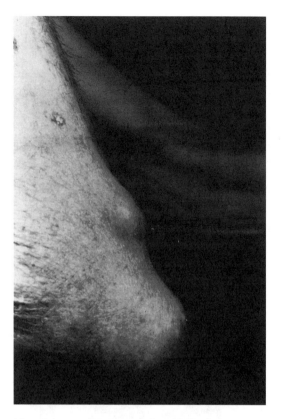

Fig. 6-17. Rheumatoid nodules on the ulnar surface of the forearm.

Courtesy Marilynne McKay, M.D., Department of Dermatology, Emory University School of Medicine, Atlanta, Ga. From Goldfarb MS, Gaspari AA, Sturm RL: The skin and the heart. In Hurst JW, editor: *Clinical essays on the heart*, vol 5, New York, 1985, McGraw-Hill, p 236. The copyright has been transferred from the publisher to me.

Young patients may have a transient rash of pink macules and papules on the face, palms, and soles in association with a small degree of temperature elevation months or years before arthritis is noted.[61] In adults with long-standing rheumatoid arthritis, rheumatoid nodules occur (Fig. 6-17).[62] These firm, movable, subcutaneous nodules are 1 to several centimeters in size and are not painful. They may be found on bony prominences anywhere in the body, and their predilection for the elbows and knees is most likely related to trauma.

Raynaud phenomenon may occur, and palmar erythemia, purpura, and ulcerations of the skin due to arteritis may be seen.[63] Pericarditis, including cardiac tamponade and constrictive pericarditis, may also occur.[64] In addition, nodules may develop on the aortic and mitral valves, and valvular insufficiency may occur.[65] Myocarditis is rare, but cardiomyopathy due to amyloid infiltration of the myocardium may occur. Conductive system disease of the heart may occur but is also rare.[66] Coronary arteritis may also occur and may, on rare occasions, lead to myocardial infarction.[67]

Polyarteritis nodosa. Polyarteritis nodosa is a type of vasculitis that involves all layers of the small and midsize arteries. Numerous body systems may be involved, including the skin and heart.[68]

The skin lesions consist of erythema, vesicular eruptions, urticaria, erythema nodosum, and macular and papular rashes. Lesions usually occur on the lower legs and feet. Macular lesions may ulcerate at their center; a small scar with a brown halo may remain as these lesions heal. Gangrene of the fingers and toes may develop.

Patients may have hypertension, left ventricular hypertrophy, pericarditis, and coronary artery disease.[68] The epicardial coronary arteries may exhibit areas of dilatation, including aneurysms. Coronary thrombosis and infarction may occur. The smaller coronary arteries may be involved, and atrioventricular block and intraventricular conduction abnormalities may occur.

Kawasaki disease. This childhood disease produces fever, lymphadenopathy, hepatitis, arthritis, meningitis, gastroenteritis, arteritis, and lesions of the skin (Fig. 6-18).[69] Its cause is unknown. A generalized erythematous exanthem develops a few days after fever begins. The skin lesions are composed of red nodules that may re-

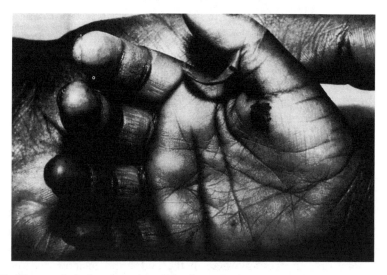

Fig. 6-18. Characteristic desquamation of the fingertips in a child with Kawasaki disease (mucocutaneous lymph node syndrome).

Courtesy Mary K. Spraker, M.D., Department of Dermatology, Emory University School of Medicine, Atlanta, Ga. From Goldfarb MS, Gaspari AA, Sturm RL: The skin and the heart. In Hurst JW, editor: *Clinical essays on the heart*, vol 5, New York, 1985, McGraw-Hill, p 239. The copyright has been transferred from the publisher to me.

semble early erythema multiforme. The feet and hands become edematous, and the palms and soles become purplish red. This phase of the disease lasts 5 to 15 days; desquamation of the skin occurs 2 to 3 weeks later.[69] Transverse lines in the nails may be seen in a few weeks. Red eyes occur in almost all cases, and the red color is caused by engorgement of the bulbar vessels[70]; it is not caused by conjunctivitis. The pharynx appears redder than normal, the tongue takes on the appearance of a ripe strawberry, and the lips become dry and cracked.

Pericarditis, myocarditis, and conduction abnormalities may occur.[70] Many patients have abnormal Q waves in the electrocardiogram.[71] Mitral regurgitation may be caused by papillary muscle dysfunction. Coronary artery aneurysms and stenosis occur in one fifth of the patients who are studied by coronary arteriography.[72] Myocardial infarction occurs as a result of coronary thrombosis. It is likely that isoembolism occurs in the coronary arteries. Although the disease is, to a degree, reversible, the coronary aneurysms may persist.

Hereditary hemorrhagic telangiectasia. Hereditary hemorrhagic telangiectasia was first described by Osler, Weber, and Rendu. The telangiectasia occurs on the lips, mucous membranes, face, trunk, and palms (Fig. 6-19).[73] The first clinical presentation is usually an episode of epistaxis.

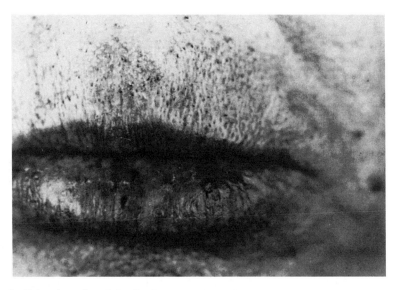

Fig. 6-19. Telangiectasias of the lips in a patient with Osler-Weber-Rendu syndrome. Similar vascular lesions may occur in CREST syndrome.

Courtesy Lynn A. Drake, M.D., Department of Medicine, Emory University School of Medicine, Atlanta, Ga. From Goldfarb MS, Gaspari AA, Sturm RL: The skin and the heart. In Hurst JW, editor: *Clinical essays on the heart*, vol 5, New York, 1985, McGraw-Hill, p 240. The copyright has been transferred from the publisher to me.

The lesions are actually arteriovenous fistulas. These lesions may occur in several organs, and the result may be high-output heart failure. Pulmonary arteriovenous fistulas may produce cyanosis and clubbing,[74] and gastrointestinal lesions may produce periodic gastrointestinal bleeding.

Exfoliative erythroderma. The generalized red, scaly rash may be due to a variety of disorders.[75] Atrophic eczema, contact dermatitis, drug eruptions, psoriasis, and, rarely, an internal malignancy may all precipitate exfoliative erythroderma (red, peeling skin). The disease usually starts with small patches of erythema and scaling, which gradually enlarge and spread, becoming generalized.

Small areas of the skin may desquamate, or the peeling may occur in large sheets. Body temperature is elevated during the entire process, because the patient cannot sweat, and shaking chills are common. Itching of the skin may be severe, and scratch marks are often evident. Nails may be lost, and hair loss may be generalized; lymphadenopathy is common. Hyperpigmentation and/or hypopigmentation may occur.

Patients may develop high-output cardiac failure.[76] Edema of the lower extremities is common, because there is an increase in capillary permeability.

Psoriasis. The characteristic papulosquamous lesions may be located on large areas of the body. Arthritis of the small joints of the fingers may be apparent. When the skin lesions are extensive (exfoliative erythroderma), high-output cardiac failure may develop.[76]

Scars. See later discussion on auscultation over scars.

Behçet syndrome. Behçet syndrome includes vasculitis of the skin, uveitis, ulcerations of the mucous membranes of the mouth and genitalia in both sexes, and synovial membrane inflammation.[77] The cause is unknown. Oral ulcers with a yellow base and red border may become as large as 1 cm; they require 1 to 2 weeks to heal. These patients exhibit pathergy, the development of a papule or pustule after a needle prick.[78]

Patients with Behçet syndrome may have pericarditis or myocarditis. Superficial thrombophlebitis or deep vein thrombosis may develop. Some patients develop obstruction of the superior or inferior vena cava.[79] Arterial aneurysms or thrombosis may occur in any major artery.[80]

Reiter syndrome. Reiter syndrome comprises dermatitis, conjunctivitis, urethritis, and polyarthritis (Fig. 6-20).[81] The condition may follow sexual intercourse and may be caused by *Chlamydia trachomatis, Ureaplasma urealyticum, Shigella flexneri, Salmonella,* or *Yersinia* infection. Keratoderma blennorrhagicum occurs in most patients. This condition is characterized by small vesicles and papules with a red base on the palms, soles, and nail beds. Some patients have a small vesicle with a red base located near the urethral meatus. A crusted lesion may appear on the glans penis. Ulcers may also appear in the oropharynx.

Patients with Reiter syndrome may develop pericarditis and conduction abnormalities in the heart. Later there may be evidence of aortitis caused by obstruction

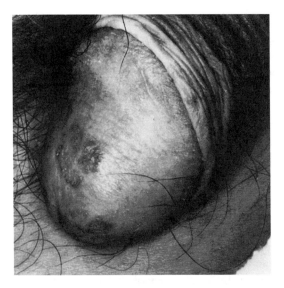

Fig. 6-20. Typical scaly plaques on the glans penis of a patient with Reiter syndrome. This eruption on the penis is called balanitis circinata.

Courtesy Marilynne McKay, M.D., Department of Dermatology, Emory University School of Medicine, Atlanta, Ga. From Goldfarb MS, Gaspari AA, Sturm RL: The skin and the heart. In Hurst JW, editor: *Clinical essays on the heart,* vol 5, New York, 1985, McGraw-Hill, p 245. The copyright has been transferred from the publisher to me.

of the vasa vasorum, which may be followed by aortic regurgitation.[82] The disease process may extend into the ventricular septum and mitral valve annulus.

Malignant melanoma. A cutaneous mole that changes color, size, surface texture, shape, or consistency, or a mole that itches, becomes painful, or is tender to pressure may indicate malignant melanoma.[83] The malignant skin mole may be located anywhere on the body.

Malignant melanoma commonly metastasizes to the heart. There may be a small speck of melanoma in the heart, or the heart may be so laden with the neoplasm that it is called a "charcoal" heart. Pericarditis, pericardial effusion, cardiac tamponade, cardiac arrhythmias, QRS complex conduction abnormalities, and heart failure may occur.[84]

Carcinoid syndrome. In addition to the transient red flush that is so characteristic of carcinoid syndrome (see earlier discussion on skin color), the skin may exhibit permanent changes in the capillaries of the skin, so that telangiectasia develops,[30] giving certain areas of the skin a bluish red appearance. Patients with the carcinoid syndrome may have tryptophan deficiency, and the skin lesions of pellagra may develop. Accordingly, there may be hyperpigmented scaly dermatitis of the skin after it is persistently exposed to light. Some patients develop scleromatous changes in the skin. On rare occasions there is an increase in production of ectopic adrenocorticotropic hormone (ACTH), creating a cushingoid state.

Whipple disease. Patients with intestinal lipodystrophy (Whipple disease) may exhibit hyperpigmentation and purpura of the skin.[85] These patients may have pericarditis, mitral regurgitation, and heart failure.[86]

Polycythemia vera. Patients with polycythemia vera have a ruddy appearance of the skin and mucous membranes and may have arterial or venous thrombosis. The fingers and toes may exhibit transient ischemia, which on rare occasions may result in gangrene. Pyoderma gangrenosum, consisting of ulcers that begin as pustules or nodules, may occur on the calves, thighs, buttocks, and face. Many patients with polycythemia vera have severe pruritus after a hot bath.[87]

Coronary thrombosis and infarction occur with increased frequency in patients with polycythemia vera, as compared with subjects who do not have the disease.[88]

Glycogen storage disease (type III). Glycogen storage disease (type III), known as Cori disease, is caused by a deficiency of the enzyme amylo-1,6-glucosidase. The skin becomes slightly yellow, and xanthomas may be found on the buttocks and tendons.

The heart becomes infiltrated with polysaccharide, which may lead to heart failure and sudden death.[89] The QRS voltage in the electrocardiogram may be enormous. The heart may also be involved in type II glycogen storage disease (Pompe disease) or type IV glycogen storage disease (Andersen disease).

Ochronosis. Alcaptonuria is caused by an inherited error in tyrosine metabolism due to a deficiency in the enzyme homogentisic acid oxidase. Ochronosis is produced by the deposition of pigment in the cartilage, sclerae, skin, and heart. The cartilage of the ears becomes a slate-gray color, as do the sclerae. The hair follicles in the pubic and axillary areas develop a bluish color.[90]

The ochronotic bluish pigment may impregnate the endocardium and heart valves. Aortic stenosis has been described.[91]

Fabry disease. Fabry disease is an inherited condition that appears predominantly in males and is caused by a deficiency of lysosomal enzyme α-galactosidase A, which permits the accumulation of glycosphingolipid in vascular endothelium.[92] Angiokeratomas develop in the skin (Fig. 6-21). These lesions are small ectatic vessels of the upper dermis that bulge upward into the epidermis. Numerous small reddish blue papules may appear on the trunk. They may appear on the scrotum, genitalia, thighs, and buttocks. The lesions may later appear on the lips and mucous membrane of the mouth. They are never as numerous in females as in males. Sweating is less common than usual in such patients.

Glycosphingolipid is deposited in the lysosomes of the endothelial cells and cardiac myocytes, which may lead to angina or myocardial infarction because the coronary arteries cannot dilate normally. The myocytes cannot function normally, and

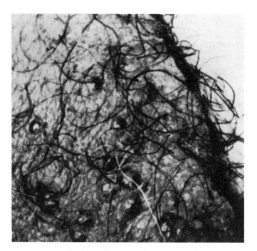

Fig. 6-21. Angiokeratoma of the scrotum (Fordyce spots). This is a normal variant. The occurrence of these vascular papules in a disseminated manner is an indication of Fabry disease.
Courtesy Marilynne McKay, M.D., Department of Dermatology, Emory University School of Medicine, Atlanta, Ga. From Goldfarb MS, Gaspari AA, Sturm RL: The skin and the heart. In Hurst JW, editor: *Clinical essays on the heart,* vol 5, New York, 1985, McGraw-Hill, p 223. The copyright has been transferred from the publisher to me.

heart failure develops. Conduction disturbances of the QRS complex may occur, as may increased QRS voltage in the electrocardiogram.[93]

Tuberous sclerosis. Tuberous sclerosis is a congenital disorder that is characterized by hypopigmented white macules, usually occurring on the trunk in infancy.[94] Later, by the age of 2 to 5 years, pinkish, dome-shaped angiofibromas cluster around the nose and malar areas of the face (Fig. 6-22). These lesions, misnamed adenoma sebaceum, are hamartomas composed of vascular and fibrous tissue. They may involve the chin, scalp, and forehead. "Garlic clove" fibromas may develop under or around the fingernails and on the gums. Rough, elevated plaques that have the appearance of leather (shagreen patches) often appear near the lumbar spine.

Many patients with tuberous sclerosis have rhabdomyomas of the heart. The tumors may be obstructive and may cause death.[95]

Ehlers-Danlos syndrome. Ehlers-Danlos syndrome is characterized by extraordinarily fragile skin (pseudoxanthoma elasticum) and hypermobile joints.[96] There are at least seven different subtypes of this collagen disorder. The skin is quite elastic and can be stretched a great distance from the body (Fig. 6-23); it scars easily because of defects in subcutaneous collagen. Subcutaneous fat may bulge through thin "cigarette paper" scars.

The root of the aorta and sinuses of Valsalva may be involved with the process,

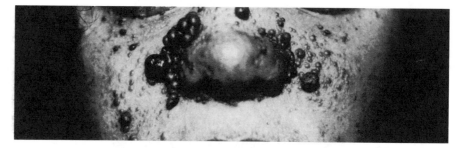

Fig. 6-22. Characteristic flesh-colored papules of tuberous sclerosis on the cheeks and in na-
solabial folds.

Courtesy Marilynne McKay, M.D., Department of Dermatology, Emory University School of Medicine,
Atlanta, Ga. From Goldfarb MS, Gaspari AA, Sturm RL: The skin and the heart. In Hurst JW, editor:
Clinical essays on the heart, vol 5, New York, 1985, McGraw-Hill, p 221. The copyright has been trans-
ferred from the publisher to me.

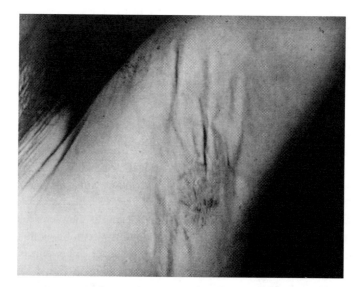

Fig. 6-23. Pseudoxanthoma elasticum in a patient with Ehlers-Danlos syndrome. The skin is
crepelike, lax, redundant, and elastic.

Reproduced with permission from Logue RB, Hurst JW: General inspection of the patient with cardiovascular disease. In Hurst JW, Logue RB, editors: *The heart*, ed 1, New York, 1966, McGraw-Hill, p 57.

resulting in aortic regurgitation. The aorta and other arteries may become calcified and rupture.[97] Mitral valve prolapse and conduction abnormalities of the QRS complex have been reported to occur in patients with this condition.[98] Hypertension and gastrointestinal hemorrhage may also occur in these patients.

Multiple lentigines syndrome. The acronym LEOPARD is useful in remembering the components of this inherited syndrome: *L*entigines, *E*lectrocardiographic abnormalities, *O*cular hypertelorism, *P*ulmonary valve stenosis, *A*bnormalities of genitalia, *R*etardation of growth, and *D*eafness.[99] The skin may be covered with numerous small tan to brown macules. These lesions are present at birth or soon after birth and increase in number as the child grows.

Pulmonary valve stenosis occurs commonly in these patients[100] and may be accompanied by aortic valve stenosis. Obstructive cardiomyopathy, as well as sudden death, has been reported.[101] Conduction defects may be seen in the QRS complex, and endocardial fibrosis and left atrial myxomas have been reported to occur in patients with lentigines.

Marfan syndrome. Marfan syndrome is discussed later in the chapter under skeletal abnormalities. The skin lesions include a decrease in subcutaneous fat; atrophic striae on the abdomen, thighs, buttocks, and pectoral and deltoid regions; and small horny papules on the neck.

Hemochromatosis. Idiopathic hemochromatosis is caused by a genetic abnormality that causes the intestine to absorb large amounts of iron and allows the reticuloendothelial cells to release large amounts of iron to the plasma.[102] Hemochromatosis may occur when patients ingest excessive amounts of iron or receive multiple transfusions for anemia or hemophilia. The iron deposits in the tissue can cause cirrhosis, diabetes mellitus, arthritis, hypogonadism, and cardiomyopathy.

The skin may be a bronze color as a result of hypermelanosis or a slate-gray color as a result of hemosiderin.[103] The exposed skin is more likely to exhibit the color change, as may scars, the nipples, and genitalia. The mucous membrane of the mouth may be involved. The skin may become dry and scaly. The hair may become sparse, and "spooning" of the nails may occur.

Restrictive cardiomyopathy may develop in patients with hemochromatosis.[104] The iron becomes more concentrated in the myocytes of the epicardium than in those of the endocardium. Heart failure may develop, cardiac arrhythmias are common, and the electrocardiogram may show low voltage of the QRS complexes.

Hypereosinophilia syndrome. Hypereosinophilia syndrome is characterized by skin lesions, eosinophilia, and Loeffler myocarditis.[105] The skin lesions consist of red, hyperpigmented macules or papules, as well as urticaria, angioedema, and perifollicular papules. Dermatographism may occur. The skin itches, and scratch marks may be evident.[106,107]

Myocarditis is common. Arteritis of the small coronary arteries may lead to myocardial necrosis, and mural thrombi are common. Restrictive cardiomyopathy due to major involvement of the endocardium may develop, and heart failure is common.[108]

Tertiary syphilis. Tertiary syphilis has been seen rarely in the United States in recent years. However, there has been a dramatic increase in the incidence of primary and secondary syphilis; thus the incidence may change with time. The gumma is the major skin lesion associated with tertiary syphilis (Fig. 6-24). The gumma, a granulomatous lesion, is caused by a hypersensitivity to *Treponema pallidum.* It begins as a small nodule that grows in size, leaving an ulcerated gummy center that eventually scars. The lesions may erode the nose, tongue, and hard palate. Carcinoma of the tongue may follow a gummatous ulceration. Smaller, but similar, lesions known as a nodular syphilids may occur.

Cardiovascular disease may occur in patients with acquired, untreated syphilis.[109] Obliterative endarteritis of the vasa vasorsum may develop and is usually detected in the ascending aorta. The disease is more intense around the sinuses of Valsalva and coronary arteries and in the aortic valve annulus. This process does not involve the aortic valve leaflets. Angina pectoris due to coronary ostial disease may develop, and aortic valve regurgitation due to dilatation of the aortic valve annulus may occur. A tambour second heart sound may be heard, and a cooing diastolic murmur of aortic regurgitation due to a retroverted aortic valve cusp may make its appearance. A saccular aneurysm may develop in the ascending aorta. The aneurysm may attain a huge size and erode the sternum and other bony structures, as well as adjacent soft tissue.

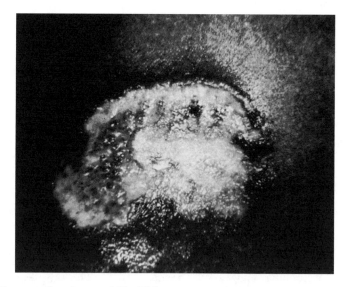

Fig. 6-24. Gumma of tertiary syphilis. This asymptomatic ulcerative plaque appeared on the back of a patient 10 years after a penile chancre had healed.

Courtesy Sidney Olansky, M.D., Professor Emeritus of Dermatology, Emory University School of Medicine, Atlanta, Ga. From Goldfarb MS, Gaspari AA, Sturm RL: The skin and the heart. In Hurst JW, editor: *Clinical essays on the heart,* vol 5, New York, 1985, McGraw-Hill, p 204. The copyright has been transferred from the publisher to me.

Endocarditis. Endocarditis is caused by bacteria or fungi that enter the bloodstream and attack the heart valves.[7] Emboli from the aortic and mitral valve vegetations may involve any area of the body: eyes, kidneys, myocardium, brain, arteries to the arms, legs, etc. The skin lesions that may be seen in patients with endocarditis are of two types: skin lesions such as infected wounds or furuncles that serve as the source for bacteremia and subsequent endocarditis, and skin lesions that are secondary to the endocarditis itself. The latter include petechial hemorrhages of the skin, mucous membranes, and inner surface of the lower and upper eyelids (see Fig. 6-3, *A*); Roth spots in the retinas; Osler nodes; Janeway lesions; splinter hemorrhages under the fingernails; and clubbing of the fingertips.

Osler nodes are painful, erythematous nodules located in the pulp of the fingertip.[110] They are probably due to small emboli. *Janeway lesions* are small, flat, red spots located on the palms and soles. They do not blanch with pressure and are probably due to circulating immune complexes. *Splinter hemorrhages* found beneath the fingernails are probably embolic.[111] They are not specific for endocarditis and are commonly due to trauma or renal failure (see Fig. 6-3, *B*); they may rarely be due to trichinosis (see Fig. 6-3, *C*). *Clubbing of the fingers* may occur in patients with endocarditis but is rarely seen today. The base of the nail is softer in patients with recently acquired clubbing than it is in patients with long-standing clubbing.

The murmurs of congenital heart disease, including patent ductus arteriosus, interventricular septal defect, bicuspid aortic valve stenosis, pulmonary valve stenosis, ostium primum septal defect, and coarctation of the aorta, may be present. The murmur of mitral valve prolapse may be found, and the murmurs of acquired aortic or mitral valve disease may be evident.[7] Drug addicts who "mainline" their drugs may have tricuspid and/or pulmonary valve endocarditis.[7] Artificial valves are particularly prone to infection.[7]

These patients are all at risk for peripheral emboli. Coronary emboli followed by myocardial infarction may occur, especially when the endocarditis involves the aortic valve. Aortic valve abscesses may develop and may tunnel into the right atrium or produce complete heart block. Of course, new heart murmurs may develop, such as aortic valve regurgitation or mitral valve regurgitation. The latter may occasionally be due to the rupture of the chordae tendineae of the mitral valve.

Lyme disease. Lyme disease is an inflammatory systemic disease that is caused by the spirochete *Borrelia burgdorferi,* which is transmitted by the bite of deer ticks, such as *Ixodes dammini,* that have lived on infected deer. The tick bite causes a papule that enlarges, clearing in the center and becoming annular.[112]

Cardiac abnormalities follow the skin lesions and arthropathy in about 3 weeks.[113] Atrioventricular block, including complete heart block, may develop and may cause syncope. There may be evidence of myopericarditis with poor cardiac function. The condition must be differentiated from rheumatic fever, Rocky Mountain spotted fever, *Yersinia enterocolitica* infection, and viral diseases that are associated with a rash.

The myocarditis subsides without evidence of chronic cardiomyopathy.[113] Although no permanent heart valve damage has been described, I believe it would be wise to follow patients with Lyme disease for chronic valvular abnormalities, because some of the features of the acute stage of the disease are similar to those observed in patients with acute rheumatic fever.

Herpes zoster. Herpes zoster (shingles) is a viral disease that produces small vesicles along the path of an intercostal nerve. The skin of the involved area is exquisitely sensitive, tender, and painful. The pain may be mistaken for myocardial ischemia.

Acquired immunodeficiency syndrome. Acquired immunodeficiency syndrome (AIDS) is caused by HIV infection and invariably results in death within a few years.[114] Patients die of intercurrent infections that involve virtually every organ of the body. Chronic lymphadenopathy is common, and patients are subject to infections with *Pneumocystis carinii*, *Mycobacterium avium*, tuberculosis, syphilis, and numerous viruses. Kaposi sarcoma and other malignances of lymphoid tissue may occur in AIDS patients.

The Kaposi sarcoma that is associated with AIDS begins with what appears to be a simple bruise or nevus that follows the skin lines.[115] There may be papules or macules (Fig. 6-25).

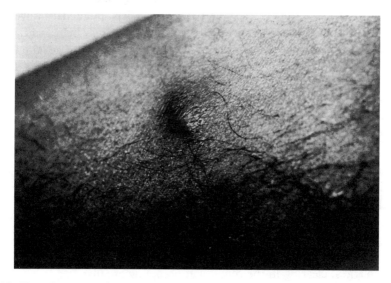

Fig. 6-25. Kaposi sarcoma: innocent-appearing violaceous nodule on the arm of a homosexual man.

Courtesy Mark Holzberg, M.D., Department of Dermatology, Emory University School of Medicine, Atlanta, Ga. From Goldfarb MS, Gaspari AA, Sturm RL: The skin and the heart. In Hurst JW, editor: *Clinical essays on the heart*, vol 5, New York, 1985, McGraw-Hill, p 209. The copyright has been transferred from the publisher to me.

Kaposi sarcoma may involve the subepicardial fat tissue of the heart.[116] Myopericarditis may occur in patients with AIDS; it is most likely due to a concomitant viral infection but may be caused by the AIDS virus.

Diabetes mellitus. Skin abnormalities are common in patients with diabetes mellitus. The rarest of these is *necrobiosis lipoidica diabeticorum*, which occurs without diabetes in almost half of the cases.[117] Lesions begin as small red papules overlying the tibias and gradually enlarge. The lesions gradually become atrophic with a red border and yellow center; telangiectasias may develop. *Diabetic dermopathy* is characterized by pigmented atrophic scars located in the pretibial areas.[118] *Bullous diabeticorum* occurs on the hands, feet, lower legs, and forearms (Fig. 6-26).[119] These large bullous lesions are filled with bloody fluid; they heal in a few weeks without scarring. *Eruptive xanthomas* can be seen in diabetic patients with hyperlipidemia and elevated serum triglyceride levels (Fig. 6-27). These small pinkish yellow papules with a red base erupt on the buttocks and extensor surface of the forearms. Vitiligo occurs more commonly in diabetic patients as compared with a controlled population.[120] Small areas of *lipodystrophy* may develop at the injection sites where insulin has been given.

Patients with diabetes mellitus are more likely to develop atherosclerotic coronary artery disease than are nondiabetic persons. It is important to be aware that

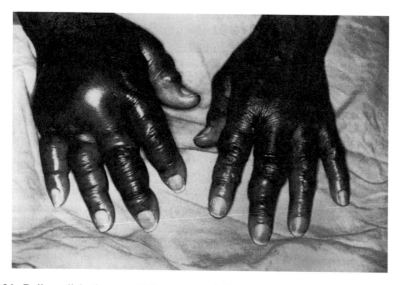

Fig. 6-26. Bullous diabeticorum. This tense, noninflammatory, painless blister formed spontaneously on the dorsum of the hand of this diabetic patient.

Courtesy Marilynne McKay, M.D., Department of Dermatology, Emory University School of Medicine, Atlanta, Ga. From Goldfarb MS, Gaspari AA, Sturm RL: The skin and the heart. In Hurst JW, editor: *Clinical essays on the heart*, vol 5, New York, 1985, McGraw-Hill, p 210. The copyright has been transferred from the publisher to me.

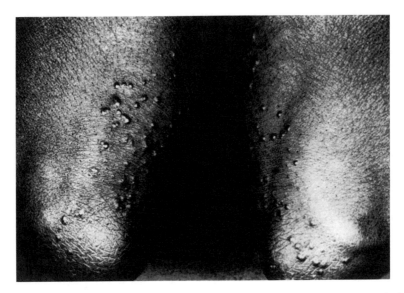

Fig. 6-27. Eruptive xanthomas. Yellow papules on an erythematous base appeared abruptly in crops over the elbows in this diabetic patient whose serum glucose level was poorly controlled.

Courtesy Marilynne McKay, M.D., Department of Dermatology, Emory University School of Medicine, Atlanta, Ga. From Goldfarb MS, Gaspari AA, Sturm RL: The skin and the heart. In Hurst JW, editor: *Clinical essays on the heart*, vol 5, New York, 1985, McGraw-Hill, p 225. The copyright has been transferred from the publisher to me.

myocardial ischemia, including myocardial infarction, may occur in a patient with diabetes mellitus wherein the patient remains asymptomatic. Heart failure is more likely to appear in diabetic patients than in nondiabetic persons, even when the coronary lesions do not appear sufficiently severe to cause it. There is increasing evidence that diabetic patients may have a specific type of cardiomyopathy. Newborn infants of diabetic mothers may have hypertrophic cardiomyopathy.

Hyperlipidemia. Xanthomatous lesions are composed of localized infiltrations of lipid-containing macrophages that are located within the tendons and skin.[121] The plaques and nodules are usually found within the Achilles tendons, within the tendons of the hands, or in the fascia near the elbows (Fig. 6-28). These lesions are attached to the tendon; they are not freely mobile. Xanthomas are found most often in patients with familial hyperlipidemia (types II and III). These patients are highly likely to develop advanced atherosclerosis, including coronary atherosclerosis.

Eruptive xanthomas are small, pinkish yellow papules that occur on the buttocks and extensor surface of the elbows.[122] They are associated with familial hyperlipidemia (types I, IV, and V) or with diseases such as diabetes, myxedema, pancreati-

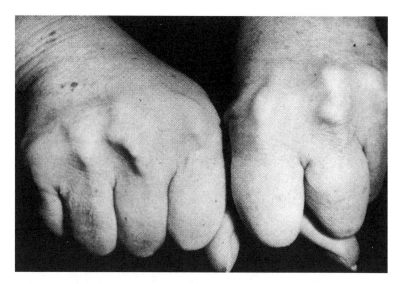

Fig. 6-28. Xanthomatous nodules on the tendons of the hands.

Reproduced with permission from Logue RB, Hurst JW: General inspection of the patient with cardio-vascular disease. In Hurst JW, Logue RB, editors: *The heart*, ed 1, New York, 1966, McGraw-Hill, p 63.

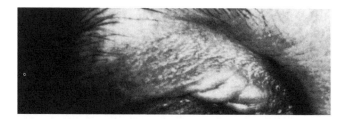

Fig. 6-29. Xanthelasma palpebrarum.

Courtesy Hiram M. Sturm, M.D., Clinical Professor of Dermatology, Emory University School of Med-icine, Atlanta, Ga. From Goldfarb MS, Gaspari AA, Sturm RL: The skin and the heart. In Hurst JW, editor: *Clinical essays on the heart*, vol 5, New York, 1985, McGraw-Hill, p 224. The copyright has been transferred from the publisher to me.

tis, nephrosis, and glycogen storage disease (see Fig. 6-27). These patients are highly likely to develop atherosclerosis.

Soft tuberous xanthomas may occur on the extensor surfaces of the elbows, knees, and dorsum of the hands and feet. They later become fibrotic and firm. These lesions usually occur in patients with hypertriglyceridemia.[123] These patients are likely to develop atherosclerosis.

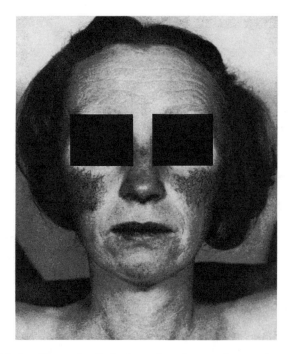

Fig. 6-30. Mitral facies. The malar flush shown here is more intense than usual.

Reproduced with permission from Cleland W, Goodwin J, McDonald L, Ross D: *Medical and surgical cardiology*, Oxford, UK, 1969, Blackwell Scientific Publications, facing p. 4.

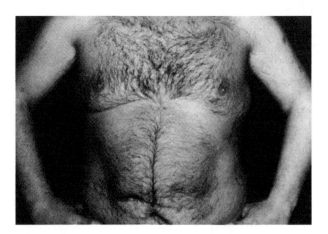

Fig. 6-31. Cushing syndrome. The striae on the lateral aspects of the upper portion of the abdomen suggest the diagnosis. This patient did not exhibit "moon facies."

Reproduced with permission from Logue RB, Hurst JW: General inspection of the patient with cardiovascular disease. In Hurst JW, Logue RB, editors: *The heart*, ed 1, New York, 1966, McGraw-Hill, p 59.

Xanthelasma may appear on the eyelids, palms, neck, and upper part of the chest (Fig. 6-29). About one fourth of patients with these lesions have hypercholesterolemia, type II_a or II_b. These skin lesions are more likely to be associated with an elevated serum cholesterol value when they are observed in young people. Such patients are likely to develop atherosclerosis.

Mitral stenosis. A malar flush occurs in some patients with mitral stenosis (Fig. 6-30). The cause is unknown.

Ebstein anomaly. A malar flush occurs in some patients with Ebstein anomaly. The cause is unknown.

Cushing syndrome. The hypertensive patient may exhibit a "buffalo hump," "moon facies," and abdominal striae (Fig. 6-31).

EXAMINATION OF THE BONES*

Kyphoscoliosis[124]

Kyphoscoliosis is obvious on inspection of the chest (Fig. 6-32). The deformity may interfere with pulmonary and cardiac function and often produces confusing abnormalities found on physical examination and in the electrocardiogram.

Abnormal cardiac pulsations may be felt on the surface of the chest, and abnormal systolic murmurs may be heard. Pulmonary hypertension leads to right ventricular hypertrophy and heart failure. The electrocardiogram is likely to be abnormal because of the abnormal position of the heart relative to the abnormality of the chest wall.

Straight back syndrome

Straight back syndrome is characterized by the loss of the normal kyphotic curve of the upper portion of the spine (Fig. 6-33).[125] The anteroposterior diameter of the chest is also commonly diminished in these patients as compared with the average subject without this syndrome.

The pulmonary artery may be palpable in the second left intercostal space near the sternum.[126] A few patients will exhibit a precordial pulsation located to the left of the midportion of the sternum. Wider than normal splitting of the second heart sound may occur with inspiration, and the split may not close normally with expiration. The tricuspid valve closure sound may be delayed, mimicking a pulmonary ejection sound. A systolic murmur may be heard in the second left intercostal space adjacent to the sternum and is due to compression of the pulmonary artery. The elec-

---

*Most of this section is abstracted from Battey LL: The heart and the bones. In Hurst JW, editor: *Clinical essays on the heart*, vol 5, New York, 1985, McGraw-Hill, p 113. The copyright has been transferred by the publisher to me. Dr. Lewis Battey, the author of the original text, has given me permission to abstract the original material.

Fig. 6-32. Kyphoscoliosis in an adolescent patient with Friedreich ataxia. This young boy developed marked cardiac enlargement of the type seen in Friedreich ataxia before kyphoscoliosis developed.

Reproduced with permission from Logue RB, Hurst JW: General inspection of the patient with cardiovascular disease. In Hurst JW, Logue RB, editors: *The heart,* ed 1, New York, 1966, McGraw-Hill, p 59.

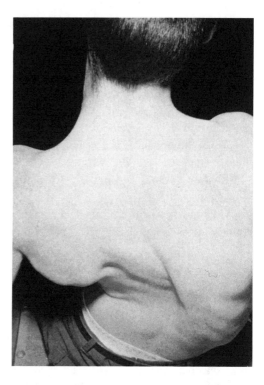

Fig. 6-33. Posterior view of a patient with straight back syndrome demonstrating the straight vertebral column between the scapulae.

From deLeon A, Perloff J, Twigg H, Majd M: The straight back syndrome—clinical cardiovascular manifestations, *Circulation* 32:193, 1965. Reproduced by permission of the American Heart Association, Inc.

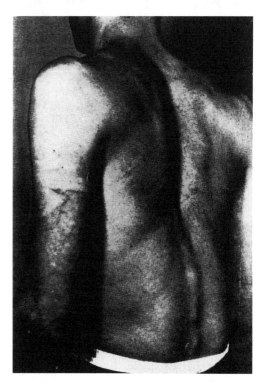

trocardiogram is usually normal, but the mean QRS vector may be directed vertically.

Most patients have no physiologic abnormalities detected on cardiac catheterization, but a few abnormalities have been reported, including a small pressure gradient across the pulmonary valve and exercise-induced mild pulmonary hypertension.[127] I also suspect that mitral valve prolapse is more common in patients with straight back syndrome.

Pectus excavatum[128]

Pectus excavatum is an abnormality of the anterior chest wall that is characterized by depression of the lower portion of the sternum (Fig. 6-34). The central tendon of the diaphragm is shortened, permitting abnormal traction to be exerted on the xiphisternal region of the sternum.

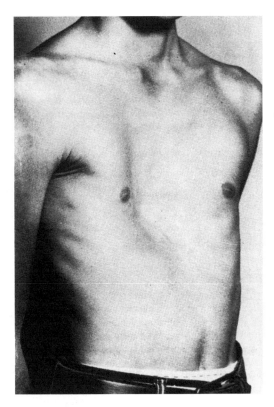

Fig. 6-34. Severe pectus excavatum in a young man.

Reproduced with permission from Guller B, Hable K: Cardiac findings in pectus excavatum in children: review and differential diagnosis, *Chest* 66:165, 1974.

This bony abnormality can produce physical findings that simulate those caused by heart disease. The cardiac apex impulse is displaced leftward, and the first and second heart sounds may be widely split. A systolic murmur may be heard in the second and third interspaces adjacent to the sternum. The heart may appear to be enlarged in the chest x-ray film. The electrocardiogram is abnormal in many patients.[129]

No hemodynamic abnormalities are detected in most patients, but a few exhibit a small pressure gradient across the tricuspid and pulmonary valves, as well as signs similar to those of constrictive pericarditis.[130]

This chest wall deformity may be associated with mitral valve prolapse, straight back syndrome, and connective tissue disorders.

Tietze syndrome

Tietze syndrome is characterized by a tender, painful swelling of the costosternal and sternoclavicular joints (Fig. 6-35).[131] Its cause is unknown.[132] The pain may be confused with the pain of myocardial ischemia, but otherwise the condition is benign and self-limiting.

Mondor disease

Thrombophlebitis of the veins in the chest wall in the precordial area is called Mondor disease.[133] The cause is unknown. Tender, dilated veins are visible. The condition is self-limiting but may be mistaken for myocardial ischemia.

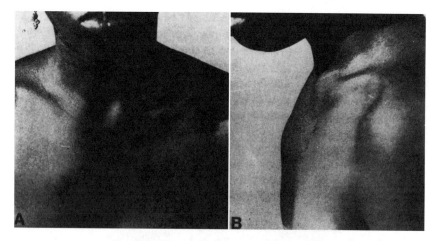

Fig. 6-35. Frontal, **A,** and lateral, **B,** views of a young woman with Tietze syndrome. Note the discrete area of swelling at the left sternoclavicular joint.

Reproduced with permission from Kayser H: Tietze's syndrome: a review of the literature, *Am J Med* 21:982, 1956.

Thoracic outlet syndrome

Thoracic outlet syndrome is caused by compression of the lower cervical and upper thoracic spinal nerves.[134] These nerves innervate the serratus, pectoral, and intercostal muscles. The condition is caused by osteoarthritis, degeneration of intervertebral disks, trauma, and postural strain. Pressure on the spine produces radiation of the pain. Pressure applied to the top of the head with the head tilted to the side may reproduce the pain. The pain may be reproduced by having the patient inhale deeply while the neck is flexed toward a shoulder and the arms are stretched across the chest. Thoracic outlet syndrome can also be identified by eliciting arm pain and a diminution of the strength of radial artery pulsation when the arm is elevated above the head. This type of pain may be confused with myocardial ischemia.

Skeletal abnormalities sometimes associated with mitral valve prolapse

Mitral valve prolapse is common and has been claimed to be associated with many other conditions. The bony abnormalities include those of Marfan disease and bony deformities, including pectus excavatum, straight back syndrome, scoliosis, and a decrease in anteroposterior diameter of the chest.[135-137]

Paget disease

Paget disease is the result of excessive osteoclastic bone resorption.[138] The cause is unknown. The patient may experience pain and swelling in the bones of the lower extremities, skull, pelvis, and/or spine. The patient may also develop a hearing loss, kidney stones, fractures of the bones, and/or sarcoma.

Patients with Paget disease may develop cardiac enlargement and high–cardiac output failure.[139] The pulse pressure may become greater than normal. This situation occurs because the bone marrow is initially replaced by vascular fibrous connective tissue and then by dense, poorly organized, trabecular bone.

Fibrous dysplasia

The cause of fibrous dysplasia of the bones is unknown.[140] The condition is seen in both males and females, but only females show sexual precocity. Brown macules appear in the skin, and fractures of the bones are common.

These patients may develop a high–cardiac output syndrome, presumably as a result of small arteriovenous fistulas located in the areas of the dysplasia. Heart failure has been reported.

Osteogenesis imperfecta[141]

The bones of the patient with osteogenesis imperfecta are easily fractured. There may be bowing of the long bones, kyphoscoliosis, deformities of the vertebrae, and bossing of the frontal and parietal bones. The patient may be deaf, and the sclerae are usually blue.[142]

The patient may have aortic regurgitation as a result of dilatation of the aortic annulus. The mitral leaflets may become redundant and the mitral annulus may dilate, resulting in mitral regurgitation.[143] The chordae tendineae of the mitral valve may occasionally rupture.

Ehlers-Danlos syndrome

Ehlers-Danlos syndrome is discussed earlier under skin abnormalities. The patient may exhibit hyperextensible joints, kyphoscoliosis, pectus excavatum or pectus carinatum, and looseness of the sternal ends of the clavicles. In addition to the hyperelastic skin, the retinas may show angioid lines.[144]

Aortic regurgitation, aortic dissection, mitral valve prolapse, and tricuspid valve prolapse may occur in these patients.[145]

Marfan syndrome

Marfan syndrome is discussed earlier in relation to the eyes, mouth, and skin. In addition to the ectopic lens, tremulous iris, high-arched palate, and skin lesions, the patient may have several bony abnormalities.[146] The fingers of the patient with Marfan syndrome are long, slender, and tapering. The joints are lax, and the long bones are longer than usual (Fig. 6-36). The patient is usually, but not always, tall and slender.[147]

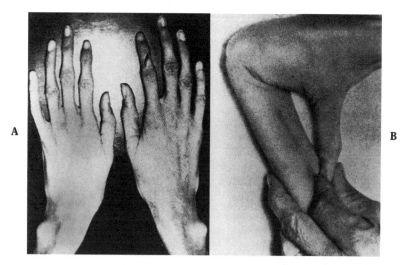

A   B

Fig. 6-36. Characteristic abnormalities in Marfan syndrome. **A**, Long, slender, tapering fingers (arachnodactyly). **B**, Lax joints.

Reproduced with permission from Silverman ME, Hurst JW: The hand and the heart, *Am J Cardiol* 22:723, 1968.

Patients with Marfan syndrome have aortic dilatation, aortic regurgitation, mitral regurgitation, mitral valve prolapse, and cardiomyopathy.[148]

Hurler syndrome

Hurler syndrome is a genetically determined disorder of mucopolysaccharide metabolism that results in an increase in collagen and cells containing acid mucopolysaccharide in the myocardium, endocardium, and coronary arteries.[149] Dwarfism, mental retardation, and enlargement of the liver and spleen, as well as skeletal abnormalities, characterize these patients (Fig. 6-37).

These patients have aortic and mitral regurgitation.[149] Mitral stenosis has also been reported. The coronary arteries are narrowed because of fibrous tissue and acid mucopolysaccharides, but myocardial infarction is rare.[150] Systemic and pulmonary arterial hypertension may occur. Restrictive cardiomyopathy and heart failure are common.

Sickle cell anemia

Pain in the bones may occur in patients with sickle cell crisis. Joint swelling may occur. Ulcers of the skin and osteomyelitis may be present.

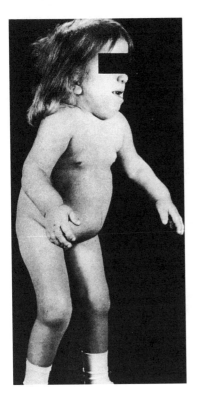

Fig. 6-37. Characteristic facial features and body configuration in a child with Hurler syndrome.
Courtesy Dr. L.J. Krovetz. Reproduced with permission from Taylor J: Genetics and the cardiovascular system. In Hurst JW, Logue RB, editors: *The heart*, ed 1, New York, 1966, McGraw-Hill, p 13.

The heart may be large, and atrial and ventricular gallop sounds may be heard. Severe anemia causes a high–cardiac output state. A systolic murmur due to mitral regurgitation and a mitral diastolic rumble may be heard. Myocardial damage may occur because of occlusion of the smaller coronary arteries.[151]

Chest deformities due to heart disease

Young patients with right ventricular hypertrophy and dilatation from congenital heart disease may exhibit a precordial bulge to the left of the mid and lower sternal region (Fig. 6-38).[152] Fig. 6-39 shows a left parasternal bulge in an adult with a secundum atrial septal defect. A syphilitic aortic aneurysm may erode the sternum and produce an obvious, pulsating bulge (Fig. 6-40).

Patients with coarctation of the aorta may appear more muscular in the upper body and arms than they do in the legs. Patients with ovarian agenesis (Turner syndrome) may have a shieldlike chest and "webbing" of the neck (Fig. 6-41). Patients with Turner syndrome commonly have coarctation of the aorta.

Hand abnormalities

Holt-Oram syndrome is an inherited autosomal condition with abnormalities of the hands and the heart.[153] The thumb may be long and broad or resemble a finger (Fig. 6-42). Other skeletal abnormalities may be present, but the "fingerized" thumb is the best-known anomaly. These patients usually have a secundum type of atrial septal defect.[154]

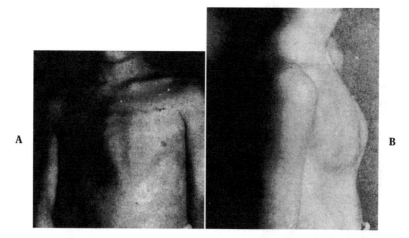

Fig. 6-38. A, Bilateral upper sternal protrusion and, **B,** increased anteroposterior chest diameter in a child with congenital heart disease and pulmonary hypertension.

Reproduced with permission from Davies H, Williams J, Wood P: Lung stiffness in states of abnormal pulmonary blood flow and pressure, *Br Heart J* 24:129, 1962.

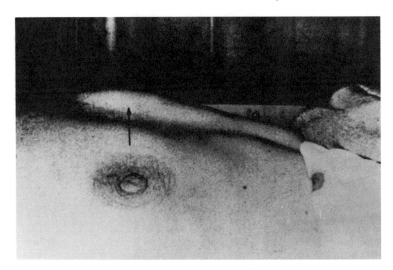

Fig. 6-39. Left parasternal bulge *(arrow)* in an adult with a secundum atrial septal defect.
Reproduced with permission from Silverman ME, Hurst JW: Inspection of the patient. In Hurst JW, editor: *The heart*, ed 2, New York, 1970, McGraw-Hill, p 164.

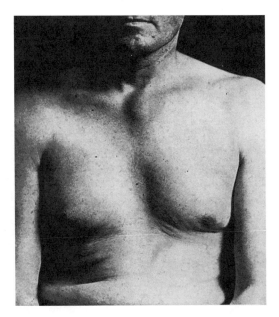

Fig. 6-40. Chest deformity due to a syphilitic aortic aneurysm bulging through the upper sternum.
Reprinted with the permission of Macmillan Publishing Company from *Heart Disease* by Dr. Paul Dudley White, p 51. Copyright 1931 Macmillan Publishing Company; copyright renewed © 1959 Paul Dudley White.

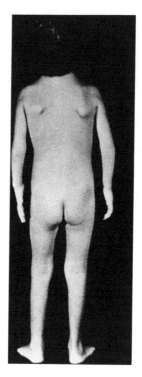

Fig. 6-41. Webbing of the neck and an increased carrying angle of the elbows led to the diagnosis of ovarian agenesis (Turner syndrome) in this girl.

Reproduced with permission from Taylor J: Genetics and the cardiovascular system. In Hurst JW, Logue RB, editors: *The heart*, ed 1, New York, 1966, McGraw-Hill, p 6.

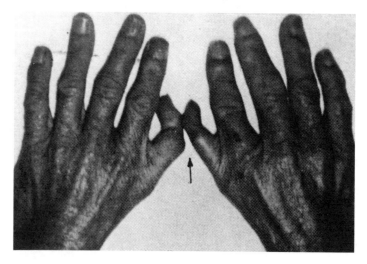

Fig. 6-42. Fingerized thumb *(arrow)* of Holt-Oram syndrome.

Reproduced with permission from Silverman ME, Hurst JW: Inspection of the patient. In Hurst JW, editor: *The heart*, ed 2, New York, 1970, McGraw-Hill, p 156.

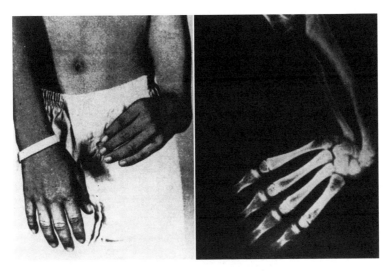

Fig. 6-43. Absent left thumb and hypoplastic radius in an adolescent with ventriculoradial dysplasia.

Reproduced with permission from Harris L, Osborne W: Congenital absence or hypoplasia of the radius with ventricular septal defect: ventriculoradial dysplasia, *J Pediatr* 68:625, 1966.

The thumbs may be small or absent in patients with *ventriculoradial dysplasia* (Fig. 6-43). This syndrome is characterized by radial hypoplasia and a ventricular septal defect.[155]

Whenever there is an unusual abnormality of the bones of the hands, it is wise to search for congenital heart disease.

Infants with *E_1 trisomy (group 16 to 18) syndrome* have a peculiar posturing of the hands (Fig. 6-44). Such patients may have a variety of serious types of congenital heart disease.

Clubbing of the fingers occurs in patients with congenital heart disease and a right-to-left shunt (Fig. 6-45). The toes may be clubbed as well. When the toes of both feet are more clubbed and more cyanotic than the right hand, the patient has a patent ductus arteriosus with Eisenmenger physiology; the blood flow in the ductus is reversed.

Shoulder-hand syndrome

Shoulder-hand syndrome is characterized by pain in the left or right shoulder. The shoulder pain usually precedes the abnormalities of the hand by days or weeks. The hand becomes stiff, and the joints of the fingers may become swollen (Fig. 6-46). Pain may occur when the fingers are flexed in an effort to close the hand. Dupuytren-like contraction may occur, as may Raynaud phenomenon.

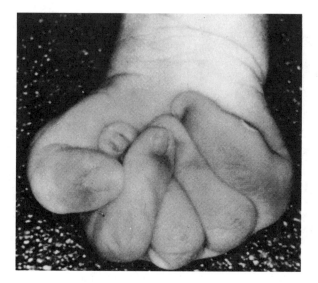

Fig. 6-44. E_1 trisomy (group 16 to 18) syndrome. Typical posturing of the hands occurs in these patients.

Reproduced with permission from Logue RB, Hurst JW: General inspection of the patient with cardiovascular disease. In Hurst JW, Logue RB, editors: *The heart*, ed 1, New York, 1966, McGraw-Hill, p 58.

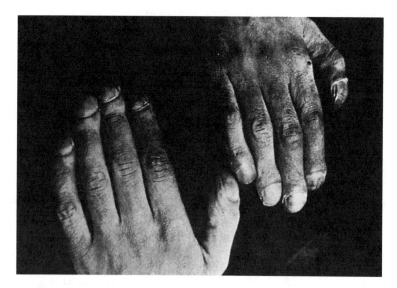

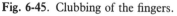

Fig. 6-45. Clubbing of the fingers.

Reprinted with the permission of Macmillan Publishing Company from *Heart Disease* by Dr. Paul Dudley White, p 61. Copyright 1931 Macmillan Publishing Company; copyright renewed © 1959 Paul Dudley White.

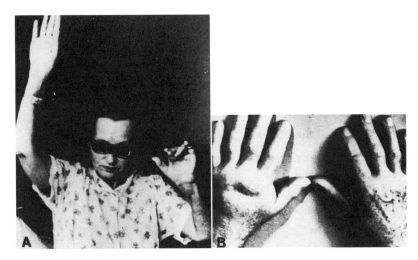

Fig. 6-46. Patient with shoulder-hand syndrome with, **A,** limitation of shoulder movement and, **B,** pitting edema of the left hand.

From McCarty DJ: *Arthritis and allied* conditions: a textbook of rheumatology, ed 9, Philadelphia, 1979, Lea & Febiger. p 1111. Reprinted with permission.

The syndrome, sometimes referred to as reflex sympathetic dystrophy, may be associated with many conditions, including ischemic heart disease,[156,157] trauma, cerebrovascular disease, spinal cord lesions, and cervical spine abnormalities, and may appear after myocardial infarction.[158,159] It has also been seen prior to signs of coronary artery disease and after the development of angina pectoris. The condition, it seems to me, is rarely seen today, because the rehabilitation of patients with infarction is much more aggressive today than it was formerly.

Joint swelling

Rheumatoid arthritis produces permanent joint abnormalities and may be associated with heart disease (see earlier discussion under skin abnormalities). Acute rheumatic fever produces arthritis in multiple joints, but permanent arthritis does not occur. Jacoud "arthritis" is not really arthritis. In this condition the hands appear to be deformed, as they are with rheumatoid arthritis, but the ulnar deviation of the fingers can be voluntarily corrected. The condition is due to lax connective tissue surrounding the joints of the fingers that resulted from recurrent joint effusion associated with recurrent episodes of rheumatic fever. Jacoud arthritis is rarely seen, because rheumatic fever is seen less often now than it was several decades ago. The heart is commonly involved.

Lupus erythematosus and progressive systemic sclerosis may produce nonpermanent joint swelling and heart disease. Lyme disease may also produce joint swelling and heart disease.

A single "hot" joint may be due to sepsis. A common cause is gonococcus arthritis, in which small skin papules may also occur. This condition may be associated with gonococcal endocarditis.

Gross enlargement of the bones

Acromegaly may be characterized by enlargement of the feet; the development of large, spadelike hands and a large jaw; and prominence of the supraorbital regions of the frontal bone (Fig. 6-47). The patient may develop cardiomyopathy and accelerated coronary atherosclerosis.[160]

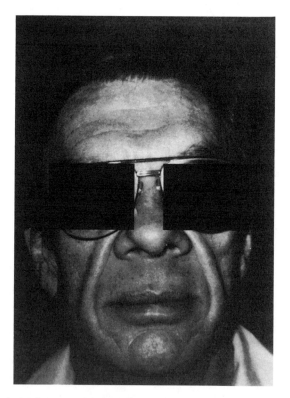

Fig. 6-47. Coarse facial features, folds of skin, and prognathism, characteristic of acromegaly.

From Silverman ME: Visual clues to diagnosis, *Prim Cardiol* 13(2):45, 1987. Reprinted with permission from Physicians World Communications Group.

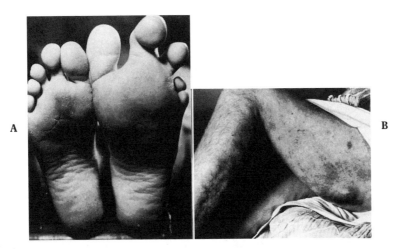

Fig. 6-48. Congenital peripheral arteriovenous fistulas. **A,** The grotesque enlargement of the toes and left foot is obvious. **B,** Note the peculiar location of the "masses" due to dilatation of the veins on the lateral aspect of the lower leg and on the posterior surface of the upper leg. In addition, this young woman had multiple pulmonary emboli.

Reproduced with permission from Logue RB, Hurst JW: General inspection of the patient with cardiovascular disease. In Hurst JW, Logue RB, editors: *The heart*, ed 1, New York, 1966, McGraw-Hill, p 64.

Congenital peripheral arteriovenous fistulas. Congenital peripheral arteriovenous fistulas may result in hemihypertrophy, a large hand or finger, or a large foot with asymmetric large toes (Fig. 6-48). Such patients may have port-wine nevi, varicose veins, and pulmonary emboli.[161]

EXAMINATION OF THE CARDIOVASCULAR SYSTEM

Physical examination of the arteries

Measurement of blood pressure. The blood pressure should be measured while the patient is lying down. Normally, the systolic blood pressure measured in the arms should be 145 mm Hg or less, and the diastolic blood pressure should be 85 mm Hg or less. The blood pressure should be measured in both arms and, if elevated, should be measured in the legs. A large cuff should be wrapped around the thigh, and the blood pressure should be measured by placing the head of the stethoscope over the popliteal artery when the patient is in the prone position. When a large cuff is not available, the usual cuff may be placed around the calf with the head of the stethoscope placed over the posterior tibial artery.

The blood pressure measured in the legs is normally higher than the pressure measured in the arms, because the muscle mass that must be compressed by the inflated cuff is greater in the legs than it is in the arms and the peak intraarterial systolic pressure is normally a little higher in the legs than it is in the arms (the intraarterial mean pressure is, of course, lower in the legs than it is in the arms).

Coarctation of the aorta and severe peripheral arterial disease due to atherosclerosis of the iliac or femoral arteries are the usual causes of the blood pressure measurement in the legs being lower than the blood pressure measurement in the arms.[162] Dissection of the aorta and embolization of the terminal portion of the aorta are causes of acute obstruction of the blood flow and a decrease in pressure in the arteries of the lower extremities. Pseudocoarctation of the aorta is caused by the buckling of an elongated thoracic aorta due to medial sclerosis.

The blood pressure should be measured in the arms with the patient supine and with the patient standing. The blood pressure should not fall more than a few millimeters when the patient is standing as compared with the blood pressure measured with the patient lying down. If the blood pressure falls 10 mm or more when the patient assumes the upright position, it is important to record the pulse rate. With hypovolemia the pulse rate increases; with postural hypotension, because of autonomic dysfunction, the heart rate may not increase.

Hill's sign may be useful in estimating the amount of aortic regurgitation in patients with the murmur of aortic regurgitation. When the systolic blood pressure measured in the legs exceeds that measured in the arms by less than 20 mm Hg, the aortic regurgitation is mild. When the systolic blood pressure measured in the legs exceeds that measured in the arms by 20 to 40 mm Hg, the aortic regurgitation is moderate. When the systolic blood pressure measured in the legs exceeds that measured in the arms by more than 60 mm Hg, the aortic regurgitation is severe.[163]

Pulsus paradoxus occurs in patients with cardiac tamponade, but hypotension may prevent its identification.[164] It may also be present in patients with constrictive pericarditis, but it is less likely to occur than it is when there is cardiac tamponade. The most common cause of pulsus paradoxus is obstructive lung disease. Pulsus paradoxus is identified by measuring the systolic blood pressure during expiration and during inspiration. Normally, the difference between the two measurements should be no more than 10 mm Hg (Fig. 6-49). Pulsus paradoxus is identified when the difference between the two is more than 10 mm Hg.

Magnitude of pulsation of the peripheral arteries. Each of the accessible peripheral arteries should be palpated, and the magnitude of pulsation should be graded as 0 to 4. Pulsations that are graded as 3 are considered normal. Pulsations that are graded as 4 are considered abnormal. Such hyperdynamic pulsation may be caused by aortic regurgitation, patent ductus arteriosus, a peripheral arteriovenous fistula, anemia, thyrotoxicosis, temperature elevation, or anxiety. The pulsation of the carotid artery may be hyperdynamic in patients with tetralogy of Fallot or truncus arteriosus and hyperdynamic to a lesser degree in patients with mitral regurgitation or idiopathic hypertrophic subaortic stenosis. A femoral artery pulsation that is diffi-

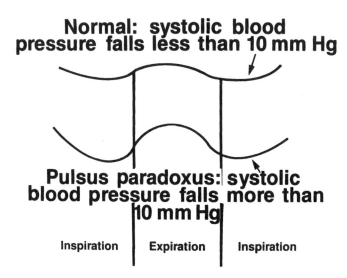

Fig. 6-49. Pulsus paradoxus. The effect of inspiration and expiration on the systolic blood pressure of a person without cardiopulmonary disease is shown in the upper diagram. The effect of inspiration and expiration on the systolic blood pressure of a patient with cardiac tamponade is shown in the lower diagram. Note that the systolic pressure falls more than 10 mm Hg during inspiration when pulsus paradoxus is present.

Reproduced with permission from Hurst JW: The examination of the heart: the importance of initial screening, *Dis Mon* 36(5):278, 1990.

cult to feel in a young person is almost always caused by coarctation of the aorta. When the femoral artery pulsation is felt but is delayed slightly beyond the radial artery pulsation in a young individual, the cause is usually coarctation of the aorta.[165] In middle-aged and elderly patients the magnitude of femoral artery pulsation may be less than normal (grade 0 to 2) because of obstructive atherosclerotic disease of the terminal portion of the aorta, iliac arteries, or femoral arteries. A decrease in pulsation of the popliteal and posterior tibial arteries usually signifies obstructive atherosclerotic disease. The dorsalis pedis arteries may be congenitally absent. Therefore the absence of pulsation of the dorsalis pedis arteries cannot be used to identify acquired peripheral vascular disease. A radial artery may be congenitally displaced, so that it courses on the outside of the radius, and a casual examination may not detect it. The brachial arteries may pulsate less than normal because of more proximal obstructive atherosclerotic disease.

Allen's sign. Allen's sign may be positive when there is obstruction of the radial or ulnar artery.[166] This sign is elicited as follows. The examiner uses one of his or her thumbs to compress the radial artery and the other thumb to compress the region of the ulnar artery. The patient is then instructed to repeatedly open and close his or her hand until the palm of the hand becomes white. The examiner then removes the thumb from the radial artery. Normally, the entire palm of the patient's hand will become red. In fact, it will become redder than normal because of reactive hyperemia. However, when the radial artery is obstructed by atherosclerosis, there will be a delay in the development of palmar erythema. Following the test for radial artery competence, the entire process is repeated (with the examiner removing the thumb from the ulnar artery) to test the patency of the ulnar artery. Allen's sign is not elicited routinely, but if the history suggests intermittent claudication of the hands, it should be used to identify obstructive arterial disease of the radial or ulnar artery. Obstruction of the radial or ulnar artery may be caused by atherosclerosis, embolus, arteritis, trauma, or surgery.

Acute arterial obstruction. Any artery may become occluded suddenly by an embolus. The source of the embolus may be a mural thrombus in the left ventricle secondary to myocardial infarction, a thrombus in the left ventricle of a patient with dilated cardiomyopathy, a thrombus in the left atrium in a patient with atrial fibrillation, a clot in the left atrium of a patient with mitral stenosis with or without atrial fibrillation, a left atrial myxoma, a clot on an atheromatous plaque in the aorta, cholesterol emboli from the aorta, or a clot from the veins of the legs that passes through a foramen ovale.

Three of these causes deserve emphasis, because they are more common than previously thought. A stroke, or evidence of a peripheral embolus, in a young person without evidence of heart disease may be from a *crossed embolus*.[167] That is, the embolus may have originated in the leg veins and passed to the systemic arterial circulation through a foramen ovale. The first sign of a *left atrial tumor* may be an arterial embolus. If the embolus is removed, it must be examined for evidence of a myxoma.[168] There may be numerous *atheromatous lesions in the aorta*. Referred to as a "shaggy" aorta, this condition may lead to repeated embolic episodes due to cholesterol emboli.[169]

Any artery may become occluded suddenly by dissection of the aorta or its branches.[170]

Pulsus alternans. Pulsus alternans[171] should be searched for in every patient. The patient's rhythm must be normal in order for the sign to be detected. The examiner feels the femoral artery to determine if the magnitude of the arterial pulsation changes every other beat (alternating between strong and weak) (Fig. 6-50). I believe the abnormality should be searched for in the femoral artery, because the pulsation in the femoral artery is so easily detected as compared with the pulsation in the radial artery. Pulsus alternans can be detected more readily following a premature ventricular contraction and when the patient stands. Pulsus alternans indicates severe left ventricular dysfunction except when it is observed in a patient with atrial tachycardia who has no other evidence of heart disease. It correlates with a left ventricular

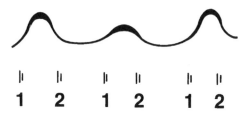

1 2 1 2 1 2

Fig. 6-50. Pulsus alternans. Note that the magnitude of the arterial pulsation alternates with every other beat. The heart sounds are illustrated in the lower portion of the figure. The thick portion of the line that illustrates the arterial pulse indicates the part of the pulse that the examiner feels.

Reproduced with permission from Hurst JW: The examination of the heart: the importance of initial screening, *Dis Mon* 36(5):278, 1990.

ejection fraction of about 30% or less when there is no valve disease.[172] When pulsus alternans is severe, alternate arterial pulsation may be completely eliminated, because left ventricular contraction is only able to open the aortic valve every other heartbeat. The electrocardiogram may show a heart rate of 100 ventricular depolarizations per minute and an arterial pulse rate of 50 pulsations per minute in such patients, representing electrical-mechanical dissociation every other beat.

Pulsus alternans is an easily detected sign of advanced heart failure and is commonly felt in patients with heart muscle disease, such as dilated cardiomyopathy of any cause, including multiple myocardial infarcts due to atherosclerotic coronary heart disease.

Magnitude of the arterial pulsation following a premature beat. When there is a systolic heart murmur, suggesting left ventricular outflow tract obstruction, it is useful to study the magnitude of the arterial pulsation that occurs following a premature contraction of the heart. The pulsation following a premature contraction is larger than the pulsation preceding the premature contraction when there is aortic valve stenosis. The pulsation following a premature cardiac contraction may be less than the pulsation preceding the premature contraction when there is idiopathic hypertrophic subaortic stenosis.[173]

Contour of the carotid artery pulsation. The examiner should feel the carotid artery for abnormalities of the pulse contour but must not obstruct the blood flow in the artery and must not compress the carotid sinus. The examiner should feel the upstroke of the carotid artery pulsation for 1 or 2 beats and then stop. Next the examiner should feel the top of the carotid artery pulsation for 1 or 2 beats and then stop. The examiner should then feel the downstroke of the carotid artery pulsation for 1 or 2 beats. At no time should the carotid artery be occluded in a middle-aged or older patient. The contour of the normal carotid pulsation is shown in Fig. 6-51. The heart sounds should be used as reference points.

Delay of the carotid artery upstroke. Normally, the upstroke of the carotid artery is abrupt. The upstroke is delayed, however, when there is aortic valve stenosis (Fig. 6-52).[174] This sign occurs with severe aortic valve stenosis and may not be perceived

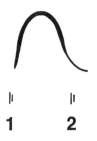

1   2

Fig. 6-51. Normal carotid pulsation. The heart sounds, which are illustrated in the lower portion of the figure, are used as reference points. Note that the upstroke is smooth, as is the top of the curve. The downstroke slows a little at the end of the curve, indicating the location of the dicrotic notch. The thick portion of the line that illustrates the carotid arterial pulse indicates the part of the pulse that the examiner feels.

Reproduced with permission from Hurst JW: The examination of the heart: the importance of initial screening, *Dis Mon* 36(5):278, 1990.

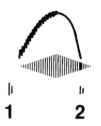

1   2

Fig. 6-52. Carotid artery pulsation associated with severe aortic valve stenosis. Note the delay in the upstroke of the carotid pulse. Note, too, the coarse vibrations that are illustrated as a thick, irregular portion of the line that represents the upstroke. The diamond-shaped murmur is characteristic of aortic valve stenosis. The lower portion of the diagram illustrates the heart sounds. The intensity of the sound is altered considerably when there is aortic valve stenosis (see text). In this illustration the second component of the second sound represents the aortic valve closure sound. It follows the pulmonary valve closure sound and is decreased in intensity. The pulmonary valve closure sound is masked by the murmur and may be difficult to hear.

Reproduced with permission from Hurst JW: The examination of the heart: the importance of initial screening, *Dis Mon* 36(5):278, 1990.

with mild to moderate aortic valve stenosis, especially if aortic valve regurgitation is present. Because of these limitations, I do not rely on this sign to determine the presence of aortic valve stenosis. When it is present, however, the abnormality indicates severe aortic valve stenosis. A shudder (thrill) may also be felt in the carotid artery when there is moderately severe valvular aortic stenosis.

Brisk carotid artery upstroke. The upstroke of the carotid artery is brisk when there is aortic regurgitation, because left ventricular systolic ejection is greater than normal (Fig. 6-53). The abnormal pulse is referred to as being hyperdynamic. The carotid artery upstroke is also brisk in patients with idiopathic hypertrophic subaortic stenosis, anemia, thyroticosis, anxiety, peripheral arteriovenous fistula, patent ductus arteriosus, tetralogy of Fallot, or truncus arteriosus.

Pulsus bisferiens. Pulsus bisferiens may be detected in the pulsation of the carotid artery.[175] The examiner concentrates on the smoothness of the pulsation at the peak of the carotid artery pulsation. Normally, it is smooth and uninterrupted. Pulsus bisferiens is identified by a bifid pulsation at the height of the carotid artery pulsation (Fig. 6-54).

A common cause of pulsus bisferiens is aortic regurgitation. The unusual pulse is the result of an aortic reflective wave that is secondary to a large systolic ejection volume. A pulsus bisferiens may also occur in normal, young, excited subjects and in patients with a dynamic arterial circulation from any cause. In addition, a pulsus bisferiens may occur in patients with idiopathic hypertrophic subaortic stenosis. In this case it results from the uneven delivery of left ventricular output of blood during left ventricular systole. The abnormal pulse contour is eliminated when the patient takes a beta-blocking drug.

Further examination of the carotid arteries. The carotid arteries should never be completely occluded by the examiner. In older patients one runs the risk of pro-

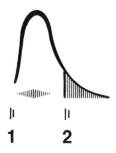

Fig. 6-53. Hyperdynamic carotid pulse. Note the prominent upstroke and downstroke, as well as the diastolic murmur following the second sound (signifying aortic regurgitation).

Reproduced with permission from Hurst JW: The examination of the heart: the importance of initial screening, *Dis Mon* 36(5):278, 1990.

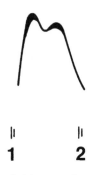

1   **2**

Fig. 6-54. Pulsus bisferiens. Note the brisk upstroke and bifid summit of the carotid pulse curve. The examiner actually feels the portion of the pulse that is indicated by the thicker part of the line.

Reproduced with permission from Hurst JW: The examination of the heart: the importance of initial screening, *Dis Mon* 36(5):278, 1990.

ducing a stroke by dislodging a small thrombus on an atheromatous plaque. Remember, in some patients one of the carotid arteries may be totally occluded, so that inadequate cerebral blood flow will develop when the examiner occludes the opposite carotid artery. Also, older patients may have a sick sinus node or a sick atrioventricular node, and carotid artery manipulation, even without carotid sinus massage, may produce asystole and subsequent ventricular fibrillation.

The bell of the stethoscope should be placed on each centimeter of each carotid artery.[176] A carotid systolic bruit may be heard, and this phenomenon commonly, but not always, identifies an atheromatous plaque in the carotid artery. Such a systolic bruit may occur in patients with anemia, thyrotoxicosis, or a dynamic circulation from other causes. A bruit may, on rare occasion, be produced by fibromuscular hyperplasia of the carotid artery.

It may be impossible to separate a carotid bruit from the transmitted systolic murmur of aortic valve stenosis. At times, the systolic murmur of aortic valve stenosis is heard only a few centimeters above the clavicle, and a separate carotid bruit may be identified higher in the neck if there is a silent area between the two murmurs.[176]

The clinician must always remember that a carotid bruit due to an atheromatous plaque not only marks the patient for a potential transient cerebral ischemic attack, but also (and more commonly) marks the patient for atherosclerotic coronary artery disease.

A localized, prominent pulsation of the carotid artery may be misinterpreted as being caused by a carotid artery aneurysm, whereas it is really caused by "buckling" of the artery.[177] The buckling is caused by elongation of the thoracic aorta and carotid arteries resulting from sclerosis of the media of the arteries. This same disease makes the thoracic aorta, as well as the brachial and temporal arteries, tortuous.

Auscultation of the peripheral arteries. Auscultation of the carotid arteries, auscultation of the distal pulmonary arteries, and auscultation over intercostal arteries are discussed later in the chapter. Bruits heard over the ribs of the back indicate the presence of coarctation of the aorta. Bruits heard in the intercostal spaces of the back may be due to coarctation of the pulmonary arteries, and on rare occasion such a bruit may be due to the increased pulmonary blood flow associated with an atrial septal defect. Bruits heard in the abdomen in the region of the kidneys may be caused by obstructive lesions in the renal arteries.[178] The obstruction may be caused by atherosclerosis or fibromuscular hyperplasia of the renal arteries.

Auscultation over scars. The head of the stethoscope should be placed on every scar in an effort to hear the continuous murmur of an arteriovenous fistula. Remember this limerick: "Don't look so very far without listening over every scar."[179] An arteriovenous fistula may be produced by laminectomy, operations on the kidneys, or other surgical procedures and may result from penetrating trauma. The examiner should also listen over any artery that has been invaded by an arterial catheter. For example, the continuous murmur of an arteriovenous fistula may be heard over the femoral arteries following coronary arteriography or coronary angioplasty.

Examination of the abdominal aorta.[180] The abdominal aorta should be examined in all patients. The examiner, who should be standing to the right of the recumbent patient, should place his or her left hand on the left lateral portion of the patient's abdomen. The examiner's left thumb is then extended toward the midline of the patient's abdomen at about the level of the umbilicus. The fingers of the right hand of the examiner should be placed on the right lateral portion of the patient's abdomen. The examiner should then press downward and inch the thumb of the left hand and fingertips of the right hand toward the midline of the patient's abdomen. The objective is to trap the aorta between the thumb of the left hand and the fingers of the right hand. The examiner tries to feel the aortic pulsations as he or she inches the thumb and finger toward the midline. Obviously, the thickness of the abdominal wall determines, to a large degree, the success of this effort. No pulsation may be detected in patients with a thick abdominal wall. If the aortic pulsation is felt, it should be no wider than 5 to 6 cm when the abdominal wall is of average thickness. At times it is easy to conclude that an abdominal aneurysm is present. This conscious effort on the part of the physician is necessary, because routine, cursory examination of the abdomen may not reveal a large abdominal aortic aneurysm.

Physical examination of the veins

Examination of the neck veins.[181] Examination of the neck veins is one of the most important acts of the entire physical examination; yet it is commonly not done or is done poorly.

The result of the examination may yield evidence of heart failure and disease or dysfunction of the right side of the heart. Two different veins should be examined:

the external jugular veins should be examined for distention, and the internal jugular veins should be examined for pulsations. The external jugular veins are easily seen, whereas the internal jugular veins themselves are not seen—only the pulsations are seen.

The examiner should adjust the patient's neck so that the neck muscles are relaxed. This is accomplished by placing a pillow under the patient's head and neck and instructing the patient to look forward.

The *external jugular veins* are always distended when the patient is recumbent. The examiner should elevate the trunk of the patient to determine the degree of elevation required to eliminate the visibility of the external jugular veins. Both sides of the neck must be visualized. Normally, the distention of the external jugular veins should disappear when the trunk of the patient is elevated 20 to 30 degrees above the recumbent position. The venous pressure is abnormally elevated if the external jugular veins are distended when the patient's trunk is elevated more than 30 degrees above the recumbent position (Fig. 6-55). Abnormal distention of the external jugular veins usually signifies the presence of heart failure. The *hepatojugular reflux* is identified when the examiner presses the abdomen (not the liver) and instructs the patient not to perform a Valsalva maneuver. Normally, the external jugular veins will not be further distended by the additional volume of blood that enters the thorax as a result of this procedure.

The pulsations of the *internal jugular veins* are commonly not identified or may be misinterpreted as being due to pulsation of the carotid artery. The pulsations can be differentiated if the examiner remembers that a large arterial pulsation in the neck will be vigorous whereas a large venous pulsation is undulating, and if the examiner compresses the neck to eliminate the venous pulsation but continues to feel the carotid artery pulsation. More definitively, when the abdomen is pressed with the palm of the hand and the patient is instructed to avoid performing a Valsalva maneuver, the internal jugular vein pulsation will become more prominent whereas the carotid artery pulsation will not change.

The pulsations of the internal jugular veins are not seen when the patient is recumbent, because the veins are overdistended. The trunk of the patient should be elevated until there is maximum pulsation of the internal jugular veins. The examiner should examine the neck by directing his or her line of vision perpendicular to the direction of the pulsating waves (a penlight is useful; its rays should be directed perpendicular to the direction of pulsation). The examiner should listen to the heart while inspecting the pulsations of the internal jugular veins, because the heart sounds can be used as the reference points signaling the onset of systole and diastole. Normally, the pulsations of the internal jugular veins are not seen when the trunk of the patient is elevated from the recumbent position by about 30 degrees.

Normal internal jugular venous pulsations. The normal pulsations of the internal jugular veins are illustrated in Fig. 6-56, and the normal waves themselves are discussed here.

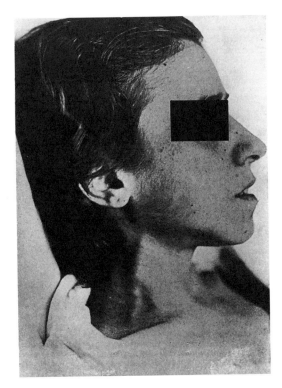

Fig. 6-55. Engorged external jugular vein in a young woman with severe congestive heart failure complicating mitral stenosis with atrial fibrillation. An abnormal pulsation of the internal jugular veins due to tricuspid regurgitation would almost always be observed in such a patient. The patient is bolstered up in bed with the thorax nearly vertical.
Reprinted with the permission of Macmillan Publishing Company from *Heart Disease* by Dr. Paul Dudley White, p 49. Copyright 1931 Macmillan Publishing Company; copyright renewed © 1959 Paul Dudley White.

A normal a wave is produced by right atrial contraction, which occurs during the end of ventricular diastole. It is the largest wave in a series of positive waves. A normal z wave occurs just after atrial contraction and is difficult to see on physical examination. It is due to relaxation of the atria before the c wave. A normal c wave is produced when right ventricular contraction produces an upward bulging of the tricuspid valve during right ventricular systole. A normal x wave is produced before the right atrium begins to be filled with blood during right atrial diastole and right ventricular systole. A normal v wave is produced as the right atrium becomes filled with blood during right atrial diastole and right ventricular systole. A normal y wave is produced as the tricuspid valve opens and blood rushes from the right atrium, which is filled with blood, into a relatively empty right ventricle, which is now actually dilating (sucking) during right ventricular diastole.

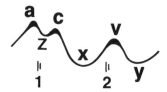

Fig. 6-56. Normal jugular venous pulse (see text for an explanation of the waves). The heart sounds are illustrated in the lower portion of the figure. NOTE: In the remainder of the figures in this chapter illustrating pulsations (with the exception of Fig. 6-59 and as indicated in the preceding figures illustrating pulsations), the thicker portions of the lines or curves illustrating the pulsations indicate the parts of the pulsations that are actually felt or seen. The heart sounds illustrated in these figures should be used as reference points indicating the onset of systole and diastole.

Reproduced with permission from Hurst JW: The examination of the heart: the importance of initial screening, *Dis Mon* 36(5):280, 1990.

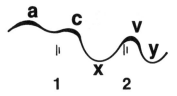

Fig. 6-57. Internal jugular venous pulse associated with a longer than normal PR interval (first-degree atrioventricular block). Note that the length of time that elapses between the a wave and the first heart sound is longer in this illustration than it is in Fig. 6-56. Although it is not illustrated here, the first heart sound will be fainter than normal in such patients.

Reproduced with permission from Hurst JW: The examination of the heart: the importance of initial screening, *Dis Mon* 36(5):280, 1990.

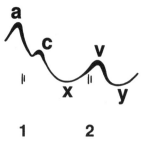

Fig. 6-58. Abnormal jugular venous pulse associated with a decreased right ventricular compliance or tricuspid stenosis. Note the abnormally large a wave (see text).

Reproduced with permission from Hurst JW: The examination of the heart: the importance of initial screening, *Dis Mon* 36(5):280, 1990.

The examiner must note the appearance of the heart sounds in relationship to the waves of the internal jugular pulse. The heart sounds are excellent reference points, because they can be used to identify the onset of ventricular systole and ventricular diastole more easily than determining the exact time of onset of these events by palpating an arterial pulse.

Abnormal internal jugular venous pulsations. The abnormal waves that can be detected in the internal jugular venous pulsations are illustrated in Figs. 6-57 through 6-62, and the abnormal waves themselves are discussed here.

An abnormal a wave is more easily seen when the PR interval is long (Fig. 6-57). The a wave may become more prominent when right ventricular compliance is decreased or in patients with tricuspid valve stenosis (Fig. 6-58). Right ventricular compliance is decreased in patients with right ventricular hypertrophy secondary to pulmonary valve stenosis, tetralogy of Fallot, pulmonary hypertension due to mitral valve stenosis, primary pulmonary hypertension, or Eisenmenger physiology. The a wave is also large when the atrium contracts against a closed tricuspid valve, such as occurs intermittently when there is complete heart block (Fig. 5-59). The large explosive wave is called a cannon wave.

An abnormal x descent becomes less apparent, and no a wave is seen when atrial fibrillation is present, because there is no atrial contraction or discrete period of prolonged atrial diastole (Fig. 6-60). The x wave becomes more prominent in patients

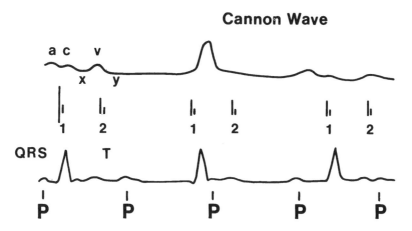

Fig. 6-59. Abnormal jugular venous pulse associated with complete heart block in a patient with normal atrial activity. When the atrium contracts against a closed tricuspid valve (which exists during right ventricular systole), the venous pulse becomes a large cannon wave. Note the regular appearance of the P waves in the electrocardiogram and the a waves in the jugular pulse. The third P wave occurs during ventricular systole in this illustration. When the atrium contracts against a closed tricuspid valve, a large cannon wave occurs in the neck.

with early-stage constrictive pericarditis, especially when it is associated with the persistence of pericardial effusion (see lower diagram in Fig. 6-61). The x wave may be eliminated in patients with tricuspid regurgitation (see following discussion).

A normal v wave occurs at the end of ventricular systole. Its most prominent point coincides with the second sound that marks the opening of the tricuspid valve. When there is tricuspid valve regurgitation, the regurgitant jet of blood created by right ventricular systole produces a large, positive wave in the internal jugular veins.

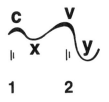

Fig. 6-60. Abnormal jugular venous pulse associated with atrial fibrillation. The a wave is not seen in patients with atrial fibrillation, because there is no atrial contraction. Also, the x wave may be less obvious, because the right atrium has no discrete period of relaxation.

Reproduced with permission from Hurst JW: The examination of the heart: the importance of initial screening, *Dis Mon* 36(5):280, 1990.

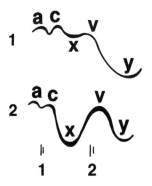

Fig. 6-61. Abnormal jugular venous pulse associated with constrictive pericarditis. The diagram shown in the upper portion of the figure illustrates the abnormal jugular venous pulse associated with chronic constrictive pericarditis. The a, c, and v waves may be seen, but it is the large negative y wave that is abnormal. The diagram shown in the lower portion of the figure illustrates the abnormal jugular venous pulse that is sometimes associated with subacute constrictive pericarditis in which pericardial effusion is still present. Note the prominent x descent and prominent y wave.

Reproduced with permission from Hurst JW: The examination of the heart: the importance of initial screening, *Dis Mon* 36(5):280, 1990.

The v wave occurs early in ventricular systole when there is severe tricuspid regurgitation (Fig. 6-62). It is this wave that is often misinterpreted as being due to carotid artery pulsation. A rare condition exists in which the v wave is actually an arterial wave. When a sinus of Valsalva ruptures into the right atrium, the systolic and diastolic aortic pressure is reflected in the right atrium and internal jugular venous system.

An extreme example of tricuspid regurgitation may be observed in the eyes.[182] When the venous pressure is extremely high, the eyes may exhibit very slight exophthalmos, and in patients with severe tricuspid regurgitation the eyeballs will move forward with each v wave when the patient is recumbent. Also when the patient is recumbent, the v wave is not seen in the internal jugular veins, because the veins are overdistended. In these patients the abnormal v wave becomes prominent when the patient is sitting upright, at which time the eye movement is not seen.

An abnormal y descent is eliminated or blunted in patients with tricuspid valve stenosis due to rheumatic or carcinoid heart disease.

The y descent may be very prominent in patients with chronic constrictive pericarditis (see upper diagram in Fig. 6-61). The a, c, and v waves become equally prominent and more confluent, producing a rather prominent wave, which in turn is followed by a rapid y descent. The large volume of blood held in the right atrium enters the right ventricle in a very abrupt manner.

Examination of the leg veins

Varicose veins. Varicose veins occur in about one sixth of the adult population. They occur in women more often than in men, and some families seem to be more

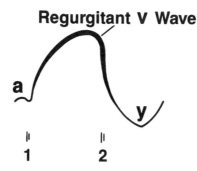

Regurgitant V Wave

Fig. 6-62. Abnormal jugular venous pulse associated with tricuspid valve regurgitation. The v wave becomes so prominent that it may be misinterpreted as an arterial pulse. The technique that should be used to identify that the large positive wave is a venous pulsation is discussed in the text.

Reproduced with permission from Hurst JW: The examination of the heart: the importance of initial screening, *Dis Mon* 36(5):280, 1990.

affected than others. Varicose veins are unsightly but usually produce no symptoms.[183]

Varicose veins are easily seen. The physician may perform one of two simple physical procedures to determine if the superficial veins, the deep veins, or the communicating veins are at fault: the Tredelenburg test or the Perthe test.

The *Trendelenburg test* is performed as follows.[183] The patient is asked to lie flat on the examining table, and the physician elevates the leg with the varicose veins. The blood should drain out of the leg in about 15 seconds. A rubber tourniquet is placed around the leg just below the knee. The patient is asked to stand, and the physician notes the amount of time required for the varicose veins below the knee to become visible. If the varicose veins become evident instantly, one can conclude that the deep and communicating veins are incompetent. If the varicose veins become evident in about 30 seconds, one can conclude that the deep veins are competent but the communicating veins are incompetent. If the varicose veins fill very slowly, one can conclude that the superficial veins are at fault and that the deep veins and communicating veins are competent.

The *Perthe test* may also be used to identify which veins are incompetent.[183] While the patient is standing, a rubber tourniquet is placed below the knee of the leg showing the varicose veins. The patient is asked to elevate himself or herself on the balls of the feet repeatedly. If the varicose veins disappear, one can conclude that the communicating veins and deep veins are competent. If the varicose veins persist despite the actions of the muscles, one can conclude that the deep veins and communicating veins are incompetent.

Varicose veins can, on rare occasion, be so large that the patient may experience postural hypotension.

Thrombophlebitis. Patients with thrombophlebitis of the veins of the legs may experience pain, tenderness, and increased temperature in the region of the veins that are affected.[184]

When the gastrocnemius muscle is stretched by dorsiflexion of the foot, there is a feeling of resistance in the examiner's hand; pain in the calf may or may not occur when this test, originally described by Homan, is performed.[184] A palpable, cordlike vein may be felt in the popliteal space, and slight ankle edema may develop. The circumference of the calf may become larger.

Thrombosis of the deep veins of the legs may occur with no symptoms or physical signs.[184] Deep vein thrombosis of the legs is a common complication of surgery, especially surgery for fracture of the hip, knee replacement, or prostate surgery. It also occurs with congestive heart failure, after long plane trips in which the legs are motionless, and when there has been trauma to the legs.

Pulmonary embolism may be the first sign of deep vein thrombosis of the lower legs, which is why deep vein thrombosis is a very serious disease. In addition, there may be other complications. For example, postphlebitis syndrome, characterized by persistent edema and a gradual increase in skin pigmentation, may develop.

There are two types of severe, painful, deep-vein thrombophlebitis. *Phlegmasia alba dolens* is said to be present when the leg is edematous and blanched of color. *Phlegmasia cerulea dolens* is said to be present when the leg is edematous and blue, and the arterial pulsation is compromised. The two conditions are actually different phases of the same process: some venous flow continues with the former, and no venous flow is present with the latter. These conditions are very serious, because they can lead to amputation of the leg or death.

Inspection and palpation of precordial pulsations

The examiner should search for precordial pulsations.[185] This part of the physical examination has replaced percussion of the heart. Percussion, at its best, can only assist one in determining the size of the heart, whereas inspection and palpation of the precordium yield insight into the physiologic behavior of the heart, as well as its size.

It is important to realize that certain pulsations are seen more easily than they are felt, and vice versa. The patient should be examined in the recumbent position and, at the end of the examination, should be turned about halfway toward the left lateral recumbent position. The examiner must remember that his or her line of vision should be directed perpendicular to the direction of the pulsation. This effort is aided when the rays of a penlight are directed perpendicular to the direction of the precordial movement. The heart sounds should be used as reference points as the examiner feels or observes the precordial movements.

The examiner should concentrate on six precordial areas (Fig. 6-63).

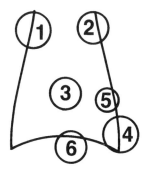

Fig. 6-63. The six areas of the anterior portion of the chest that should be inspected and palpated. Area 1 is examined in an effort to detect abnormalities of the aorta. Area 2 is examined in an effort to detect abnormalities of the pulmonary artery. Area 3 is examined in an effort to detect abnormalities of the right ventricle. Area 4 is examined in an effort to detect abnormalities of the left ventricle. Area 5 is examined in an effort to detect an ectopic pulsation of the left ventricle. Area 6 is examined for evidence of right ventricular hypertrophy in patients with pulmonary emphysema.

Reproduced with permission from Hurst JW: The examination of the heart: the importance of initial screening, *Dis Mon* 36(5):282, 1990.

Sternoclavicular area and second right intercostal space adjacent to the sternum. Normally, there is very little pulsation seen or felt in this area (area 1 in Fig. 6-63). A slow systolic movement of the sternoclavicular joint may be palpated in patients with an acute dissection of the proximal portion of the aorta. A prominent systolic pulsation may be seen or felt in the second right intercostal space adjacent to the sternum in patients with an aortic aneurysm and in patients with aortic regurgitation.

A thrill may be felt in this area in patients with aortic valve stenosis.

Second left intercostal space adjacent to the sternum. Normally, very little pulsation is detected in this area (area 2 in Fig. 6-63). An abnormal systolic pulsation of the pulmonary artery that is detected in this area may be due to an increase in pulmonary artery pressure or to pulmonary artery blood flow. In the first case the pulmonary hypertension may be from any cause, such as primary pulmonary hypertension, Eisenmenger syndrome, or mitral stenosis. Characteristic of a systolic pressure–induced pulsation, the pulsation is prolonged and forceful, but its onset and offset are not abrupt (Fig. 6-64). A pulsation that is prominent with an abrupt onset and offset is commonly due to an increase in systolic volume. This type of pulsation occurs in patients with atrial septal defect.

There may be a palpable pulsation in this area in patients with pulmonary valve stenosis if the pulmonary artery is sufficiently dilated. In such a case the pulsation is not prominent, and its onset and offset are gradual.

A thrill may be felt in this area in patients with pulmonary valve stenosis or tetralogy of Fallot. The pulmonary valve closure sound may be felt when there is pulmonary artery hyptertension.

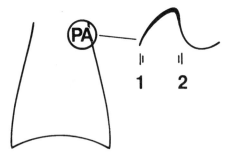

Fig. 6-64. Abnormal systolic pulsation in the second left intercostal space, which is characteristic of an increase in pulmonary artery *(PA)* pressure; the onset and offset of the pulsation are gradual (see text). Note in the illustration that the second component of the second heart sound is depicted as being louder than normal. This also indicates pulmonary artery hypertension.

Reproduced with permission from Hurst JW: The examination of the heart: the importance of initial screening, *Dis Mon* 36(5):282, 1990.

Pulsation of the anterior portion of the precordium. A short outward systolic pulsation may be felt in this area (area 3 in Fig. 6-63) in normal thin subjects and is followed by a visible inward pulsation (see upper diagram in Fig. 6-65). A prominent anterior systolic pulsation with a relatively slow onset and offset is felt in this area when there is right ventricular systolic hypertension (see upper diagram in Fig. 6-66). Characteristic of a pressure overload in the right ventricle, this pulsation occurs with pulmonary valve stenosis, tetralogy of Fallot, and pulmonary artery hypertension due to primary pulmonary artery hypertension, Eisenmenger physiology, or mitral stenosis.

A prominent anterior systolic pulsation with a rapid onset and offset may be felt in this area (see upper diagram in Fig. 6-67). This type of movement is characteristic of volume overload of the right ventricle such as occurs with a secundum type of atrial septal defect.

Severe mitral regurgitation may produce an anterior lift of the sternum and the precordial area just to the left of it. This occurs because the left atrium is located posteriorly in the central region of the chest between the spine and the remainder of the heart. Therefore, when the left atrium expands, it forces the entire heart forward. The anterior pulsation occurs almost simultaneously with the first heart sound, whereas the anterior lift secondary to right ventricular hypertrophy occurs slightly after the first sound.

A thrill may be felt in this area in patients with a congenital or acquired interventricular septal defect. The thrill of aortic valve stenosis may also be felt in this area.

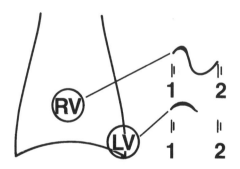

Fig. 6-65. Pulsations of the normal right ventricle and normal left ventricle. The normal pulsation of the right ventricle *(RV)* is illustrated in the upper curve. Note that the brief outward pulsation is followed by a longer inward pulsation. The normal apex impulse of the left ventricle *(LV)* is illustrated in the lower curve. Note that the outward pulsation occupies about one third of systole.

Reproduced with permission from Hurst JW: The examination of the heart: the importance of initial screening, *Dis Mon* 36(5):282, 1990.

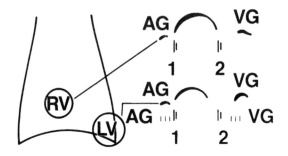

Fig. 6-66. Pulsations due to systolic pressure overload of the right and left ventricles. Right and left atrial gallop movements and right and left ventricular gallop movements are shown. *Upper curve:* The long, outward, systolic pulsation is caused by pressure overload of the right ventricle *(RV)*. The right atrial gallop movement *(AG)* is caused by a decrease in right ventricular compliance. The right ventricular gallop movement *(VG)* indicates right ventricular dysfunction. *Lower curve:* The long, outward systolic pulsation is caused by pressure overload of the left ventricle *(LV)*. In addition, the apex impulse is larger than a 25-cent piece. A bifid systolic pulsation may be produced by idiopathic hypertrophic subaortic stenosis. The left atrial gallop movement *(AG)* is caused by a decrease in left ventricular compliance. The left ventricular gallop movement *(VG)* indicates left ventricular dysfunction. *Bottom portion of figure:* This diagram shows the first and second heart sounds, the right and left atrial gallop sounds *(AG)*, and the right and left ventricular gallop sounds *(VG)*.

Reproduced with permission from Hurst JW: The examination of the heart: the importance of initial screening, *Dis Mon* 36(5):262, 1990.

The precordial movement associated with a right atrial gallop sound may be felt in this area (see upper diagram in Fig. 6-66). The precordial movement associated with a right ventricular gallop sound may also be felt in this area (see upper diagram in Fig. 6-66). An atrial gallop movement felt in the anterior portion of the chest indicates poor compliance of the right ventricle. A ventricular gallop felt in this area signifies right ventricular dysfunction.

Apex impulse. The normal apex impulse is usually seen and felt in the fifth left intercostal space near the midclavicular line. The examiner should inspect and palpate the impulse while listening to the heart sounds. Caused by movement of the left ventricle, the impulse is normally seen and felt as an outward movement that occupies the first third of systole (see lower diagram in Fig. 6-65). The normal apex impulse is the size of a circle with a diameter of about 2 cm. No other movements are felt normally.

When the apex impulse is larger than 2 to 3 cm or is located to the left of the left midclavicular line, the examiner should consider the probability of left ventricular hypertrophy. In such cases careful attention must be paid to the nature of the pulsation itself. Systolic pressure overload, such as produced by aortic valve stenosis or

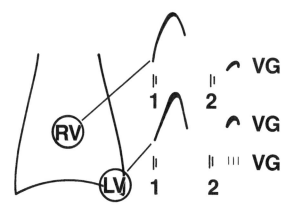

Fig. 6-67. Abnormal pulsations due to volume overload of the right and left ventricles. Right and left ventricular gallop movements are shown. *Upper curve:* The prominent systolic pulsation with its abrupt onset is characteristic of volume overload of the right ventricle *(RV)*. This type of pulsation may be produced by a secundum atrial septal defect. A right ventricular gallop *(VG)* movement may be felt. *Lower curve:* The prominent pulsation with its abrupt onset is characteristic of volume overload of the left ventricle *(LV)*. This type of pulsation may be produced by aortic regurgitation or mitral regurgitation. A left ventricular gallop movement *(VG)* may be felt. *Bottom portion of figure:* This diagram shows the first and second heart sounds and the right and left ventricular gallop sounds *(VG)*.

Reproduced with permission from Hurst JW: The examination of the heart: the importance of initial screening, *Dis Mon* 36(5):282, 1990.

hypertension, produces a prominent systolic pulsation that lasts one half or more of systole. The pulsation (see lower curve in Fig. 6-66) has a relatively gradual onset and offset as compared with the pulsation caused by volume overload of the left ventricle (see lower curve in Fig. 6-67). Volume overload of the left ventricle produces a prominent systolic pulsation that has a brisk onset and offset. Such a pulsation is produced by aortic or mitral valve regurgitation (see lower curve in Fig. 6-67).

The systolic pulsation may be bifed in patients with idiopathic hypertrophic subaortic stenosis and correlates with the pulsus bisfiriens that is felt in the carotid artery.

A left atrial gallop sound can be seen or palpated just before the first heart sound in patients in whom left ventricular compliance is diminished (see lower curve in Fig. 6-66). This commonly occurs in patients with coronary artery disease, systemic hypertension, aortic valve stenosis, or hypertrophic cardiomyopathy and may also occur in patients with aortic or mitral valve regurgitation. A left ventricular gallop movement may be seen or felt in patients with the same conditions just mentioned (see lower curve in Fig. 6-66). A palpable left ventricular gallop movement indicates left ventricular dysfunction except when it is caused by mitral regurgitation. Note

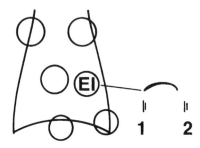

Fig. 6-68. Abnormal systolic ectopic impulse *(EI)*. No pulsation should be felt in this area in normal patients.

Reproduced with permission from Hurst JW: The examination of the heart: the importance of initial screening, *Dis Mon* 36(5):262, 1990.

that a left atrial gallop movement or a left ventricular gallop movement is not felt in patients with isolated mitral stenosis.

A systolic thrill may be palpated at the apex in patients with severe mitral regurgitation. A diastolic thrill and loud first heart sound may be palpated in patients with mitral stenosis.

Ectopic impulse. An ectopic impulse is defined as a pulsation that is not located in one of the areas described previously (Fig. 6-68). The most common location for such a pulsation is area 5 in Fig. 6-63. A systolic pulsation in this area may be produced by a ventricular aneurysm or a dysdynamic area of infarcted left ventricular myocardium. Another cause for such a pulsation is dilated cardiomyopathy.

Epigastric area. The palm of the examiner's right hand should be placed on the upper portion of the abdomen of the patient, and the fingertips should be placed under the midportion of the rib cage (area 6 in Fig. 6-63). This maneuver is useful for the detection of right ventricular hypertrophy in patients with pulmonary emphysema. The right ventricle strikes the tips of the fingers in such patients, and the aortic pulsation strikes the front of the fingers and palms.

Auscultation of the heart, arteries, and veins
The stethoscope
Origin of the stethoscope and its use. René T.H. Laennec was the first person to create an instrument to be used to examine the heart and lungs. Prior to his invention physicians placed an ear directly on the chest in order to hear the sounds made by the heart and the lungs. The following account of Laennec's discovery was translated from Laennec's original report[186] by Paul Dudley White[187]:

I was consulted in 1816 by a young woman who presented general symptoms of heart disease and in whose case the application of the hand and percussion gave little information because of her obesity. Since the age and the sex of the patient forbade my using the method of examination already described (that is, immediate auscultation) I happened to recall a well known acoustic phenomenon: if one applies the ear to the end of a beam, one hears very distinctly a pin scratch at the other end. I thought that I could profit by this physical property in the case of the patient under discussion. I took a sheet of paper, rolled it up tightly, applied one end of this cylinder on the precordial region, and, placing my ear against the other end I was as surprised as pleased to hear the heart beat in a manner much more clear and distinct than I had ever done by applying the ear immediately to the chest. . . .

I use at present a cylinder of wood pierced in its centre by a tube three lines in diameter and divided in the middle by a screw-joint in order to make it more portable.*

Initially the stethoscope was not accepted by every physician, just as new instruments are not initially accepted by everyone today. This is as it should be, because not all new instruments are valuable. Although the stethoscope was invented in 1816, many years passed before the mechanisms responsible for the normal and abnormal heart sounds and murmurs were understood. The understanding occurred as physicians correlated the heart sounds and murmurs with the abnormalities found at autopsy, phonocardiography, cardiac catheterization, and echocardiography. Now, regrettably, beginners believe that an echocardiogram is always needed to identify the presence of a murmur and its cause. Although echocardiography is commonly needed, it has not as yet replaced the routine use of the stethoscope, a discerning ear, and a thoughtful brain as the initial step in the identification of abnormal heart sounds and murmurs. Actually, auscultation of the heart is the most cost-effective method of identifying murmurs, and the predictive value of the observations made by a skilled examiner is excellent. In addition, a physician who suspects a certain auscultatory abnormality is better able to advise the echocardiographer about the problem he or she is trying to solve. In other words, excellent auscultation leads to excellent echocardiography and vice versa if the appropriate correlations are made.

Structure of the modern stethoscope. Whereas there are various prices attached to many different stethoscopes, there are relatively few requirements for an excellent instrument. There should be two earpieces and two tubes leading from the head of the stethoscope. The tubes should be as short as possible while remaining sufficiently long for the examiner's comfort while listening to the heart. The head of the instrument must have both a bell and a diaphragm. The examiner should apply the bell of the instrument to the skin with light pressure in order to hear low-pitched sounds and murmurs and should apply the specially designed diaphragm to the skin with firm pressure in order to hear high-pitched sounds and murmurs.

---

*Reprinted with the permission of Macmillan Publishing Company from *Heart Disease*, third edition, by Dr. Paul Dudley White, p 56. Copyright 1946 Macmillan Publishing Company; copyright renewed © 1974 Paul Dudley White.

Placement of the head of the stethoscope on the chest and elsewhere. The head of the stethoscope should be placed in the second right intercostal space adjacent to the sternum; in the second left intercostal space adjacent to the sternum; along the left sternal border and, at times, the right sternal border; and at the cardiac apex. Certain murmurs may radiate from the site of maximum intensity, and the listener must learn to identify the path of radiation. Finally, bruits or murmurs may be heard in the neck, back, over scars, in the abdomen, over the sacrum, and on the surface of the head.

Timing of the heart sounds. The first and second heart sounds must be identified with certainty. The first and second heart sounds can almost always be identified when the diaphragm of the stethoscope is placed in the second right intercostal space adjacent to the sternum; the second sound is normally louder than the first sound in this area of the chest. Whenever the first sound is louder than the second sound, one can deduce that there must be a condition that makes the first sound louder than usual or a condition that makes the second sound fainter than usual (see subsequent discussion).

It is possible to hear ten heart sounds. Four of these sounds are normal (but may become abnormal secondary to certain diseases), and six are almost always abnor-

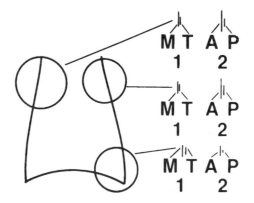

Fig. 6-69. The normal heart sounds. The first sound *(1)* is produced by mitral valve closure *(M)* followed by tricuspid valve closure *(T)*. The second heart sound *(2)* is produced by aortic valve closure *(A)* followed by pulmonary valve closure *(P)*. Note that the second sound is louder than the first sound when one is listening in the second intercostal space adjacent to the sternum. This is due to loudness of the aortic valve closure *(A)*. Note, also, that the pulmonary valve closure sound *(P)* is louder in the second intercostal space adjacent to the sternum than it is at the cardiac apex. In normal subjects the pulmonary closure sound is not heard at the apex, or it is only barely heard.

Reproduced with permission from Hurst JW: *The examination of the heart: the importance of initial screening, Dis Mon* 36(5):294, 1990.

mal. The four normal sounds are the first heart sound, which is composed of the mitral valve closure sound followed by the tricuspid valve closure sound, and the second heart sound, which is composed of the aortic valve closure sound followed by the pulmonary valve closure sound (Fig. 6-69). (These sounds may become abnormal with certain diseases). The six abnormal sounds, in addition to the normal heart sounds, are shown in Fig. 6-70. (These sounds are almost always abnormal.)

Normal heart sounds.[188-190] Physicians commonly write and state, "The heart sounds are normal." At times, when pressed to describe the characteristics of normal heart sounds, they may have some difficulty. The characteristics of normal heart sounds are described in this section.

Second right intercostal space adjacent to the sternum. As previously stated, the auscultatory process should begin by placing the diaphragm of the stethoscope in the second right intercostal space adjacent to the sternum. The normal heart sounds are illustrated in Fig. 6-69. The second heart sound in normal individuals is always louder than the first heart sound in this area (Fig. 6-71). The first component of the first heart sound is caused by mitral valve closure, and the second component of the first heart sound is produced by tricuspid valve closure but is seldom identified when listened for at this auscultatory area.

The two components of the second heart sound may be heard when listening in this area. The aortic valve closure sound and the pulmonary valve closure sound may be heard. When the two components are heard in normal subjects, the aortic valve closure sound is louder than the pulmonary valve closure sound. The interval of time

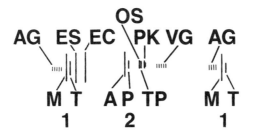

Fig. 6-70. The four normal and six abnormal heart sounds. *AG,* Atrial gallop; *M,* mitral valve closure; *T,* tricuspid valve closure; *ES,* ejection sound; *EC,* ejection click; *A,* aortic valve closure; *P,* pulmonary valve closure; *OS,* opening snap of the mitral valve; *PK,* pericardial knock; *VG,* ventricular gallop. A pericardial friction rub (not shown here) may have three components that coincide with heart movements: a rub when the atria contract, a rub associated with ventricular systole, and a rub associated with ventricular diastole. (See text for a discussion of normal and abnormal heart sounds.)

Reproduced with permission from Hurst JW: The examination of the heart: the importance of initial screening, *Dis Mon* 36(5):284, 1990.

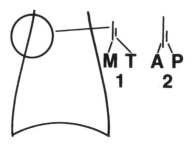

Fig. 6-71. The normal heart sounds in the second right intercostal space adjacent to the sternum. Note that the aortic valve closure sound is the loudest component of the heart sounds. Reproduced with permission from Hurst JW: The examination of the heart: the importance of initial screening, *Dis Mon* 36(5):264, 1990.

between the two sounds is short. However, this is not the ausculatory area where it is useful to study the splitting of the second sound (see subsequent discussion).

There should be no additional gallop sounds or clicks heard in this area in normal subjects.

Second left intercostal space adjacent to the sternum. The second sound is studied in this area. The diaphragm of the stethoscope should be used. The normal heart sounds are illustrated in Fig. 6-69. The second sound is composed of the aortic valve closure sound followed by the pulmonary valve closure sound. The pulmonary valve closure sound is always fainter than the aortic valve closure sound in normal subjects. Furthermore, the normal pulmonary valve closure sound diminishes in intensity as one moves the stethoscope to the cardiac apex (see subsequent discussion). The effect of inspiration and expiration on the "splitting" of the second sound must always be determined. At this point in the discussion it is adequate to point out that the small auscultatory gap that separates the aortic valve closure sound from the pulmonary valve closure sound during inspiration becomes almost imperceptible during expiration in normal subjects (Fig. 6-72).

There should be no additional gallop sounds or clicks heard in this area in normal subjects.

Left sternal border and precordial area. The diaphragm and the bell of the stethoscope should be "inched" along the left sternal border. The second heart sound is louder than the first heart sound, but as one approaches the apex, this relationship may change in normal subjects.

There should be no additional gallop sounds or clicks heard in this area in normal subjects.

Cardiac apex. The apex impulse must be identified as the first step in auscultation of the apex, because the diaphragm and the bell of the stethoscope should be placed at that spot on the chest. The first sound listened to with the diaphragm is composed of the mitral valve closure sound and the tricuspid valve closure sound

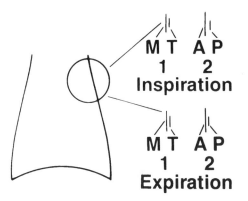

Fig. 6-72. Effect of inspiration and expiration on the splitting of the normal second heart sound, which is heard by placing the diaphragm of the stethoscope in the second intercostal space near the sternum. *Upper diagram:* Note the degree of splitting of the second heart sound during inspiration. *Lower diagram:* Note that the duration of the gap between the sound made by aortic valve closure *(A)* and the sound made by pulmonary valve closure *(P)* is less than it is during inspiration. In fact, in normal subjects the second sound commonly becomes single during expiration in most normal subjects.

Reproduced with permission from Hurst JW: The examination of the heart: the importance of initial screening, *Dis Mon* 36(5):284, 1990.

and may be louder than, fainter than, or equal to the intensity of the second sound (see Fig. 6-69). The listener must judge, however, whether the first sound is louder than usual or fainter than usual and if it is abnormally split. The second sound, composed of the aortic valve closure sound followed by the pulmonary valve closure sound, should be listened to carefully with the diaphragm in order to determine if the pulmonary valve closure sound is heard. Normally, the pulmonary valve closure sound is not heard or is only barely detected at the apex. A pulmonary valve closure sound that is easily heard indicates pulmonary hypertension (see later discussion).

The bell of the stethoscope is then applied with light pressure to the cardiac apex in an effort to hear low-pitched sounds such as a left atrial gallop sound or a left ventricular gallop sound. A low-pitched third heart sound may be heard in early diastole in normal children. It occurs during the rapid filling phase of ventricular diastole.

Normal heart murmurs.[188-190] A faint systolic murmur may be heard when the stethoscope is placed in the second left intercostal space adjacent to the sternum in normal children. The term *physiologic* is sometimes used to describe such a murmur, but since all normal and abnormal murmurs are physiologic, the term should be abandoned. The murmur should be referred to as a normal murmur.

A normal continuous murmur may be heard in the neck in young children when the cervical area is listened to with the child in the sitting position. This murmur may be heard in the upper portion of the chest and, at times, is confused with the continuous murmur produced by a patent ductus arteriosus. This interesting normal murmur, called a venous hum, is discussed in detail later in the section on continuous murmurs.

Several normal murmurs may be heard in pregnant women during the last few months of pregnancy. A systolic murmur may be heard in the second left intercostal space adjacent to the sternum, and a bruit may be heard in systole over the mammary arteries.

A systolic murmur may be heard in this area in anemic patients; such a murmur should be referred to as a hemic murmur.

Abnormal heart sounds[188-190]

Second right intercostal space adjacent to the sternum. When the first heart sound is louder than, or equal to, the loudness of the second sound in the second intercostal space adjacent to the sternum, one can conclude that something is causing the first heart sound to be louder than normal or that something is causing the second heart sound to be fainter than normal.

Mitral stenosis is the most common cause of a louder than normal first heart sound. The diastolic rumble is never heard in the second intercostal space adjacent to the sternum, but the loud first sound is widely distributed and is heard in this area of the chest. Accordingly, the intensity of the first heart sound is equal to or louder than the second heart sound in the second right intercostal space; it is a signal to listen at the cardiac apex with the bell of the stethoscope, after the patient has exercised to increase the heart rate, in an effort to hear the diastolic rumble of mitral stenosis.

The most common cause of a second heart sound that is fainter than normal (equal to the intensity of the first heart sound or fainter than the first heart sound) is aortic valve stenosis. The absence of a systolic murmur heard while listening in this area virtually excludes aortic valve stenosis as a cause of a second sound that is fainter than the first sound.

The listener should determine whether there is normal or abnormal splitting of the second heart sound. However, this area is not the best location to listen to the splitting of the second heart sound; the best location is the second left intercostal space adjacent to the sternum (see Fig. 6-72). Accordingly, the abnormal second heart sound will be discussed in the following section. It is mentioned here because, at times, the clinician may believe that the second heart sound is abnormally split when he or she is listening at the second right intercostal space adjacent to the sternum. In such cases it may be the opening snap of mitral valve stenosis that has been misinterpreted as the second component of the second sound because the opening snap of mitral valve stenosis is widely distributed.

An ejection sound may occasionally be heard just after the first heart sound; this same sound is usually detected at the cardiac apex, where it is much louder (see Fig.

6-70). It is commonly due to a bicuspid aortic valve, and the systolic or diastolic murmur associated with this congenital abnormality enables the listener to determine the cause of the ejection sound. In such patients it is the opening snap of an abnormal aortic valve. Such a sound may also be heard in patients with acquired aortic valve regurgitation. In these patients the sound is probably due to an aortic wall snap resulting from the large systolic ejection volume.

Atrial and ventricular gallop sounds are not usually heard in the second intercostal space adjacent to the sternum.

Second left intercostal space adjacent to the sternum. An ejection sound may be heard just after the first heart sound (see Fig. 6-70). The ejection sound may be associated with pulmonary valve stenosis; in such a case it is due to an "opening snap" of the abnormal pulmonary valve. A systolic murmur is heard in such cases. An ejection sound may also be heard when right ventricular systolic ejection volume is greater than normal, as it is in patients with a secundum atrial septal defect. In such patients the sound is a pulmonary artery wall snap.

An enormous amount of information can be obtained by studying the second heart sounds in this area. The clinician should determine if pulmonary artery hypertension is present and if abnormal splitting of the second sound suggests a particular type of cardiac abnormality.

Identifying pulmonary artery hypertension. Whenever the intensity of the second component of the second sound, which is due to pulmonary valve closure, is equal to or louder than the first component of the second sound, which is due to aortic valve closure, it is highly likely that pulmonary artery hypertension is present. The pres-

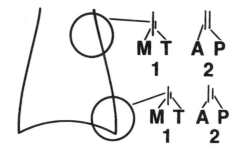

Fig. 6-73. Abnormally loud pulmonary valve closure (*P*) sound due to pulmonary artery hypertension. *Upper diagram:* The pulmonary valve closure sound (*P*) is as loud as the aortic valve closure sound (*A*); this is abnormal and suggests pulmonary artery hypertension. *Lower diagram:* The pulmonary valve closure sound (*P*) is easily heard at the apex and is louder than usual; this is virtually diagnostic of pulmonary artery hypertension.

Reproduced with permission from Hurst JW: The examination of the heart: the importance of initial screening, *Dis Mon* 36(5):284, 1990.

ence of pulmonary artery hypertension is even more likely when the second component of the second sound is easily heard at the cardiac apex (Fig. 6-73).

Normal splitting of the second sound. The two components of the second heart sound
are almost superimposed during expiration; there is very little or no gap between
them (see Fig. 6-72). Normally, during the last phase of inspiration the two components of the second sound separate, and both components of the sound are heard.
The split is caused, for the most part, by the delay in pulmonary valve closure. This
delay occurs because inspiration enhances the inflow of blood into the right ventricle, thus prolonging ventricular mechanical systole, which delays pulmonary valve
closure by about 0.08 second.

Abnormally wide splitting of the second sound. Abnormally wide splitting of the second sound can be caused by the following cardiac abnormalities.

FIXED SPLITTING OF THE SECOND SOUND. The term *fixed splitting of the second heart
sound* implies that the two components of the second heart sound are separated in
time more than normal and that there is no change in the interval between them
with inspiration and expiration.

The most common cause of this abnormality is congenital secundum atrial septal
defect (Fig. 6-74). Fixed splitting of the second heart sound occurs in patients with
this defect because during expiration a large amount of blood enters the right atrium
through the defect and a normal amount of blood enters the right atrium from the

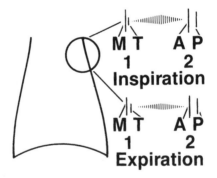

Fig. 6-74. Fixed, wide splitting of the second heart sound during inspiration and expiration,
characteristic of a secundum atrial septal defect. The abnormally large lapse of time between
the aortic *(A)* and pulmonary *(P)* valve closure sounds remains constant during inspiration
and expiration. Note the systolic diamond-shaped pulmonary artery murmur that is caused by
a large right ventricular stroke volume. Also note that the pulmonary valve closure sound is
louder than normal in the second left intercostal space and at the apex, because the pulmonary artery pressure may be slightly or moderately elevated.

Reproduced with permission from Hurst JW: The examination of the heart: the importance of initial
screening, *Dis Mon* 36(5):284, 1990.

venae cavae. Because of this combination of sources, a larger than normal amount of blood enters the right ventricle, resulting in a prolonged right ventricular systole and a delay in the sound made by pulmonary valve closure. During inspiration the volume of blood entering the right atrium and, in turn, the right ventricles is derived from the same two sources. The amount of blood entering the right atrium from the venae cavae is increased during inspiration as compared with its volume during expiration, but the left-to-right shunt through the secundum atrial septal defect is decreased during this period as compared with its volume during expiration. The combined sources are, however, always greater than normal. In summary, in patients with a secundum atrial septal defect the volume of blood entering the right ventricle is greater than normal and is about the same during inspiration and expiration. Accordingly, right ventricular mechanical systole is prolonged about the same amount of time during inspiration and expiration. As a result, the two components of the second sound remain widely separated from each other during inspiration and expiration. The cause, for the most part, is the delay in the closure of the pulmonary valve during inspiration and expiration.

ABNORMALLY SPLIT SECOND HEART SOUND THAT BECOMES MORE WIDELY SPLIT DURING INSPIRATION. When the second heart sound is more widely split than normal on expiration and the separation increases with inspiration, it is highly likely that right bundle-branch block will be found in the electrocardiogram and vice versa (Fig. 6-75). The pulmonary valve closure sound will be fainter than the aortic valve closure sound unless pulmonary artery hypertension is present.

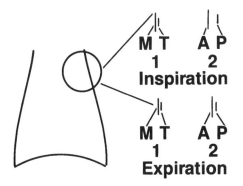

Fig. 6-75. Splitting of the second heart sound in patients with right bundle-branch block. *Lower diagram:* During expiration the aortic valve closure sound *(A)* and the pulmonary valve closure sound *(P)* are separated from each other by an interval of time that is greater than normal (see text for explanation). *Upper diagram:* During inspiration the interval of the time between the aortic valve closure sound *(A)* and the pulmonary valve closure sound *(P)* is increased beyond that observed during expiration (see text for explanation).

The causes of right bundle-branch block include coronary atherosclerotic heart disease; cardiomyopathy; primary disease of the conduction system (Lenegre disease); Lev disease; cardiac surgery; and conditions causing right ventricular hypertrophy, such as primary pulmonary hypertension, cor pulmonale, Eisenmenger syndrome, pulmonary emboli, and pulmonary valve stenosis.

Wide splitting of the components of the second heart sound during expiration and further separation on inspiration are due to the following physiologic mechanisms. Right ventricular depolarization is slightly delayed when there is right bundle-branch block, and this delay produces a delay in right ventricular myocardial contraction. Accordingly, during expiration and inspiration the pulmonary valve closure sound is delayed. The pulmonary valve closure sound is additionally delayed during inspiration, as it is normally, because right ventricular mechanical systole is prolonged in order to expel the increased volume of blood that entered the right ventricle during inspiration.

Wide splitting of the second heart sound with further separation on inspiration does not occur in every patient who has right bundle-branch block. For example, a patient with a secundum atrial septal defect may have right bundle-branch block in the electrocardiogram, but fixed splitting of the second sound is usually present because of a greater than normal volume of blood entering the right ventricle during inspiration and expiration. Wide splitting of the second heart sound with further separation on inspiration may not be detected when right bundle-branch block is caused by right ventricular hypertrophy due to pulmonary valve stenosis or right ventricular outflow tract obstruction; when right bundle-branch block is caused by these conditions, the pulmonary valve closure sound is usually difficult to hear. Wide splitting of the second heart sound with further separation on inspiration may not be detected in patients with right bundle-branch block associated with pulmonary emphysema, because the heart sounds may be difficult to hear during inspiration; only the louder of the two components of the second sound may be heard. The increase in splitting of the second sound during inspiration may not occur if the right ventricle is so damaged that mechanical systole is abnormally prolonged during both inspiration and expiration. Accordingly, I believe that patients with right bundle-branch block who have severe heart failure, such as occurs with cardiomyopathy, may not exhibit further separation of the components of the second heart sound during inspiration. At times, for unknown reasons, the second heart sound may not be widely split on expiration or may fail to split further on inspiration in patients with right bundle-branch block.

PARADOXICAL SPLITTING OF THE SECOND HEART SOUND. When the two components of the second heart sound are separated during expiration and become less separated during inspiration, the splitting is said to be paradoxical, because this behavior is opposite of normal (Fig. 6-76). This abnormal response of the second sound to inspiration and expiration is usually observed in patients who exhibit left bundle-branch

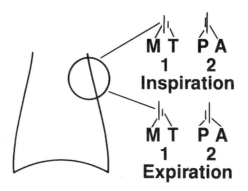

Fig. 6-76. Paradoxical splitting of the second heart sound caused by left bundle-branch block. *Lower diagram:* During expiration the aortic valve closure sound *(A)* is delayed because of left bundle-branch block. Accordingly, the aortic valve closure sound may appear after the pulmonary valve closure sound *(P)*. *Upper diagram:* During inspiration the pulmonary closure sound *(P)* is delayed, as it is normally, until it almost coincides with the aortic valve closure sound *(A)*.

Reproduced with permission from Hurst JW: *The examination of the heart: the importance of initial screening, Dis Mon* 36(5):284, 1990.

block in the electrocardiogram, but it may occasionally be observed in patients with severe aortic valve stenosis.

Paradoxical splitting of the second sound associated with left bundle-branch block is produced by the following mechanisms. Depolarization of the left ventricle is delayed because of left bundle-branch block, producing a delay in the onset of left ventricular contraction and a delay in the aortic valve closure sound during expiration, so that it occurs after the pulmonary valve closure sound. During inspiration the right ventricular mechanical systole is prolonged, as it is normally, because it must expel the increased volume of blood that has entered the right ventricle as a result of inspiration. Accordingly, the pulmonary closure sound is delayed and becomes superimposed on the aortic valve closure sound that has been delayed because of the left ventricular conduction abnormality.

Patients with severe aortic valve stenosis may have paradoxical splitting of the second sound because the aortic valve obstruction prolonged left ventricular systole and during expiration the aortic valve closure sound occurs after the pulmonary valve closure sound. During inspiration the pulmonary valve closure sound is delayed, because right ventricular mechanical systole is prolonged in order to expel the increase in the volume of blood that has entered the right ventricle during inhalation. Therefore the second heart sound becomes almost single during inspiration.

The causes of left bundle-branch block include coronary atherosclerotic heart disease; cardiomyopathy; primary disease of the conduction system (Lenegre disease); sclerosis of the cardiac skeleton (Lev disease); and left ventricular hypertrophy due to aortic valve stenosis, aortic regurgitation, mitral regurgitation, or idiopathic hypertrophy.

Paradoxical splitting of the second sound may not always occur when there is left bundle-branch block. For example, when the left bundle-branch block is associated with severe aortic valve stenosis, the aortic valve closure sound may not be heard, because it is often faint or inaudible in such patients. The entire second sound may be inaudible in such patients because the aortic closure sound may not be heard and the pulmonary valve closure sound may be buried in the end of the systolic murmur of aortic valve stenosis. Also, it may be difficult to hear both components of the second sound when there is considerable pulmonary emphysema; only the louder of the two components may be heard.

Left sternal border and precordium. Abnormal heart sounds may be heard along the left sternal border and precordium. Some of the abnormalities that are heard in the right and left second intercostal spaces are also heard at the upper portion of the left sternal border. These include an abnormally loud first heart sound, an abnormally loud pulmonary valve closure sound, an abnormally split second heart sound, an aortic or pulmonary ejection sound, and the opening snap of mitral stenosis. As the listener inches the stethoscope along the left sternal border and toward the cardiac apex impulse, some of these sounds diminish in intensity and certain new sounds may be heard.

The abnormal sounds listed in the preceding paragraph can be identified more easily by using the diaphragm of the stethoscope. The bell of the stethoscope should be applied with light pressure to the middle of the left sternal border, over the precordium to the left of this area, and at the apex in order to hear low-pitched atrial and ventricular gallop sounds.

A right atrial gallop may be heard along the middle portion of the left sternal border and over the precordium (Fig. 6-77). Being low pitched, it is usually separated from the higher-pitched first heart sound without difficulty. A right atrial gallop sound increases in intensity during inspiration, whereas a left atrial gallop sound decreases with inspiration. The sound is produced within the right ventricle; it is produced by the volume of blood that is propelled rapidly into the right ventricle, as a result of right atrial contraction, in patients with a decrease in right ventricular compliance. A decrease in right ventricular compliance occurs in patients with right ventricular hypertrophy from any cause and in patients with cardiomyopathy of any type.

A right ventricular gallop may be heard along the middle portion of the left sternal border and over the precordium (Fig. 6-78). The sound occurs after the second heart sound and is heard at about the one-third point in ventricular diastole. It is lower pitched than the opening snap of mitral stenosis that occurs earlier in diastole

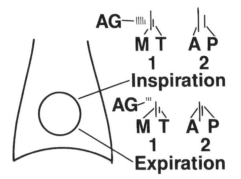

Fig. 6-77. Right atrial gallop sound. *Lower diagram:* During expiration the low-pitched, atrial gallop sound *(AG)* is heard just prior to the mitral valve closure sound *(M)*. *Upper diagram:* During inspiration the atrial gallop sound *(AG)* increases in intensity. The mechanisms involved in the production of the atrial gallop sound are discussed in the text.

Reproduced with permission from Hurst JW: The examination of the heart: the importance of initial screening, *Dis Mon* 36(5):284, 1990.

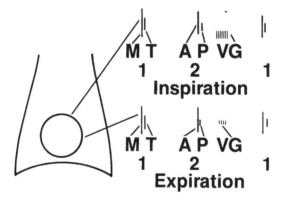

Fig. 6-78. Right ventricular gallop sound. *Lower diagram:* During expiration the low-pitched ventricular gallop sound *(VG)* occurs at about the one-third point in ventricular diastole. *Upper diagram:* During inspiration the ventricular gallop sound *(VG)* increases in intensity as compared with its loudness during expiration. The mechanisms responsible for the ventricular gallop sound are discussed in the text.

Reproduced with permission from Hurst JW: The examination of the heart: the importance of initial screening, *Dis Mon* 36(5):294, 1990.

and the pericardial knock of constrictive pericarditis that occurs at about the same time in diastole. The intensity of a right ventricular gallop sound increases with inspiration, whereas a left ventricular gallop sound decreases with inspiration. A right ventricular gallop sound is a sign of right ventricular dysfunction. When such a sound is heard in adults, it is always abnormal.

The opening snap of tricuspid valve stenosis may be heard at the end of the sternum, and a pericardial friction rub may be heard in the precordial area. These abnormal sounds are discussed later in the section on abnormal heart murmurs in the left sternal border and end of the sternum.

Cardiac apex. The first heart sound should be studied carefully when one is listening to the cardiac apex; the diaphram should be used for this purpose. The sound is composed of mitral valve closure followed by tricuspid valve closure (see Fig. 6-69). The mitral component is the louder of the two sounds, and the listener should think in terms of the mitral valve and left ventricular events when listening to the first sound.

The intensity of the first heart sound at the cardiac apex is determined by three factors:

- The interval of time that occurs between atrial contraction and ventricular contraction is the major factor determining the intensity of the first heart sound at the cardiac apex. This duration is reflected in the PR interval in the electrocardiogram. When the PR interval is 0.20 second or more, the time interval between atrial contraction and ventricular contraction is longer than usual and the first heart sound will be fainter than normal. This occurs because the mitral valve leaflets have time to float toward a closed position before left ventricular contraction occurs; the result is decreased intensity of the second heart sound (Fig. 6-79).

  When the PR interval is short (in the range of 0.14 to 0.16 second), the time interval between atrial contraction and ventricular contraction is short; this is associated with a louder than usual first heart sound. When atrial contraction varies in its relationship to ventricular contraction, as it does in complete heart block, the first heart sound at the apex will vary in intensity from beat to beat (Fig. 6-80). In such patients the loud first heart sound is referred to as a cannon sound.

- The structural integrity of the mitral valve influences the intensity of the first heart sound. When the leaflets of the mitral valve are partially destroyed, such as occurs with rheumatic mitral valve disease with regurgitation, there may be inadequate mitral valve tissue to coapt sufficiently to produce a loud first sound. Accordingly, the first heart sound may be faint.

  When the mitral valve is thicker and stiffer than normal, mitral valve closure is delayed slightly, because a higher level of left ventricular pressure is needed to close the valve. The result is a loud "snapping" first heart sound

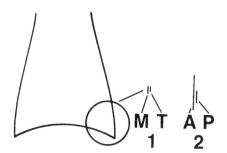

Fig. 6-79. Faint first heart sound heard at the cardiac apex. The most common cause of a faint first heart sound is an abnormal period of time elapsing between atrial contraction and ventricular contraction in association with a long PR interval in the electrocardiogram. One should visualize the mitral valve closing and the left ventricle contracting when listening to the first component of the second sound.

Reproduced with permission from Hurst JW: The examination of the heart: the importance of initial screening, *Dis Mon* 36(5):284, 1990.

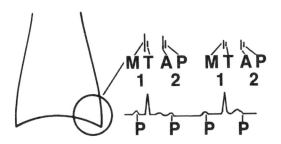

Fig. 6-80. Varying intensity of the first heart sound—varying relationship of atrial contraction to ventricular contraction—associated with complete atrioventricular heart block. Note that the first component of the first heart sound is loud in the first heart cycle and that it is faint in the second heart cycle, because the P wave and atrial contraction occur nearer the QRS complex and ventricular systole in the first heart cycle than they do in the second heart cycle.

Reproduced with permission from Hurst JW: The examination of the heart: the importance of initial screening, *Dis Mon* 36(5):284, 1990.

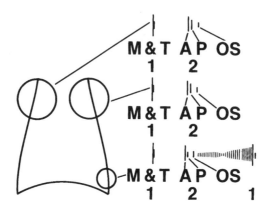

Fig. 6-81. Opening snap, as well as other auscultatory features, of mitral stenosis. *Upper diagram:* Note the abnormally loud mitral *(M)* component of the first heart sound when one is listening in the second right intercostal space. It is louder than the second sound. The pulmonary valve closure sound *(P)* may be heard. The opening snap *(OS)* of the mitral valve is also heard in this area. *Middle diagram:* The first heart sound is louder than normal, and an opening snap *(OS)* is heard when one is listening in the second left intercostal space. The pulmonary valve closure sound *(P)* is often heard. *Lower diagram:* The first sound is loud. An opening snap is heard. A low-pitched, rumbling murmur of mitral stenosis is heard. Note that the diastolic rumble of mitral stenosis is heard only at the cardiac apex, whereas the loud first sound and opening snap are widely transmitted.

Reproduced with permission from Hurst JW: The examination of the heart: the importance of initial screening, *Dis Mon* 36(5):284, 1990.

(Fig. 6-81). When the mitral valve leaflets are densely calcified, the first sound may not be loud, because it is almost immobile and cannot buckle.

- The strength of left ventricular contraction affects the intensity of the first heart sound; the more forceful the contraction, the louder the first sound. When left ventricular contraction is weak, as it is with cardiomyopathy, it closes the mitral valve more gently; when it is strong, such as occurs in patients with thyrotoxicosis, it closes the mitral valve with vigor. However, the strength of left ventricular contraction influences the intensity of the first heart sound less than the first two factors listed.

Two different abnormal sounds may be heard in systole at the cardiac apex. They should be listened for by using the diaphragm of the stethoscope. The ejection sound of a congenital bicuspid aortic valve may be louder at the cardiac apex than it is at the second right intercostal space adjacent to the sternum. It is an aortic valve opening snap (see Fig. 6-70).

Mitral valve prolapse may produce a midsystolic ejection click or clicks (see Fig. 6-70). These high-pitched sounds move closer to the first heart sound when the patient stands. The click may be followed by a murmur (see following section on abnormal murmurs). The systolic click (or clicks) is caused by the abrupt tensing of slack chordae tendineae and ballooning mitral valve leaflets. The mitral valve leaflets may be normal or may exhibit myxomatous degeneration.

Normally the pulmonary closure sound is not heard, or is barely heard, at the cardiac apex. Accordingly, when it is easily heard, it is often associated with pulmonary valve hypertension.

The opening snap of mitral valve stenosis is a high-pitched sound occurring about 0.08 to 0.12 second after the aortic valve closure sound (see Fig. 6-81). Because the opening snap is high pitched, it is more easily heard by using the diaphragm. It is differentiated from a ventricular gallop sound because the gallop sound occurs slightly later in diastole and is lower pitched than the opening snap. The precordial knock, which is associated with constrictive pericarditis, is high pitched rather than low pitched but occurs slightly later in diastole than the opening snap (see Fig. 6-70). The tumor plop of a left atrial tumor may simulate the opening snap of mitral stenosis.

A left atrial gallop sound may be heard at the cardiac apex (Fig. 6-82) and is more easily heard with the bell of the stethoscope. It does not increase in intensity with inspiration. A left atrial gallop sound signifies that the compliance of the left ventricle is less than normal. The sound may be heard in patients with aortic valve stenosis, hypertrophic cardiomyopathy, systemic hypertension, or atherosclerotic coronary heart disease; during an episode of angina; etc. It may occur with rupture of the chordae tendineae of the mitral valve, because the volume of blood expelled by the left atrium into a normal left ventricle is much greater than normal.

A left ventricular gallop sound may be heard at the cardiac apex (Fig. 6-83) and is more easily heard with the bell of the stethoscope. It occurs during the rapid filling

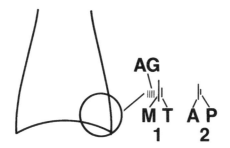

Fig. 6-82. Left atrial gallop sound. Heard at the cardiac apex, the left atrial gallop sound (*AG*), is low pitched and immediately precedes the high-pitched first heart sound. With a few exceptions it is a sign of decreased left ventricular compliance (see text).

Reproduced with permission from Hurst JW: *The examination of the heart: the importance of initial screening, Dis Mon* 36(5):284, 1990.

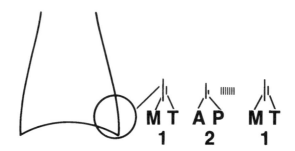

Fig. 6-83. Left ventricular gallop sound. Heard in ventricular diastole, the left ventricular gallop sound is low pitched and occurs at about the one-third point in diastole. With a few exceptions it is a sign of left ventricular dysfunction.

Reproduced with permission from Hurst JW: The examination of the heart: the importance of initial screening, *Dis Mon* 36(5):284, 1990.

phase of left ventricular filling and does not become louder with inspiration. A left ventricular gallop sound is a sign of left ventricular dysfunction with a few exceptions. A similar sound is heard in normal children and is referred to as a normal third sound. Such a sound does not necessarily indicate left ventricular dysfunction in patients with thyrotoxicosis or mitral regurgitation, or in pregnant patients. Gallop rhythm is said to be present when an atrial or ventricular gallop sound is heard in a patient with tachycardia. When the heart rate is fast, the cadence of the heartbeats, including the gallop sounds, resembles the gallop of a horse. At times the atrial and ventricular gallop sounds occur at the same time, creating a summation gallop. This situation occurs when the heart rate is rapid, the PR interval is longer than usual, and there is poor ventricular compliance and dysfunction.

A pericardial friction rub occurs when the heart moves (Fig. 6-84). Therefore a rub is heard when atrial systole occurs, when ventricular systole occurs, and when ventricular diastole occurs. Three high-pitched, scratchy sounds heard at the apex, or over the precordium, are virtually diagnostic of pericarditis. When two scratchy sounds are heard, they are likely to be caused by pericarditis. When only one scratchy sound is heard, it may or may not be due to pericarditis.

Abnormal heart murmurs.[188-190] There are three general types of heart murmurs: systolic murmurs, diastolic murmurs, and continuous murmurs. These murmurs are described here as one hears them in the auscultatory locations described earlier in this discussion.

Freeman and Levine[191] devised the system that is used to grade the intensity of heart murmurs:

Grade 1: The murmur is not heard easily. It is not heard immediately; the listener must "tune in" and listen to several heart cycles to hear the murmur.

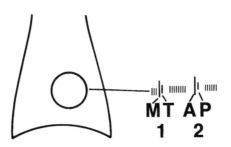

Fig. 6-84. Pericardial friction rub. Three components of the pericardial friction rub, which is commonly heard over the precordial area, are shown here. The high-pitched, scratchy sound is commonly heard when the heart moves during atrial systole, ventricular systole, and ventricular diastole.

Reproduced with permission from Hurst JW: The examination of the heart: the importance of initial screening, *Dis Month* 36(5):284, 1990.

Grade 2: The murmur is easily heard immediately, but it is only slightly louder than a grade 1 murmur.

Grade 3: The murmur is moderately loud.

Grade 4: The murmur is louder than a grade 3 murmur. It is not heard when only a portion of the rim of the stethoscope touches the chest wall.

Grade 5: The murmur is heard when only a portion of the rim of the stethoscope touches the chest wall. It is not heard when the stethoscope is not touching the chest wall.

Grade 6: The murmur is heard when the stethoscope is not touching the chest wall.

Murmurs that are classified as grade 1, 4, 5, or 6 are easily labeled. Experience is needed to classify murmurs as grade 2 or 3. Also, the grading system can be used to describe systolic murmurs more accurately than it can be used to describe diastolic murmurs.

The pitch of a murmur should always be determined and recorded. Pitch is determined by the number of sound vibrations that occur per second. The pitch and intensity of a murmur are determined by the velocity of blood flow.

A murmur is produced when there is a pressure gradient across a heart valve or across an abnormal hole, such as a ventricular septal defect or patent ductus. The diastolic pressure gradient across a stenosed mitral valve is small, resulting in a low velocity of blood flow. Accordingly, the diastolic murmur of mitral stenosis is low pitched and is usually classified as grade 1 or 2. The systolic pressure gradient across an incompetent mitral valve is great, resulting in a high velocity of blood flow. Accordingly, the murmur is high pitched, and the intensity of the murmur is roughly proportional to its severity.

Second right intercostal space adjacent to the sternum. Aortic valve sclerosis develops as patients grow older. The stiff aortic valve leaflets may or may not obstruct the aortic blood flow during ventricular systole.

The diaphragm of the stethoscope should be used to listen for the grade 1 or 2 systolic murmur, which is somewhat diamond shaped. The second sound remains normal, and the murmur is not widely distributed.

Aortic valve stenosis may be caused by a congenital unicuspid or bicuspid aortic valve. The diaphragm of the stethoscope should be used to listen for the grade 2 or 4 systolic murmur (Fig. 6-85). During early life the systolic murmur is introduced with a systolic ejection sound, which is caused by the aortic valve attempting to open. The ejection sound is often louder at the cardiac apex. The more severe the stenosis (obstruction to blood flow), the more likely it is that the peak of the diamond-shaped murmur will be delayed in systole (Figs. 6-86 and 6-87). Also, the more severe the stenosis, the more likely it is that the aortic valve closure sound will be diminished in intensity, and the more likely it is that there will be paradoxical splitting of the second heart sound, although these observations are better made in the second left intercostal space adjacent to the sternum (see Fig. 6-87).

When the murmur of aortic valve stenosis is heard at ages 40 to 50, it may be due to a congenital bicuspid aortic valve that is beginning to calcify, or it may be due to rheumatic heart disease. It is not possible, from auscultation alone, to diag-

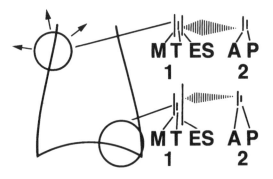

Fig. 6-85. Aortic valve stenosis due to a congenital bicuspid valve. *Upper diagram:* When one is listening in the second right intercostal space near the sternum, the first sound may be louder than the second sound, because the second sound may be fainter than usual. A high-pitched ejection sound *(ES)* may be heard immediately after the first heart sound. The aortic valve closure sound *(A)* remains normal unless the stenosis is severe. With midstenosis the peak of the systolic murmur occurs early in systole. *Lower diagram:* The ejection sound *(ES)* may be louder at the apex than it is in the second right intercostal space.

Reproduced with permission from Hurst JW: The examination of the heart: the importance of initial screening, *Dis Mon* 36(5):285, 1990.

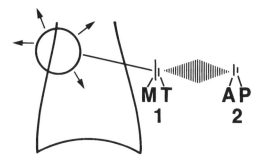

Fig. 6-86. Murmur of moderately severe aortic valve stenosis. Note that the first sound is louder than the second sound, because the normal mitral valve closure sound *(M)* is louder than the aortic valve closure sound *(A)*, which is diminished in intensity. The peak of the systolic diamond murmur occurs in midsystole.

Reproduced with permission from Hurst JW: The examination of the heart: the importance of initial screening, Dis Mon 36(5):285, 1990.

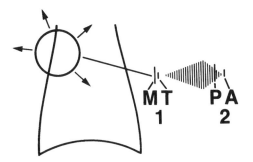

Fig. 6-87. Murmur of severe aortic valve stenosis. The aortic valve closure sound *(A)* is delayed and is faint or inaudible. The pulmonary valve closure sound *(P)* may be masked by the end of the murmur, even when it is louder than normal because of heart failure and mild pulmonary artery hypertension. Commonly, neither component of the second heart sound is heard. If both components of the second sound are heard, there may be paradoxical splitting of the second heart sound. The peak of the coarse systolic murmur appears late in systole, and the murmur is transmitted into the neck, right shoulder, and upper part of the right arm.

Reproduced with permission from Hurst JW: The examination of the heart: the importance of initial screening, *Dis Mon* 36(5):285, 1990.

nose rheumatic heart disease as the cause unless there are mitral murmurs that can be attributed to rheumatic heart disease. When the systolic murmur is heard for the first time at age 60 and beyond, it is usually due to calcific aortic valve stenosis of the elderly. Regardless of the cause, it is important to estimate the likelihood that the aortic valve disease is causing significant obstruction to blood flow. This judgment is made as follows (see Figs. 6-86 and 6-87). Significant obstruction is likely when the murmur is coarse; the diamond-shaped murmur peaks late in systole; the aortic valve closure sound is faint; there is paradoxical splitting of the second heart sound; neither component of the second sound is heard, because the aortic valve closure sound is not audible and the pulmonary valve closure sound is masked by the late portion of the systolic murmur; and there is wide distribution of the murmur into the neck, right arm, and cardiac apex.

A faint or loud systolic murmur may occur in this area in patients who have moderate to severe aortic regurgitation from any cause. The systolic murmur is caused by the larger than normal quantity of blood that is ejected by the left ventricle during systole.

The high-pitched *decrescendo murmur of aortic valve regurgitation* may be heard in this area, but it is better heard along the left sternal border and cardiac apex. Aortic regurgitation and its causes are discussed later in the section on abnormal murmers in the left sternal border and end of the sternum. At this point it should be emphasized that slight to moderate aortic regurgitation may accompany aortic valve stenosis.

Second left intercostal space adjacent to the sternum. A faint systolic murmur may be heard in this area in normal children and adolescents.

A systolic, diamond-shaped murmur may be heard in this area when the right ventricular systolic stroke volume is greater than normal, as it is in patients with a secundum atrial septal defect (see Fig. 6-74).

The *systolic murmur of pulmonary valve stenosis* is also heard in this area. The diaphragm of the stethoscope should be used. The diamond-shaped systolic murmur may be ushered in with a pulmonary valve ejection sound. When pulmonary valve stenosis is severe, the peak intensity of the murmur may be delayed, the pulmonary valve closure sound may be delayed and decreased in intensity, and the aortic valve closure sound may be masked by the late phase of the systolic murmur (Fig. 6-88).

A systolic murmur associated with tetralogy of Fallot may be heard in this area. The murmur is due, for the most part, to the right-to-left shunt that is produced because the aorta overrides the upper portion of the interventricular septum. The pulmonary closure sound and a pulmonary ejection sound are not heard in patients with tetralogy of Fallot.

Pulmonary valve stenosis is almost always congenital in origin; it may rarely occur with carcinoid heart disease. The systolic murmur associated with carcinoid pulmonary valve stenosis is composed of high- and low-pitched vibrations—it defies de-

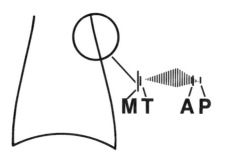

Fig. 6-88. Murmur of moderately severe pulmonary valve stenosis. The pulmonary valve closure sound *(P)* is delayed and is fainter than normal. The aortic valve closure sound *(A)* may be masked by the end of the diamond-shaped systolic murmur, because right ventricular ejection is prolonged. Therefore the second sound may be fainter than the normal first sound. The peak of the diamond-shaped murmur appears in midsystole or a little later. An early systolic ejection sound (not shown here) may be present.

Reproduced with permission from Hurst JW: The examination of the heart: the importance of initial screening, *Dis Mon* 36(5):285, 1990.

scription, but it is different from the murmur of congenital pulmonary valve stenosis.

The diaphragm should be used to listen for the high-pitched *decrescendo murmur of aortic valve regurgitation or pulmonary valve regurgitation.* Although these murmurs are heard in this area, they are better studied by listening along the left sternal border (see following discussion). As discussed later, it is not always possible to distinguish between these two murmurs. The loudness of the pulmonary valve closure sound must be assessed by listening for it in this area, because when it is louder than normal, there is an increased probability that the high-pitched decrescendo diastolic murmur is due to pulmonary valve regurgitation secondary to pulmonary artery hypertension.

Left sternal border and end of the sternum. The diaphragm of the stethoscope should be used to listen for the systolic diamond-shaped systolic murmurs of aortic valve stenosis and pulmonary valve stenosis. These murmurs may be heard at the upper portion and midportion of the left sternal border. The murmur of aortic valve stenosis is more likely to be transmitted to the end of the sternum and cardiac apex than is the murmur of pulmonary valve stenosis.

The *systolic murmur of idiopathic hypertrophic subaortic stenosis* may be heard to the left of the midportion of the sternum and near the apex (Fig. 6-89). The listener may initially have difficulty determining whether the murmur is due to aortic valve stenosis or mitral regurgitation. The murmur tends to be diamond shaped, and the second sound is usually normal in patients with idiopathic hypertrophic subaortic

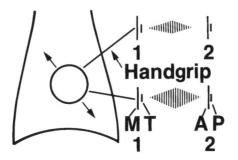

Fig. 6-89. Systolic murmur associated with idiopathic hypertrophic subaortic stenosis. The intensity of the murmur increases with handgrip isometric exercise. It becomes louder when the patient stands from a squatting position.

Reproduced with permission from Hurst JW: The examination of the heart: the importance of initial screening, *Dis Mon* 36(5):285, 1990.

stenosis. The murmur becomes fainter with handgrip-induced isometric exercise and louder when the patient stands up from a squatting position.

The *systolic murmur of atrial septal defect* is due to the increase in pulmonary blood flow. It may be heard in the second and third left intercostal spaces adjacent to the sternum. There is fixed splitting of the second sound in such patients (see Fig. 6-74).

The *systolic murmur of interventricular septal defect* due to congenital heart disease, trauma, or a ruptured septum secondary to myocardial infarction is usually located to the left of, and over, the midportion of the sternum (Fig. 6-90). The systolic murmur usually lasts throughout systole. The murmur may taper a little near its end as the right ventricular cavity fills with blood from the left-to-right shunt. Fixed splitting of the second heart sound does not occur under these circumstances, as it does with a secundum atrial septal defect, although there is an increase in pulmonary blood flow. The reason is that the left-to-right shunt that is due to an interventricular septal defect may not be as large as the left-to-right shunt that is due to an atrial septal defect. In addition, the right ventricular conduction delay, as observed in the electrocardiogram, occurs in almost all cases of secundum atrial septal defect but rarely occurs with an interventricular septal defect.

The *systolic murmur of tricuspid valve regurgitation* is heard at the lower end of the sternum (Fig. 6-91). The murmur becomes louder during inspiration because of the increase in blood flow into the right side of the heart during inhalation (Carvallo sign). Tricuspid regurgitation is common and is not always accompanied by a systolic murmur. A more reliable sign of tricuspid valve regurgitation is a positive v wave in the deep jugular veins.

Most tricuspid regurgitation is secondary to disease of the left side of the heart

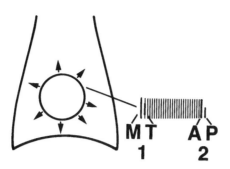

Fig. 6-90. Systolic murmur of interventricular septal defect. The murmur usually lasts throughout systole; it may taper a little at its end as the right ventricle becomes filled with blood.

Reproduced with permission from Hurst JW: The examination of the heart: the importance of initial screening, *Dis Mon* 36(5):285, 1990.

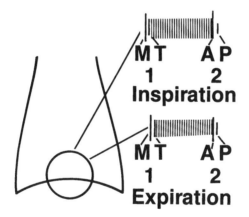

Fig. 6-91. Systolic murmur of tricuspid valve regurgitation. The murmur increases in intensity during inspiration *(upper diagram)*.

Reproduced with permission from Hurst JW: The examination of the heart: the importance of initial screening, *Dis Mon* 36(5):285, 1990.

and heart failure. Accordingly, patients with heart failure due to aortic or mitral valve disease, cardiomyopathy, coronary atherosclerotic heart disease, or systemic hypertension may develop sufficient right ventricular dilatation and tricuspid valve incompetence to produce tricuspid regurgitation. Patients with idiopathic pulmonary hypertension, repeated pulmonary emboli, pneumoconiosis, Eisenmenger syndrome, or pulmonary valve stenosis may also develop tricuspid regurgitation. Primary causes of tricuspid valve regurgitation include rheumatic heart disease, Epstein anomaly of the tricuspid valve, carcinoid syndrome, and infective endocarditis in addicts who "mainline" their drugs.

The tricuspid valve annulus is not as well formed as the mitral valve annulus. Accordingly, tricuspid regurgitation occurs with a lower ventricular pressure than is required to produce mitral regurgitation. For example, the mitral valve may remain competent even though the systolic pressure in the left ventricle may be 200 mm Hg because of aortic valve stenosis. The tricuspid valve, however, may become incompetent when the systolic pressure in the right ventricle is only moderately elevated to a level of 70 mm Hg in patients with an atrial septal defect. This is best explained by the fact that the tricuspid valve orifice is larger than the mitral valve orifice and the tricuspid valve annulus does not encircle the valve as the mitral valve annulus does.

The diaphragm of the stethoscope should be used to listen for a high-pitched diastolic decrescendo murmur along the upper portion of the left sternal border. The murmur is more easily heard when the patient is sitting and leaning forward. Such a murmur may be caused by aortic valve regurgitation or pulmonary valve regurgitation. It is not always possible to determine which of the two causes is present or if both causes are operative.

The *diastolic murmur of aortic valve regurgitation* may be heard along the left sternal border, at the end of the sternum, and at the cardiac apex; the pulmonary closure sound is not loud; and there are peripheral signs of aortic valve regurgitation (Fig. 6-92).

Aortic valve regurgitation may be caused by systemic hypertension, rheumatic heart disease, a congenital bicuspid aortic valve, endocarditis, an interventricular septal defect with a poorly supported aortic valve, aortic valve stenosis of the elderly, myxomatous degeneration of the aortic valve, annuloaortic ectasia, a congenital fixed-

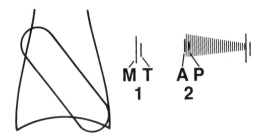

Fig. 6-92. High-pitched distolic murmur of aortic valve regurgitation. The murmur is heard with maximum intensity along the left sternal border when the patient is sitting and leaning forward.

Reproduced with permission from Hurst JW: The examination of the heart: the importance of initial screening, *Dis Mon* 36(5):285, 1990.

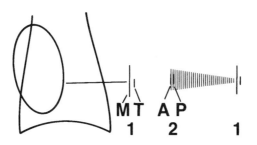

Fig. 6-93. The diastolic murmur of aortic valve regurgitation due to aortic root disease may be heard with maximum intensity along the right sternal border (see text).
Reproduced with permission from Hurst JW: The examination of the heart: the importance of initial screening, *Dis Mon* 36(5):285, 1990.

orifice subaortic membrane, aortic dissection, trauma, syphilis, or Marfan disease of the aorta. When the murmur of aortic regurgitation is louder along the right sternal border than it is along the left sternal border, an aortic root abnormality is likely to be the cause of the murmur (Fig. 6-93). Aortic regurgitation that produces a "cooing" type of murmur signifies a retroverted aortic valve cusp due to syphilis, myxomatous degeneration of the valve, a hole in the cusp due to endocarditis, or a tear in a prosthetic tissue valve. The murmur of aortic regurgitation decreases in intensity during the late stage of pregnancy because of the decrease in peripheral systemic resistance associated with the gravid state. The murmur will increase in intensity in the pregnant patient when she squats, because this increases the peripheral systemic resistance.

The *diastolic murmur of pulmonary valve regurgitation* may be considered when the pulmonary valve closure sound is loud, signifying pulmonary artery hypertension, and when there are other cardiac or peripheral clues indicating conditions that could be responsible for pulmonary artery hypertension or an increased pulmonary blood flow. For example, a prominent vigorous systolic pulsation in the second left intercostal space suggests a dilated pulmonary artery that could be caused by a larger than normal pulmonary blood flow. When there is also an anterior precordial systolic pulsation, suggesting right ventricular hypertrophy, the palpable pulsation of the pulmonary artery should be interpreted as an indication of either increased pulmonary artery pressure from some cause or an increased pulmonary blood flow, such as occurs with secundum atrial septal defect. When the systolic precordial pulsation is dynamic, the cause is more likely to be an increased pulmonary blood flow.

Pulmonary valve regurgitation can be caused by the following conditions:
- Pulmonary valve regurgitation due to an increase in pulmonary artery blood flow. A secundum atrial septal defect is the most common cause of this abnormality. The left-to-right shunt at the atrial level can cause a huge increase in

pulmonary artery blood flow and right ventricular dilatation. The pulmonary artery pressure may be normal, slightly increased, moderately increased, or markedly increased (Eisenmenger physiology). The intensity of the pulmonary valve closure sound may be normal or increased, depending on the level of the pulmonary artery pressure. Fixed splitting of the second heart sound is almost always present. Other causes of an increase in pulmonary blood flow and pressure are interventricular septal defect, patent ductus arteriosus, and ostium primum atrial septal defect with cleft mitral valve.

- Pulmonary valve regurgitation due to pulmonary artery hypertension. I suspect that the most common cause of pulmonary valve regurgitation today is primary pulmonary hypertension (Fig. 6-94). Formerly the most common cause was rheumatic heart disease with mitral valve stenosis. It was in this setting that Graham Steele identified pulmonary valve regurgitation. Other causes of an increase in pulmonary artery pressure without an increase in pulmonary blood flow are repeated pulmonary emboli, pneumoconiosis, and Eisenmenger syndrome. Initially, of course, in patients with Eisenmenger syndrome there is an increase in pulmonary blood flow due to a left-to-right shunt at the atrial or ventricular level, or through a ductus arteriosus; however, as pulmonary arteriolar disease develops, the pulmonary artery pressure increases and the pulmonary flow decreases, and the left-to-right shunt is replaced with a right-to-left shunt. The pulmonary valve closure sound is increased in all of these patients.
- Pulmonary valve stenosis as a cause of pulmonary valve regurgitation. The valve leaflets of pulmonary valve stenosis may not completely close the pulmonary valve orifice during diastole. Accordingly, the faint murmur of pulmonary valve regurgitation may follow the systolic murmur due to pulmonary valve stenosis. Here we have an unusual situation in which pulmonary artery hypotension,

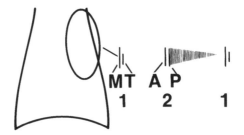

Fig. 6-94. Pulmonary valve regurgitation due to pulmonary hypertension. Note the increase in intensity of the pulmonary valve closure sound (*P*).

Reproduced with permission from Hurst JW: The examination of the heart: the importance of initial screening, *Dis Mon* 36(5):285, 1990.

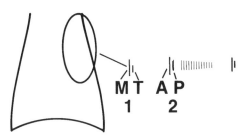

Fig. 6-95. Diastolic murmur due to pulmonary valve regurgitation associated with pulmonary valve dysplasia or absence of a pulmonary valve leaflet. The murmur may be lower pitched than the high-pitched diastolic murmur associated with pulmonary hypertension. The murmur follows the second sound by a short interval.

Reproduced with permission from Hurst JW: The examination of the heart: the importance of initial screening, *Dis Mon* 36(5):285, 1990.

rather than hypertension, is associated with pulmonary valve regurgitation. Under these circumstances the decrescendo diastolic murmur of pulmonary valve regurgitation seems to be slightly delayed after the appearance of the second heart sound, and the murmur is less high pitched than it is when it is associated with pulmonary artery hypertension.

- Congenital pulmonary valve regurgitation. This rare condition, due to pulmonary valve dysplasia or absence of a pulmonary valve leaflet, produces a low-pitched diastolic murmur that follows the second heart sound by a short interval (Fig. 6-95).

There is an additional, rare cause of a high-pitched, decrescendo murmur that may be heard along the upper portion of the left sternal border. Young patients with any of the four types of truncus arteriosus may have *truncal regurgitation*, because the valve leaflets may be incompetent and because the truncal pressure is at systemic levels. The second sound is always single in these patients; splitting of the second sound is not possible, because there are no separate aortic and pulmonary valves.

The bell of the stethoscope should be used to hear a low-pitched *diastolic rumble at the end of the sternum*. This murmur can be caused by rheumatic tricuspid valve stenosis or carcinoid plaque. When the murmur is due to rheumatic tricuspid valve stenosis, a loud first sound and opening snap of the tricuspid valve may be heard.

The diastolic rumble of secundum atrial septal defect may be heard at the lower end of the sternum; it is fainter at the cardiac apex. The first sound may be loud in such patients, and an opening snap of the tricuspid valve may be heard. The loud first sound is due to an increase in right ventricular contraction, and the diastolic rumble and opening snap are due to the larger than normal blood volume entering the right ventricle during diastole. This explains why a secundum atrial septal defect can be misdiagnosed as tricuspid or mitral valve stenosis.

Cardiac apex. Systolic murmurs are high pitched and should be listened for by using the diaphragm of the stethoscope. Mitral regurgitation may be due to primary disease of the mitral valve apparatus or secondary to aortic valve disease or left ventricular disease.

The mitral valve apparatus is composed of the mitral valve annulus, mitral valve leaflets, chordae tendineae, papillary muscles, and the left ventricular myocardium to which the papillary muscles are attached. Mitral regurgitation may be caused by an abnormality, or a combination of several abnormalities, of these structures.

Calcification of the mitral valve annulus may be associated with a systolic murmur that lasts throughout systole or occurs late in systole. Presumably, the sphincterlike action of the mitral valve annulus is diminished, and there is calcification of the outer reaches of the mitral valve leaflets. Although the exact cause of the murmur is unknown, it is likely that the calcification of the undersurfaces of the mitral valve leaflets near the annulus lift them upward, so that they do not coapt. This condition occurs in elderly individuals and can be identified in the chest x-ray film (see Fig. 8-29) or by echocardiography. The condition rarely produces severe mitral regurgitation.

The *systolic murmur of mitral valve regurgitation due to rheumatic fever* is caused by scarring and shrinking of the valve leaflets and shortening and thickening of the chordae tendineae (Fig. 6-96). The murmur may be faint or loud. It usually lasts through-

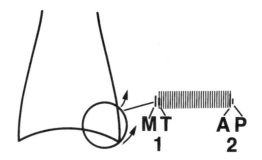

Fig. 6-96. Systolic murmur of mitral regurgitation due to rheumatic fever. Note that the mitral valve closure sound is decreased in intensity because the mitral valve leaflets are damaged and do not coapt properly, and that the murmur lasts throughout systole. This murmur may have several different configurations; the first sound may be normal or even increased in intensity if it is sufficiently scarred by the rheumatic process.

Reproduced with permission from Hurst JW: The examination of the heart: the importance of initial screening, *Dis Mon* 36(5):285, 1990.

out systole, but the louder it is, the more widely it is transmitted. It is usually transmitted laterally to the left side of the thorax.

The *systolic murmur of mitral valve regurgitation due to endocarditis* usually lasts throughout systole. A loud murmur is transmitted laterally. Endocarditis commonly involves valves that have been previously damaged or that function abnormally. Accordingly, the systolic murmur of rheumatic mitral valve damage or mitral valve prolapse may have preceded the murmur created by the damage of endocarditis. Thus the new murmur may be slightly different in configuration, duration, or loudness. It should be emphasized that endocarditis may be present and that there may be no change in a previously identified murmur.

A *left atrial myxoma* may beat against the mitral valve until it damages the leaflets, causing mitral regurgitation to develop. This "wrecking ball" effect occurs during ventricular diastole when the myxoma is forced into the mitral orifice by atrial systole and during systole when the left ventricle extrudes the tumor from the mitral orifice back into the left atrium. As discussed later, a diastolic rumble is produced by the tumor, and a "tumor plop" is sometimes heard in diastole (see Fig. 6-70). Accordingly, the murmurs may simulate the murmurs of rheumatic mitral stenosis and regurgitation.

The most common cause of mitral valve regurgitation is *mitral valve prolapse* (Fig. 6-97). This systolic murmur is usually ushered in with an ejection click and may be faint or loud. As suggested by Woodfin Cobbs,[192] the murmur may seem to increase in intensity during the last part of systole, but this may be because it increases in frequency at the end, which gives it the illusion of being louder. This occurs because the chordae tendineae and leaflets become more redundant as the left ventricle

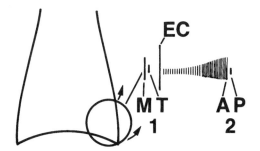

Fig. 6-97. Systolic murmur and ejection click of mitral valve prolapse. There may be multiple systolic ejection clicks, and the murmur may vary in configuration from the one illustrated here. The increase in intensity of the murmur illustrated here may be more apparent than real (see text).

Reproduced with permission from Hurst JW: The examination of the heart: the importance of initial screening, *Dis Mon* 36(5):285, 1990.

becomes smaller. The click and murmur occur earlier in systole and become louder when the patient stands. Loud murmurs are transmitted laterally. A systolic click, or a click with a faint systolic murmur, is common and is often benign. In such patients there may be no progression of the condition involving the mitral valve apparatus; the cords are somewhat slack and the leaflets are somewhat large, but the condition does not change over time. Such patients, however, may need prophylaxis against bacterial endocarditis.

Severe, progressive mitral regurgitation due to mitral valve prolapse is usually caused by myxomatous degeneration of the mitral valve leaflets and chordae tendineae. The chordae tendineae may rupture in some patients (see following discussion). Some patients with mitral valve prolapse will need mitral valve replacement. Such patients have heart failure or cardiac arrhythmias, including ventricular tachycardia and fibrillation. Unfortunately, mitral valve replacement may not eliminate the rhythm disturbance. The echocardiogram is useful in identifying mitral valve prolapse, but it is probably overused. An echocardiogram is not needed when there is only an ejection click. An echocardiogram should be obtained when there is a click and murmur, but the procedure should not be repeated unless the murmur increases in loudness.

Rupture of the chordae tendineae may be due to myxomatous degeneration, endocarditis, or trauma. Many patients with rupture of the chordae tendineae have mitral valve prolapse prior to the rupture. On rare occasions the thick, but weak and scarred, chordae tendineae that result from rheumatic fever may rupture. One of two clinical syndromes may be caused by rupture of the chordae tendineae of the mitral valve.

When a ruptured cord to the mitral valve occurs in a heart that was otherwise normal except for mild mitral valve prolapse, the patient develops abrupt, severe mitral regurgitation and pulmonary edema. The heart size remains normal and the rhythm usually remains normal in such patients. A loud left atrial gallop sound may be audible. The systolic murmur is virtually diagnostic. It is heard at the cardiac apex, and it lasts throughout systole. It is transmitted laterally and is often heard over the spine. It may radiate to the cervical spine and sacrum. It may even be heard on top of the patient's head. The murmur may radiate to the second right intercostal space or to the right or left of the midsternal area. When this occurs, the murmur may simulate the murmur of aortic valve stenosis. It was formerly believed that rupture of the cords that are attached to the anterior leaflet of the mitral valve caused the murmur to be transmitted up and down the spine and that rupture of the cords to the posterior leaflet of the mitral valve caused the murmur to radiate to the base of the heart. My experience has been that some of the cords to both leaflets are usually ruptured.

When there is considerable mitral valve regurgitation, a large heart, and atrial fibrillation prior to the rupture of the chordae tendineae of the mitral valve, there may be an increase in the already existing heart failure. The murmur of mitral regurgitation may change and assume the characteristics of the murmur described in the preceding paragraph; a ventricular gallop sound or mitral diastolic flow rumble may be heard in such patients.

Rupture of a left ventricular papillary muscle is caused by myocardial infarction due to coronary atherosclerosis or trauma. Infarction of the tip of a papillary muscle will disengage the attachment of a small number of the chordae tendineae of the mitral valve, whereas rupture of the entire belly of a papillary muscle will disengage a larger number of the chordae tendineae. Accordingly, the degree of mitral regurgitation depends on the number of disengaged chordae tendineae. There may be a moderately loud systolic murmur at the apex when the disengagement of a few chordae tendineae result in a flail mitral valve. When a large number of chordae tendineae are disengaged from the papillary muscle, a major part of the mitral valve may become flail. This does not necessarily produce a louder systolic murmur at the apex. In fact, because of hypotension and a wide-open mitral valve during ventricular systole, there may be no murmur.

Papillary muscle dysfunction may be responsible for a systolic murmur at the apex. Almost any shape of systolic murmur may develop, but the murmur is seldom very loud. In most instances it is due to infarction of the myocardium at the base of a papillary muscle; the myocardium is dyskinetic, and the papillary muscle is unable to tense the chordae tendineae as it does normally. The result is mitral regurgitation. The papillary muscle may also become damaged by infarction but may not rupture. Accordingly, the papillary muscle may be unable to contract normally, resulting in mitral regurgitation.

The diamond-shaped systolic murmur produced by *aortic valve stenosis* may be heard at the cardiac apex. It is higher pitched there than it is in the second right intercostal space or along the left sternal border. The murmur is not transmitted beyond the cardiac apex.

The murmur of *idiopathic hypertrophic subaortic stenosis* may also be heard at the apex, but it is usually louder to the right of and superior to the cardiac apex.

A loud, cooing type of systolic murmur may be heard at the cardiac apex when endocarditis destroys a portion of the mitral valve or when there is a tear in a prosthetic tissue valve.

The only high-pitched diastolic murmur heard at the cardiac apex is the transmitted murmur of aortic regurgitation. All other diastolic murmurs heard at the cardiac apex are low pitched and emanate from the mitral valve. The bell of the stethoscope, applied to the chest wall with light pressure, should be used to hear these murmurs.

Low-pitched *diastolic murmurs produced by the mitral valve* are heard at the cardiac apex, usually in a small, circumscribed area. Low-pitched diastolic murmurs are often referred to as rumbles. At times, especially when one is listening for the diastolic rumble of mitral stenosis, the cardiac apex should be listened to with the patient in the left lateral recumbent position after performing a sit-up exercise, which increases the heart rate and increases the blood flow across the restricted mitral valve opening.

Low-pitched rumbles are produced when the flow of blood passes through a smaller than normal mitral valve opening or when a larger than normal quantity of blood passes through a relatively normal mitral valve opening.

The most common cause of mitral valve stenosis is rheumatic fever (Fig. 6-98; see also Fig. 6-81). The valve leaflets and chordae tendineae become scarred, relatively rigid, and calcified some years after the episode of rheumatic fever. Other, rare causes of mitral stenosis are a left atrial tumor, congenital mitral stenosis, ergot medication, a normally functioning prosthetic tissue valve, sclerosis and calcification of a tissue valve, and malfunction and clotting of a mechanical valve.

The diastolic murmur of mitral stenosis is localized at the cardiac apex. It is easy to miss, and there are situations wherein experienced observers fail to detect its presence. For example, in patients with aortic valve stenosis, the diastolic pressure in the left ventricle may eventually become elevated, and when this occurs, the pressure gradient between the left atrium and the left ventricle during diastole decreases to the point where diastolic blood flow is slowed, and the mitral diastolic rumbling murmur of mitral stenosis may disappear. The diastolic rumble may also be difficult to hear in patients with pulmonary emphysema. The auscultatory abnormalities produced by mitral stenosis are as follows: the first heart sound is louder than normal; the second sound may be normal, but the pulmonary valve closure sound may be loud when pulmonary hypertension is present; and the opening snap of the mitral valve is usually heard. The time interval of the second sound—opening snap—is brief when there is severe mitral stenosis, because the pressure in the left atrium is

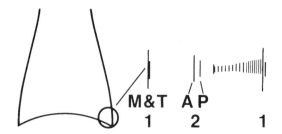

Fig. 6-98. Diastolic murmur of mitral stenosis. The first sound is loud because the mitral valve closure sound *(M)* is usually louder than normal. The opening snap occurs in early diastole. The snap is followed by a low-pitched, rumbling, murmur that becomes louder and higher pitched just before the loud first sound. The pulmonary valve closure sound *(P)* is louder than normal, signifying pulmonary artery hypertension (see text).

Reproduced with permission from Hurst JW: The examination of the heart: the importance of initial screening, *Dis Mon* 36(5):285, 1990.

higher in patients with severe obstruction of the mitral valve. Accordingly, it is useful for the listener to estimate the time interval between the opening snap of the mitral valve and the aortic valve closure sound. The diastolic rumble begins after the opening snap and persists throughout diastole. The presystolic accentuation of the rumble is produced by the enhancement of blood flow through the mitral valve as a result of atrial contraction.

The diastolic rumble produced by a left atrial tumor is similar to that of rheumatic mitral valve stenosis, and the "tumor plop" simulates the opening snap of mitral stenosis (see Fig. 6-70). The first heart sound is not louder than normal, however, because the mitral valve leaflets are either normal or damaged by the wrecking ball effect of the left atrial tumor.

A middiastolic mitral rumble may be heard in patients who have a prosthetic tissue valve in the mitral position. Even the normally functioning prosthetic tissue valve may produce a diastolic rumble, because the pressure gradient across the mitral valve during diastole is sufficient to produce the murmur. The opening snap is not heard and the first sound is not louder than normal unless the leaflets of the prosthetic tissue valve have become scarred and partially calcified. A clot may form on a mechanical valve and prevent proper opening during diastole, resulting in a diastolic rumble.

A diastolic rumble may be heard rarely at the cardiac apex in patients with *hypertrophic cardiomyopathy*. The murmur is due to the obstruction to blood flow presented by the large papillary muscles and a small left ventricular cavity.

The *Austin Flint rumble* is heard at the cardiac apex. It is similar to the murmur of mitral valve stenosis, although the opening snap of mitral stenosis and a louder than normal first heart sound do not occur. The murmur is produced because the aortic valve regurgitation forces the anterior leaflet of the mitral valve toward a closed position, thus impeding the inflow of blood from the left atrium into the left ventricle during diastole. It is, in fact, a type of obstruction to blood flow. In addition, the blood entering the left ventricle from the left atrium collides with the volume of blood regurgitated from the aorta into the left ventricle during diastole. These two mechanisms conspire to produce a diastolic rumble. Obviously, the presence of an Austin Flint rumble indicates a moderate degree of aortic regurgitation.

A mitral diastolic rumble can be produced when a larger than normal quantity of blood passes through a relatively normal mitral valve opening. This occurs secondary to mitral valve regurgitation from any cause, because the volume of blood that must pass through the mitral orifice is composed of the normal amount of blood that enters the left atrium from the pulmonary veins plus the amount of blood that is regurgitated into the left atrium during ventricular systole. An opening snap of the mitral valve may be heard, because the large volume of blood rushes against abnormally thick mitral valve leaflets. The first heart sound is not unusually loud; the damaged leaflets cannot coapt normally.

Other causes of a mitral diastolic rumble due to a larger than normal quantity of blood passing through a normal mitral valve opening are an interventricular septal defect and a patent ductus arteriosus. The increase in pulmonary blood flow in both conditions enters the pulmonary veins and left atrium. The intensity of the diastolic rumble is roughly proportional to the amount of left-to-right shunt. A mitral diastolic rumble may be heard in patients with severe anemia because of the increase in velocity of blood flow. Such a murmur is especially likely to occur when there is sickle cell anemia, in which case there is likely to be cardiac dilatation.

A *tricuspid valve diastolic rumble* due to the larger than normal blood flow across the tricuspid valve occurs in patients with secundum atrial septal defects. This murmur is usually heard at the end of the sternum but may also be heard at the cardiac apex; the right ventricular dilatation associated with this condition rotates the heart clockwise (as viewed in the transverse plane) in the chest, so that the rumble may be heard in the region of the cardiac apex. An opening snap of the tricuspid valve may be heard, and the first sound may be loud because of the onrush of a large volume of blood during diastole and an increase in force of right ventricular systolic contraction, respectively.

Continuous murmurs. A continuous murmur is said to be present when a murmur occupies systole and diastole. The murmur does not always occupy *all* of systole and diastole, but the unique feature of a continuous murmur is that it continues from systole into diastole without interruption. Actually, the murmur builds up in intensity in systole; encompasses and almost masks the second heart sound; and continues into, but decreases in intensity, in diastole.

A *venous hum* is heard in the neck of all normal children at some time in their life. The normal venous hum is heard in the child's neck when the child is sitting up

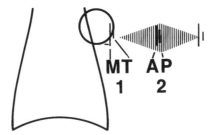

Fig. 6-99. Continuous murmur of patent ductus arteriosus. Note that the murmur builds up in intensity at the end of ventricular systole, envelops the second heart sound, and then continues into ventricular diastole. It is almost always louder in the second left intercostal space near the sternum.

Reproduced with permission from Hurst JW: The examination of the heart: the importance of initial screening, *Dis Mon* 36(5):286, 1990.

but is not heard when the child is lying down. Light pressure on the neck will eliminate the murmur, and turning the neck to the side may alter the pitch of the murmur. A venous hum may be heard in adults with a rapid circulation due to thyrotoxicosis or severe anemia.

The most common cause of a continuous murmur is a *patent ductus arteriosus* (Fig. 6-99). It is heard best when the diaphragm is placed in the second left intercostal space adjacent to the sternum. Shortly after birth the murmur may not be continuous, because the pulmonary artery pressure is elevated. Later the murmur may not be continuous in patients who develop Eisenmenger physiology (pulmonary hypertension). The pulmonary valve closure sound is louder than normal in patients with pulmonary artery hypertension. A diastolic rumble may be heard at the cardiac apex when the left-to-right shunt through the ductus is large, and pulmonary valve regurgitation may be heard in patients with pulmonary artery hypertension.

An *aortic septal defect* may produce a continuous murmur that is located in the second right intercostal space adjacent to the sternum. The murmur may, however, be located in the same area as the murmur produced by a patent ductus arteriosus.

When a continuous murmur is heard in a region of the precordium other than the second left intercostal space (where a patent ductus arteriosus is heard), a condition other than patent ductus arteriosus is the cause; a *congenital coronary arteriovenous fistula* or a *ruptured sinus of Valsalva* is highly likely (Fig. 6-100). When the murmur appears suddenly for the first time, it is obviously a rupture of a sinus of Valsalva into the right atrium or right ventricle. In such a patient, if the deep jugular veins exhibit a large positive wave, it indicates that the rupture is into the right atrium.

Exploring with the stethoscope. The clinician should place the head of the stethoscope over the length of the carotid arteries in search for bruits that would indicate a narrow segment of the artery due to atherosclerosis or fibromuscular hy-

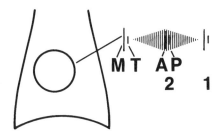

Fig. 6-100. Continuous murmur produced by the rupture of a sinus of Valsalva. Note that the murmur builds up in intensity and envelops the second heart sound.

Reproduced with permission from Hurst JW: The examination of the heart: the importance of initial screening, *Dis Mon* 36(5):286, 1990.

perplasia. The head of the stethoscope should also be placed over the right and left lateral aspects of the abdomen in search of renal artery bruits due to atherosclerotic lesions of fibromuscular hyperplasia of the renal arteries. The clinician should listen over every scar for the continuous murmur of an arteriovenous fistula. In fact, it is wise to listen for a continuous murmur over every artery that has ever been used for cardiac catheterization even if the scar is barely visible.

Systolic bruits may be heard over the ribs of the posterior portion of the thorax in patients with coarctation of the aorta. These bruits are due to the large and tortuous intercostal arteries. The systolic murmur of the coarctated segment itself can be heard in the interscapular area. The systolic murmur associated with ruptured chordae tendineae may be heard up and down the spine, over the sacrum, and on the top of the head (see earlier discussion). Systolic murmurs may be heard over the back in patients with secundum atrial septal defects. The murmurs are due to the enormous amount of blood flow in the pulmonary arteries. Continuous murmurs may be heard over the back in patients with coarctation of the pulmonary arteries. The systolic murmur of mitral regurgitation may be heard in the left lung base posteriorly, and the systolic murmur of an interventricular septal defect is often heard over the spine in the middle of the back. The continuous murmur of a cerebral arteriovenous malformation may be heard in the head.

Key Points

- The physical examination begins when the physician first sees the patient, hears the patient talk, watches the patient walk, and feels the patient's hand as they greet each other with a handshake.
- The physician collects data during the history by organizing the task according to body systems. The physician collects data by performing the physical examination by examining the patient according to an anatomic arrangement. That is, the physician examines the patient from the "head to the feet." When the physical examination is complete, however, I recommend that the physician arrange the data that he or she has collected along the lines of body systems. In this way the data collected during the history and the data collected by physical examination can be clustered together. All the data that relate to the cardiovascular system, including the information gleaned from the history, physical examination, electrocardiogram, chest x-ray film, and routine laboratory tests, can then be viewed as a unit. The same applies to the gastrointestinal system, the neurologic system, etc. When this is done, the process of correlation becomes easier and the physician is less likely to forget to include even the smallest diagnostic clue in his or her thinking process.
- The cardiovascular data that must be collected on every patient must be defined

before the patient is examined. The abnormalities must be sought on every patient who is examined. The cardiovascular data that must be collected by the physical examination are described in this chapter.

- The physical findings collected from the cardiovascular system should be recorded in the patient's medical record. Diagrams are very useful for this purpose. Crude diagrams similar to those used in this chapter should be created on each patient. Accordingly, it is useful to diagram the contour of the carotid pulsation, the pulsation of the deep jugular pulse, the precordial movements, and the heart sounds and murmurs. This approach generates considerable self-discipline; when a diagram cannot be drawn, the physician should return to examine the patient again and, following his or her reexamination, try again to diagram the cardiovascular movements and sounds.

- Many cardiovascular physical findings are diagnostic of specific disease processes. For example, the classic rumble of mitral stenosis is rarely simulated by other conditions, such as a left atrial tumor. The presence of systemic hypertension is identified by recording the blood pressure in the arms. When the arterial pressure is lower in the legs than in the arms in young patients, the physician diagnoses coarctation of the aorta. And so it goes. The physical examination provides many clues for detecting the presence of cardiovascular disease. One must never forget, however, that the most common cardiac disease—atherosclerosis of the coronary arteries—is usually associated with a normal physical examination.

REFERENCES

1. White PD: *Heart disease*, New York, 1931, Macmillan, p 38.
2. Jervell A, Lange-Nielsen F: Congenital deaf-mutism, functional heart disease with prolongation of the QT interval, and sudden death, *Am Heart J* 54(1):59, 1957.
3. Nugent EW, Plauth WH Jr, Edwards JE, Williams WH: The pathology, abnormal physiology, clinical recognition, and medical and surgical treatment of congenital heart disease. In Hurst JW, editor-in-chief: *The heart*, ed 7, New York, 1990, McGraw-Hill, pp 660-661.
4. Roberts WC, Honig H: The spectrum of cardiovascular disease in the Marfan syndrome: a clinicomorphologic study of 18 necropsy patients and comparison to 151 previously reported necropsy patients, *Am Heart J* 104:115, 1982.
5. Alexander JK: The heart and obesity. In Hurst JW, editor-in-chief: *The heart*, ed 7, New York, 1990, McGraw-Hill, pp 1538-1543.
6. Houpt JL: Anorexia nervosa. In Hurst JW, editor-in-chief: *Medicine for the practicing physician*, ed 2, Boston, 1989, Butterworth, p 50.
7. Rimland D: Infective endocarditis. In Hurst JW, editor-in-chief: *Medicine for the practicing physician*, ed 3, Boston, 1992, Butterworth, p 299.
8. Clements SD, Hurst JW: Diagnostic value of electrocardiographic abnormalities observed in subjects accidentally exposed to cold, *Am J Cardiol* 29:729, 1972.
9. Pinnell S, Murad S: Disorders of collagen. In Stanbury JB, Wyngaarden J, Fredrickson D, Goldstein J, Brown M, editors: *The metabolic basis of inherited diseases*, ed 5, New York, 1983, McGraw-Hill, p 1425.
10. Turner JS: Fluctuant hearing loss. In Hurst JW, editor-in-chief: *Medicine for the practicing physician*, ed 3, Boston, 1992, Butterworth, p 1726.
11. Nagant de Deuxchaisnes C, Krane S: Paget's disease of bone: clinical and metabolic observations, *Medicine* 43:233, 1964.
12. Paget J: On a form of chronic inflammation of bones (osteitis deformans), *Trans Med-Chir Soc Lond* 60:37, 1877.

13. Elliot WJ: Ear lobe crease and coronary artery disease, *Am J Med* 75:1024, 1983.
14. Loomis EA, Hardy LB, Ford EJ: Mental retardation. In Hurst JW, editor-in-chief: *Medicine for the practicing physician,* ed 3, Boston, 1992, Butterworth, p 54.
15. Parker F: Hyperlipoproteinemia and xanthomatosis. In Callen JP, editor: *Cutaneous aspects of internal disease,* St Louis, 1981, Mosby, p 473.
16. Nugent EW, Plauth WH Jr, Edwards JE, Williams WH: The pathology, abnormal physiology, clinical recognition, and medical and surgical treatment of congenital heart disease. In Hurst JW, editor-in-chief: *The heart,* ed 7, New York, 1990, McGraw-Hill, p 713.
17. Coles WH: Senile cataract. In Hurst JW, editor-in-chief: *Medicine for the practicing physician,* ed 3, Boston, 1992, Butterworth, p 1790.
18. Stone JH: Ectopia lentis, cardiology, and "the sign of the tremulous iris," *Am Heart J* 72(4):466, 1966.
19. Wright AD, Hill DM, Lowy C et al: Mortality in acromegaly, *Q J Med* 39:1, 1970.
20. Roberts WC, Waller BF: Cardiac amyloidosis causing cardiac dysfunction: analysis of 54 necropsy patients, *Am J Cardiol* 52:137, 1983.
21. Silverman ME, Hurst JW: Inspection of the patient. In Hurst JW, editor-in-chief: *The heart,* ed 5, New York, 1982, McGraw-Hill, p 175.
22. Christianson HB: Cutaneous manifestations of hypothyroidism, including purpura and ecchymosis, *Cutis* 17:45, 1976.
23. Scoggins RB, Hardan WR Jr: Cutaneous manifestations of hyperlipidemia and uremia, *Postgrad Med* 41:537, 1967.
24. Personal observation.
25. McLaren GD, Muir QA, Kellermeyer RW: Iron overload disorders: natural history, pathogenesis, diagnosis, and therapy, *Crit Rev Clin Lab Sci* 19:205, 1984.
26. Rietschel RL: Nail change. In Hurst JW, editor-in-chief: *Medicine for the practicing physician,* ed 3, Boston, 1992, Butterworth, p 761.
27. Arsura E, Lichstein E, Guadagnino V et al: Methemoglobin levels produced by organic nitrates in patients with coronary artery disease, *J Clin Pharmacol* 24:160, 1984.
28. Akiyama T: Atrioventricular (AV) block (first-degree heart block). In Hurst JW, editor-in-chief: *Medicine for the practicing physician,* ed 3, Boston, 1992, Butterworth, p 1075.
29. Fulk CS: Primary disorders of hyperpigmentation, *J Am Acad Dermatol* 10:1, 1984.
30. Hurst JW, Whitworth HB, O'Donoghue S et al: Heart disease due to ovarian carcinoid: successful replacement of the pulmonary and tricuspid valves with porcine heterografts and removal of the tumor. In Hurst JW, editor: *Clinical essays on the heart,* vol 5, New York, 1985, McGraw-Hill, p 177.
31. Berlin W: Diagnosis and classification of the polycythemias, *Semin Hematol* 12:339, 1975.
32. Porter JM, Rivers SP, Anderson CJ, Baur GM: Evaluation and management of patients with Raynaud's syndrome, *Am J Surg* 142:183, 1981.
33. Gossling HR, Pellegrini VD Jr: Fat embolism syndrome: a review of the pathophysiology and physiological basis of treatment, *Clin Orthop* 165:68, 1982.
34. Kyle RA, Greipp PR: Amyloidosis (AL): clinical and laboratory features in 229 cases, *Mayo Clin Proc* 58:665, 1983.
35. Goltz RW: Systematized amyloidosis: a review of the skin and mucous membrane lesions and a report of two cases, *Medicine* 31:381, 1952.
36. Hall WD, Wollam GL, Tuttle EP: Diagnostic evaluation of the patient with hypertension. In Hurst JW, editor-in-chief: *The heart,* ed 7, New York, 1990, McGraw-Hill, p 1165.
37. Stollerman GH, Markowitz M, Taranta A, Wannamaker LW: Jones criteria (revised) for guidance in the diagnosis of rheumatic fever, *Circulation* 32:664, 1965.
38. Luria MN, Asper SP Jr: Onycholysis in hyperthyroidism, *Ann Intern Med* 49:102, 1958.
39. Woeber KA: Thyrotoxicosis and the heart, *N Engl J Med* 327(2):94, 1992.
40. Braverman IM: *Skin signs of systemic disease,* ed 2, Philadelphia, 1981, WB Saunders, p 633.
41. DeGroot LJ, Larson PR, Refetoff S et al: Adult hypothyroidism. In *Thyroid and its disease,* ed 5, New York, 1984, John Wiley & Sons, p 546.
42. Vanhaelst L, Neve P, Chally P, Bastenie PA: Coronary artery disease in hypothyroidism, *Lancet* 2:800, 1967.
43. Blum A, Aviram A: Splinter hemorrhages in patients receiving regular hemodialysis, *JAMA* 239:47, 1978.
44. Hudson JB, Dennis AJ: Transverse white lines in the fingernails after acute and chronic renal failure, *Arch Intern Med* 117:276, 1966.
45. Lindsay PG: The half-and-half nail, *Arch Intern Med* 71:129, 1969.
46. Silverberg S, Oreopoulos DG, Wise DJ et al: Pericarditis in patients undergoing long term hemodialysis and peritoneal dialysis, *Am J Med* 63:874, 1977.
47. Rosen H, Freedman SA, Raizner AE, Geistmann K: Azotemic arteriopathy, *Am Heart J* 84:250, 1972.

48. Schever J, Stezoski SW: The effects of uremic components on cardiac function and metabolism, *J Mol Cell Cardiol* 5:287, 1973.
49. Braverman IM: *Skin signs of systemic disease*, ed 2, Philadelphia, 1981, WB Saunders, p 256.
50. Klacsmann PG, Bulkley BH, Hutchins GM: The changed spectrum of pericarditis: an 86 year autopsy experience in 200 patients, *Am J Med* 63:666, 1977.
51. Libman E, Sacks B: A hitherto undescribed form of valvular and mural endocarditis, *Arch Intern Med* 33:701, 1924.
52. Morris DC, Hurst JW, Logue RB: Myocardial infarction in young women, *Am J Cardiol* 38:299, 1976.
53. Braverman IM: *Skin signs of systemic disease*, ed 2, Philadelphia, 1981, WB Saunders, p 315.
54. Sabini R, Rodnan GP, Leon DF, Shaver JA: Pulmonary hypertension in the CREST syndrome variant of PSS (scleroderma), *Ann Intern Med* 86:394, 1977.
55. Bulkey BH, Ridolfi RL, Salyer WR, Hutchins GM: Myocardial lesions of PSS, *Circulation* 53:483, 1976.
56. Braverman IM: Dermatomyositis and polymyositis. In Demis DJ, editor: *Clinical dermatology*, vol 1, ed 11, sect 5-4, Philadelphia, 1984, Harper & Row, p 1.
57. Muller SA, Winkelmann RK, Brunsting LA: Calcinosis in dermatomyositis, *Arch Dermatol* 79:669, 1959.
58. Rook A, Wilkinson DS, Ebling FJG: *Textbook of dermatology*, ed 3, London, 1979, Blackwell Scientific Publications, p 1236.
59. Reid MM, Murdoch R: Polymyositis and complete heart block, *Br Heart J* 41:628, 1979.
60. Braverman IM: *Skin signs of systemic disease*, ed 2, Philadelphia, 1981, WB Saunders, p 359.
61. Calabro JJ, Marchesano JM: Rash associated with juvenile rheumatoid arthritis, *J Pediatr* 72:611, 1968.
62. Rodnan GP, Schumacher HR, Zvaifler NJ, editors: Rheumatoid arthritis. In *Primer on the rheumatic diseases*, ed 8, Atlanta, 1983, Arthritis Foundation, p 38.
63. Short CL, Bauer W, Reynolds WE: *Rheumatic arthritis*, Cambridge, Mass, 1957, Harvard University Press.
64. Thadini V, Iveson JMI, Wright V: Cardiac tamponade, constrictive pericarditis and pericardial resection in rheumatoid arthritis, *Medicine* 54:261, 1975.
65. Roberts WC, Dangel JC, Bulkley GH: Nonrheumatic valvular cardiac disease: a clinicopathologic survey of 27 different conditions causing valvular dysfunction, *Cardiovasc Clin* 5:333, 1973.
66. Lev M, Bharati S, Hoffman F, Leight L: The conduction system in rheumatoid arthritis with complete atrioventricular block, *Am Heart J* 90:78, 1975.
67. Swezey RL: Myocardial infarction due to rheumatoid arthritis, *JAMA* 199:191, 1967.
68. Cohen RD, Conn DL, Distrup DM: Clinical features, prognosis and response to treatment in polyarteritis, *Mayo Clin Proc* 55:146, 1980.
69. Fujiwara H, Hamashima Y: Pathology of the heart in Kawasaki disease, *Pediatrics* 61:1, 1978.
70. Fukushige J, Nihill MR, McNamara DG: Spectrum of cardiovascular lesions in mucocutaneous lymph node syndrome: analysis of eight cases, *Am J Cardiol* 45:98, 1980.
71. Fujiwara H, Chen CH, Fujiwara T et al: Clinicopathologic study of abnormal Q waves in Kawasaki disease, *Am J Cardiol* 45:797, 1980.
72. Hiraishi S, Yashiro K, Oguchi K et al: Clinical course of cardiovascular involvement in the mucocutaneous lymph node syndrome, *Am J Cardiol* 47:323, 1981.
73. Braverman IM: *Skin signs of systemic disease*, ed 2, Philadelphia, 1981, WB Saunders, p 532.
74. Dines DE, Arms RA, Bernatz PE, Gomes MG: Pulmonary arteriovenous fistulas, *Mayo Clin Proc* 49:460, 1974.
75. Scollay DA, Sibrack LA: Systemic manifestations of exfoliative dermatitis. In Callen JP, editor: *Aspects of internal medicine*, St Louis, 1981, Mosby, p 635.
76. Voigt GC, Kronthal HL, Crounse RG: Cardiac output in erythrodermic skin disease, *Am Heart J* 72:615, 1966.
77. France R, Buchanan RN, Wilson MW et al: Relapsing iritis with recurrent ulcers of the mouth and genitalia (Behçet's syndrome), *Medicine* 30:335, 1951.
78. Tuzun Y, Yzaici H, Parzarh B et al: The usefulness of nonspecific skin hyperreactivity (the pathergy test) in Behçet's disease in Turkey, *Acta Derm Venereol* 59:77, 1978.
79. Kansu E, Ozer FL, Akalin E et al: Behçet's syndrome with obstruction of the vena cava, *Q J Med* 41:151, 1972.
80. Little AG, Zarino CK: Abdominal aortic aneurysm and Behçet's disease, *Surgery* 91:359, 1982.
81. Hancock J: Surface manifestations of Reiter's disease in the male, *Br J Vener Dis* 36:36, 1960.
82. Paulus HE, Pearson CM, Pitts W Jr: Aortic insufficiency in five patients with Reiter's syndrome: a detailed clinical-pathologic study, *Am J Med* 53:464, 1972.
83. Gumport SL, Harris MN, Kopf A: Diagnosis and management of common skin cancers, *Cancer* 24:218, 1974.
84. Glancy DL, Roberts WC: The heart in malignant melanoma: a study of 70 autopsy cases, *Am J Cardiol* 21:555, 1968.
85. Chears WC, Hargrove MD, Verner JV et al: Whipple's disease, *Am J Med* 30:226, 1961.
86. McAllister HA Jr, Fenoglio JJ: Cardiac involvement in Whipple's disease, *Circulation* 52:152, 1975.
87. Braverman IM: *Skin signs of systemic disease*, ed 2, Philadelphia, 1981, WB Saunders, p 193.

88. Yeager SB, Freed MD: Myocardial infarction as a manifestation of polycythemia in cyanotic heart disease, *Am J Cardiol* 53:953, 1984.

89. Olson LJ, Reeder GS, Noller KL et al: Cardiac involvement in glycogen storage disease III: morphologic and biochemical characterization with endo-myocardial biopsy, *Am J Cardiol* 53:980, 1984.

90. Goldfinger SE: Cutaneous changes in errors of amino acid metabolism: alcaptonuria. In Fitzpatrick TB, Eisen AZ, Wolff K et al, editors: *Dermatology in general medicine*, New York, 1979, McGraw-Hill, p 1048.

91. Gould L, Reddy CVR, DePalma D et al: Cardiac manifestations of ochronosis, *J Thorac Cardiovasc Surg* 72:708, 1976.

92. VonGemminger G, Kierland RR, Optiz JM: Angiokeratoma corporis diffusum (Fabry's disease), *Arch Dermatol* 91:206, 1965.

93. Ferrans VJ, Hibbs RG, Burda CD: The heart and Fabry's disease: a histologic and electron microscopic study, *Am J Cardiol* 24:95, 1969.

94. Hurwitz S, Braverman IM: White spots in tuberous sclerosis, *J Pediatr* 77:587, 1970.

95. Fenoglio JJ, Jr, McAllister HA, Ferrans VJ: Cardiac rhabdomyomas: a clinicopathologic and electron microscopic study, *Am J Cardiol* 38:241, 1976.

96. Braverman IM: *Skin signs of systemic disease*, ed 2, Philadelphia, 1981, WB Saunders, p 715.

97. McFarland W, Fuller D: Mortality in Ehlers-Danlos syndrome due to spontaneous rupture of large arteries, *N Engl J Med* 271:1309, 1964.

98. Cupo LN, Pyerrty RE, Olson JL et al: Ehlers-Danlos syndrome with abnormal collagen fibrils, sinus of Valsalva aneurysm, myocardial infarction, panacinar emphysema, and cerebral heterotopias, *Am J Med* 71:1051, 1981.

99. Gorlin RJ, Anderson RD, Blow M: Multiple lentigines syndrome, *Am J Dis Child* 117:652, 1969.

100. Voron DA, Hatfield HH, Kalkhoff RK: Multiple lentigines syndrome: case report and review of the literature, *Am J Med* 60:447, 1976.

101. Polani PE, Moynahan EJ: Progressive cardiomyopathic letiginosis, *Q J Med* 41:205, 1972.

102. Bothwell TH, Charlton RW, Motulsky AG: Idiopathic hemochromatosis. In Stanbury JB, Wyngaarden JB, Fredrickson DS et al, editors: *The metabolic basis of inherited disease*, ed 5, New York, 1983, McGraw-Hill, p 1269.

103. Chevrant-Breton J, Simon M, Bourel M, Ferrand B: Cutaneous manifestations of idiopathic hemochromatosis, *Arch Dermatol* 113:161, 1977.

104. Cutler DJ, Isner JM, Bracey AW et al: Hemochromatosis heart disease: an unemphasized cause of potentially reversible restrictive cardiomyopathy, *Am J Med* 69:923, 1980.

105. Roberts WC, Liegler DC, Carbone PP: Endomyocardial disease and eosinophilia: a clinical and pathologic spectrum, *Am J Med* 46:28, 1968.

106. Kazmierowski JA, Chusid MJ, Parrillo JE et al: Dermatologic manifestations of the hypereosinophilic syndrome, *Arch Dermatol* 114:531, 1978.

107. Pincus SH, Wolff SM: Dermatologic diseases associated with eosinophilia. In Fitzpatrick TB, Eisen AZ, Wolff K et al, editors: *Update: dermatology in general medicine*, New York, 1983, McGraw-Hill, p 14.

108. Parrillo JE, Boer JS, Henry WL et al: The cardiovascular manifestations of the hypereosinophilia syndrome, *Am J Med* 67:572, 1979.

109. Kampmeier RH: Manifestations of late syphilis, *South Med Bull* 53:17, 1965.

110. Alpert JS, Krons HF, Dalen JE et al: Pathogenesis of Osler's nodes, *Ann Intern Med* 85:471, 1976.

111. Kilpatrick ZM, Greenberg PA, Sanford JP: Splinter hemorrhages: their clinical significance, *Arch Intern Med* 115:730, 1965.

112. Steere AC, Broderick TF, Malavista SE: Erythema chronicum migrans and Lyme arthritis: epidemiologic evidence for a tick vector, *Am J Epidemiol* 108:312, 1978.

113. Steere AC, Batsford WP, Weinberg M et al: Lyme carditis: cardiac abnormalities of Lyme disease, *Ann Intern Med* 93:8, 1980.

114. Spira TJ: Human immunodeficiency virus infection and the acquired immunodeficiency syndrome. In Hurst JW, editor-in-chief: *Medicine for the practicing physician*, ed 3, Boston, 1992, Butterworth, p 474.

115. Friedman-Kien AE, Laubenstein LJ, Rubinstein P et al: Disseminated Kaposi's sarcoma in homosexual men, *Ann Intern Med* 96(6):693, 1982.

116. Silver MS, Macher AM, Reichert CM et al: Cardiac involvement by Kaposi's sarcoma in acquired immune deficiency syndrome (AIDS), *Am J Cardiol* 53:983, 1984.

117. Muller SA, Winkelmann RK: Necrobiosis lipoidica diabeticorum: a clinical and pathologic investigation of 171 cases, *Arch Dermatol* 93:272, 1966.

118. Melin H: An atrophic circumscribed skin lesion in the lower extremities of diabetics, *Acta Med Scand* Suppl 423:1, 1964.

119. Dobozy A, Husa S, Schneider I, Szabo E: Bullous dermatosis associated with latent diabetes: a case report, *Dermatologica* 144:283, 1972.

120. Lerner AB: Vitiligo, *J Invest Dermatol* 32:285, 1950.

121. Scott PJ, Winterbourn CC: Low density lipoproteins accumulate inactively growing xanthomas, *J Atheroscler Res* 7:207, 1967.
122. Parker F: Xanthomas. In Demis DJ, McGuire J, editors: *Clinical dermatology*, ed 11, vol 2, unit 12-1, Philadelphia, 1984, Harper & Row, p 1.
123. Parker F: Hyperlipoproteinemia and xanthomatosis. In Callen JP, editor: *Cutaneous aspects of internal disease*, St Louis, 1981, Mosby, p 473.
124. Fishman A, Turino G, Bergofsky E: Disorders of the respiration and circulation in subjects with deformities of the thorax, *Mod Concepts Cardiovasc Dis* 27:449, 1958.
125. Rawlings M: The "straight back" syndrome: a new cause of pseudoheart disease, *Am J Cardiol* 5:333, 1960.
126. deLeon A, Perloff J, Twigg H, Majd M: The straight back syndrome: clinical cardiovascular manifestations, *Circulation* 32:193, 1965.
127. Matsuo S, Yoshioka M, Yano K, Hashiba K: Straight back syndrome: clinical and hemodynamic study of 9 cases, *Am Heart J* 86:828, 1973.
128. Wachtel F, Ravitch M, Grishman A: The relation of pectus excavatum to heart disease, *Am Heart J* 52:121, 1956.
129. Reusch C: Hemodynamic studies in pectus excavatum, *Circulation* 24:1143, 1961.
130. Lyons H, Zuhdi M, Kelly J: Pectus excavatum (funnel breast), a cause of impaired ventricular distensibility as exhibited by right ventricular pressure pattern, *Am Heart J* 50:921, 1955.
131. Tietze A: Ueber eine eigenartige Haufung van fallen mit dystrophie der rippenknorpel, *Klin Wochenschr* 58:829, 1921.
132. Kayser H: Tietze's syndrome: a review of the literature, *Am J Med* 21:982, 1956.
133. Mondor H: Tronculite sous-cutanee subaigue de la paroi thoracique antero-laterale, *Mem Acad Chir* 65:1271, 1939.
134. Machleder HI: Thoracic outlet disorders. In Wilson SE, Veith FJ, Hobson RW et al, editors: *Vascular surgery principles and practice*, New York, 1987, McGraw-Hill, p 687.
135. DeLeon AC Jr, Ronan JA Jr: Thoracic bony abnormalities with the click and late apical systolic murmur syndrome, *Circulation* 43(suppl 2):157, 1971 (abstract).
136. Bon Tempo CP, Ronan JA Jr, DeLeon AC Jr, Twigg HL: Radiographic appearance of the thorax in systolic click–late systolic murmur syndrome, *Am J Cardiol* 36:27, 1975.
137. Salomon J, Shah PM, Heinle RA: Thoracic skeletal abnormalities in idiopathic mitral valve prolapse, *Am J Cardiol* 36:32, 1975.
138. Krane S: Paget's disease of bone. In Petersdorf R, Adams R, Braunwald E et al, editors: *Harrison's principles of internal medicine*, ed 10, New York, 1983, McGraw-Hill, p 1960.
139. Holling HE: Paget's disease: cardiovascular aspects, *Heart Bull* 13:68, 1964.
140. Albright F, Butler A, Hampton A, Smith P: Syndrome characterized by osteitis fibrosa disseminating areas of pigmentation and endocrine dysfunction with precocious puberty in females, *N Engl J Med* 216:727, 1937.
141. Heppner R, Babitt H, Bianchine J, Warbasse JR: Aortic regurgitation and aneurysm of sinus of Valsalva associated with osteogenesis imperfecta, *Am J Cardiol* 31:654, 1973.
142. Pinnell S, Murad S: Disorders of collagen. In Stanbury JB, Wyngaarden J, Fredrickson D et al, editors: *The metabolic basis of inherited diseases*, ed 5, New York, 1983, McGraw-Hill, p 1425.
143. Criscitiello M, Ronan J, Besterman E, Schoenwetter W: Cardiovascular abnormalities in osteogenesis imperfecta, *Circulation* 31:255, 1965.
144. Fialkow P: Disorders of connective tissue. In Petersdorf R, Adams R, Braunwald E et al, editors: *Harrison's principles of internal medicine*, ed 10, New York, 1983, McGraw-Hill, p 574.
145. Leier C, Call T, Fulkerson P, Wooley C: The spectrum of cardiac defects in the Ehlers-Danlos syndrome, types I and III, *Ann Intern Med* 92(part I):171, 1980.
146. Come P, Fortuin N, White R, McKusick V: Echocardiographic assessment of cardiovascular abnormalities in the Marfan syndrome: comparison with clinical findings and with roentgenographic estimation of aortic root size, *Am J Med* 74:465, 1983.
147. Hirst A, Gore I: Marfan's syndrome: a review, *Prog Cardiovasc Dis* 16:187, 1973.
148. Roberts WC, Honig H: The spectrum of cardiovascular disease in the Marfan syndrome: a clinicomorphologic study of 18 necropsy patients and comparison to 151 previously reported necropsy patients, *Am Heart J* 104:115, 1982.
149. Renteria V, Ferrans V, Roberts WC: The heart in the Hurler syndrome: gross, histologic and ultrastructural observations in five necropsy cases, *Am J Cardiol* 38:487, 1976.
150. Brosius F, Roberts WC: Coronary artery disease in the Hurler syndrome: qualitative and quantitative analysis of the extent of coronary narrowing at necropsy in six children, *Am J Cardiol* 47:649, 1981.
151. Hardison J, Rogers CM: Cardiovascular manifestations of sickle-cell anemia. In Hurst JW, editor: *Update I: the heart*, New York, 1979, McGraw-Hill, p 185.

152. Maxwell G: Chest deformity in children with congenital heart disease, *Am Heart J* 54:368, 1957.
153. Holt M, Oram S: Familial heart disease with skeletal malformations, *Br Heart J* 22:236, 1960.
154. Silverman M, Copeland A, Hurst JW: The Holt-Oram syndrome: the long and the short of it, *Am J Cardiol* 25:11, 1970.
155. Harris L, Osborne W: Congenital absence or hypoplasia of the radius with ventricular septal defect: ventriculo-radial dysplasia, *J Pediatr* 68:265, 1966.
156. Osler W: *Lectures on angina pectoris and allied states,* New York, 1897, Appleton, p 50.
157. Howard T: Cardiac pain and periarthritis of the shoulder, *Med J Rec* 131:364, 1930.
158. Askey J: The syndrome of painful disability of the shoulder and hand complicating coronary occlusion, *Am Heart J* 22:1, 1941.
159. Steinbrocker O, Spitzer N, Friedman HH: The shoulder hand syndrome in reflex dystrophy of the upper extremity, *Ann Intern Med* 29:22, 1948.
160. Hejtmancik MR, Bradfield JY Jr, Herrmann GR: Acromegaly and the heart: a clinical and pathologic study, *Ann Intern Med* 34:1445, 1951.
161. Hurst JW: Some disconnected odds and ends of cardiology, *Trans Am Clin Climatol Assoc* 72:159, 1960.
162. Lutz JF, Schlant RC: Coarctation of the aorta. In Hurst JW, editor-in-chief: *Medicine for the practicing physician,* ed 3, Boston, 1992, Butterworth, p 1106.
163. Frank MJ, Casanegra T, Levinson GE: Evaluation of aortic insufficiency, *Circulation* 28:723, 1963.
164. Fowler NO: Pericardial disease, *Heart Dis Stroke* 1(2):85, 1992.
165. McNamara DG: Is prevention of all cardiovascular birth defects a feasible goal? *Heart Dis Stroke* 1(4):176, 1992.
166. Allen EV: Thromboangiitis obliterans, *Am J Med Sci* 178:237, 1929.
167. Lechat P, Mass JL, Lascault G et al: Prevalence of patent foramen ovale in patients with stroke, *N Engl J Med* 318(18):1148, 1988.
168. Peters MN, Hall RJ, Cooley DA et al: The clinical syndrome of atrial myxoma, *JAMA* 230:694, 1974.
169. Hollier LH, Kazmier FJ, Ochsner J et al: "Shaggy" aorta syndrome with atheromatous embolization to visceral vessels, *Ann Vasc Surg* 5(5):439, 1911.
170. Lindsay J Jr: Aortic dissection, *Heart Dis Stroke* 1(2):69, 1992.
171. Gleason WL, Braunwald E: Studies on Starling's law of the heart. VI. Relationships between left ventricular end-diastolic volume and stroke volume in man with observations on the mechanics of pulsus alternans, *Circulation* 25:841, 1962.
172. Personal observation.
173. Braunwald E, Lambrew CT, Rockoff SD et al: Idiopathic hypertrophic subaortic stenosis, *Circulation* 30(suppl 4):1, 1964.
174. Wood P: Aortic stenosis, *Am J Cardiol* 1:553, 1958.
175. Wigle ED: The arterial pressure pulse in muscular subaortic stenosis, *Br Heart J* 25:97, 1963.
176. Hurst JW, Hopkins LC, Smith RB III: Noises in the neck, *N Engl J Med* 302:862, 1980.
177. Wood P: *Diseases of the heart and circulation,* ed 2, Philadelphia, 1956, JB Lippincott, p 31.
178. Hall WD, Wollam GL, Tuttle EP Jr: Diagnostic evaluation of the patient with hypertension. In Hurst JW, editor-in-chief: *The heart,* ed 7, New York, 1990, McGraw-Hill, p 1158.
179. Hurst JW: Unpublished limerick.
180. Hurst JW: Unpublished observation.
181. Hurst JW, Schlant RC: Examination of the veins. In Hurst JW, Logue RB, editors: *The heart,* ed 1, New York, 1966, McGraw-Hill, pp 81-91.
182. Earnest DL, Hurst JW: Exophthalmos, stare, increase in intraocular pressure and systolic propulsion of the eyeballs due to congestive heart failure, *Am J Cardiol* 26:351, 1970.
183. Dodson TF: Varicose veins. In Hurst JW, editor-in-chief: *Medicine for the practicing physician,* ed 3, Boston, 1992, Butterworth, p 1206.
184. Dodson TF: Thrombophlebitis of the lower extremity. In Hurst JW, editor-in-chief: *Medicine for the practicing physician,* ed 3, Boston, 1992, Butterworth, p 1203.
185. Hurst JW: The examination of the heart: the importance of initial screening, *Dis Mon* 36(5), 1990.
186. Laennec RTH: *Traite de l'auscultation mediate,* ed 2, Paris, 1826, Brosson et Chaude.
187. White PD: *Heart disease,* ed 3, New York, 1946, Macmillan, p 56.
188. Leatham A: *An introduction to the examination of the cardiovascular system,* ed 2, Oxford, 1978, Oxford University Press.
189. Levine SA, Harvey WP: *Clinical auscultation of the heart,* ed 2, Philadelphia, 1959, WB Saunders.
190. Shaver JA, Salerni R: Auscultation of the heart. In Hurst JW, editor-in-chief: *The heart,* ed 7, New York, 1990, McGraw-Hill, pp 175-242.
191. Freeman AR, Levine SA: Clinical significance of systolic murmurs: study of 1000 consecutive "non-cardiac" cases, *Ann Intern Med* 6:1371, 1933.
192. Cobbs BW Jr: Personal communication.

CHAPTER 7

The electrocardiogram

The interpretation of the electrocardiogram is not merely a matter of memorizing a few characteristic pictures; there are many unusual variations and combinations of electrocardiographic phenomena which must be studied, analyzed, and correlated one with another and with other available data before any definite conclusion is possible. These situations demand some acquaintance with the electrical and physiologic principles by which they are determined. . . .

FRANK N. WILSON 1952[1]*

DEFINITION

The electrocardiogram is the graphic recording of the electrical activity produced by the heart. The normal sequential contractions of the atria and ventricles would not take place unless the working myocytes of the atria and ventricles were stimulated by the organized electrical activity of the heart. The biologic components that are uniquely involved in the creation of the electrical activity of the heart are, however, quite different from those that are responsible for the mechanical activity of the heart.[3]

COMPONENTS OF THE ELECTROCARDIOGRAM

A diagram of the electrocardiographic waves that are produced by the electrical activity of the heart is shown in Fig. 7-1.

The size and duration of the waves, as well as the intervals between them, can be altered by disease processes. Accordingly, when there is a change in the size, shape, or duration of the waves, when the interval between the waves is shorter or longer than normal, or when there is a change in the relationship of one wave to another, physicians are challenged to create an electrical differential diagnosis as to the cause

---

Most of what I know about spatial vector electrocardiography was taught to me by Dr. Robert Grant, who, while working at Emory University in Atlanta, Ga., in the late 1940s and early 1950s, created the vector approach to electrocardiography.[2]

*Reproduced with permission from Wilson FN: Foreword. In Barker JM: *The unipolar electrocardiogram: a clinical interpretation*, New York, 1952, Appleton-Century-Crofts, pp xi-xii.

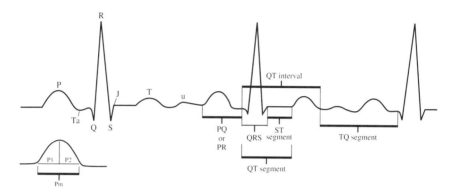

Fig. 7-1. Waves and intervals of the electrocardiogram. The waves are shown in the lefthand portion of the illustration. The *P wave (P)* is produced by depolarization of the atria and is divided into *P1* and *P2*. P1 is produced by depolarization of the right atrium, and P2 is produced by depolarization of the left atrium. The letters *Pm* (mean of the P) are used to represent the entire P wave. The letters *Ta* are used to designate the wave that is produced by repolarization of the atria. The *QRS complex* is due to depolarization of the ventricles. The *Q wave* is the initial downward deflection of the QRS complex. The *R wave* is the initial upward deflection of the QRS complex. A second upward deflection of the QRS complex may be present and is designated as an *R prime (R')* wave. The *S wave* is the terminal downward deflection of the QRS complex. The *T wave (T)* is due to repolarization of the ventricles. The cause of the *U wave* is controversial (see text).

The intervals are shown in the righthand portion of the illustration. The *PR interval,* or preferably the *PQ interval,* is measured from the beginning of the P wave to the beginning of ventricular depolarization (the beginning of the Q wave should be used when there is a Q wave; the beginning of the R wave should be used when there is no Q wave). The *duration of the QRS complex* is measured from the beginning of the QRS complex to the end of the QRS complex. The *ST segment* is defined as the segment that begins with the end of the S wave and ends with the beginning of the T wave. The *QT interval* is measured from the beginning of the Q wave to the end of the T wave. The *QT segment* is measured from the beginning of the Q wave to the beginning of the T wave. The *TQ segment* is measured from the end of the T wave to the beginning of the QRS complex.

Redrawn with permission from Hurst JW: *Ventricular electrocardiography,* New York, 1991, Gower, fig 5.2.

of the abnormalities and to speculate regarding the clinical conditions that might cause them.

At the outset it should be stated that serious cardiac diseases can be present while the electrocardiogram remains normal. For example, patients with advanced coronary artery disease commonly have normal resting electrocardiograms. Equally important, certain abnormalities may be seen in the electrocardiogram when there is no other evidence of heart disease. Such abnormalities are often proved to be benign by the long-term follow-up of the patient.

The electrocardiogram is commonly used as a diagnostic and prognostic tool. In fact, a physician cannot state that the heart is normal without recording and interpreting the electrocardiogram.

ESSENTIAL BACKGROUND INFORMATION

To understand the deflections created by the electrical activity of the heart, it is necessary to be familiar with certain aspects of cardiac anatomy and electrophysiology. Such knowledge should not be memorized and detached from the analysis of each electrocardiogram but should be used to interpret each electrocardiogram. The vector approach to electrocardiography requires that the interpreter use such knowledge when he or she attempts to analyze each electrocardiogram, whereas pattern interpretation, as used by many individuals, does not require the use of anatomic or electrophysiologic knowledge. This is the major reason why this chapter emphasizes the vector approach to interpretating electrocardiograms.

Location of the heart chambers and interventricular septum

The heart rests on the diaphragm. The anatomic long axis of the *left ventricle* is directed inferiorly, to the left, and slightly anteriorly (Fig. 7-2, *A* and *C*). The base of the left ventricle is thicker than the apex.

The *right ventricle* is located anteriorly; it is not located on the right as its name implies (Fig. 7-2, *B* and *C*).

The *left atrium* is located posteriorly in a central position; it is not located on the left as its name implies (Fig. 7-2, *C*). The superior portion of the left atrium abuts the inferior portion of the left bronchus, and the posterior portion of the left atrium abuts the esophagus and spine.

The *right atrium* is named correctly; it is located on the right, anterior to the left atrium (Fig. 7-2, *A* and *C*).

The *interventricular septum* is often depicted inaccurately in diagrams; it is commonly illustrated as a vertical structure that separates the left ventricle from the right ventricle. This inaccurate depiction is perpetuated because it is difficult to create a diagram of the heart, which is a three-dimensional structure, on a two-dimensional surface. It must be appreciated that the interventricular septum is part of the left

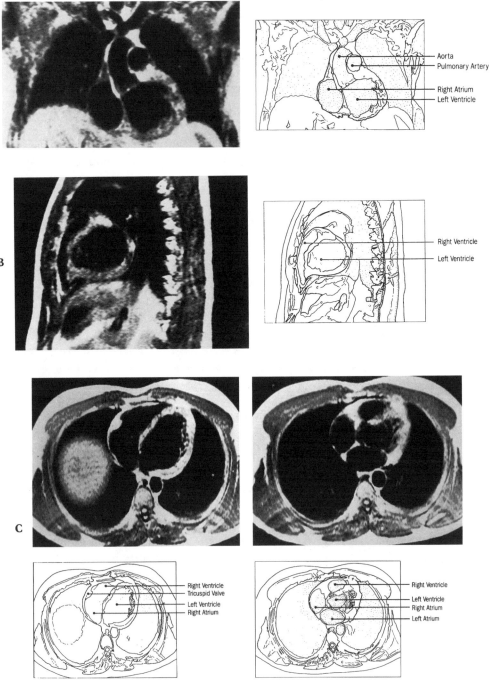

Fig. 7-2

ventricle (Fig. 7-2, *C*)—that part of the left ventricle that is located predominantly anteriorly. The right ventricle is located anterior to the ventricular septum. In fact, the posterior portion of the right ventricle is the interventricular septum (Fig. 7-2, *C*).

Origin and spread of electrical activity within the heart

The *electrical impulse* originates normally in the *sinoatrial node*, which is located where the superior vena cava enters the left atrium (Fig. 7-3). The electrical activity spreads from atrial cell to atrial cell; there are no identifiable conduction pathways that are composed of cells that differ anatomically from the functioning atrial myocytes. However, there are *preferential conduction pathways*. These pathways exist, according to Becker,[4] because the atrial myocytes are crowded together as they are forced to circumvent the "holes" in the right and left atria. The holes in the right atrium are produced by the entrance of the superior vena cava and the inferior vena cava into the right atrium, the tricuspid valve, and the fossa ovale. The holes in the left atrium are produced by the entrance of the pulmonary veins into the left atrium and the mitral valve.

The spread of electrical activity within the atria is called *atrial depolarization* and normally leads to atrial contraction. Atrial depolarization is caused by the loss of electrical charges on the surface of the atrial myocytes. The wave of atrial depolarization is guided by the preferential conduction pathways. It spreads anteriorly and inferiorly in the right atrial wall and then spreads posteriorly and inferiorly in the left atrial wall. The electrical impulse reaches the atrioventricular node before it completes its spread in the left atrial wall.[5] The depolarization of the right and left atria produces the *P wave* in the electrocardiogram. The first half of the P wave is produced by right atrial depolarization, and the second half of the P wave is produced by left atrial depolarization.

Repolarization of the atria occurs when the electrical charges are rebuilt on the surface of the atrial myocytes. The new wave that is created is referred to as the T of the P, or *Ta wave*. This wave is seen only occasionally in the electrocardiogram.

There is a tendency to ignore the P wave abnormalities in the electrocardiogram. This is unfortunate, because P wave abnormalities commonly reflect abnormalities

---

Fig. 7-2. Location of the four heart chambers. The technique of magnetic resonance imaging can be used to show the frontal view, **A,** left lateral view, **B,** and transverse view, **C,** of the heart. The various cardiac chambers are labeled in the diagrams that accompany the magnetic resonance images. These views of the heart must be kept in mind as one analyzes the electrical forces of the heart.

Courtesy Mark Lowell, M.D., Roderic I. Pettigrew, M.D., and the Radiology Department of Emory University School of Medicine and Hospital, Atlanta, Ga. Reproduced with permission from Hurst JW: *Ventricular electrocardiography,* New York, 1991, Gower, figs 4.5, 4.6, 4.7.

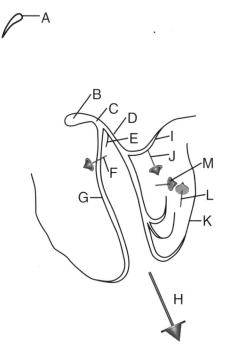

Fig. 7-3. Diagrammatic representation of the sinoatrial node, the atrioventricular node, and the left and right bundle branches. *A,* Sinoatrial node—responsible for the creation of electrical impulses that initiate depolarization of the atria. *B,* Atrioventricular node—slows and channels electrical activity to the bundle of His. *C,* Bundle of His—channels electrical activity to the right and left bundle branches. *D,* Left bundle branch. *E,* Twig of the left bundle branch—responsible for the early depolarization of the interventricular septum. *F,* Electrical force (represented by arrow) produced by depolarization of the first part of the septum. *G,* Right bundle branch. *H,* Electrical forces (represented by arrow) created by depolarization of the endocardial layer of the left and right ventricles. *I,* Left anterosuperior division (LASD) of the left bundle branch. *J,* Mean of the electrical forces (represented by arrow) created by the myocytes that are stimulated by the electrical impulse that is guided by the LASD of the left bundle branch. *K,* Left posteroinferior division (LPID) of the left bundle branch. *L,* Mean of the electrical forces (represented by arrow) created by the myocytes that are stimulated by the electrical impulse that is guided by the LPID of the left bundle. *M,* Vector sum of arrows *K* and *L;* the electrical forces responsible for *K* and *L* occur almost simultaneously, although the forces responsible for *L* may occur a little later than the forces responsible for *K.*

This figure illustrates three consecutive electrical fields: the vector (arrow) *F* creates the first electrical field; the vector (arrow) *H* creates the second electrical field; and the vector (arrow) *M* creates the third electrical field. As discussed and illustrated later, the QRS complex is produced by a series of different electrical fields.

of the ventricles, as well as abnormalities of the atria. In fact, the P waves yield more clues to ventricular disease than they do to primary atrial disease.

The *atrioventricular node, bundle of His, right and left bundle branches,* and *Purkinje fibers* are identifiable structures (see Fig. 7-3). The atrioventricular node is located in the right atrium in the lower portion of the atrial septum. This unique structure slows the speed of electrical activity that reaches it as the result of depolarization of the right atrium. This delay is the major cause of the *PR interval* in the electrocardiogram (see Fig. 7-1). However, the interval is more accurately visualized as a PQ interval, because it actually represents the time from the beginning of atrial depolarization to the beginning of ventricular depolarization. During this interval the electrical activity travels through the atrial myocytes, the atrioventricular node, the bundle of His, the left and right bundle branches, and the Purkinje fibers to reach the ventricular myocytes. The electrical activity travels about 200 mm/sec in the atrioventricular node and 4000 mm/sec in the bundle branches and their Purkinje fibers.[6] Accordingly, most, but not all, of the delay of the transmission of electrical activity that originates in the sinus node and travels to the ventricular myocytes occurs in the atrioventricular node. When the ventricular myocytes are stimulated to undergo depolarization, the wave is slowed to the rate of 1000 mm/sec.[6]

The electrical activity in the atrioventricular node, the bundle of His, the bundle branches, and the Purkinje fibers is too small to be recorded in the surface electrocardiogram. The working myocytes depolarize when the ventricles are stimulated by the electrical activity presented to them by the Purkinje fibers of the right and left bundle branches. That is, the ventricular myocytes lose the electrical charges that are located on the surface of the cells. It is the *depolarization of the ventricular myocytes* that produces the QRS complex in the electrocardiogram (see Fig. 7-1). The depolarization process begins normally in the myocytes located in the ventricular endocardium and proceeds toward the myocytes in the ventricular epicardium. After a short delay, the electrical charges are rebuilt on the surface of the ventricular myocytes. This *repolarization of the ventricular myocytes* creates the *T wave* in the electrocardiogram (see Fig. 7-1). The repolarization process, as discussed later, begins normally in the epicardium and proceeds toward the endocardium. Note that the direction of the repolarization process is opposite to the direction of the depolarization process (the reason for this is discussed later).

The *U wave* is believed by some individuals to be due to late repolarization activity of the ventricular myocytes located in the papillary muscles or to repolarization of the Purkinje fibers (see Fig. 7-1). Others, however, believe it is due to the late depolarization of isolated myocytes.[7]

Certain aspects of the left and right bundle branches deserve additional emphasis:

- A small branch of the initial portion of the left bundle branch initiates depolarization of the left superior portion of the interventricular septum. This is the first portion of the ventricles to depolarize (see Fig. 7-3). Recall the exact location of the interventricular septum (see Fig. 7-2, *C*).

- The left bundle branch divides into the left anterosuperior division and the left posteroinferior division (see Fig. 7-3). These divisions of the left bundle branch deliver electrical impulses to the left ventricular myocytes in a unique manner; their importance will become apparent later in the discussion. The right bundle is long and does not divide into smaller branches until it reaches the right ventricle (see Fig. 7-3).

The first portion of the ventricles to undergo depolarization is the left upper portion of the ventricular septum (see Fig. 7-3). This depolarization process is usually directed slightly anteriorly. It may be directed to the right or left and inferiorly or superiorly during the initial 0.01 to 0.02 second of the depolarization process (Fig. 7-4, *A*). It is important to appreciate the shape and location of the septum in order to understand how a slight change in its position or shape can alter the direction of that portion of the depolarization process of the ventricles. During the next 0.03 to 0.055 second the depolarization process is directed normally inferiorly and leftward, because it is produced by depolarization of the endocardial layer of the right and left ventricles (Fig. 7-4, *B*). The terminal 0.01 to 0.02 second of the depolarization process takes place in the posterobasilar portion of the left ventricle (Fig. 7-4, *C*).[8] This occurs because the normal left ventricle is thicker than the right ventricle and because the left posteroinferior division branch of the left bundle branch delivers electrical stimuli to that area of the left ventricle, whereas there is no such arrangement

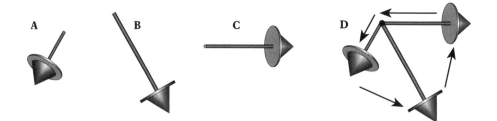

Fig. 7-4. Diagrammatic representation of the depolarization sequence responsible for the QRS complex (see text). **A,** An arrow representing the electrical forces (vectors) produced by the initial depolarization of the septum is directed anteriorly and to the right. **B,** An arrow representing the electrical forces (vectors) produced by depolarization of the endocardial layer of the left and right ventricles is directed inferiorly and slightly to the left and, in this illustration, is parallel with the frontal plane. **C,** An arrow representing the electrical forces (vectors) produced by depolarization of the posterolateral portion of the left ventricle is directed to the left and posteriorly. **D,** A crude QRS loop is created when the origin of the electrical forces is assumed to arise from a common point and when a line (the loop) is drawn around the termini of the electrical forces.

in the right ventricle. These electrical forces can be visualized as originating from a common source (Fig. 7-4, *D*). A line drawn around the termini of these electrical forces (vectors) creates a QRS loop.

In summary, the configuration of the ventricular complexes (QRS and T waves) in the electrocardiogram is determined by the location and structure of the ventricles (including the location and shape of the ventricular septum); the sequence of depolarization, which is controlled by the conduction system; and the sequence of repolarization, which, in the normal subject, is predetermined by the sequence of depolarization.

VECTORS

The depolarization and repolarization processes create measurable electrical forces, and it is useful to conceive of these forces as vectors. The mathematical symbol used to represent a vector is an arrow. Although we were all exposed to vectors in high school and college mathematics, it is usually necessary for beginners in electrocardiography to refresh their memories of vectors. Only a few points are made here; greater detail is presented in the section dealing with the atrial and ventricular electrocardiogram.

Any force, be it mechanical or electrical, can be conceived of as a vector. A vector, in turn, can be symbolized as an arrow (Fig. 7-5).[2] A vector has magnitude, direction, and sense. The *magnitude* (size) of a vector can be illustrated by the length

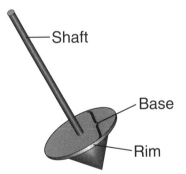

Fig. 7-5. An arrow (the symbol for a vector) has three parts: the shaft, the base of the arrowhead, and the rim of the arrowhead. The base of the arrowhead represents the zero potential plane. The rim of the arrowhead represents the transitional pathway (see Fig. 7-7). The length of the shaft represents the magnitude of the electrical force. The inclination of the arrow represents the orientation of the electrical force in space. The arrowhead indicates the polarity (the sense) of the force, which, taken along with its inclination, indicates the direction of the force.

of the arrow; the *direction* refers to the inclination of the vector in space; and the *sense*, or polarity, is symbolized by the location and orientation of the arrowhead. It must be appreciated, too, that any force, be it mechanical or electrical, exerts its influence in three dimensions. That is, a force is directed up or down, right or left, and toward the front or back.

The electrocardiogram can be interpreted in terms of the size, direction, and sense of the electrical forces (vectors) that produce it.[2] In addition, when vectors (arrows) are used to represent electrical forces, the relationship of one electrical force (vector) to another can be discerned easily.[2] For example, it is important to identify the relationship of the direction of the vector representing the entire T wave (mean T vector) with the vector representing the entire QRS complex (mean QRS vector). No other method of interpreting surface electrocardiograms enables the physician to es-

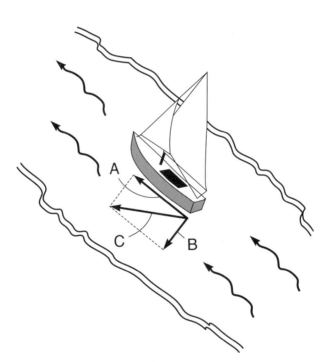

Fig. 7-6. Summation of forces using the concept of a parallelogram. Suppose the current of a river moves a boat at the rate of 2 miles/hr in the direction shown by arrow *A*. Imagine that the wind blows the sail of the boat at right angles to the direction of the current at the rate of 1 mile/hr as depicted by arrow *B*. Note that arrow *B* is half as long as arrow *A*. The forces can be added by creating a parallelogram. The diagonal of the parallelogram, represented by arrow *C*, indicates the direction the boat would take during the hour of observation. The length of arrow *C* indicates the distance that the boat would move. The actual distance can be deduced by measuring arrow *C* and using the same units of distance used in arrows *A* and *B*.

tablish the relationship of one electrical force (vector) to another as accurately as the Grant method of analysis.[2]

Vectors can be added together by constructing a parallelogram.[2] See Fig. 7-6 for an example of a mathematical problem that can be solved using vectors.

TRANSMISSION OF ELECTRICAL ACTIVITY PRODUCED BY THE HEART

To understand how the electrical activity created in the heart is transmitted throughout the body, it is useful to consider the transmission of a single electrical force (vector) in the body. In Fig. 7-7 a single electrical force (vector), originating in the cen-

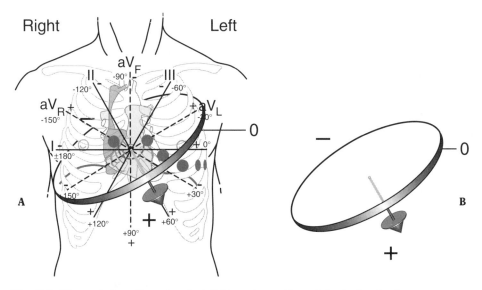

Fig. 7-7. Transmission of an electrical field to the surface of the body. **A,** An arrow representing the electrical force (vector) originating in the center of the heart is directed at +60 degrees and 30 to 40 degrees posteriorly. The zero potential plane is perpendicular to the direction of the arrow and divides the body into a negative area (in this example the negative portion of the electrical field is located superior to the zero potential plane) and a positive area (in this example the positive portion of the electrical field is located inferior to the zero potential plane). When the zero potential plane extends to the body surface (the skin), it creates the transitional pathway. In this example, the electrocardiograph machine will record a negative deflection superior to the transitional pathway, a positive deflection inferior to the transitional pathway, and zero potential along the transitional pathway. **B,** The length of the arrow indicates the magnitude of the electrical force; the direction and sense of the electrical force is illustrated by the inclination of the arrow and the location of the arrowhead. The arrowhead itself has considerable meaning (see Fig. 7-5).

ter of the heart, which is located in the center of the chest, is represented by an arrow that is directed inferiorly, to the left, and slightly posteriorly. An electrical field surrounds the electrical force (vector) and is transmitted throughout the body. The electrical field is also distributed to the body surface (skin). One portion of the electrical field is produced by negative charges, and another portion of the electrical field is produced by positive charges. In between the negative and positive portions of the electrical field there is a *zero potential plane* that is perpendicular to the electrical force (vector) that created it. The zero potential plane intersects the surface of the body and creates the *transitional pathway* (Fig. 7-7, *A*). Accordingly, if the appropriate measuring device is applied to the skin, it is possible to determine the distribution of the area of negativity, the area of positivity, and the location of the transitional pathway. Obviously, it should be possible to deduce the direction, magnitude, and sense of the electrical force (vector) by identifying the location of the transitional pathway and the distribution of the negative and positive portions of the electrical field on the chest.

See Fig. 7-7, *B*, for an explanation of how the arrow itself symbolizes the electrical force.

MEASURING DEVICE

Electrocardiograph machine

The electrocardiograph machine produces a graph that is created by the electrical forces generated by the heart. The machine itself has been designed to detect a small amount of electric current. Einthoven was stimulated by Waller's work and improved Ader's galvanometer.[9] Einthoven's galvanometer had two poles: a positive pole and a negative pole. Einthoven connected a wire to each pole of the galvanometer and connected the other end of each wire to the patient. As discussed later, the attachment to the patient was achieved by the use of buckets of saline. The machine was cumbersome to use and required a photographic recording system, which delayed immediate access to the record.

Modern electronic electrocardiograph machines were created in parallel with the development of high technology that uses electricity. The modern direct-writing machine is easy to use and yields an immediate recording of the electrocardiogram, although it is no more accurate than Einthoven's galvanometer.

Paper and paper speed

The paper speed is 25 mm/sec. A special grid is imprinted on the paper that allows one to measure the length of time required to inscribe a specified portion of the electrocardiographic tracing (Fig. 7-8). The machine is programmed so that 1 cm of movement of the writing arm (stylus) equals 1 mV of electrical potential (Fig. 7-8).

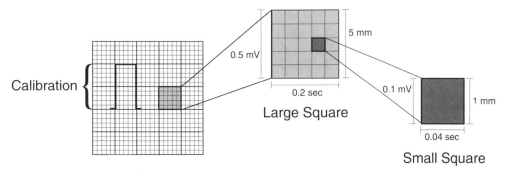

Fig. 7-8. Paper used to record electrocardiograms.

Electrodes

The machine is connected to wires that are, in turn, connected to electrodes. The electrodes, which are attached to the skin, sense the electrical potential on the surface of the body. The current is transmitted by the wires to the machine, and a recording is made.

Electrode attachments and leads

The development of simple electrodes was, for some unexplained reason, difficult and slow. The first "electrodes" consisted of buckets of saline. Each arm and one foot were placed in separate buckets of saline, and each of the buckets was connected to the galvanometer. Obviously, this crude arrangement delayed the development of chest leads, which require that the electrodes be placed on the surface of the chest itself.

Today, small metal electrodes are attached to the skin surface by suction cups. Excellent skin contact is ensured by the use of special paste, and the anatomic locations of the electrodes have been defined (see subsequent discussion).

Bipolar leads

Einthoven's bipolar extremity leads.[10] Einthoven connected the wire that was attached to the negative pole of the galvanometer to the right arm and the wire that was attached to the positive pole of the galvanometer to the left arm to create lead I (Fig. 7-9, *A*). He connected the wire that was attached to the negative pole of the galvanometer to the left arm and the wire that was attached to the positive pole of the galvanometer to either leg to create lead III. He connected the wire that was attached to the negative pole of the galvanometer to the right arm and the wire that was attached to the positive pole of the galvanometer to the leg to create lead II.

Einthoven visualized the axis of lead I as a line drawn between the attachments to the right and left arms, the axis of lead II as a line drawn between the attachments to the right arm and the leg, and the axis of lead III as a line drawn between the attachments to the left arm and the leg (Fig. 7-9, *A*). He recognized that when recording lead I, the galvanometer measured the difference between the electrical potential of the right and left arms; that when recording lead II, the galvanometer measured the difference in electrical potential between the right arm and the leg; and that when recording lead III, the galvanometer measured the difference in electrical potential between the left arm and the leg. Accordingly, these leads are called *bipolar leads.* They are also considered *frontal plane leads,* because the leads are influenced by electrical forces (vectors) that are directed superiorly and inferiorly and to the right or left but are not influenced by electrical forces (vectors) that are directed only anteriorly or posteriorly.

Einthoven also created the *electrical equilateral triangle* (Fig. 7-9, *B*). He reasoned that the electrode attachments to the right arm, left arm, and either leg were electrically equidistant from the origin of electrical potential produced by the heart even though, from an anatomic viewpoint, the attachment to the leg was located a greater distance from the heart than were the attachments to the arms. This being true, if the electrode attachments to each arm and one leg are electrically equidistant from

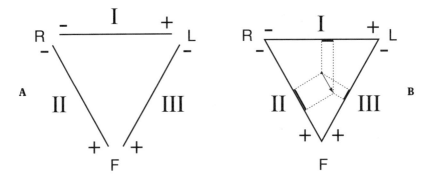

Fig. 7-9. Einthoven's bipolar extremity leads. **A,** Einthoven created lead I by attaching a wire from the right arm to the negative pole of the galvanometer and a wire from the left arm to the positive pole of the galvanometer. He created lead II by attaching a wire from the right arm to the negative pole of the galvanometer and a wire from one leg to the positive pole of the galvanometer. He created lead III by attaching a wire from the left arm to the negative pole of the galvanometer and a wire from the leg to the positive pole of the galvanometer. (He originally used buckets of saline for electrodes.) **B,** Einthoven viewed the bipolar extremity lead hookup between the patient and the electrocardiograph machine as an electrical equilateral triangle, because the "electrodes" recorded the electrical potential at points that were located a great distance from its origin (see text). He pointed out that electrical forces were projected onto the lead axes as shown here. Note how the arrow "projects" its "shadow" onto each of the lead axes.

the origin of electrical potential produced by the heart, they are electrically equidistant from each other. It follows, then, that lead axes I, II, and III create an electrical equilateral triangle. This concept can be confirmed by moving the modern electrodes from the wrist to the elbow or from the ankle to the thigh; the waves of the electrocardiogram will not change in size or contour.

When an electrical force (vector) is represented by an arrow, it is possible to visualize how the vector influences the bipolar extremity leads; the arrow can be "projected" onto the lead axes as shown in Fig. 7-9, B.

Einthoven knew that the difference in electrical potential that existed between the right and left arms, the left arm and one leg, and the right arm and one leg would, when added together, equal zero if the polarity of the electrode attachment to the machine and to the patient remained consistent. In such a case the deflection in lead I, plus the deflection in lead II, plus the deflection in lead III should equal zero. Legend holds that Einthoven preferred upright QRS complexes and reversed the polarity of lead II in order to achieve an upright deflection more often. To accomplish this, he attached the wire from the leg to the positive pole of the galvanometer and the wire from the right arm to the negative pole of the galvanometer, whereas to be consistent with the attachments of the wires used to create leads I and III, he would have attached the wire from the leg to the negative pole of the galvanometer and the wire from the right arm to the positive pole of the galvanometer. When the attachments of the wires are rearranged as he preferred, the deflection in lead I plus the deflection in lead III equals the deflection in lead II. The formula becomes:

$$I + (-II) + III = 0 \text{ or } I + III = II$$

This is now known as Einthoven's law.

Bayley's triaxial system.[11] Bayley created a more usable figure than Einthoven's electrical equilateral triangle by moving the axes of leads I, II, and III so that they passed through the electrical center of the heart (Fig. 7-10). Note that the orientation of the lead axes is no different from that shown in Einthoven's triangle and that an arrow representing an electrical force (vector) projects the same amount on Bayley's lead axes as it does on the lead axes of Einthoven's equilateral triangle.

Bipolar chest leads. Chest leads were not used for many years following the initial use of the electrocardiograph machine. The delay in their use occurred because, during the early years, buckets of saline were used as "electrodes" that connected the patient to the electrocardiograph machine. Later, when modern electrodes were developed, a single bipolar chest lead was used. This was accomplished by placing the exploring electrode on the chest and connecting it to the positive pole of the galvanometer, and connecting the other electrode, which was attached to the negative pole of the galvanometer, to either arm or leg. The chest lead was labeled either CR, CL, or CF. The letter *C* referred to the chest; the letter *R* referred to the right arm; and the letter *L* referred to the left arm. The letter *F* was used to designate the elec-

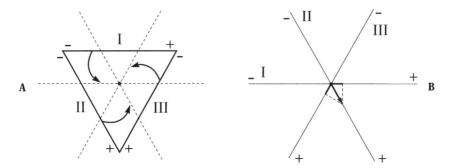

Fig. 7-10. Bayley's triaxial system. **A,** Bayley moved lead axes I, II, and III so that they pass through the same central point (considered the origin of the electrical forces). He maintained the same orientation of the lead axes as in Einthoven's electrical equilateral triangle (see Fig. 7-9, *B*). **B,** The same electrical force shown in Fig. 7-9 is reproduced in this figure. Note that the arrow projects the same amount on lead axes I, II, and III of Bayley's triaxial system as it did on the leads of Einthoven's electrical equilateral triangle.

trode that was attached to the negative pole of the machine and placed on the leg because the letter *L* had already been used to designate the lead in which the electrode was attached to the left arm. The letter *F* referred to the foot. These were bipolar chest leads, and the machine reflected the difference in the electrical potential of the two sites. Still later, six precordial bipolar chest leads were created by placing the electrode at six specified sites on the chest (see subsequent discussion).

By the late 1940s these bipolar chest leads were abandoned in favor of the Wilson unipolar chest leads.

Unipolar leads. Wilson created the unipolar lead system.[12] Using the concept that the difference in electrical potential recorded between each of the arms and between each arm and a leg adds up to zero at any point in time, he connected the wires from each arm and one leg to a central terminal. He then connected the wire from the central terminal to the negative pole of the electrocardiograph machine and connected the exploring electrode to the positive pole of the electrocardiograph machine. When it is connected to the body, the machine measures the difference in potential between the central terminal and the exploring electrode; however, because the central terminal records almost zero potential, the result is a unipolar lead that records the electrical potential wherever the exploring electrode is placed on the body (Fig. 7-11). Wilson used the unipolar lead to record the electrical potential on the extremities and on the surface of the chest.

Wilson's unipolar extremity leads.[12] The electrocardiographic deflections recorded from the extremities using Wilson's unipolar lead system were smaller than the deflections recorded using Einthoven's bipolar extremity lead system. Because of

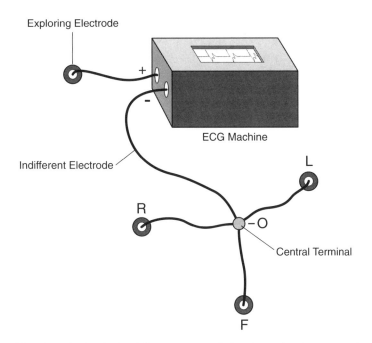

Fig. 7-11. Wilson's unipolar leads. Wilson connected the electrodes that were placed on the right arm, left arm, and one leg to a central terminal. He then connected the central terminal to the negative pole of the electrocardiograph machine. He connected the exploring electrode to the positive pole of the machine. When the exploring electrode was placed on the chest, it was referred to as a V lead. When the exploring electrode was placed on the extremities, it was referred to as VR, VL, and VF.

Slightly modified with permission from Hurst JW: *Ventricular electrocardiography*, New York, 1991, Gower, fig 4.20.

this, a mathematical relationship could not be established between the two systems. To solve this problem, Wilson increased the size of the unipolar complexes by placing amplifiers in the unipolar lead system. The leads were labeled V_R when the exploring electrode was placed on the right arm, V_L when the exploring electrode was placed on the left arm, and V_F when the exploring electrode was placed on either leg. V_F was used to identify the lead when the exploring electrode was placed on the leg, because the letter L was already used to designate the left arm. The letter F refers to the foot.

Goldberger's augmented unipolar extremity leads.[13] The unavailability of amplifiers for electrocardiographic investigation during World War II led to the search for a method that would increase the size of the deflections recorded from the extremities using Wilson's unipolar concept. Goldberger discovered that when he broke the connection from an extremity to the central terminal when the exploring electrode was placed on that extremity, the deflections were augmented but the contour of the deflection changed very little as compared with the deflection recorded using Wilson's unipolar lead.[13] Goldberger's leads are used today and are labeled aV_R, aV_L, and aV_F (Fig. 7-12). The *a* stands for augmented. Goldberger's extremity lead axis can be visualized by drawing a line that bisects the angles of Bayley's triaxial system.

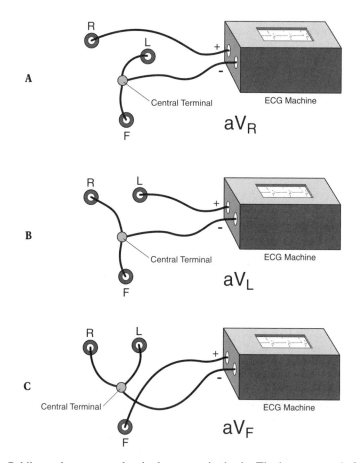

Fig. 7-12. Goldberger's augmented unipolar extremity leads. The letter *a* stands for the word *augmented*. **A,** Lead aV_R is created by disconnecting the wire from the right arm to Wilson's central terminal when the exploring electrode is placed on the right arm. **B,** aV_L is created by disconnecting the wire from the left arm to Wilson's central terminal when the exploring electrode is placed on the left arm. **C,** aV_F is created by disconnecting the wire from the leg to Wilson's central terminal when the exploring electrode is placed on the leg.

Slightly modified with permission from Hurst JW: *Ventricular electrocardiography*, New York, 1991, Gower, fig 4.24.

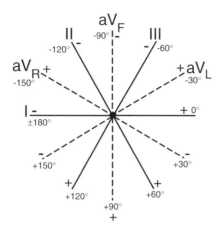

Fig. 7-13. Hexaxial reference system. The unipolar extremity lead axes bisect the angles produced by Bayley's triaxial system to create the hexaxial reference system. The direction of the vectors used to represent electrical forces can be designated as the number of degrees from the horizontal line created by lead I. Note that the 0-degree point is located at the left-hand end of lead axis I and the ±180-degree point is located at the right-hand end of lead axis I.

This figure is called the *hexaxial reference system* (Fig. 7-13). Note the circular scale shown in Fig. 7-13; this scale is used to designate the number of degrees the frontal plane projection of an electrical force (vector), which is represented by an arrow, deviates from position zero.

Wilson's unipolar chest leads.[12] When Wilson developed the unipolar extremity lead system, it was apparent that the lead axes bisected the angles of Bayley's triaxial display system, creating the hexaxial display system. Goldberger's modification of Wilson's unipolar lead system did not change that arrangement. The exploring electrodes of the unipolar extremity lead system simply viewed the electrical forces (vectors) from a slightly different vantage point than did the bipolar leads. Accordingly, both the bipolar and the unipolar extremity leads were retained, because they gave different views of the electrical field produced by the heart. Wilson's unipolar chest leads, however, completely replaced the bipolar chest leads; they give a more accurate view of the electrical field produced by the heart, because the deflections recorded by Wilson's unipolar chest leads are not contaminated by the electrical potential of either arm or leg, as are the deflections recorded by the bipolar chest leads.

It is not necessary to amplify or augment the deflections recorded with Wilson's unipolar chest leads; the deflections are sufficiently large, because the electrodes are near the heart and because one is not trying to establish a mathematical relationship with a bipolar lead system, as is the case with the extremity leads.

The seven chest electrode positions are determined by anatomic landmarks and are labeled with the letter *V*, which is the symbol for *potential* (Fig. 7-14).

V_1: The V_1 electrode position is located in the fourth right intercostal space adjacent to the sternum.

V_2: The V_2 electrode position is located in the fourth left intercostal space adjacent to the sternum.

V_3: The V_3 electrode position is located at the halfway point on an imaginary line connecting the V_2 and V_4 electrode positions.

V_4: The V_4 electrode position is located in the fifth intercostal space at the left midclavicular line.

V_5: The V_5 electrode position is located at the anterior axillary line on the left at the same horizontal level as the V_4 electrode position.

V_6: The V_6 electrode position is located at the midaxillary line on the left at the same horizontal level as the V_4 and V_5 electrode positions.

V_{3R}: V_{3R} is used in children and occasionally in adults. It is located as described for electrode position V_3 but is located on the right side of the chest.

The lead axis of each precordial unipolar chest lead can be visualized by drawing a line from the electrode position through the origin of the electrical force, which is located in the center of the heart, to the opposite side of the body.

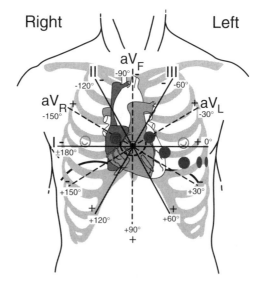

Fig. 7-14. Location of the chest electrodes (see text). This figure also illustrates the relationship of the bipolar and unipolar extremity leads to the body and to each other. The heart is shown in its anatomically correct position. The semicircle indicates the location of the left atrium. The dot in the center of the heart represents the approximate location of the origin of the electrical forces.

DETERMINING THE DIRECTION OF AN ELECTRICAL FORCE (VECTOR) IN THREE DIMENSIONS

Determining the direction of an electrical force (vector) in the frontal plane

Prior to Grant's work it was difficult to compute the direction of electrical forces of the heart.[2] Accordingly, those interested in electrocardiography attempted to memorize the *patterns* of the normal and abnormal deflections created by the electrical forces of the heart rather than determine the direction, magnitude, and sense of the electrical forces that produce them. When pattern recognition only is used, observers will soon disregard and forget the basic mechanisms that are responsible for the deflections. In addition, observers will have difficulty interpreting electrocardiograms that they have not seen previously.

Grant pointed out that the frontal plane direction of electrical forces (vectors) could be computed instantly by identifying the smallest and largest deflections in the six extremity leads. He taught that when an electrical force (vector) is parallel with a given extremity lead axis, the largest electrocardiographic deflection appears in that lead, and when an electrical force (vector) is perpendicular to a given extremity lead axis, the smallest electrocardiographic deflection appears in that lead (Fig. 7-15).[2]

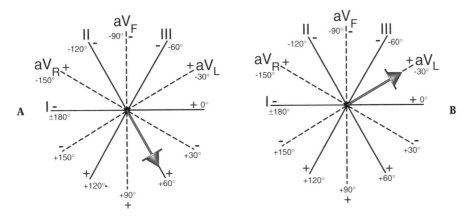

Fig. 7-15. Calculation of the direction of an electrical force (vector) in the frontal plane. **A,** When a deflection is largest in lead II, it can be represented by a vector (arrow) that is directed parallel with lead axis II. The deflection will simultaneously be smaller, but equally large, in leads I and III and smallest in lead aV_L, because the arrow will be perpendicular to lead axis aV_L. When the deflection is upright in lead II, the vector (arrow) will be directed toward the electrode of lead II that is attached to the positive pole of the electrocardiograph machine. **B,** When a deflection is smallest in lead II, it can be represented by an arrow that is perpendicular to lead axis II. The deflection will simultaneously be largest in lead aV_L, because the arrow will be parallel with lead axis aV_L. Furthermore, the deflection will be upright in lead aV_L when the vector (arrow) is directed toward the electrode that is attached to the positive pole of the electrocardiograph machine.

When the hexaxial reference system is used and when careful attention is paid to the polarity (negativity or positivity) of the deflection in each lead, it is possible to determine the frontal plane projection of an electrical force (vector) within 5 degrees of the accuracy computed by more cumbersome methods. The vectors are represented by arrows.

Determining the anteroposterior direction of an electrical force (vector)

The six extremity lead axes are influenced by the projection of electrical forces (vectors) that are directed superiorly or inferiorly and to the right or left. The first four of the six precordial lead axes are, for the most part, influenced by the projection of electrical forces (vectors) that are directed anteriorly or posteriorly. Leads V_5 and V_6 are influenced by the projection of electrical forces (vectors) that are directed anteriorly or posteriorly and by the projection of electrical forces (vectors) that are directed to the right or left and up or down. This is why a deflection in V_6 tends to resemble a deflection recorded in lead I.

Unfortunately, the same technique of determining the frontal plane direction of an electrical force (vector) cannot be used to determine the anterior or posterior direction of an electrical force (vector). This is true because the extremity lead electrodes are located a great distance from the heart and are influenced equally by the electrical activity produced by all parts of the heart. The chest electrodes are located much nearer the heart than are the extremity lead electrodes and, as a result, are influenced by the electrical activity of the portion of the heart that is nearest the electrode. Accordingly, the magnitude of a unipolar chest lead deflection cannot be used to determine that an electrical force (vector) is directed parallel with its axis.[2] In addition, there is a lack of uniformity in the size and shape of individuals. These factors conspire to prevent a mathematical relationship of the chest leads with each other and with the extremity leads. Grant emphasized that the transitional pathway of an electrical force (vector) recorded on the surface of the chest could be used to determine the anterior or posterior direction of the electrical force (vector).[2] Keep in mind that the transitional pathway on the chest is produced by the zero potential plane, which is perpendicular to the electrical force (vector). Accordingly, one can visualize the direction of an electrical force (vector) by identifying the location of the transitional pathway, which is not dependent on the size of the electrical force (Fig. 7-16). This led to the concept that there are two steps required to identify the direction of an electrical force (vector) in space:

Step 1: Determine the direction of the frontal plane of the electrical force (vector) as described in the preceding section.

Step 2: Identify the chest lead electrode position in which zero (or resultantly zero) potential is recorded. Such a deflection identifies the location of the transitional pathway on the chest; the transitional pathway is the "edge" of the zero potential plane. Deflections recorded from the electrode positions located to

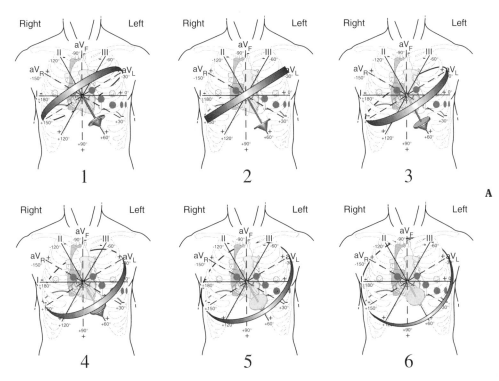

Fig. 7-16. Calculation of the anterior or posterior direction of an electrical force (vector). **A,** Assume that the frontal plane direction of an electrical force (vector) represented by an arrow is largest and positive in lead axis II. The arrow representing the electrical force (vector) would be directed parallel with lead axis II; it would be directed toward the electrode that is attached to the positive pole of the electrocardiograph machine and away from the electrode that is attached to the negative pole of the electrocardiograph machine. *1,* When the transitional pathway passes through electrode position V_1, the electrical force (vector) represented by an arrow is directed about 10 to 20 degrees anteriorly. *2,* When the transitional pathway passes through electrode position V_2, the electrical force (vector) represented by an arrow is parallel with the frontal plane. *3,* When the transitional pathway passes through electrode position V_3, the electrical force (vector) represented by an arrow is directed about 20 to 30 degrees posteriorly. *4,* When the transitional pathway passes through electrode position V_4, the electrical force (vector) represented by an arrow is directed 40 to 50 degrees posteriorly. *5,* When the transitional pathway passes through electrode position V_5, the electrical force (vector) is directed 60 to 70 degrees posteriorly. *6,* When the transitional pathway passes through electrode position V_6, the electrical force (vector) represented by an arrow is directed 80 to 90 degrees posteriorly. *Continued.*

B

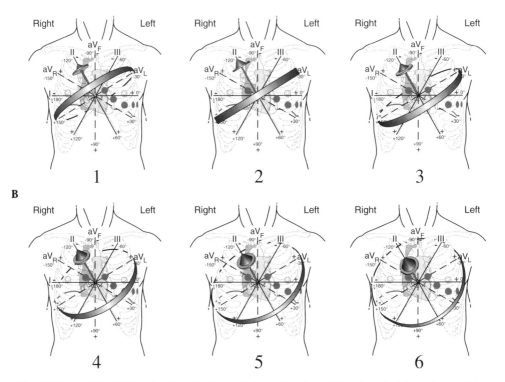

Fig. 7-16, cont'd. B, Imagine that the frontal plane direction of the electrical force (vector) is largest but negative in lead axis II. The arrow would be directed parallel to lead axis II; it is directed away from the electrode that is attached to the positive pole of the electrocardiograph machine. *1,* When the transitional pathway passes through electrode position V_1, the electrical force (vector) represented by an arrow will be directed 10 to 20 degrees posteriorly. *2,* When the transitional pathway passes through electrode position V_2, the electrical force (vector) represented by an arrow will be directed parallel with the frontal plane. *3,* When the transitional pathway passes through electrode position V_3, the electrical force (vector) represented by an arrow will be directed about 20 to 30 degrees anteriorly. *4,* When the transitional pathway passes through electrode position V_4, the electrical force (vector) represented by an arrow will be directed 40 to 50 degrees anteriorly. *5,* When the transitional pathway passes through electrode position V_5, the electrical force (vector) represented by an arrow will be directed 60 to 70 degrees anteriorly. *6,* When the transitional pathway passes through electrode position V_6, the electrical force (vector) represented by an arrow will be directed 80 to 90 degrees anteriorly.

the right of the transitional complex will record either a positive or a negative deflection, and deflections recorded from the electrode positions located to the left of the transitional complex will have an opposite polarity (Fig. 7-16).

With the frontal plane direction of an electrical force (vector) clearly in mind, one should mentally rotate the electrical force (vector) anteriorly or posteriorly until the edge of the zero potential plane (the transitional pathway) passes through the precordial electrode position where the electrocardiographic deflection is zero (isoelectric) or resultantly zero (Fig. 7-16). It is believed that the anteroposterior direction of an electrical force (vector) can be estimated within ± 15 degrees of the actual direction.

Caveat. Never execute step 2 without initially executing step 1.

THE GOAL RESTATED

Let us not forget the goal—to identify the distribution of a series of electrical fields located on the surface of the body and, by studying them, determine the characteristics of the electrical forces (vectors) that produce them. As discussed later, there is a different electrical field produced by each electrical force (vector) generated during each millisecond of each cardiac cycle.

An electrical field can be identified by placing a unipolar lead on each centimeter of the body surface. Until recently this was difficult to accomplish. Modern body surface mapping, however, is now being used to accomplish this feat.[14] The subject wears a vest that is laden with numerous unipolar electrodes, and the recording device is programmed to record the electrical field for each millisecond of the P, QRS, and T waves. The electrical fields are displayed on a screen so that the areas of negativity and positivity and the transitional pathway located on the front and back of the chest can be easily viewed. This technique is not as yet used routinely, but as discussed in Chapter 1, it is another example of how high technology has taught us more about low technology.

In reality, the extremity lead electrode positions and the chest lead electrode positions can be viewed as sample sites in our effort to identify the characteristics of the electrical field created by the heart. A paradigm for this might be a Gallop poll that is made prior to an election in an effort to decide who will be the winner of a national political contest. Gallop statisticians determine how many sample sites are needed and where in the country the samples should be taken. For the most part, a Gallop poll is remarkably accurate. The same is true for the 12 conventional electrode positions—they are excellent sample sites and can be used to calculate the series of electrical fields that occur during each heart cycle.

Thus far the discussion has dealt predominantly with the background information required to understand the electrical forces of the heart and how to measure them. Much more detail regarding the identification of the heart rate and rhythm, as well as the normal and abnormal atrial and ventricular electrocardiograms, is provided in the subsequent sections.

CARDIAC RHYTHM, RATE, AND CONDUCTION ABNORMALITIES

The usual cardiac arrhythmia is not complex and is commonly identified on the routine 12-lead electrocardiogram. However, it is useful to have a 12-lead electrocardiogram *and* a long rhythm strip recorded on lead II in order to decipher the more complex cardiac arrhythmias. At times, an observer should request a long rhythm strip recorded on the lead that he or she believes, from examining the 12 routine leads, will reveal the P waves more readily.

The following steps are used to identify the heart rhythm, the atrial and ventricular rates, and conduction abnormalities:

- *Identify the P waves, QRS complexes, and T waves.* Determine if each QRS complex is preceded by a P wave and if the RR intervals are consistently the same.
- *The heart rate should be determined.* It is possible to estimate the ventricular rate per minute by dividing 300 by the number of large squares, and increments of

Table 7-1 Relation between cycle length and minute heart rate

1	2	1	2	1	2
77.5	77.5	56	107	34	176
77	78	55	109	33	182
76	79	54	111	32	187
75	80	53	113	31	193
74	81	52	115	30	200
73	82	51	117.5	29	207
72	83	50	120	28	214
71	84.5	49	122.5	27	222
70	86	48	125	26	230
69	87	47	127.5	25	240
68	88	46	130	24	250
67	89.5	45	133	23	261
66	91	44	136	22	273
65	92.5	43	139	21	286
64	94	42	143	20	300
63	95	41	146	19	316
62	97	40	150	18	333
61	98.5	39	154	17	353
60	100	38	158	16	375
59	101.5	37	162	15	400
58	103	36	166.5	14	428
57	105	35	171.5	13	461

From Ashman R, Hull E: *Essentials of electrocardiography*, ed 2, New York, 1941, Macmillan, p 346. The copyright was transferred to the authors in 1956. The authors are deceased.

large squares, that are contained within one RR interval. If more precision is needed, the length of the RR interval can be matched with the heart rate in a table created for this purpose (Table 7-1).

When there is normal rhythm, a P wave precedes each QRS complex. The normal ventricular rate is 60 to 90 depolarizations each minute. A rate below 60 that originates in the sinus node is called *sinus bradycardia;* a rate above 90 that originates in the sinus node is called *sinus tachycardia.*

• *The PR interval should be measured.* The duration of the PR interval should be the same before each QRS complex in the normal subject. It is more accurate to measure the PQ interval, because when the PR interval is measured, the observer may include an isoelectric portion of the QRS complex in the computation. This may erroneously prolong the interval by 0.02 to 0.04 second. The duration of the PR interval of a normal adult is less than 0.20 second. The PR interval is influenced by the heart rate. Table 7-2 indicates the normal PR interval that is associated with various RR intervals. As stated earlier, the RR interval is used to determine the heart rate. A consistently long PR interval does not produce an arrhythmia. The condition is a conduction abnormality in which the QRS complex does not follow the P wave within the expected normal amount of time. An abnormally long PR interval indicates that the electrical impulse does not traverse the atrioventricular node, bundle branches, and Purkinje branches in the normal amount of time. The condition is referred to as 1-degree atrioventricular block. More advanced degrees of atrioventricular block, and the arrhythmias they produce, are discussed later.

Atrioventricular block may be caused by digitalis medication, myocarditis, cardiomyopathy, coronary disease, "degenerative" disease of the atrioventricular node, or endocarditis of the aortic valve with valve ring abscess.

• *Identify the duration of the QRS complex.* Conduction abnormalities within the ventricles manifest themselves as abnormalities of the QRS complex. The abnormalities are commonly associated with ventricular disease and are discussed later. The QRS complex may also be altered when the arrhythmogenic focus is

Table 7-2 Upper limits of the normal PR intervals

Rate	Below 70	71-90	91-110	111-130	Above 130
Large adults	0.21	0.20	0.19	0.18	0.17
Small adults	0.20	0.19	0.18	0.17	0.16
Children ages 14-17	0.19	0.18	0.17	0.16	0.15
Children ages 7-13	0.18	0.17	0.16	0.15	0.14
Children ages 1½ to 6	0.17	0.165	0.155	0.145	0.135
Children ages 0 to 1½	0.16	0.15	0.145	0.135	0.125

From Ashman R, Hull E: *Essentials of electrocardiography,* ed 2, New York, 1941, Macmillan, p 341. The copyright was transferred to the authors in 1956. The authors are deceased.

located in the ventricles, such as occurs when there is complete heart block or ventricular tachycardia. It is now customary to speak in terms of a wide–QRS complex tachycardia or a narrow–QRS complex tachycardia.

A *wide–QRS complex tachycardia* may be due to ventricular tachycardia, supraventricular tachycardia with aberrant conduction of the QRS complex, supraventricular tachycardia with preexistent bundle-branch block, or supraventricular tachycardia in a patient with preexcitation of the ventricles such as occurs with Wolff-Parkinson-White syndrome. Wolff-Parkinson-White syndrome is characterized by a short PR interval, a delta wave, and episodes of atrial tachycardia or atrial fibrillation.

A *narrow–QRS complex tachycardia* is usually due to supraventricular tachycardia but may, on rare occasion, be due to ventricular tachycardia.[15] In such cases the arrhythmogenic focus is located in the septum.

Table 7-3   Normal QT intervals and the upper limits of normal

Cycle lengths (sec)	Heart rate (per min)	Men and children (sec)	Women (sec)	Upper limits of normal Men and children (sec)	Upper limits of normal Women (sec)
1.50	40	0.449	0.461	0.491	0.503
1.40	43	0.438	0.450	0.479	0.491
1.30	46	0.426	0.438	0.466	0.478
1.25	48	0.420	0.432	0.460	0.471
1.20	50	0.414	0.425	0.453	0.464
1.15	52	0.407	0.418	0.445	0.456
1.10	54.5	0.400	0.411	0.438	0.449
1.05	57	0.393	0.404	0.430	0.441
1.00	60	0.386	0.396	0.422	0.432
0.95	63	0.378	0.388	0.413	0.423
0.90	66.5	0.370	0.380	0.404	0.414
0.85	70.5	0.361	0.371	0.395	0.405
0.80	75	0.352	0.362	0.384	0.394
0.75	80	0.342	0.352	0.374	0.384
0.70	86	0.332	0.341	0.363	0.372
0.65	92.5	0.321	0.330	0.351	0.360
0.60	100	0.310	0.318	0.338	0.347
0.55	109	0.297	0.305	0.325	0.333
0.50	120	0.283	0.291	0.310	0.317
0.45	133	0.268	0.276	0.294	0.301
0.40	150	0.252	0.258	0.275	0.282
0.35	172	0.234	0.240	0.255	0.262

From Ashman R, Hull E: *Essentials of electrocardiography*, ed 2, New York, 1941, *Macmillan*, p 344. The copyright was transferred to the authors in 1956. The authors are deceased.

The QRS duration in a normal adult is usually about 0.08 to 0.10 second. The QRS duration is, of course, much shorter in infants (0.05 to 0.06 second).

- *The QT interval should be measured.* The QT interval varies with the heart rate. It is usually about 0.36 second when the rhythm is normal. The QT interval can be looked up in a table created for that purpose (Table 7-3). Short and long QT intervals are discussed in the section dealing with the ventricular electrocardiogram.

  A long QT interval may occur in patients with coronary disease, myocardial disease, or congenital prolongation of the QT interval[16-18] and may be caused by drugs such as quinidine and electrolyte abnormalities (see later discussion). A short QT interval is produced by digitalis medication and hypercalcemia associated with hyperparathyroidism.

- *Determine the possible causes of the arrhythmia or conduction abnormality and its seriousness.* Each time an abnormal rhythm or conduction abnormality is identified, it is necessary for the physician to think in terms of the clinical conditions that might cause it and to consider the seriousness of the abnormality.

Examples of common arrhythmias

The following examples of cardiac arrhythmias (Figs. 7-17 through 7-52) have been chosen because they are common. The legends of the figures emphasize certain basic principles that are used to interpret cardiac arrhythmias. The reader is referred to books devoted solely to arrhythmias for a more detailed discussion of complex cardiac rhythm abnormalities.

Text continued on p. 238.

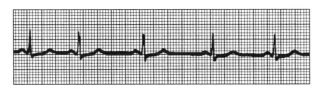

Fig. 7-17. Sinus arrhythmia. There is a normal sinus node mechanism of impulse formation, normal atrioventricular conduction, and normal ventricular response. In this tracing there is a variation in the rate of sinus node impulse formation that is greater than 0.12 second between the longest and shortest cycles (longest cycle = 0.97 second; shortest cycle = 0.70 second; therefore the variation = 0.27 second). The lack of variation in P wave morphology and in the PR interval differentiates sinus arrhythmia from a wandering atrial pacemaker.

From Hurst JW, Myerburg RJ: *Introduction to electrocardiography,* ed 2, New York, 1932, McGraw-Hill, p 232. The copyright has been transferred from the publisher to me.

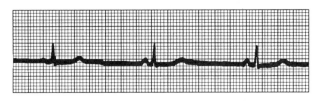

Fig. 7-18. Sinus bradycardia. The rhythm is regular, the mechanism is of normal sinus origin, and the rate is less than 60 ventricular depolarizations per minute. In this tracing the PP and RR intervals are 1.31 seconds; the rate therefore is 46 ventricular depolarizations per minute. The small "wave" after the first T wave is an artifact. An RR interval of 1 second represents a rate of exactly 60 depolarizations per minute; thus an interval greater than 1 second indicates a rate of less than 60 per minute.

From Hurst JW, Myerburg RJ: *Introduction to electrocardiography*, ed 2, New York, 1973, McGraw-Hill, p 236. The copyright has been transferred from the publisher to me.

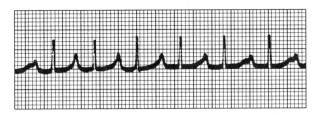

Fig. 7-19. Sinus tachycardia. The rhythm is usually regular, the mechanism is of normal sinus origin, and the rate is more than 90 depolarizations per minute. In this tracing the first, sixth, and seventh P waves can be distinguished from the preceding T waves. P waves are not ordinarily obscured by T waves at this rate (133 ventricular depolarizations per minute); however, in this case first-degree heart block (prolonged PR interval) is responsible for the obscured P waves. Slight rhythmic variation in the rate of a supraventricular tachycardia tends to favor the diagnosis of sinus tachycardia, rather than paroxysmal atrial tachycardia or atrial flutter. The rate variation in atrial fibrillation is usually erratic, rather than rhythmic.

From Hurst JW, Myerburg RJ: *Introduction to electrocardiography*, ed 2, New York, 1973, McGraw-Hill, p 238. The copyright has been transferred from the publisher to me.

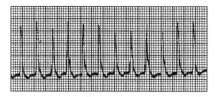

Fig. 7-20. Paroxysmal supraventricular tachycardia. A short strip of an electrocardiogram obtained during an attack of paroxysmal supraventricular tachycardia demonstrates a heart rate of 222 depolarizations per minute (RR interval = 0.27 second). The P waves cannot be discerned because of the extremely rapid rate. The duration of the QRS complex is normal.

From Hurst JW, Myerburg RJ: *Introduction to electrocardiography*, ed 2, New York, 1973, McGraw-Hill, p 239. The copyright has been transferred from the publisher to me.

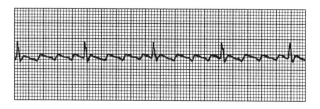

Fig. 7-21. Atrial flutter with 4:1 atrioventricular conduction. The duration of the QRS complex is normal. Typical sawtooth flutter waves and the high degree of atrioventricular block with consequent paucity of the QRS complexes make the flutter pattern easy to recognize. The atrial flutter rate is 260 per minute (PP interval = 0.23 second), and the rate of ventricular depolarization is 65 per minute (RR interval = 0.92 second). Only one of each of the four flutter waves is conducted through the atrioventricular junction to depolarize the ventricles; hence the term *4:1 atrioventricular conduction.*

From Hurst JW, Myerburg RJ: *Introduction to electrocardiography,* ed 2, New York, 1973, McGraw-Hill, p 240. The copyright has been transferred from the publisher to me.

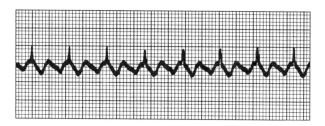

Fig. 7-22. Atrial flutter with 2:1 atrioventricular conduction. The duration of the QRS complex is normal. The atrial flutter rate is 272 per minute (PP interval = 0.22 second), and the ventricular rate is 136 ventricular depolarizations per minute (RR interval = 0.44 second). Sawtooth flutter waves may be less obvious in the presence of the more rapid ventricular response.

From Hurst JW, Myerburg RJ: *Introduction to electrocardiography,* ed 2, New York, 1973, McGraw-Hill, p 241. The copyright has been transferred from the publisher to me.

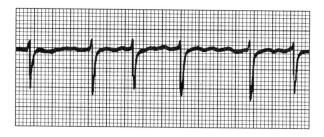

Fig. 7-23. Atrial fibrillation. The duration of the QRS complex is normal. There is a grossly irregular ventricular response, with RR intervals varying from 0.76 to 0.45 second. The baseline shows fibrillatory wave activity with some variation in the depth of the waves.

From Hurst JW, Myerburg RJ: *Introduction to electrocardiography,* ed 2, New York, 1973, McGraw-Hill, p 242. The copyright has been transferred from the publisher to me.

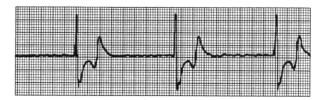

Fig. 7-24. Atrial fibrillation with complete heart block. The baseline demonstrates fine atrial fibrillation. The duration of the QRS complex is 0.12 second. However, instead of the expected gross irregularity and normal or rapid heart rate, the ventricular response is slow (36 per minute) and perfectly regular. The precise location of the ventricular pacemaker was difficult to determine in this case. Atrial fibrillation with a slow and regular ventricular response indicates the presence of a high degree of atrioventricular block, which may be either pathologic or drug induced.

From Hurst JW, Myerburg RJ: *Introduction to electrocardiography*, ed 2, New York, 1973, McGraw-Hill, p 243. The copyright has been transferred from the publisher to me.

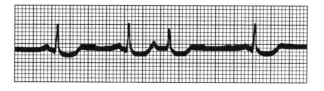

Fig. 7-25. Premature atrial depolarizations. The third QRS complex arrives early; the configuration of the complex is almost the same as that of the other complexes. The duration of the QRS complex is normal. The differential diagnosis lies between premature atrial depolarization and premature atrioventricular nodal depolarization. There is an abrupt upward deflection at the end of the T wave of the complex preceding the premature QRS complex. This deflection is not present in the T waves of the other complexes on the tracing and represents the superimposed P wave of the premature atrial depolarization. The pause following the premature QRS complex is noncompensatory (less than two full-cycle lengths), which is characteristic of premature atrial depolarizations. The PR interval of the premature complex is prolonged because of residual refractoriness in parts of the atrioventricular conduction system at the time of the early atrial depolarization.

From Hurst JW, Myerburg RJ: *Introduction to electrocardiography*, ed 2, New York, 1973, McGraw-Hill, p 245. The copyright has been transferred from the publisher to me.

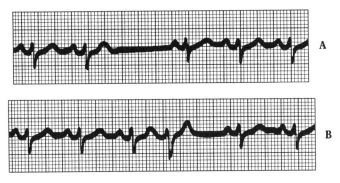

Fig. 7-26. Premature atrial depolarizations, conducted and nonconducted. **A,** The T wave of the second QRS complex on the tracing is slightly deformed by the P wave of the premature atrial depolarization. The premature atrial depolarization is not conducted to the ventricles; thus there is no QRS complex following it. **B,** The fourth atrial depolarization is premature and alters the shape of the T wave. It is conducted, but the QRS complex shows slight aberration of ventricular conduction. There is a P wave in the fourth T wave (note the difference in shape as compared with the other T waves). This P wave is not conducted.

From Hurst JW, Myerburg RJ: *Introduction to electrocardiography*, ed 2, New York, 1973, McGraw-Hill, p 246. The copyright has been transferred from the publisher to me.

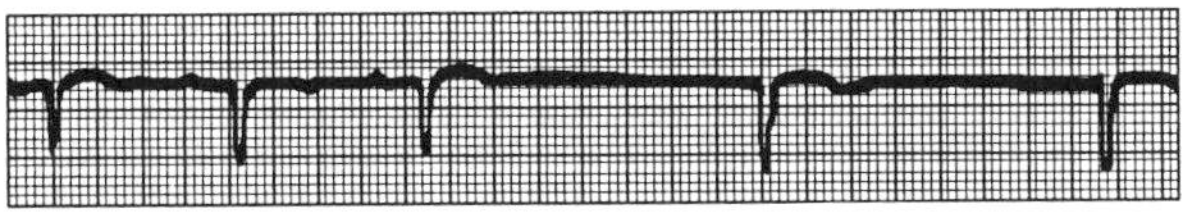

Fig. 7-27. Sinus pause or arrest with junctional escape. The first three complexes show normal sinus rhythm. The duration of the QRS complex is normal. A long pause (1.54 seconds) follows the third complex and is terminated by an escape beat. The junction escaped several times before a normal sinus mechanism returned. The escape QRS complexes have the same QRS configuration as the sinus beats.

From Hurst JW, Myerburg RJ: *Introduction to electrocardiography*, ed 2, New York, 1973, McGraw-Hill, p 249. The copyright has been transferred from the publisher to me.

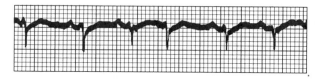

Fig. 7-28. Junctional premature depolarizations. The duration of the QRS complex is normal. The fourth depolarization is premature. This depolarization occurs early and has the same configuration as the QRS complexes of the sinus beats. In addition, the premature depolarization is preceded by an inverted P wave beginning 0.04 second before the QRS complex. Since the PR interval is less than 0.12 second, it may be concluded that the P waves are conducted retrograde from the focus of the junctional pacemaker. Since the P wave precedes the QRS complex, the site of the pacemaker is probably high in the atrioventricular junction. The PR intervals of the sinus impulses are constant at 0.14 second, and the premature junctional beats are followed by a fully compensatory pause.

From Hurst JW, Myerburg RJ: *Introduction to electrocardiography*, ed 2, New York, 1973, McGraw-Hill, p 251. The copyright has been transferred from the publisher to me.

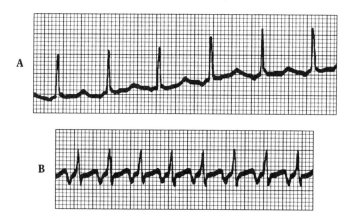

Fig. 7-29. Junctional tachycardia. **A,** The duration of the QRS complex is normal. A relatively slow junctional tachycardia is demonstrated, the rate being approximately 111 ventricular depolarizations per minute. The rhythm is perfectly regular. Since the lead is standard lead II and each QRS complex is preceded by an inverted P wave with a PR interval of 0.09 second, the assumption may be made that retrograde activation of the atria from the junctional pacemaker is occurring. **B,** A rapid junctional tachycardia is shown. The duration of the QRS complex is normal. The rhythm is perfectly regular, and the rate is about 182 ventricular depolarizations per minute. Lead II is shown here, and the QRS complexes are preceded by inverted P waves with a PR interval of 0.10 second, indicating retrograde atrial activation from the junctional pacemaker.

From Hurst JW, Myerburg RJ: *Introduction to electrocardiography*, ed 2, New York, 1973, McGraw-Hill, p 256. The copyright has been transferred from the publisher to me.

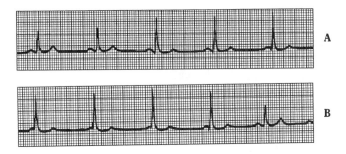

Fig. 7-30. Atrioventricular dissociation due to sinus bradycardia and junctional escape. **A,** The first two complexes are initiated in the sinus node. The atrioventricular conduction is normal. The duration of the QRS complex is normal. The heart rate is just below 60 depolarizations per minute. The third depolarization is a junctional escape beat with a slightly different QRS morphology and shorter interval between the onset of the P wave and the onset of the QRS complex than the preceding depolarizations. **B,** The sinus node rate slows a little more during the next few cycles, and the junctional escape rate remains relatively constant, perpetuating the atrioventricular dissociation. As the sinus node rate increases, the P waves emerge from the QRS complexes and finally recapture the ventricles (last complex). The atrial (higher) pacemaker is slower than the junctional (lower) pacemaker during the period of dissociation, permitting the atrioventricular dissociation to occur.

From Hurst JW, Myerburg RJ: *Introduction to electrocardiography,* ed 2, New York, 1973, McGraw-Hill, p 257. The copyright has been transferred from the publisher to me.

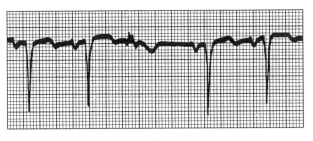

Fig. 7-31. Premature ventricular depolarizations. There is normal sinus rhythm. The third QRS complex occurs early and has a markedly different configuration from that of the normal QRS complexes. It has a QRS duration in excess of 0.12 second and is not preceded by a discernible P wave. It is followed by a full compensatory pause. These characteristics favor the diagnosis of a premature ventricular depolarization. Finally, it could be positively demonstrated in a longer rhythm strip that the sinus node cycle was not interrupted.

From Hurst JW, Myerburg RJ: *Introduction to electrocardiography,* ed 2, New York, 1973, McGraw-Hill, p 260. The copyright has been transferred from the publisher to me.

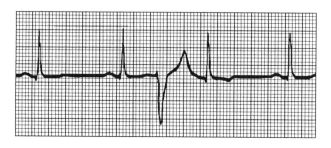

Fig. 7-32. Interpolated premature ventricular depolarization. The P waves and QRS complexes on the tracing are quite constant at a rate of about 60 depolarizations per minute. There is a wide, abnormally configured premature QRS complex located between the second and third sinus impulses, and the premature depolarization does not interrupt the sinus rhythm. The P wave of the fourth QRS complex (the one following the premature depolarization) is difficult to identify in the descending limb of the T wave of the premature depolarization, but its presence can be inferred from the fact that the QRS complex following the premature depolarization is normal in configuration and does not break the sinus cycle sequence. Finally, note the phenomenon of postextrasystolic T wave inversion in the first normal QRS complex following the premature depolarization.

From Hurst JW, Myerburg RJ: *Introduction to electrocardiography*, ed 2, New York, 1973, McGraw-Hill, p 262. The copyright has been transferred from the publisher to me.

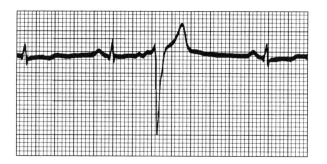

Fig. 7-33. Premature atrial impulse with aberrant ventricular conduction. The first two complexes on the tracing are produced by normal sinus impulses. The P waves, QRS complexes, and PR intervals are normal, and the rate is 67 depolarizations per minute. The T wave of the second complex is deformed by an abnormal, biphasic, early P wave, which is followed by a QRS complex of a distinctly abnormal configuration. Because of the presence of the premature P wave coupled to the abnormal QRS complex by a normal PR interval, the diagnosis of a premature atrial impulse with aberration of ventricular conduction may be made. This occurs because of refractiveness of parts of the atrioventricular junction at the time when the premature impulse arrives, causing an abnormal pathway of conduction. In the case of a premature atrioventricular junctional depolarization with aberrant conduction, the differentiation from premature ventricular depolarization may be more difficult or impossible, depending on the P wave relationship.

From Hurst JW, Myerburg RJ: *Introduction to electrocardiography*, ed 2, New York, 1973, McGraw-Hill, p 263. The copyright has been transferred from the publisher to me.

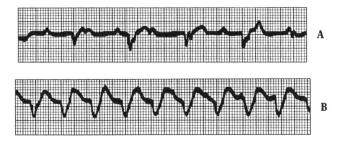

Fig. 7-34. Accelerated ventricular rhythm, ventricular tachycardia, and complete heart block. **A,** The duration of the QRS complex is 0.11 second. Atrioventricular dissociation is present, as manifested by the absence of any relationship between the P waves and QRS complexes and an idioventricular rhythm. The rate of the idioventricular rhythm, however, is much more rapid than the normal escape rate of a ventricular pacemaker (PR interval of basic rhythm = 0.86 second; rate = 70 depolarizations per minute). Therefore, even though the rate does not conform to the usual definition of tachycardia (rate = 100), it is abnormal for this pacemaker and is called an accelerated ventricular rhythm. **B,** Ventricular tachycardia with a rate of 136 depolarizations per minute (recorded from the same patient as in **A**). Complete heart block is present, and some of the P waves are easily seen. Since the PP intervals are quite constant, the presence of the other P waves is inferred. The P waves and QRS complexes are completely independent of each other because of the complete heart block.
From Hurst JW, Myerburg RJ: *Introduction to electrocardiography,* ed 2, New York, 1973, McGraw-Hill, p 265. The copyright has been transferred from the publisher to me.

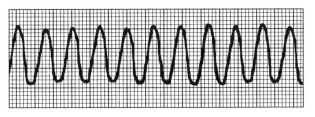

Fig. 7-35. Ventricular flutter. This rhythm forms a clinical bridge between ventricular tachycardia and ventricular fibrillation. There are very smooth, regular wave forms at a rate of 207 depolarizations per minute. The patient still had a cardiac output at the time of this event, but it was markedly reduced. This rhythm rarely lasts more than a few seconds to a minute, tending to progress rapidly to ventricular fibrillation or to revert to ventricular tachycardia or another rhythm.
From Hurst JW, Myerburg RJ: *Introduction to electrocardiography,* ed 2, New York, 1973, McGraw-Hill, p 267. The copyright has been transferred from the publisher to me.

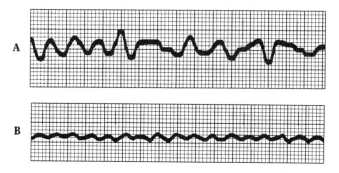

Fig. 7-36. Ventricular fibrillation. This rhythm is incompatible with life, since it represents uncoordinated ventricular activity with no cardiac output. It is, however, frequently treatable, with the success of treatment depending on the setting in which it occurs. **A,** Coarse ventricular fibrillation. Note the irregular wave form activity. **B,** Fine ventricular fibrillation. This type of pattern frequently precedes the complete cessation of electrical activity at the time of biologic death of the heart and is very difficult to defibrillate.

From Hurst JW, Myerburg RJ: *Introduction to electrocardiography*, ed 2, New York, 1973, McGraw-Hill, p 268. The copyright has been transferred from the publisher to me.

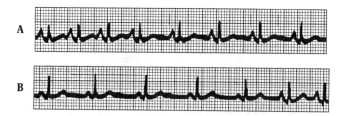

Fig. 7-37. Response of sinus tachycardia to carotid sinus pressure. **A,** Carotid sinus pressure was applied at the beginning of this rhythm strip, and the heart rate slowed progressively. **B,** When the carotid sinus pressure was discontinued during the time this tracing was recorded, the heart rate progressively increased until it reached the original rate of 136 depolarizations per minute. Note in the strip the shortening of the P waves and PR intervals as the rate decreases. They return to their original voltage and duration after the release of the carotid sinus pressure.

From Hurst JW, Myerburg RJ: *Introduction to electrocardiography*, ed 2, New York, 1973, McGraw-Hill, p 273. The copyright has been transferred from the publisher to me.

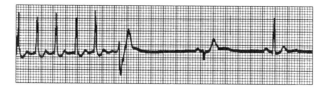

Fig. 7-38. Response of paroxysmal atrial tachycardia to carotid sinus pressure. This is a continuous tracing (lead II) recorded during a typical attack of paroxysmal atrial tachycardia in a 9-year-old girl without evidence of organic heart disease. The rate is over 200 ventricular depolarizations per minute, and P waves are not identifiable. The QRS duration and morphology are normal. The paroxysmal atrial tachycardia is terminated abruptly when carotid sinus pressure occurs. An extrasystole follows the last depolarization of the tachycardia and is followed by a pause terminated by a fusion beat (fusion between a conducted sinus impulse and an escape impulse). A normal sinus mechanism then resumes as seen in the rest of the rhythm strip.

From Hurst JW, Myerburg RJ: *Introduction to electrocardiography*, ed 2, New York, 1973, McGraw-Hill, p 275. The copyright has been transferred from the publisher to me.

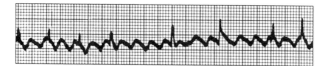

Fig. 7-39. Response of atrial flutter with 2:1 conduction to carotid sinus pressure. The effect of carotid sinus pressure in the presence of atrial flutter is demonstrated. Before the application of carotid pressure *(left portion of tracing)*, the interval between successive flutter waves is 0.22 second. The flutter rate speeds up slightly (interval is about 0.20 second) during the application of pressure. A decrease in atrioventricular node conduction is present with consequent temporary slowing of the ventricular response as a result of the increased vagal tone produced by carotid sinus pressure. The decrease in conduction is frequently a whole-number multiple of the basic flutter wave intervals. During the period of slower ventricular rate, the flutter pattern becomes more obvious.

From Hurst JW, Myerburg RJ: *Introduction to electrocardiography*, ed 2, New York, 1973, McGraw-Hill, p 276. The copyright has been transferred from the publisher to me.

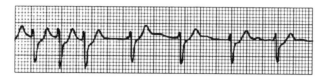

Fig. 7-40. Response of atrial fibrillation with a rapid ventricular response to carotid sinus pressure. Lead II was recorded in an attempt to make a diagnosis on this patient with tachycardia. The first three QRS complexes in the electrocardiogram demonstrate a rate of about 180 ventricular depolarizations per minute with slight irregularity. No P waves are visible, and atrial fibrillation with a rapid ventricular response was suspected. Carotid sinus massage was performed, and the ventricular rate slowed markedly, to the range of 90 to 100 depolarizations per minute. An irregular ventricular response and the absence of P waves can be seen in the strip during the period of the slower rate. Soon after the carotid sinus pressure was stopped, the ventricular rate returned to about 180 depolarizations per minute.

From Hurst JW, Myerburg RJ: *Introduction to electrocardiography*, ed 2, New York, 1973, McGraw-Hill, p 277. The copyright has been transferred from the publisher to me.

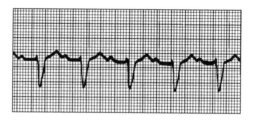

Fig. 7-41. First-degree atrioventricular block. The PR interval is constant and prolonged to 0.27 second. When the heart rate is rapid in the presence of first-degree atrioventricular heart block, the P waves may be buried in the T waves of the preceding complexes.

From Hurst JW, Myerburg RJ: *Introduction to electrocardiography*, ed 2, New York, 1973, McGraw-Hill, p 279. The copyright has been transferred from the publisher to me.

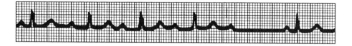

Fig. 7-42. Second-degree heart block, type I (Wenckebach phenomenon). The characteristics of the Wenckebach phenomenon are (1) progressively increasing PR intervals with (2) progressively decreasing RR intervals and (3) a pause due to a dropped ventricular depolarization, the pause being less than twice the length of the last RR interval (usually the shortest) in the period. The greatest increment in the PR interval occurs between the first and second complexes of any period, and the increment progressively decreases through the period. Thus in the first Wenckebach period in the electrocardiogram, the first PR interval is 0.20 second and the second PR interval is 0.30 second, giving an increment of $0.30 - 0.20 = 0.10$ second; the next increment is $0.33 - 0.30 = 0.03$ second; and the last increment is $0.35 - 0.33 = 0.02$ second. The RR intervals decrease from 0.92 to 0.84 second. The last RR interval before the pause should also decrease but does not do so in this case because of the presence of the concomitant sinus rate variation. The duration of the pause due to the dropped ventricular depolarization is 1.63 seconds, which is less than twice the RR interval of the last cycle of the period ($0.85 \times 2 = 1.70$).

From Hurst JW, Myerburg RJ: *Introduction to electrocardiography*, ed 2, New York, 1973, McGraw-Hill, p 280. The copyright has been transferred from the publisher to me.

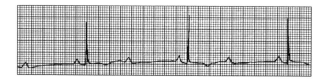

Fig. 7-43. Second-degree heart block, type II. The first, third, and fifth atrial depolarizations (P waves) are blocked. The second, fourth, and sixth atrial depolarizations are conducted with a normal PR interval. The patient has 2:1 atrioventricular block.

From Hurst JW, Myerburg RJ: *Introduction to electrocardiography*, ed 2, New York, 1973, McGraw-Hill, p 281. The copyright has been transferred from the publisher to me.

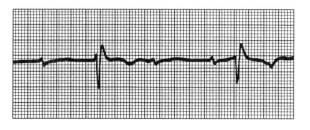

Fig. 7-44. Complete heart block. The duration of the QRS complex is 0.16 second. The ventricular rate is 32 depolarizations per minute, and the ventricular rhythm is regular. There is no fixed relationship between the P waves and QRS complexes. Some of the P waves fall within the QRS complexes or T waves and may be difficult to discern. A longer rhythm strip revealed some variation in the PP intervals. Note in this short strip that the P wave irregularity has a definite pattern; namely, the PP interval tends to be shorter when a QRS complex falls between the two P waves and tends to be longer when the two P waves fall between two QRS complexes. This phenomenon is called ventriculophasic sinus arrhythmia, a common finding in complete heart block with normal atrial activity.

From Hurst JW, Myerburg RJ: *Introduction to electrocardiography*, ed 2, New York, 1973, McGraw-Hill, p 282. The copyright has been transferred from the publisher to me.

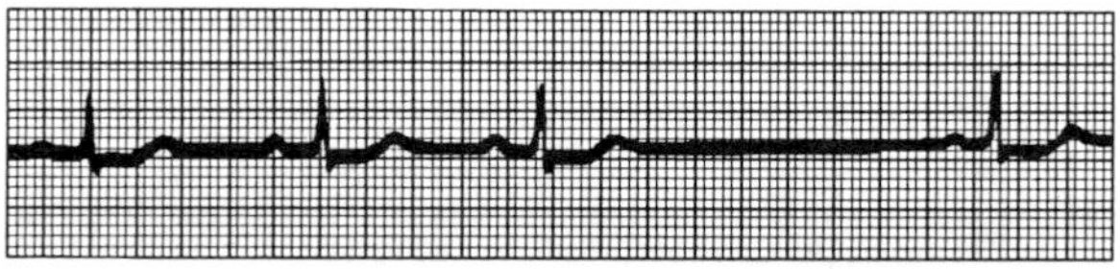

Fig. 7-45. Intermittent second-degree sinoatrial block (type II). The first three complexes on the tracing are normal sinus beats at a rate of approximately 60 ventricular depolarizations per minute. These are followed by a pause approximately equal to two cycle lengths. No P wave is seen during this pause. Since the pause is equal to two cycle lengths, it is inferred that the normal pacemaker function of the sinus node has not been interrupted and that the block, therefore, must have occurred between the sinus node and the atrial tissue (sinoatrial junction). A second pause was observed later in the rhythm strip. It was terminated by a junctional escape depolarization, because the pause was long enough to allow the escape of the intrinsic junctional pacemaker. The clue indicating the escape mechanism was the short PR interval of the escape depolarization, indicating that the atrioventricular node escaped before the atrial impulse could be conducted through the atrioventricular node.

From Hurst JW, Myerburg RJ: *Introduction to electrocardiography*, ed 2, New York, 1973, McGraw-Hill, p 287. The copyright has been transferred from the publisher to me.

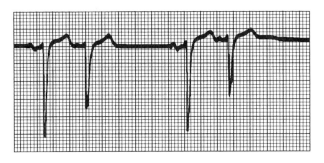

Fig. 7-46. Atrial bigeminy. The first and third P-QRS complexes on the tracing are normal sinus depolarizations. Each is followed by a premature atrial depolarization, which is followed by slightly aberrant ventricular conduction, and there is a pause after each premature depolarization. Therefore the characteristic feature is groups of two depolarizations—one normal and one premature—followed by a pause. The coupling interval—the interval between the sinus P wave and the ectopic P wave—is constant at 0.55 second. The pattern is designated as atrial bigeminy because the coupled ectopic beats are atrial in origin.

From Hurst JW, Myerburg RJ: *Introduction to electrocardiography*, ed 2, New York, 1973, McGraw-Hill, p 289. The copyright has been transferred from the publisher to me.

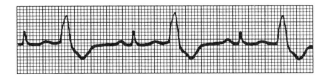

Fig. 7-47. Ventricular bigeminy. The first, third, and fifth complexes on the electrocardiogram are normal sinus depolarizations. Each of these is followed by an ectopic ventricular depolarization of abnormal configuration and a QRS complex prolongation beyond 0.12 second. No P waves precede these ectopic beats. (NOTE: The positive deflections preceding the ectopic beats are the T waves of the preceding sinus depolarizations.) The ectopic depolarizations are coupled to the preceding sinus depolarizations by a fixed coupling interval of 0.48 second, as measured from the onset of the sinus-induced QRS to the onset of the ectopic QRS. A pause then occurs; therefore the depolarizations are occurring in groups of two (bigeminy). Because the ectopic ventricular depolarizations fulfill the criteria for ventricular ectopic depolarizations, and because the pattern occurs in groups of two depolarizations, the rhythm is called ventricular bigeminy.

From Hurst JW, Myerburg RJ: *Introduction to electrocardiography*, ed 2, New York, 1973, McGraw-Hill, p 290. The copyright has been transferred from the publisher to me.

Fig. 7-48. Reciprocal depolarizations. The last depolarization of ventricular origin on this tracing (fourth QRS complex) is followed by an inverted P wave (at the end of the T wave). The inverted P wave is then coupled to a normal QRS complex by a PR interval of about 0.22 second. The impulse originates in the ventricles and is conducted retrogradely through the atrioventricular junction. It then depolarizes the atria retrogradely and reenters the atrioventricular junction to discharge the ventricles again.

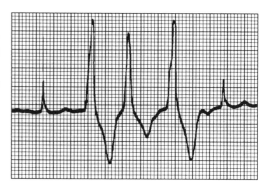

From Hurst JW, Myerburg RJ: *Introduction to electrocardiography*, ed 2, New York, 1973, McGraw-Hill, p 299. The copyright has been transferred from the publisher to me.

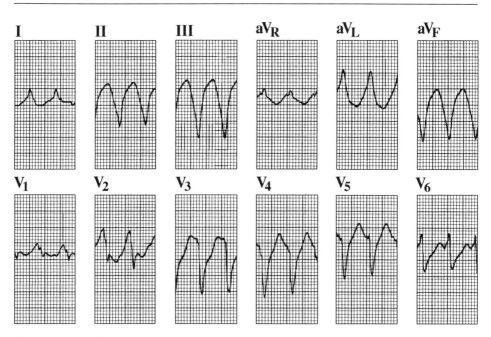

Fig. 7-49. Ventricular tachycardia (proved with electrophysiologic studies; recorded from a patient with idiopathic dilated cardiomyopathy). It is not always possible to identify ventricular tachycardia by examining a surface electrocardiogram, since there are many other causes of a wide–QRS complex tachycardia. For example, a patient with sinus tachycardia or supraventricular tachycardia who has right bundle-branch block, left bundle-branch block, or preexcitation of the ventricles may have an electrocardiogram that simulates ventricular tachycardia. In addition, a patient with supraventricular tachycardia may develop aberrant ventricular conduction, and the abnormal QRS complexes may mimic ventricular tachycardia. Most troublesome of all is that a narrow QRS complex tachycardia may occasionally be ventricular in origin; the impulse originates in the upper portion of the septum (see Fig. 7-51). The following points should be made regarding ventricular tachycardia:

- When the duration of the QRS complex is 0.14 second or more with a right bundle-branch block pattern, or greater than 0.16 second with a left bundle-branch block pattern, the diagnosis is usually ventricular tachycardia. When the QRS duration is 0.12 second during an episode of tachycardia in a patient whose QRS complex was normal prior to the episode, supraventricular tachycardia with ventricular aberrancy or ventricular tachycardia may be the cause. Ventricular tachycardia may be present when the QRS duration is only 0.11 second; this, however, is uncommon (see Fig. 7-51).
- The ventricular rate of ventricular tachycardia is usually about 150 to 200 depolarizations per minute; however, it may be above 200. A ventricular rate of less than 100 depolarizations per minute is called accelerated ventricular rhythm. The ventricular rate cannot be used to distinguish supraventricular tachycardia with aberrancy from ventricular tachycardia.
- The rhythm of ventricular tachycardia is usually regular when the tachycardia is sustained. The rhythm may be slightly irregular when the ventricular tachycardia is not sustained and may be difficult to distinguish from atrial fibrillation with aberrant ventricular conduction.
- When the P waves are easily seen and have no relationship to the abnormally wide QRS complexes, ventricular tachycardia is present. When inverted P waves follow the QRS complexes, they are considered to be retrograde P waves; this may occur in ventricular tachycardia. Unfortunately, it is not always possible to identify the P waves with certainty.
- Tachycardia that is preceded by a fusion beat is usually due to ventricular tachycardia.
- The shape of the QRS complex provides perhaps the most important means of distinguishing ventricular tachycardia from supraventricular tachycardia with aberrant ventricular conduction: the QRS complex recorded at electrode position V_1 has a larger R wave than the R$'$ wave when there is ventricular tachycardia, whereas a small initial R wave followed by a larger R$'$ wave indicates supraventricular tacycardia with aberrant conduction. When the QRS deflection recorded at each of the precordial electrode positions is negative or positive, the rhythm is usually ventricular tachycardia.
- Physical signs of ventricular tachycardia include a first heart sound that may vary in intensity from beat to beat because the relationship of atrial contraction to ventricular contraction varies from beat to beat. This sign is not present when atrial fibrillation occurs in conjunction with ventricular tachycardia. Also, the pulsation of the internal jugular veins may be erratic, because the right atrium may occasionally contract against a closed tricuspid valve in patients with ventricular tachycardia.
- Based on the clinical setting, a patient with a fresh myocardial infarct is more likely to have ventricular tachycardia than supraventricular tachycardia with aberrant ventricular conduction, whereas a young woman who has no other apparent cardiac disease is more likely to have supraventricular tachycardia with aberrant ventricular conduction than ventricular tachycardia.
- Accelerated ventricular rhythm is usually not as serious as ventricular tachycardia but is occasionally the forerunner of more serious ventricular arrhythmias.
- Bidirectional ventricular tachycardia is usually due to digitalis intoxication.
- When the rhythm cannot be identified with certainty, it should be managed as ventricular tachycardia.
- If the rhythm is believed to be supraventricular tachycardia with ventricular aberrancy, adenosine should be administered. Verapamil should be avoided for treatment of a wide-complex tachycardia.

Courtesy Sina Zaim, M.D., Emory University School of Medicine, Atlanta, Ga.

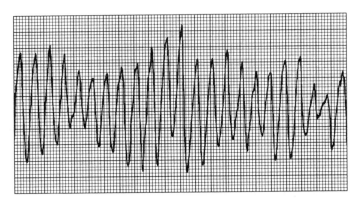

Fig. 7-50. Ventricular tachycardia showing torsades de pointes. The words *torsades de pointes* mean "turning on a point." This rhythm occurred in this 48-year-old man several days after coronary bypass surgery. He probably had an intraoperative myocardial infarction.

Courtesy Sina Zaim, M.D., Emory University School of Medicine, Atlanta, Ga.

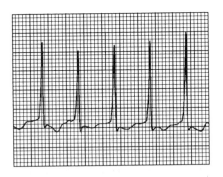

Fig. 7-51. Narrow-complex ventricular tachycardia (only lead V_6 is shown). There are 150 ventricular depolarizations per minute. The QRS duration is 0.08 second. P waves cannot be identified with certainty. This patient had inferior infarction due to total obstruction of the right coronary artery and episodes of rapid heart beat that were proved by electrophysiologic testing to be narrow-complex ventricular tachycardia.

Courtesy Steve Clements, M.D., and Sina Zaim, M.D., Emory University School of Medicine, Atlanta, Ga.

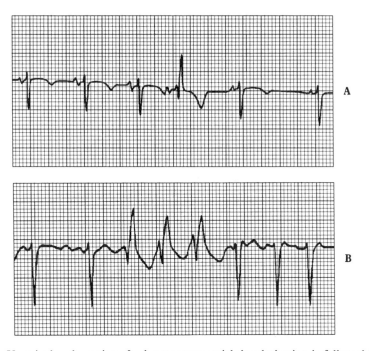

Fig. 7-52. Ventricular aberration. **A,** A premature atrial depolarization is followed by a ventricular depolarization that has a different shape than the preceding ventricular complexes. The shape is different because the electrical impulse occurs so early that a certain part of the ventricles is still refractory. Accordingly, the ventricles are depolarized in an aberrant manner. The altered QRS complex commonly simulates the complexes that are characteristic of right bundle-branch block. **B,** Ashman phenomenon is identified in patients with atrial fibrillation. It is a special type of aberrant conduction. The refractory period of the ventricles is determined by the length of the RR interval. Stated another way, the refractory period adjusts to the heart rate. When the rate is slow, the refractory period is long; when the rate is rapid, the refractory period is short. The varying RR interval associated with atrial fibrillation causes varying refractory periods. Accordingly, whenever an impulse arrives early and follows a complex with a preceding long RR interval, it sets the stage for aberrant ventricular depolarization. Note here that the RR interval preceding the first aberrant complex is short and that it follows the long RR interval of the previous ventricular depolarization. The shape of the third, fourth, and fifth QRS complexes is altered because of aberrant conduction in the ventricles.

A from Stein E: *Electrocardiographic interpretation: a self-study approach to clinical electrocardiography*, Philadelphia, 1991, Lea & Febiger, p 609. Reprinted with permission. **B** from Fox W, Stein E: *Cardiac rhythm disturbances: a step-by-step approach*, Philadelphia, 1983, Lea & Febiger, p 179. Reprinted with permission.

DIAGNOSTIC OPTIONS WHEN THE ELECTROCARDIOGRAM IS NORMAL

The physician who engages in patient care uses the electrocardiogram as a diagnostic tool. Thus it must be emphasized that many patients with heart disease have normal electrocardiograms. Because of this, it seems wise to discuss the diagnostic options that should be considered when the electrocardiogram is normal before discussing the characteristics of the normal electrocardiogram.

When the electrocardiogram is normal, the physician should consider the following possibilities:
- The heart may actually be normal.
- Serious atherosclerotic coronary heart disease may be present even though the resting electrocardiogram is normal.
- The normal electrocardiogram may have been recorded from another patient if there is abundant evidence of severe cardiac valve disease or marked cardiac enlargement in the patient being examined.
- The patient could have mild aortic or mitral valve disease with the electrocardiogram remaining normal.
- Dilated, hypertrophic, or restrictive cardiomyopathy is unlikely when the electrocardiogram is normal.
- The normal electrocardiogram does not exclude pericardial disease.
- Chronic congestive heart failure is not likely to be present when the electrocardiogram is normal, because heart failure occurs in patients with severe heart disease due to valve disease or cardiomyopathy, which is more likely to be associated with an abnormal electrocardiogram. A common exception to this rule is that diastolic cardiac dysfunction due to coronary disease is often associated with a normal electrocardiogram.
- Congenital heart disease such as atrial septal defect, pulmonary valve stenosis, tetralogy of Fallot, tricuspid atresia, transposition of the great arteries, or Ebstein anomaly, as well as many other types of complex congenital heart disease, is unlikely to be present when the electrocardiogram is normal. However, the electrocardiogram may be normal in patients with a small patent ductus arteriosus, a small interventricular defect, mild bicuspid aortic valve stenosis, or coarctation of the aorta.
- The patient may have attacks of cardiac arrhythmia with the electrocardiogram returning to normal between attacks.
- Preexcitation of the ventricles may not be present in every electrocardiogram that is recorded from a patient with preexcitation of the ventricles.

REPORT FORM

Note the headings in the legends of the electrocardiograms used to illustrate this text (beginning with Fig. 7-68). The headings are used for the following reasons. The completion of the report form used to communicate the electrocardiographic interpretation should engender a discipline that assures the interpreter that he or she has omitted nothing important. It should also demand the use of a thought process that encourages further development of the skill required to analyze electrocardiograms.

The report form should include four items:

- *Rhythm, rate, and intervals.* Measure and record the heart rhythm and rate, and the duration of the PR interval, QRS complex, and QT interval. A clinical differential diagnosis should be considered from these data.
- *Vector diagrams.* Diagram the arrows representing the mean of the electrical forces (vectors) responsible for the P waves, QRS complexes, ST segments, and T waves. When needed, arrows should be created that represent the mean of the electrical forces (vectors) responsible for the first half of the P wave, the second half of the P wave, and the initial 0.04 second and terminal 0.04 second of the QRS complexes. The interpreter should then judge whether the arrows are directed normally or abnormally and whether each arrow is related properly or improperly to the other arrows. The interpreter should, at this point, have a mental image of the conduction pathways, location of the cardiac chambers, depolarization sequence, and repolarization sequence in the normal heart and in the heart being studied.
- *Electrophysiologic considerations.* When the electrocardiogram is considered abnormal, the interpreter should create an electrophysiologic differential diagnosis to explain the abnormalities. This step is important, because it reminds the interpreter that there are usually several basic electrophysiologic causes for an abnormality and that none of the reasons should be forgotten.
- *Clinical differential diagnosis.* The final step in interpreting the electrocardiogram is to establish a clinical differential diagnosis. This is the goal of the entire endeavor and is accomplished by considering the data derived from the first three items.

CORRELATION OF APPROPRIATE DATA

The electrocardiographic interpretation should be correlated with the clinical data obtained from interpreting the abnormalities found in the history, physical examination, chest x-ray film, and routine examination of the blood and urine. Only the clinician who is responsible for the patient's care can make this correlation. Clinicians who correlate all of the data they collect become more confident in their diagnostic skills and learn more from each patient they examine.

ATRIAL ELECTROCARDIOGRAM

The atrial electrocardiogram is emphasized here because it is not generally appreciated that an alteration of P wave morphology is commonly associated with, and is often due to, disease of the ventricles. At times a P wave abnormality, when added to a minor or questionable abnormality of the QRS complex, may clarify a diagnostic problem.

Normal atrial electrocardiogram

Depolarization of the atria spreads through the atrial myocytes, guided by the three preferential conduction pathways, to reach the atrioventricular node. This produces the P wave.

Amplitude and duration of the normal P wave. The amplitude of the normal P wave is usually measured in lead II; it should be less than 3 mm in height. The duration of the normal P wave is less than 0.12 second (Fig. 7-53, *A*).

Direction of an arrow representing the mean of the electrical forces (vectors) responsible for the normal P wave. An arrow representing the mean of the electrical forces (vectors) responsible for the normal P wave is directed at about +50 to +70 degrees in the frontal plane. It is directed parallel with the frontal plane, or 10 to 15 degrees anteriorly or posteriorly (Fig. 7-53, *B*).

Direction of an arrow representing the mean of the electrical forces (vectors) responsible for the first half of the normal P wave. The first half of the normal P wave is produced by depolarization of the right atrium (Fig. 7-54, *A, 1*). An arrow representing the mean of the electrical forces (vectors) produced during the first half of the normal P wave is usually directed at about +60 to +70 degrees in the frontal plane (Fig. 7-54, *A, 2*). It is usually directed anteriorly about 15 degrees and is always anterior to an arrow representing the electrical forces (vectors) produced by normal left atrial depolarization.

Direction of an arrow representing the mean of the electrical forces (vectors) responsible for the second half of the normal P wave. The second half of the nor-

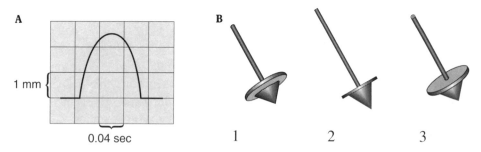

Fig. 7-53. Normal P wave. **A,** The amplitude of the P wave should be less than 3 mm; the duration should be less than 0.12 second. **B,** An arrow representing the mean of the electrical forces (vectors) responsible for the P wave may be directed at about +60 degrees in the frontal plane; it may be directed *(1)* 10 to 15 degrees anteriorly, *(2)* parallel with the frontal plane, or *(3)* 10 to 15 degrees posteriorly.

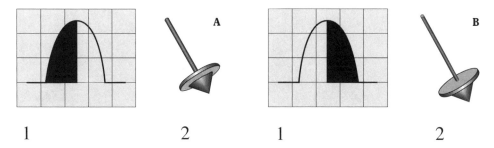

Fig. 7-54. **A,** First half of the P wave. *1,* The first half of the P wave is produced by depolarization of the right atrium. *2,* An arrow representing the mean of the electrical forces (vectors) responsible for the first half of the P wave is directed at about +60 to +70 degrees in the frontal plane; it is usually directed 10 to 15 degrees anteriorly. **B,** Last half of the P wave. *1,* The last half of the P wave is produced by depolarization of the left atrium. *2,* An arrow representing the mean of the electrical forces (vectors) responsible for the last half of the P wave is directed at about +50 to +70 degrees in the frontal plane; it is usually directed 10 to 15 degrees posteriorly.

mal P wave is produced by depolarization of the left atrium (Fig. 7-54, *B, 1*). An arrow representing the mean of the electrical forces (vectors) produced during the second half of the normal P wave is usually directed at +50 to +70 degrees in the frontal plane (Fig. 7-54, *B, 2*). When viewed in the frontal plane, the angle between an arrow representing the mean of the electrical forces (vectors) produced during the first half of the normal P wave and an arrow representing the mean of the electrical forces (vectors) produced during the second half of the normal P wave is usually 10 to 15 degrees or less. The arrow representing the mean of the electrical forces (vectors) produced during the second half of the normal P wave is always 10 to 15 degrees posterior to an arrow representing the mean of the electrical forces (vectors) produced during the first half of the P wave. The second half of the P wave recorded in lead V_1 is usually less than -0.03 mm/sec.[19,20] This measurement is made by multiplying the depth of the second half of the P wave times the width of the second half of the P wave (Fig. 7-55).

Ta wave. The repolarization process of the atria is called the Ta wave. An arrow representing the mean of the electrical forces (vectors) produced by repolarization of the atria is directed opposite to an arrow representing the mean of the electrical forces (vectors) produced by depolarization. The Ta wave is rarely seen. When it is seen, it may not be identified in a sufficient number of leads to enable one to diagram the spatial orientation of a vector that represents it. The normal Ta wave may occasionally be seen when the PR interval is long; this may simulate the abnormally displaced PQ segment associated with pericarditis (Fig. 7-56, *A*). The normal Ta wave may

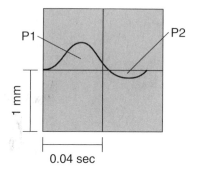

Fig. 7-55. Configuration of the P wave at electrode position V_1, according to Morris et al.[19] The first half of the P wave is usually upright (positive) when it is recorded at electrode position V_1. The last half of the P wave is usually recorded as a downward deflection (negative) when it is recorded at electrode position V_1. The normal size of the last half of the P wave can be determined by multiplying its duration by its depth. The normal measurement is about -0.03 mm/sec. In this illustration it is about 0.01 mm/sec.

Redrawn with permission from Hurst JW: *Ventricular electrocardiography*, New York, 1991, Gower, fig 5.5.

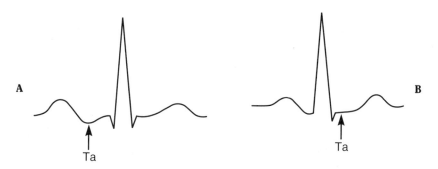

Fig. 7-56. Repolarization of the atria (Ta wave). **A,** The Ta wave due to atrial repolarization can be seen occasionally following the P wave. It is more likely to be seen when the PR interval is long or when P waves are unrelated to the QRS complex, as in patients with complete heart block. **B,** When the PR interval is short (in the range of 0.12 second), the Ta wave due to atrial repolarization may displace the ST segment downward. Such a displacement may become evident with the tachycardia associated with exercise; it may be misinterpreted as being an "ischemic" response to exercise.

Redrawn with permission from Hurst JW: *Ventricular electrocardiography*, New York, 1991, Gower, fig 5.6.

displace the ST segment after exercise in subjects with a short PR interval; this may simulate the ST segment displacement of subendocardial injury (Fig. 7-56, *B*).

VENTRICULAR ELECTROCARDIOGRAM

The QRS complexes and T waves are produced by depolarization and repolarization of the ventricular myocytes. The sequence of depolarization is determined by the unique arrangement of the conduction system and the anatomy of the ventricles and septum. As discussed later, the sequence of repolarization in normal subjects is predetermined by the sequence of depolarization.

The P waves, QRS complexes, and T waves are composed of an infinite number of sequentially generated electrical forces (vectors) that are directed either to the left or right, superiorly or inferiorly, and anteriorly or posteriorly. The contours of the deflections depend on the projection of the instantaneous electrical forces (vectors) onto specified lead axes. The creation of the QRS loop and its projection onto lead axes I, aV_F, V_1, and V_6 are shown in Fig. 7-57.

Normal QRS complex

Direction of the components of the normal QRS complex. The electrical forces (vectors) produced during the initial 0.01 to 0.02 second of the QRS complex are generated by depolarization of the left, posterosuperior portion of the ventricular septum. The septum is located anteriorly and is part of the left ventricle; it is, of course, posterior to the right ventricle. An arrow representing the mean of the electrical forces (vectors) responsible for this portion of the QRS complex is usually directed to the right, inferiorly, and slightly anteriorly (Fig. 7-58, *A*). This electrical force (vector) may, however, be directed anywhere in the frontal plane, because a slight anatomic change in the location of the septum may produce a marked change in the direction of the electrical forces (vectors) produced during this period of ventricular depolarization. Regardless of the frontal plane projection of the electrical forces (vectors) produced by depolarization of the left upper portion of the septum during the initial 0.01 to 0.02 second of the QRS complex, it is usually directed slightly anteriorly.

The electrical forces (vectors) produced by the ventricular myocytes during the next 0.02 to 0.04 second are generated by depolarization of the remaining portion of the septum and the endocardial portions of the left and right ventricles. An arrow representing the mean of these electrical forces (vectors) is directed inferiorly at about +60 degrees and is parallel with the frontal plane (Fig. 7-58, *B*).

The electrical forces (vectors) produced by the ventricular myocytes during the next 0.04 to 0.06 second are generated by depolarization of the outer layer of the right and left ventricles. An arrow representing the mean of these electrical forces (vectors) is directed inferiorly at about +50 degrees and slightly posteriorly (Fig. 7-58, *C*).

The electrical forces (vectors) produced by the ventricular myocytes during the next 0.06 to 0.08 second of the QRS complex are produced by the posterobasilar portion of the left ventricle. An arrow representing the mean of the electrical forces (vectors) produced by depolarization of this portion of the left ventricle is usually directed more toward the left and more posteriorly than any of the other electrical forces (vectors) (see darker arrow in Fig. 7-58, D). At times it may be directed superiorly, to the right, and posteriorly, because in some normal subjects the poster-

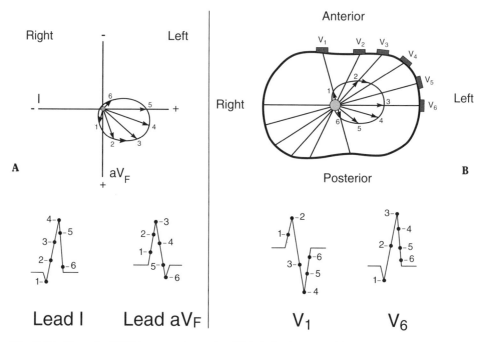

Fig. 7-57. How the QRS loop produces the QRS deflections. **A,** The upper diagram shows a QRS loop superimposed on lead axes I and aV$_F$. Note that the arrows representing the instantaneous electrical forces (vectors) are numbered from 1 to 6. The lower diagram shows the QRS deflections recorded in leads I and aV$_F$. Note how the arrows representing the instantaneous electrical forces (vectors) shown in the loop project onto the lead axes to produce the QRS deflections. The numbers on the QRS deflections correspond to the numbers assigned to the instantaneous electrical forces (vectors) shown in the upper diagram. **B,** The upper diagram shows the transverse view of the QRS loop shown in **A** as viewed from the feet. The six precordial lead axes are shown. The QRS loop and the arrows representing the six instantaneous electrical forces (vectors) are shown. The lower diagram shows the QRS deflections recorded in leads V$_1$ and V$_6$. Note how the arrows representing the instantaneous electrical forces (vectors) shown in the loop project onto the lead axes to produce the QRS deflections. The numbers on the QRS deflections correspond to the numbers assigned to the instantaneous electrical forces (vectors) shown in the upper diagram.

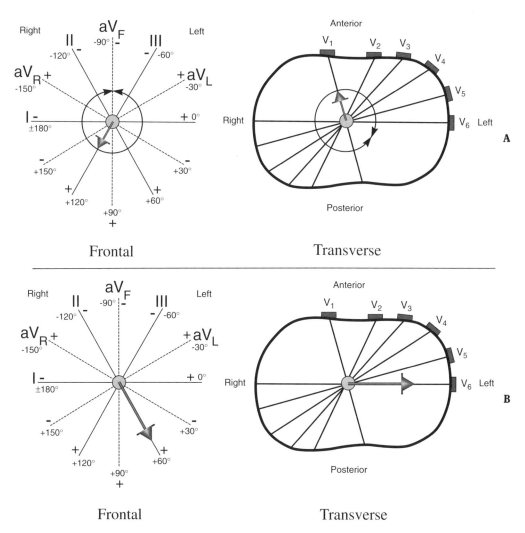

Fig. 7-58. Direction of the instantaneous QRS electrical forces (vectors) in three dimensions. **A,** The mean of the electrical forces (vectors) that are generated during the initial 0.01 to 0.02 second of the QRS complex is illustrated by the arrows shown here. The diagram on the left illustrates the direction of this vector in the frontal plane. The arrow indicates the usual direction of the electrical force (vector), and the circle implies that it can be directed anywhere within 360 degrees. The diagram on the right indicates the direction of this vector in the transverse plane. Here, too, the arrow indicates its usual direction, and the circle implies that it can be directed anywhere within 360 degrees. **B,** The mean of the electrical forces (vectors) that are generated during the 0.02 to 0.04 second of the QRS complex is illustrated by the arrows shown here. The diagram on the left illustrates the direction of this vector in the frontal plane. The diagram on the right illustrates the direction of this vector in the transverse plane. *Continued.*

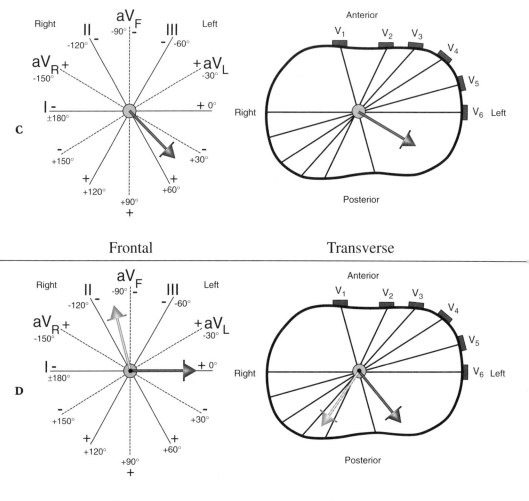

Frontal   Transverse

Frontal   Transverse

Fig. 7-58, cont'd. **C,** The mean of the electrical forces (vectors) that are generated during the 0.04 to 0.06 second of the QRS complex is illustrated by the arrows shown here. The diagram on the left illustrates the direction of this vector in the frontal plane. The diagram on the right illustrates the direction of this vector in the transverse plane. **D,** The mean of the electrical forces (vectors) that are generated during the 0.06 to 0.08 second (the terminal 0.02 second) of the QRS complex is illustrated by the arrows shown here. The diagram on the left illustrates the direction of this vector in the frontal plane. The diagram on the right illustrates the direction of this vector in the transverse plane. The dark arrows indicate the usual direction of the electrical force (vector), and the light arrows indicate the less common direction of the vector.

Redrawn from Grant RP: *Clinical electrocardiography*, New York, McGraw-Hill, 1957, p 49 (public domain).

obasilar portion of the left ventricle is located superiorly and to the right of the area designated as the location of the "origin" of electrical activity of the heart (see lighter arrow in Fig. 7-58, *D*).

Duration of the normal QRS complex. The duration of ventricular depolarization is determined by measuring from the beginning of the Q wave to the end of the S wave. Normally, the QRS duration is 0.08 to 0.09 second in adults. The duration of the QRS complex may be 0.06 second in the normal newborn.

Direction of an arrow representing the mean of the electrical forces (vectors) responsible for the QRS complex. Although the long anatomic axis of the left ventricle is directed to the left, inferiorly, and slightly anteriorly, an arrow representing the mean of the QRS electrical forces (vectors) is directed to the left, inferiorly, and posteriorly. An arrow representing the mean of the electrical forces (vectors) responsible for the entire QRS complex is directed slightly posteriorly, because the last portion of the left ventricle to depolarize is the posterobasilar portion of the left ventricle.[8] This occurs because the posteroinferior division of the left bundle-branch system directs the depolarization process posteriorly (Fig. 7-59).

The sequence in which the electrical forces (vectors) are produced by the left ventricular myocytes is controlled by the left anterosuperior division and the left posteroinferior division of the left bundle branch. During the last portion of the depolarization process the electrical forces (vectors) created by depolarization of the left ventricular myocytes that have been stimulated by electrical impulses transmitted by the left anterosuperior division are directed inferiorly, to the left, and parallel with, or slightly anterior to, the frontal plane. During almost the same time period the electrical forces (vectors) created by depolarization of the left ventricular myocytes that have been stimulated by electrical impulses transmitted by the left posteroinferior division are directed superiorly, to the left, and posteriorly. Many of the electrical forces created in this manner occur simultaneously, and the sum of the vectors determine the contour of the mean terminal 0.04 second portion of the QRS complex (Fig. 7-59, *A*). The very terminal portion of the QRS complex is, however, produced predominantly by electrical forces that are guided by the posteroinferior division of the left bundle branch. The direction of the arrow produced by the mean terminal 0.04 second vector is determined to some degree by the anatomic position of the heart. In all cases, however, it is directed posterior to the anatomic axis of the left ventricle. Accordingly, when the posterobasilar portion of the left ventricle is located superiorly, posteriorly, and at about −110 degrees, as it is occasionally, an arrow representing the mean of the electrical forces responsible for the terminal portion of the QRS complex may be directed superiorly at about −110 to −120 degrees and posteriorly (Fig. 7-59, *B*).

The sequence of depolarization described above applies to the normal *adult* subject. It must be remembered that the right ventricle of a *newborn* is thicker than the left ventricle and that the septum conforms to the shape of the right ventricle. Ac-

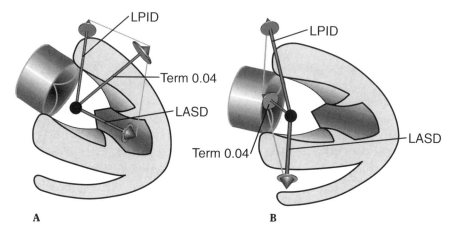

Fig. 7-59. Influence of the electrical forces (vectors) created by the ventricular myocytes stimulated by the left anterosuperior division *(LASD)* and the left posteroinferior division *(LIPD)* of the left bundle branch. This diagram, as well as all of the diagrams dealing with the conduction system, should be viewed as a teaching device only. The true picture of the effect of the electrical forces (vectors) created by the myocytes stimulated by the LASD and LPID of the left bundle branch is very complex. **A,** An intermediate position of the ventricles of the heart is shown in this illustration. Note the arrow representing the electrical forces (vectors) produced by the ventricular myocytes stimulated by the LASD of the left bundle branch. Also note the arrow representing the electrical forces (vectors) produced by the ventricular myocytes stimulated by the LPID of the left bundle branch. The vector sum of these two electrical forces is identified as the terminal 0.04 second QRS vector. It is directed horizontally to the left and posteriorly. This illustration shows why the electrical forces (vectors) responsible for the terminal portion of the QRS complex are directed to the left and posteriorly. **B,** A horizontal position of the heart is shown in this illustration. Note how this position influences the direction of the vectors. This explains why the terminal portion of the QRS complex of some hearts may be produced by electrical forces (vectors) that are directed superiorly, posteriorly, and at -110 to -120 degrees.

cordingly, the direction of an arrow representing the mean of the electrical forces (vectors) generated by depolarization of the ventricles is directed to the right and anteriorly. This represents normal right ventricular dominance of the newborn (Fig. 7-60, *A*). As the newborn ages, the left ventricle gradually gains anatomic dominance over the right ventricle as the pulmonary vascular resistance decreases and the systemic vascular resistance increases (Fig. 7-60, *A*). The normal adult exhibits normal left ventricular dominance. An arrow representing the mean of the electrical forces responsible for the entire QRS complex is usually directed inferiorly in tall individuals, in an intermediate position in individuals of average build, and horizontally in broad-chested individuals (Fig. 7-60, *B*). It is always directed slightly posteriorly in normal adults.

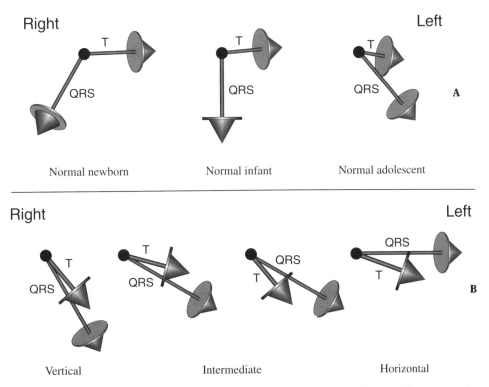

Fig. 7-60. Directions of arrows representing the mean QRS vector and mean T vector in, **A,** the normal newborn, normal infant, and normal adolescent, and, **B,** the normal adult. When the mean QRS vector in the normal adult is directed vertically, the mean T vector should be located to its left. When the mean QRS vector is directed intermediately, the mean T vector can be located to its right or left. When the mean QRS vector is directed horizontally, the mean T vector should be directed inferior to it. The normal QRS-T angle may be 60 degrees but is commonly 30 to 45 degrees or less. The mean T vector should always be anterior to the mean QRS vector.
Redrawn with permission from Hurst JW: *Ventricular electrocardiography*, New York, 1991, Gower, fig 5.9.

The first step in determining the direction of an arrow that represents the mean of the electrical forces (vectors) responsible for the QRS complex is to identify the smallest and largest deflections of the QRS complexes that are recorded in the six extremity leads.[2] This is accomplished by adding, in algebraic fashion, the area contained within each of the QRS complexes that is above the line (positive) to the area contained within the same QRS complex that is below the line (negative). The algebraic sum of these two areas is referred to as the resultant size of the complex. Errors will be made if the amplitude of the QRS complex is used. The mean electrical force (vector) can be represented as an arrow that is directed parallel to the extremity lead axis in which the resultantly largest deflection is recorded or perpendicular to the extremity lead axis in which the resultantly smallest deflection is recorded. The resultantly smallest deflection identified in the chest leads identifies the transitional pathway on the chest and is used to determine the posterior or anterior direction of the arrow representing the mean of the QRS forces (vectors). As discussed earlier, this is possible because the smallest deflection (or the deflection that is computed to be resultantly zero) is recorded from the edge of the zero potential plane that is perpendicular to the direction of the electrical forces (vectors) that produce it.

The frontal plane direction of an arrow representing the mean of the QRS forces (vectors) in normal adults is usually located from +110 to −30 degrees in the frontal plane (Fig. 7-61, A). It is more commonly directed between +30 and +60 degrees. It is rarely seen beyond +110 degrees to the right and −30 degrees to the left. The arrow representing the mean of the QRS forces (vectors) is usually directed 30 to 50

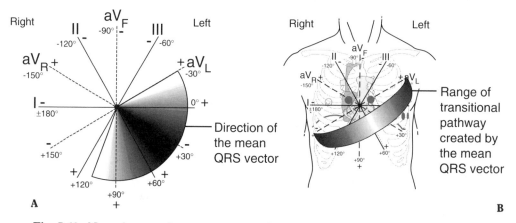

Fig. 7-61. Normal range of an arrow representing the mean of the electrical forces (vectors) responsible for the QRS complex in an adult. **A,** Although the mean QRS vector is usually directed inferiorly from +30 to +60 degrees, the vector can be directed to the right or left of this zone. The shaded areas represent the frequency distribution of the normal mean QRS vector. When an arrow representing the mean of the electrical forces (vectors) responsible for the QRS complex is directed more than +110 degrees to the right or −30 degrees to the left, the QRS complex is considered abnormal. **B,** The normal transitional pathway of an arrow representing the mean of the electrical forces (vectors) responsible for the QRS complex is located so that it passes through electrode position V$_3$ or V$_4$. The transitional pathway is produced when the zero potential plane, which is perpendicular to the direction of the mean QRS vector, is extended in all directions to intersect the surface of the chest, where it produces the transitional pathway. Accordingly, the normal mean QRS vector is directed 30 to 40 degrees posteriorly.

degrees posteriorly. The transitional QRS complex in the chest leads is usually located in lead V_3 or V_4 (Fig. 7-61, *B*).[21]

The shape of the chest influences how far posteriorly the arrow representing the mean of the QRS forces (vectors) is perceived to be directed. Note how, in a tall, thin person, the electrode sites V_2, V_3, and V_4 are located almost on a same vertical line, whereas in a broad-chested person the electrode positions V_2, V_3, and V_4 are located on a more horizontal line; this variance in chest size and shape will alter how many degrees posteriorly the arrow representing the mean of the QRS forces (vectors) is calculated to be (Fig. 7-62).

Some years ago it was common to hear a description of *axis deviation*. This term was used when referring to the QRS complexes only, and those who used it referred only to the frontal plane axis. It is more accurate to realize that each electrical force (vector) that composes the P wave, QRS complex, ST segment displacement, and T wave has an axis and that it is directed superiorly or inferiorly, to the left or right, and anteriorly or posteriorly. Accordingly, it seems wise to discontinue the use of

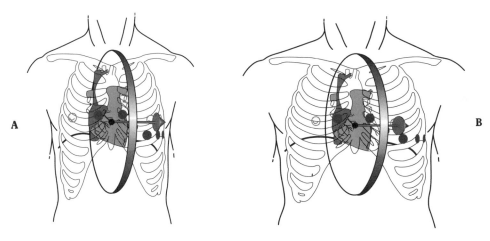

A   B

Fig. 7-62. Influence of the size and shape of the chest on calculating the direction of an electrical force (vector) and representing it with an arrow. **A,** When the patient is tall, the electrode positions V_2, V_3, and V_4 are such that each is located almost directly above or below the others. When an arrow representing an electrical force (vector) is directed at 0 degrees to the left and the transitional pathway passes through electrode position V_4, the vector will be directed about 20 to 30 degrees posteriorly. **B,** When the patient is broad chested, the electrode positions V_2, V_3, and V_4 are such that each is located a bit lateral to the others—they are located side by side rather than one above the other, as they are when the patient is tall. When an arrow representing an electrical force (vector) is directed at 0 degrees to the left and the transitional pathway passes through electrode position V_4, the vector will be directed 30 to 40 degrees or more posteriorly—a little more than is illustrated in **A.**

the term *axis deviation* to refer only to the frontal plane direction of the QRS vector. In fact, the words—*axis deviation*—are not needed when an arrow is drawn or visualized to represent the spatial orientation of the electrical force (vector).

Direction of an arrow representing the mean of the electrical forces (vectors) responsible for the initial 0.04 second of the normal QRS complex. The directions of the arrows representing the initial 0.01 to 0.02 second, the next 0.02 second, the next 0.02 second, and the last 0.02 second of the QRS complex are discussed earlier in the explanation of the creation of the contour of the QRS complex. The discussion that follows is concerned with the study of the mean initial 0.04 second of the QRS complex. This portion of the QRS complex deserves special attention because it is necessary to determine the size and direction of the vector that represents it in each electrocardiogram that is interpreted. This measurement is needed because an electrically inert area in the endocardium may alter the direction of electrical forces responsible for the initial 0.04 second of the QRS complex.

An arrow representing the mean of the electrical forces (vectors) responsible for the initial 0.04 second of the normal QRS complex should be directed to the left of a vertically directed arrow that represents the mean of the electrical forces (vectors) responsible for the entire QRS complex (Fig. 7-63, *A*). The normal mean initial 0.04 second QRS vector may be directed to the right or left of an arrow representing the mean of the electrical forces (vectors) responsible for the entire QRS complex that is directed in an intermediate location (Fig. 7-63, *B*) and should be normally directed inferior to a horizontally directed arrow representing the mean of the electrical forces (vectors) responsible for the entire QRS complex (Fig. 7-63, *C*). An arrow representing the mean of the electrical forces (vectors) responsible for the initial 0.04 second of the normal QRS complex is always directed anterior to the direction of an arrow representing the mean of the electrical forces (vectors) responsible for the entire QRS complex. The angle between these two arrows is normally less than 60 degrees and is commonly 30 to 45 degrees. The calculation of an arrow to represent the mean initial 0.04 second QRS forces (vectors) requires that the area, not the amplitude, encompassed during the initial 0.04 second of the QRS complex be used to make the measurement. It should be recalled that the electrical forces generated during the initial 0.04 second of the QRS complex are produced by depolarization of the septum and subendocardial portions of the left and right ventricles.

Direction of an arrow representing the mean of the electrical forces (vectors) responsible for the terminal 0.04 second of the normal QRS complex. The direction of the terminal 0.02 second of the QRS complex is discussed earlier in an effort to explain how the direction of the electrical forces (vectors) projected onto lead axes produce the contour of the QRS deflection. The size and direction of the vector representing the terminal 0.04 second of the QRS complex is discussed here because it should be calculated in every electrocardiogram that is interpreted. The direction of this vector is used to determine the type of conduction defect that is present.

Right   Left

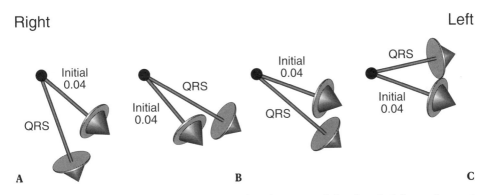

Fig. 7-63. Relationship of an arrow representing the mean of the electrical forces (vectors) responsible for the initial 0.04 second of the normal QRS complex to an arrow representing the mean of the electrical forces (vectors) responsible for the entire QRS complex. **A,** An arrow representing the mean of the electrical forces (vectors) responsible for the initial 0.04 second of the normal QRS complex should be located to the left of, and anterior to, a vertically directed arrow representing the mean of the electrical forces (vectors) responsible for the entire QRS complex. The angle between the two may be 60 degrees but is commonly 30 to 45 degrees or less. **B,** An arrow representing the mean of the electrical forces (vectors) responsible for the initial 0.04 second of the normal QRS complex can be located to the right or left of, and anterior to, an intermediately directed arrow representing the mean of the electrical forces (vectors) responsible for the entire QRS complex. The angle between the two may be 60 degrees but is commonly 30 to 45 degrees or less. **C,** An arrow representing the mean of the electrical forces (vectors) responsible for the initial 0.04 second of the normal QRS complex should be directed inferior and anterior to a horizontally directed arrow representing the mean of the electrical forces (vectors) responsible for the entire QRS complex. The angle between the two may be 60 degrees but is commonly 30 to 45 degrees or less.
Redrawn with permission from Hurst JW: *Ventricular electrocardiography*, New York, 1991, Gower, fig 5.12.

An arrow representing the mean of the electrical forces (vectors) responsible for the terminal 0.04 second of the normal QRS complex is usually directed to the right of a vertically directed arrow representing the mean of the electrical forces (vectors) responsible for the entire QRS complex (Fig. 7-64, *A*). The arrow may be directed to the right or left of an intermediately directed arrow representing the mean of the electrical forces (vectors) responsible for the entire QRS complex (Fig. 7-64, *B*) and is usually directed superior to a horizontally directed arrow representing the mean of the electrical forces (vectors) responsible for the entire QRS complex (Fig. 7-64, *C*). An arrow representing the mean of the electrical forces (vectors) responsible for the terminal 0.04 second of the QRS complex is normally directed posterior to the direction of an arrow representing the mean of the electrical forces (vectors) responsi-

Right   Left

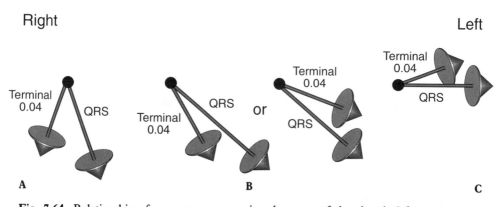

A   B   C

Fig. 7-64. Relationship of an arrow representing the mean of the electrical forces (vectors) responsible for the terminal 0.04 second of the normal QRS complex to an arrow representing the mean of the electrical forces (vectors) responsible for the entire QRS complex. **A,** An arrow representing the mean of the electrical forces (vectors) responsible for the terminal 0.04 second of the normal QRS complex should be located to the right of, and posterior to, a vertically directed arrow representing the mean of the electrical forces (vectors) responsible for the entire QRS complex. The angle between the two may be 60 degrees but is commonly 30 to 45 degrees or less. **B,** An arrow representing the mean of the electrical forces (vectors) responsible for the terminal 0.04 second of the normal QRS complex may be located on either side of, and posterior to, an intermediately directed arrow representing the mean of the electrical forces (vectors) responsible for the entire QRS complex. The angle between the two may be 60 degrees but is commonly 30 to 45 degrees or less. **C,** An arrow representing the mean of the electrical forces (vectors) responsible for the terminal 0.04 second of the normal QRS complex should be located superior and posterior to a horizontally directed arrow representing the mean of the electrical forces (vectors) responsible for the entire QRS complex. The angle between the two may be 60 degrees but is commonly 30 to 45 degrees or less.

Redrawn with permission from Hurst JW: *Ventricular electrocardiography,* New York, 1991, Gower, fig 5.13.

ble for the entire QRS complex. The angle between these two arrows is normally less than 60 degrees and is commonly 30 to 45 degrees or less.

It should be recalled that the electrical forces (vectors) generated during the terminal 0.04 second of the QRS complex are produced by depolarization of the epicardial portion of the left ventricle and that depolarization of the the posterobasilar portion of the left ventricle is responsible for the last few milliseconds of the QRS complex (see Fig. 7-59). Remember, the area encompassed within the last 0.04 second of the QRS complex, and not the amplitude, is used to make the calculation.

Amplitude of the QRS complex in the normal adult. The normal amplitude of the QRS complex is determined by the normal thickness of the ventricular muscle, the presence of normal myocytes, the presence of a normal pericardium and a normal amount of pericardial fluid, the distance the measuring electrodes are from the heart, the skin resistance, the amount of subcutaneous tissue, the relationship of the direction of the electrical force (vector) to the direction of the lead axis used to measure it, and the standardization of the machine itself.

With all of these variables to consider, it is impossible to develop rigid criteria for the amplitude of the QRS complexes in normal subjects. Accordingly, the range of normal for the amplitude of the QRS complexes is wide.[22] The criteria for left ventricular hypertrophy established by Romhilt and Estes[23] is shown in Table 7-4. Remember, too, that when the magnitude of an electrical force is determined, one uses the area of the electrocardiographic deflection being measured, whereas when the amplitude is being measured, one uses the height of the electrocardiographic deflection being measured. Obviously, when the QRS amplitude is less than that listed in Table 7-4, it falls within the range of normal. Every measurement in biology has its own sensitivity, specificity, and predictive value for determining the probability that the measurement is within the normal range or is abnormal. This concept applies to the amplitude of the QRS, as well as to any other measurement. Odum et al.[24] created the total QRS amplitude concept. They found that the total amplitude of the QRS complex was normally 80 to 185 mm in patients who later died and had normal hearts at autopsy. The amplitude of each lead is identified by adding arith-

Table 7-4 Point-score system

	Points[a]
Amplitude[b]	3
ST-T segment	
Without digitalis[c]	3
With digitalis	(1)
Left atrial involvement[d]	3
Left axis deviation[e]	2
QRS duration[f]	1
Intrinsicoid deflection[g]	1
MAXIMUM TOTAL	13

Reproduced with permission from Romhilt DW, Estes EH Jr: A point-score system for the ECG diagnosis of left ventricular hypertrophy, *Am Heart J* 75(6):752, 1968.
[a]Five points is read as LVH; four points is read as probable LVH.
[b]Positive if any one of the following is present: (1) largest R or S wave in the limb leads $\geq$ 20 mm, (2) S wave in V_1 or V_2 $\geq$ 30 mm, (3) R wave in V_5 or V_6 $\geq$ 30 mm.
[c]Positive if typical ST-T pattern of left ventricular strain is present (ST-T segment vector shifted in direction opposite to mean QRS vector).
[d]Positive if the terminal negativity of the P wave in V_1 is 1 mm or more in depth with a duration of 0.04 second or more.
[e]Positive if left axis deviation of -30 degrees or more is present in frontal plane.
[f]Positive if QRS duration is $\geq$ 0.09 second.
[g]Positive if intrinsicoid deflection in V_5 or V_6 $\geq$ 0.05 second.

metically the depth of the Q wave to the height of the R wave to the depth of the S wave and then adding together the total amplitude of the QRS complexes measured in all 12 leads of the electrocardiogram (Fig. 7-65).

It must be recalled that the range of normal amplitude for the QRS complexes is wide. Accordingly, the amplitude can be on the low side of the normal range at one point in time, then increase in size over a period of months or years but still be within the normal range. Unless the previously recorded electrocardiogram is available, it would not be possible for an observer to identify the abnormal increase in amplitude. The same is true when the amplitude is at the upper range of normal at one point in time and then as time passes becomes lower but remains within the normal range. The decrease in amplitude is abnormal but cannot be detected without comparing the recently recorded electrocardiogram with the electrocardiogram that was recorded earlier.

As discussed later, left or right ventricular hypertrophy from any cause or hypertrophic cardiomyopathy may be responsible for an abnormal increase in QRS ampli-

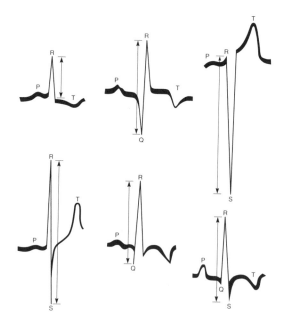

Fig. 7-65. Measurement of the total QRS amplitude. The total QRS amplitude is derived by adding the amplitude (positive and negative waves) of all of the deflections recorded in all 12 leads of the electrocardiogram.

Redrawn with permission from Siegel RJ, Roberts WC: Electrocardiographic observations in severe aortic valve stenosis: correlative necropsy study to clinical, hemodynamic, and ECG variables demonstrating relation of 12-lead QRS amplitude to peak systolic transaortic pressure gradient, *Am Heart J* 103:212, 1982.

tude, whereas other diseases, such as infiltrative cardiomyopathy, pericardial effusion, constrictive pericarditis, myxedema, anasarca, emphysema, and increased skin resistance, may be responsible for an abnormally low QRS amplitude. Exceptions to this rule include glycogen storage disease and Fabrey disease, which cause a great increase in the amplitude of the QRS complexes.

Normal intrinsicoid QRS deflection. The *intrinsic* deflection is defined as that portion of the QRS complex that is recorded from its onset to its zenith. Its height is proportional to the thickness of the heart muscle located beneath the electrode. This measurement is made when the electrode is placed directly on the heart. The *intrinsicoid* deflection is defined as that portion of the QRS complex that is recorded from its onset to its zenith when the electrode is placed on the chest wall. The duration of the intrinsicoid deflection is normally 0.04 second or less in leads V_5 and V_6 and less than 0.03 second in leads V_1 and V_2. It is longer in duration than the intrinsic deflection.[25]

Normal T wave

After the depolarization process of the ventricles is completed, the myocytes, having lost their electrical charges, remain electrically inactive until the recovery process begins. The ST segment of the electrocardiogram represents this period of time. Usually the ST segment indicates the location of the baseline of the electrocardiogram. The T wave is produced when the myocytes rebuild their electrical charges.[26] The act of rebuilding electrical charges is called the repolarization process.

The sequence of repolarization in the normal heart is predetermined by the sequence of depolarization plus certain hemodynamic factors, which are discussed subsequently.

Direction of an arrow representing the mean of the electrical forces (vectors) responsible for the normal T wave. The frontal plane direction of an arrow representing the mean of the electrical forces (vectors) responsible for the T wave is determined by identifying the smallest T wave and the largest T wave in the six extremity leads. An arrow representing the mean T force (vector) is directed parallel with the extremity lead axis in which the T wave is largest and perpendicular to the lead axis in which the T wave is not visible (or is resultantly zero). The area encompassed by the T wave is used to make the calculation. The chest lead in which the T wave is isoelectric, or resultantly the smallest, is then identified. The arrow representing the mean T force (vector) is rotated anteriorly or posteriorly until the transitional pathway, which is the edge of the zero potential plane, passes through the electrode position in which the T wave is isoelectric, or resultantly the smallest.[2]

The *depolarization* process passes predominantly from the endocardium to the epicardium and produces an electrical force (vector) that is directed in the same direction. If one assumes that each myocyte takes the same amount of time to rebuild its electrical charges that were lost during depolarization, the *repolarization* process should begin in the cells that were the first to be depolarized.[27,28] Should that happen, the repolarization process should begin, as depolarization did, in the endocardium and travel toward the epicardium. Under such circumstances, an arrow representing the mean of the electrical forces (vectors) responsible for repolarization (the T wave) would be directed opposite to an arrow representing the mean of the electrical forces (vectors) responsible for depolarization (the QRS complex). However, this does not occur in the normal adult; the repolarization process begins at the epicardium and then travels toward the endocardium. Accordingly, an arrow representing the mean of the electrical forces (vectors) responsible for the T wave is directed relatively parallel with an arrow representing the mean of the electrical forces (vectors) responsible for the QRS complex. This occurs in the normal adult heart because the myocytes located in the endocardium do not repolarize as quickly as the myocytes located in the epicardium.

The delay of the repolarization process in the endocardium as compared with that in the epicardium is presumably due to the transmyocardial pressure gradient produced during ventricular systole.[29,30] The T wave is actually inscribed during the last part of ventricular systole, and during that period of time the transmyocardial pressure gradient is higher in the endocardium of the heart than it is in the epicardium. This causes the myocytes in the endocardial area to repolarize later than those in the epicardial area. Thus the repolarization process travels from the epicardium toward the endocardium, producing electrical forces (vectors) that are directed in an opposite direction.

In the normal adult the direction of an arrow representing the mean of the electrical forces (vectors) responsible for the T wave should be located to the left of a vertically directed arrow representing the mean of the electrical forces (vectors) responsible for the QRS complex (see Fig. 7-60, B). The mean T vector may be directed to the right or left of an intermediately directed arrow representing the mean of the electrical forces (vectors) responsible for the QRS complex. The mean T vector should be directed inferior to a horizontally directed arrow representing the mean of the electrical forces (vectors) responsible for the QRS complex. An arrow representing the mean of the electrical forces (vectors) responsible for the T wave should normally be directed anterior to an arrow representing the mean of the electrical forces (vectors) responsible for the entire QRS complex. The angle between the two is less than 60 degrees and is commonly 30 to 45 degrees in the normal adult.

Normal ventricular gradient. The ventricular gradient is a measurement of the extent to which the repolarization process is dictated by the depolarization process.[31] The ventricular gradient is the diagonal of a parallelogram of which one side is an arrow representing the mean QRS force (vector) and the other side is an arrow representing the mean T force (vector). The ventricular gradient is normally directed at the left lower quadrant of the hexaxial reference system (Fig. 7-66). The ventricular gradient is directed anterior to the arrow representing the mean of the electrical forces (vectors) responsible for the QRS complex and posterior to the arrow representing the mean of the electrical forces (vectors) responsible for the T wave. The arrow representing the ventricular gradient points away from the area of the heart where the myocytes remain depolarized the longest.

It is not always possible to compute the ventricular gradient when the QRS or T waves are abnormal, but when it can be computed, it is a useful concept for distinguishing primary T wave abnormalities from secondary T wave abnormalities (see later discussion).

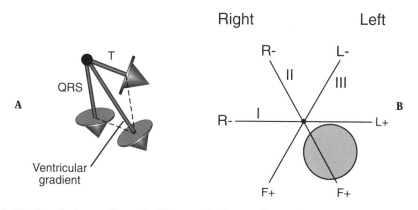

Fig. 7-66. Ventricular gradient. **A,** The ventricular gradient, when represented as a vector, indicates the relationship of the total depolarization process of the ventricles to the total repolarization process of the ventricles. The gradient is created by drawing an arrow to represent the mean QRS vector and the mean T vector; constructing a parallelogram using the arrow representing the mean QRS vector and the arrow representing the mean T vector as its sides; and drawing a diagonal arrow to illustrate the gradient. **B,** The normal gradient should be directed to the left lower quadrant of the hexaxial reference system. It should be directed posterior to the arrow representing the mean T vector and anterior to the arrow representing the mean QRS vector. The calculation of the gradient is used to distinguish secondary T wave abnormalities from primary T wave abnormalities (see text).

Redrawn from Burch G, Winsor T: *A primer of electrocardiography*, Philadelphia, 1945, Lea & Febiger, p 186. Used with permission.

Normal ST segment displacement

The ST segment of the electrocardiogram usually represents the baseline of the recording; there is no up or down displacement of the segment. Some normal subjects have rather large T waves, and at times there is an ST segment displacement due to the electrical forces (vectors) of early repolarization. When the ST segment is normally displaced, it can be illustrated by an arrow that represents the mean of the electrical forces (vectors) that are produced during that period of time. When present in a normal heart, it should be directed in the same direction as an arrow used to represent the mean of the electrical forces (vectors) responsible for the T wave (Fig. 7-67).

The repolarization of the atria produces the Ta wave. This wave, when seen, is usually displaced downward when the P wave is upright. When the PR interval is prolonged, the Ta wave may be seen following the P wave (see Fig. 7-56, *A*). At times, especially with sinus tachycardia, the Ta wave will cause the ST segment to be displaced downward when the PR interval is short and the QRS complex is upright (see Fig. 7-56, *B*). It is difficult to diagram an arrow that represents these electrical forces (vectors), because the ST segment displacement is small and may not be seen in all leads. One can usually determine, however, that an arrow representing the mean of the electrical forces (vectors) responsible for the ST segment displacement is not directed parallel with an arrow representing the mean of the electrical forces (vectors) responsible for the T wave. This, of course, is not at all characteristic of the mean ST vector caused by normal early repolarization.

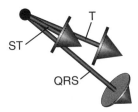

Fig. 7-67. Normal ST segment vector. An arrow representing the normal mean ST segment vector (when there is one) should be directed parallel with an arrow representing the mean T vector. At times, when there is a large mean T vector, the mean ST segment vector may also be large. This is referred to as normal early repolarization. An arrow representing a prominent mean ST segment vector that is parallel with an arrow representing a normal or abnormal mean T vector is called a secondary ST segment vector, because it is part of the repolarization process.

Normal U wave

The U wave cannot be represented by an arrow, because it is rarely seen in all of the extremity and chest leads. The U wave is never larger than the T wave in normal subjects.

Illustrations of normal electrocardiograms

Normal P waves, QRS complexes, and T waves are depicted in the electrocardiograms shown in Figs. 7-68 through 7-70. An electrocardiogram illustrating a normal vertical mean QRS vector is shown in Fig. 7-68. An electrocardiogram illustrating a normal intermediate mean QRS vector is shown in Fig. 7-69. An electrocardiogram illustrating a normal horizontal mean QRS vector is shown in Fig. 7-70.

DIAGNOSTIC OPTIONS WHEN THE ELECTROCARDIOGRAM IS ABNORMAL

An abnormal electrocardiogram may be recorded from a patient who has no other evidence of heart disease, and it is important to recall the admonitions of Frank Wilson[32]:

> In the last two decades there has been a tremendous growth of interest in electrocardiographic diagnosis and in the number and variety of electrocardiographs in use. In 1914, there was only one instrument of this kind in the State of Michigan, and this was not in operation; there were probably no more than a dozen electrocardiographs in the whole of the United States. Now there is one or more in almost every village of any size, and there are comparatively few people who are not in greater danger of having their peace and happiness destroyed by an erroneous diagnosis of cardiac abnormality based on a faulty interpretation of an electrocardiogram, than of being injured or killed by an atomic bomb.*

There are five subsets of diagnostic options in these patients:
- P wave abnormalities may exist without other evidence of heart disease. Such abnormalities are usually benign.
- T wave abnormalities may be due to former pericarditis or some unknown factor. The T wave abnormality may persist with no other evidence of heart disease becoming apparent on long-term follow-up.
- Some benign T wave abnormalities are due to normal physiologic responses and may occur intermittently.
- Ventricular conduction defects such as right ventricular conduction delay and right bundle-branch block may occur in the absence of other evidence of heart disease.

---

*Reproduced with permission from Wilson F: Foreword. In Lepeschkin E, editor: Modern electrocardiography, Baltimore, 1978, Little, Brown and Company.

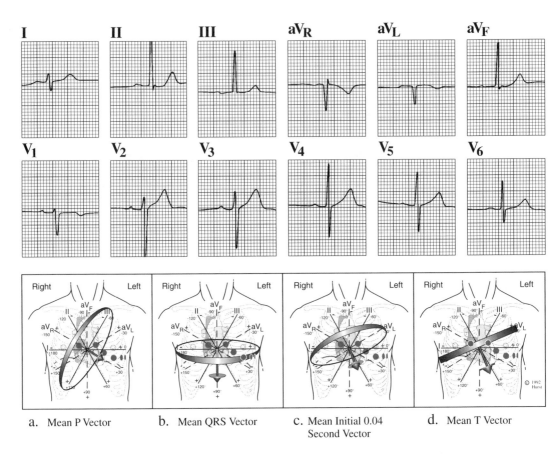

a. Mean P Vector
b. Mean QRS Vector
c. Mean Initial 0.04 Second Vector
d. Mean T Vector

Fig. 7-68

- Some T wave abnormalities and conduction defects are early markers of heart disease that has not progressed to the stage where other signs are apparent.

  The following abnormalities indicating the presence of heart disease may be identified in the ventricular electrocardiogram: certain cardiac arrhythmias, an abnormally long or short PR interval, an abnormally long or short QT interval, left or right ventricular hypertrophy, conditions causing lower than normal amplitude of the QRS complexes, left anterosuperior division block, left posteroinferior division block, uncomplicated left or right bundle-branch block, complicated left or right bundle-branch block, left bundle-branch block plus left anterosuperior division block, right

Fig. 7-68. Normal vertically directed mean QRS vector.
- *Rhythm:* Sinus bradycardia
  Rate: Undetermined in short strip
  PR interval: 0.20 second
  QRS duration: 0.08 second
  QT interval: 0.40 second
- *Vector diagrams of electrical forces:* See *a*, *b*, *c*, and *d* below the electrocardiogram.
- *Electrophysiologic considerations:*
  The mean P, QRS, initial 0.04 second QRS, and T vectors are normally directed and ex-
  hibit normal amplitude.
  The mean QRS vector is directed about +90 degrees inferiorly and about 30 degrees poste-
  riorly.
  The mean initial 0.04 second QRS vector is directed to the left of, and anterior to, the mean
  QRS vector.
  The mean T vector is directed to the left of, and anterior to, the mean QRS vector. The
  QRS-T angle is about 30 degrees.
  The size and direction of the mean vectors representing depolarization of the atria and ventricles, the initial 0.04 second of the QRS complex, and repolarization of the ventricles
  are normal.
- *Clinical differential diagnosis:* The heart may be normal, or the patient could have atherosclerotic coronary heart disease, mild valvular disease, or systemic hypertension that has
  not as yet produced left ventricular hypertrophy. The patient could have a history of arrhythmias or old pericarditis. It is unlikely that the patient has hypertrophic, dilated, or
  restrictive cardiomyopathy. Other clinical data are needed to determine which diagnosis is
  the correct one.
- *Discussion:* This electrocardiogram was recorded from a 37-year-old normal male physician
  who was an active athlete. He was tall and thin and had no evidence of heart disease.

Electrocardiogram courtesy Paul Gainey, M.D. Reproduced with permission from Hurst JW: *Ventricular electrocardiography*, New York, 1991, Gower, fig 5.25.

---

bundle-branch block plus left anterosuperior division block, right bundle-branch block plus left posteroinferior division block, myocardial ischemia, myocardial in-jury, Q wave infarction, non–Q wave myocardial infarction, pseudoinfarction, pul-monary embolism, pericarditis, abnormalities due to cerebral disease, abnormalities due to physical training (the athlete's heart), electrolyte abnormalities, and abnor-malities due to drugs and physiologic phenomena.

The prognosis of a patient exhibiting one or more of these abnormalities should not be determined by the electrocardiographic abnormality alone. All available data should be used to make a cardiac appraisal of the patient (see Chapter 4).

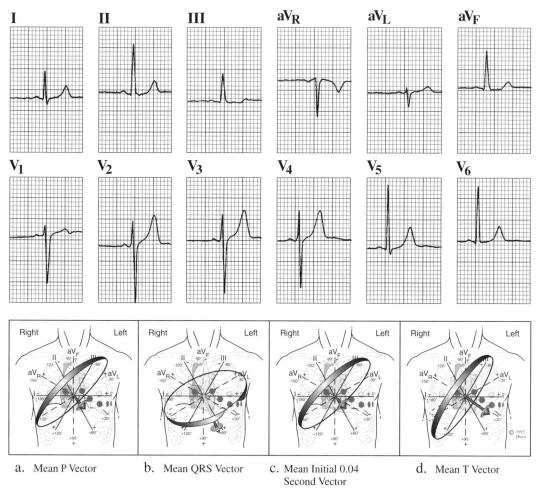

a. Mean P Vector   b. Mean QRS Vector   c. Mean Initial 0.04   d. Mean T Vector
                                                   Second Vector

Fig. 7-69

ABNORMAL ATRIAL ELECTROCARDIOGRAM AS A SIGN OF VENTRICULAR DISEASE

P wave abnormalities are often spoken of as signs of left or right atrial enlargement. Although such a correlation is occasionally possible, the premise is wrong. I believe that most abnormalities of the P waves are produced by conduction defects within the atrial walls. Accordingly, for decades now I have referred to P wave abnormalities as a left atrial abnormality, a right atrial abnormality, or biatrial abnormality. Perhaps the preferential conduction pathways of the atria do not transmit electrical impulses normally because they become "stretched," even when the atria are not definitely dilated.

Fig. 7-69. Normal intermediately directed mean QRS vector.

- *Rhythm:* Normal sinus rhythm
  Rate: Undetermined in short strip
  PR interval: 0.16 second
  QRS duration: 0.08 second
  QT interval: 0.04 second
- *Vector diagrams of electrical forces:* See *a, b, c,* and *d* below the electrocardiogram.
- *Electrophysiologic considerations:*
  The mean QRS vector is directed about +70 degrees inferiorly and about 50 degrees poste-
  riorly.
  The mean initial 0.04 second QRS vector is directed to the left of, and anterior to, the mean
  QRS vector (it may normally be directed to the right or left of an intermediately directed
  mean QRS vector).
  The QRS-T angle is 60 degrees, and the mean T vector is directed to the left of, and anterior to, the mean QRS vector. (It may normally be directed to the right or left of an
  intermediately directed mean QRS vector.)
  The size and direction of the mean vectors representing depolarization of the atria and ventricles, the initial 0.04 second of the QRS complex, and repolarization of the ventricles
  are normal.
- *Clinical differential diagnosis:* The heart may be normal, or the patient could have coronary
  atherosclerotic heart disease, mild valvular disease, or systemic hypertension that has not as
  yet produced left ventricular hypertrophy. The patient could have a history of arrhythmias
  or old pericarditis. It is unlikely that the patient has hypertrophic, dilated, or restrictive
  cardiomyopathy. Other clinical data are needed to determine which diagnosis is the correct
  one.
- *Discussion:* This electrocardiogram was recorded from a 27-year-old normal male physician.
  He was of average body build and exhibited no evidence of heart disease.

Electrocardiogram courtesy Mark Lowell, M.D. Reproduced with permission from Hurst JW: *Ventricular electrocardiography,* New York, 1991, Gower, fig 5.26.

Most atrial abnormalities are associated with ventricular disease. An elevation of
left ventricular diastolic pressure, poor compliance in the left ventricle, or mitral valve
disease may produce a left atrial abnormality, and an elevation of right ventricular
diastolic pressure, poor compliance of the right ventricle, or tricuspid valve disease
may produce a right atrial abnormality. Obviously, at times abnormalities of the P
waves correlate with the presence of congestive heart failure. Atrial infarcts may also
deform the P waves. It must be remembered, too, that there may be P wave abnormalities without any other evidence of heart disease, and in such patients the deformed P waves usually have no clinical significance.

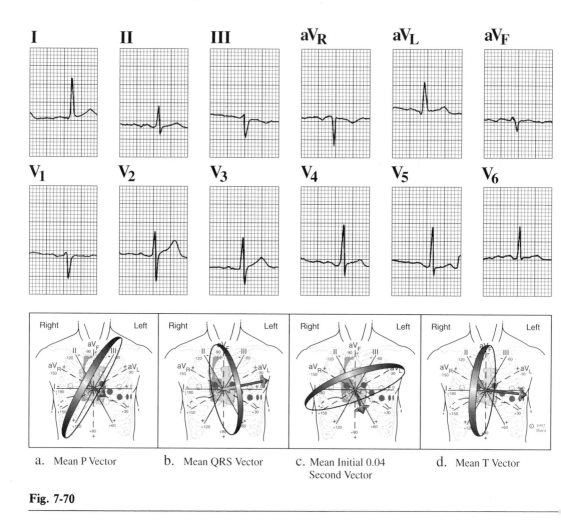

a. Mean P Vector b. Mean QRS Vector c. Mean Initial 0.04 Second Vector d. Mean T Vector

Fig. 7-70

Left atrial abnormality[19,20]

The duration of the P wave is usually 0.12 second or greater, and the amplitude of the P wave is usually less than 3 mm. The P wave tends to be notched at the halfway point.

An arrow representing the mean of the electrical forces (vectors) responsible for the second half of the P wave is commonly, but not always, directed to the left of an arrow representing the mean of the electrical forces (vectors) responsible for the first half of the P wave. It is usually directed +50 to +60 degrees inferiorly. Remember, the first half of the P wave is produced by depolarization of the right atrium, and the second half of the P wave is produced by depolarization of the left atrium. The ar-

Fig. 7-70. Normal horizontally directed mean QRS vector.

- *Rhythm:* Normal sinus rhythm
  Rate: Undetermined in short strip
  PR interval: 0.16 second
  QRS duration: 0.08 second
  QT interval: 0.33 second
- *Vector diagrams of electrical forces:* See *a, b, c,* and *d* below the electrocardiogram.
- *Electrophysiologic considerations:*
  The mean QRS vector is directed −15 degrees to the left and about 20 degrees posteriorly.
  The mean initial 0.04 second QRS vector is directed inferior and anterior to the mean QRS vector.
  The mean T vector is directed inferior and anterior to the mean QRS vector. The QRS-T angle is about 25 degrees.
  The size and direction of the mean vectors representing depolarization of the atria and ventricles, the initial 0.04 second of the QRS complex, and repolarization of the ventricles are normal.
- *Clinical differential diagnosis:* The heart may be normal, or the patient could have coronary atherosclerotic heart disease or mild valvular disease or systemic hypertension that has not as yet produced left ventricular hypertrophy. The patient could have a history of arrhythmias or old pericarditis. It is unlikely that the patient has hypertrophic, dilated, or restrictive cardiomyopathy. Other clinical data are needed to determine which diagnosis is the correct one.
- *Discussion:* This electrocardiogram was recorded from a normal 31-year-old male physician. The man was robust and broad chested and had no other evidence of heart disease.

Electrocardiogram courtesy Curtis Weaver, M.D. Reproduced with permission from Hurst JW: *Ventricular electrocardiography,* New York, 1991, Gower, fig 5.27.

---

row representing the mean of the electrical forces (vectors) responsible for the second half of the P wave is always directed posterior to the arrow representing the mean of the electrical forces (vectors) responsible for the first half of the P wave. The second half of the P wave is usually negative in lead V_1. A left atrial abnormality is likely when the last half of the P wave is negative in leads V_2 and V_3. A left atrial abnormality is more likely to be present when the second half of the P wave recorded in lead V_1 is greater than −0.03 mm/sec.[19] The greater the number, the more likely it is that there is a left atrial abnormality. For example, when this figure is −0.06 mm/sec, a left atrial abnormality is almost certainly present.

An electrocardiogram illustrating a left atrial abnormality is shown in Fig. 7-71.

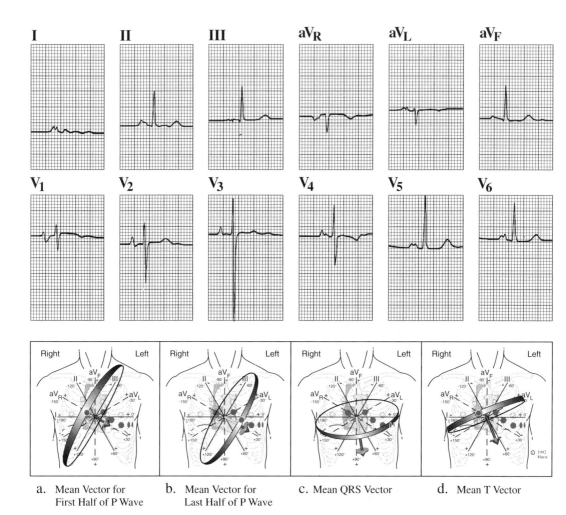

a. Mean Vector for
   First Half of P Wave

b. Mean Vector for
   Last Half of P Wave

c. Mean QRS Vector

d. Mean T Vector

Fig. 7-71

Fig. 7-71. Left atrial abnormality.

- *Rhythm:* Normal sinus rhythm

   Rate: Undetermined in short strip. There were 60 depolarizations per minute in a longer strip.

   PR interval: 0.18 second

   QRS duration: 0.08 second

   QT interval: 0.04 second

- *Vector diagrams of electrical forces:* See *a*, *b*, *c*, and *d* below the electrocardiogram.

- *Electrophysiologic considerations:*

   The P wave is 0.11 second in duration and is notched in leads I, II, aV$_L$, V$_4$, V$_5$, and V$_6$. The P waves are abnormal; they are broader than normal and abnormally notched.

   The mean vector representing the first half of the P wave is somewhat prominent, suggesting a right atrial abnormality. The mean vector representing the last half of the P wave is definitely abnormal. It is directed about +30 degrees inferiorly in the frontal plane and about 30 degrees posteriorly. The last half of the P wave in lead V$_1$ measures at least 0.08 mm/sec; this indicates a left atrial abnormality with a predictive value of 100%.

   The mean QRS vector is directed about +80 degrees inferiorly and about 50 degrees posteriorly.

   The mean T vector is directed about +70 degrees inferiorly and about 10 degrees anteriorly. The T wave is inverted in lead V$_4$.

   This electrocardiogram is abnormal. There is a definite left atrial abnormality and possibly a right atrial abnormality. The possible right atrial abnormality could indicate pulmonary artery hypertension. The vertically directed mean QRS vector could be normal, but when it is associated with a definite left atrial abnormality, it is likely to be abnormal. It may represent right ventricular hypertrophy from acquired heart disease. The cause of the isolated T wave inversion is not known.

- *Clinical differential diagnosis:* The abnormalities in this electrocardiogram are almost specific for rheumatic mitral valve stenosis. The left atrial abnormality is characteristic, and the possible right atrial abnormality indicates that the mitral stenosis is moderately severe. The following rare conditions that could cause the abnormalities include congenital mitral stenosis, left atrial tumor, and mitral stenosis due to ergot medication.

- *Discussion:* This electrocardiogram was recorded from a 35-year-old woman with rheumatic mitral stenosis. The mitral valve area was 0.7 cm, and the resting pulmonary artery pressure was 38/18 mm Hg.

Electrocardiogram courtesy Henry Hanley, M.D., University of Louisiana at Shreveport.

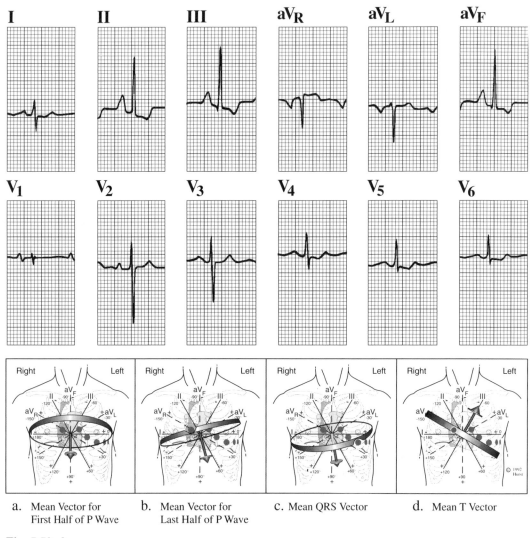

a. Mean Vector for
   First Half of P Wave

b. Mean Vector for
   Last Half of P Wave

c. Mean QRS Vector

d. Mean T Vector

Fig. 7-72, A

Right atrial abnormality

The duration of the P wave is usually less than 0.12 second. The amplitude of the P wave is commonly 3 mm or more. The first half of the P wave tends to be peaked.

The frontal plane direction of an arrow representing the mean of the electrical forces (vectors) responsible for the first half of the P wave is usually +60 to +70 degrees. It is commonly, but not always, directed to the right of an arrow representing the mean of the electrical forces (vectors) responsible for the second half of the P wave. The arrow is directed more anteriorly than normal when there is a right atrial abnormality; the first half of the P wave is usually larger in leads V_1 and V_2 than it is

Fig. 7-72. A, Right atrial abnormality.

- *Rhythm:* Sinus tachycardia

  Rate: Undetermined in short strip. There were 99 depolarizations per minute in a longer
    strip.

  PR interval: 0.16 second in lead II. Note that the PR interval in lead I is 0.13 second; the
    first half of the P wave in this lead is isoelectric.

  QRS duration: 0.07 second

  QT interval: 0.28 second

- *Vector diagrams of electrical forces:* See *a, b, c,* and *d* under the electrocardiogram.

- *Electrophysiologic considerations:*

  The P waves are abnormal. The duration of the P wave in lead II is 0.09 second, and its
    amplitude is 4 mm. The vector representing the first half of the P wave is directed about
    +90 degrees inferiorly and is anteriorly directed. These abnormalities indicate a right atrial
    abnormality with a predictive value of 100%. The last half of the P wave is normal.

  The mean QRS vector is directed about +78 degrees inferiorly and about 30 degrees poste-
    riorly. The direction of this QRS vector could be normal but is likely to be abnormal
    when a definite right atrial abnormality is present. The vertical but posterior direction of
    the vector suggests that it could be right ventricular hypertrophy from acquired heart
    disease.

  The mean T vector is directed −62 degrees to the left and is parallel with the frontal plane.
    The QRS-T angle is abnormally wide.

- *Clinical differential diagnosis:* The electrocardiogram could be produced by several diseases
    that can cause a right atrial abnormality and a vertically directed mean QRS vector that is
    posteriorly directed. These include repeated pulmonary emboli, Eisenmenger syndrome, and
    primary pulmonary hypertension. A mean QRS vector of this type is not caused by congen-
    ital heart disease such as tetralogy of Fallot or severe pulmonary valve stenosis (see text).
    This type of QRS vector is commonly seen during the early course of acquired right ven-
    tricular hypertrophy such as may occur from one of the conditions just listed.

- *Discussion:* This electrocardiogram was recorded from a 50-year-old woman with primary
    pulmonary hypertension. The systolic pressure in the pulmonary artery was 100 mm Hg.

Continued.

---

in V_6. There is an exception to this rule. When the right atrium is huge, as it is in
Ebstein anomaly or congenital tricuspid atresia, the first half of the P wave may be
normal whereas the second half is directed posteriorly, suggesting a left atrial abnormality. In reality, the P wave abnormality is produced by an extremely large right
atrium; the posterior direction of the arrow is produced by the depolarization wave
passing posteriorly in the large right atrium as the wave "ripples" toward the left
atrium.

Electrocardiograms illustrating right atrial abnormality are shown in Fig. 7-72.

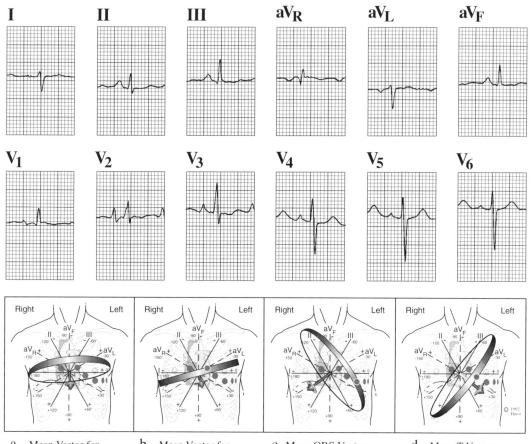

a. Mean Vector for
   First Half of P Wave

b. Mean Vector for
   Last Half of P Wave

c. Mean QRS Vector

d. Mean T Vector

Fig. 7-72, B

Fig. 7-72, cont'd. B, Right atrial abnormality in another patient.

- *Rhythm:* Sinus tachycardia

  Rate: Undetermined in short strip. There were 100 depolarizations per minute in a longer strip.

  PR interval: 0.16 second

  QRS duration: 0.08 second

  QT interval: 0.36 second

- *Vector diagrams of electrical forces:* See *a, b, c,* and *d* below the electrocardiogram.

- *Electrophysiologic considerations:*

  The mean P vector is directed about +90 degrees inferiorly and about 15 degrees anteriorly. The rightward direction of the mean P vector, especially the vector representing the first half of the P wave, is abnormal. The P waves are not large, but they are narrow and peaked in leads V_2 and V_3, because the first half of the P wave is normal and peaked. This, plus the rightward direction of the vector that produces it, indicates a right atrial abnormality.

  The mean QRS vector is directed about +145 degrees to the right and about 25 degrees anteriorly. This indicates right ventricular hypertrophy.

  The mean T vector is directed +40 degrees inferiorly and 10 to 15 degrees posteriorly. Although the slightly posterior direction of the mean T vector can be normal, it may be abnormal in this patient with right ventricular hypertrophy. The mean T vector tends to point away from the hypertrophied right ventricle.

- *Clinical differential diagnosis:* This electrocardiogram could be produced by a number of diseases that can cause a right atrial abnormality and a mean QRS vector that is directed to the right and anteriorly. These include pulmonary valve stenosis, tetralogy of Fallot, late-course Eisenmenger syndrome complicating a left-to-right shunt, and late-course primary pulmonary hypertension.

- *Discussion:* This electrocardiogram was recorded from a 29-year-old man with primary pulmonary hypertension. The pulmonary artery pressure was 100/60 mm Hg. Early in the course of right ventricular hypertrophy due to an acquired disease, the mean QRS vector shifts rightward but retains a posterior direction. Later, as in this case, the mean QRS vector shifts anteriorly. Patients with pulmonary valve stenosis rarely exhibit a posterior direction of the mean QRS vector.

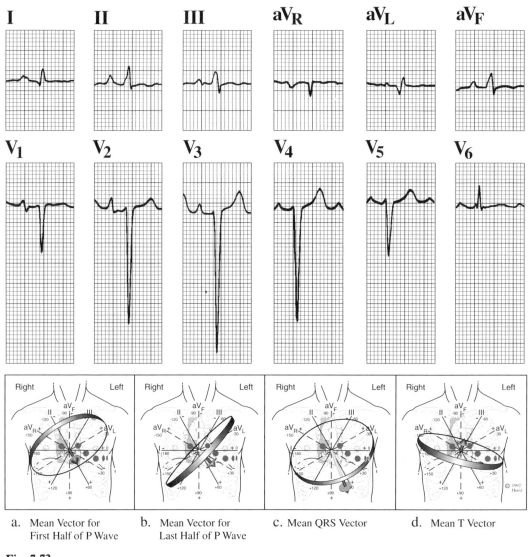

Fig. 7-73

Biatrial abnormality

The duration of the P wave is usually greater than 0.12 second. The amplitude of the P wave is commonly greater than 3 mm.

An arrow representing the mean of the electrical forces (vectors) responsible for the second half of the P wave is directed inferiorly to the left and abnormally posteriorly. The second half of the P wave is greater than −0.03 mm/sec in lead V_1. An arrow representing the mean of the electrical forces (vectors) responsible for the first half of the P wave is directed inferiorly and to an abnormal degree anteriorly. As expected, biatrial abnormalities consist of a combination of right and left atrial abnormalities.

Fig. 7-73. Biatrial abnormality.

- *Rhythm:* Sinus tachycardia
  Rate: Undetermined in short strip. There were 100 depolarizations per minute in a longer strip.
  PR interval: 0.20 second in lead I. Note that the PR interval is 0.14 second in lead aV_L. This discrepancy in the measurement occurs because the electrical forces responsible for the first portion of the P wave are perpendicular to lead axis aV_L.
  QRS duration: 0.09 second
  QT interval: About 0.36 second
- *Vector diagrams of electrical forces:* See *a*, *b*, *c*, and *d* below the electrocardiogram.
- *Electrophysiologic considerations:*
  The vector representing the first half of the P wave is perpendicular to lead axis aV_L (note that the PR interval is shorter in lead aV_L than it is in lead I; the first portion of the PR interval is isoelectric in lead aV_L). It is directed about +60 degrees inferiorly and 45 to 60 degrees anteriorly (note that the first half of the P wave in lead V_1 is larger than it is in V_6. This suggests a right atrial abnormality. The vector representing the second half of the P wave is directed about +55 degrees inferiorly and about 10 to 15 degrees posteriorly. The last half of the P wave measures about −0.04 mm/sec in lead V_1. This suggests a left atrial abnormality.
  The mean vector representing the QRS complexes is directed about +70 degrees inferiorly and about 70 to 80 degrees posteriorly. This, plus the abnormally large amplitude of the QRS complexes in leads V_2, V_3, and V_4, suggests left ventricular hypertrophy.
  The mean T vector is directed −85 degrees superiorly and about 30 degrees anteriorly. The QRS-T angle is 155 degrees; this supports the view that there is left ventricular dilatation and hypertrophy. The biatrial abnormalities indicate left ventricular disease and pulmonary hypertension.
- *Clinical differential diagnosis:* Several types of heart disease could produce these abnormalities, including severe multivalvular disease with heart failure, idiopathic dilated cardiomyopathy, ischemic dilated cardiomyopathy, and dilated cardiomyopathy due to infiltrative myocardial disease.
- *Discussion:* This electrocardiogram was recorded from a 23-year-old man with idiopathic dilated cardiomyopathy with heart failure. The abnormalities of the first and second halves of the P waves are due to left ventricular disease and pulmonary hypertension, respectively.

It is interesting to follow a patient with left ventricular disease or mitral stenosis and observe the development of a left atrial abnormality in the electrocardiogram, which, as time passes, may be followed by the development of a right atrial abnormality. When this occurs, it is sometimes possible to deduce that the patient has developed pulmonary artery hypertension and that there is poor compliance of the right ventricle.

An electrocardiogram illustrating biatrial abnormality is shown in Fig. 7-73.

ABNORMAL VENTRICULAR ELECTROCARDIOGRAM

Abnormal QT interval

Long QT interval. The length of the QT interval is influenced by the heart rate. In practice, one simply looks up the RR interval and its associated QT interval in a specially designed table (see Table 7-3). The QT interval may become prolonged as a result of Romano-Ward syndrome,[16,17] Jervell and Lange-Nielsen syndrome,[18] medications such as quinidine or procainamide, myocardial ischemia, hypocalcemia, cerebral disease such as brain tumor, subarachnoid hemorrhage, cerebral hemorrhage,[33] head injury,[34] hypothermia, or for unknown reasons. Most of these conditions prolong the ST segment and the T wave as well. Hypocalcemia prolongs the ST segment more than it prolongs the T wave. Hypokalemia may produce prominent U waves that join the preceding T wave; this union gives the appearance of a long QT interval.

When no apparent cause for a long QT interval is identified and the patient has syncope or a history of tachycardia, the patient may have Romano-Ward syndrome.[16,17] In such patients it is not wise to use a drug that is known to prolong the QT interval to treat an arrhythmia. If such a patient has congenital deafness, he or she has Jervell and Lange-Nielsen syndrome.[18]

The electrocardiogram of a patient with Romano-Ward syndrome is shown in Fig. 7-74.

Short QT interval. The QT interval may be shorter than average (0.28-0.30 second) as a result of digitalis medication or hypercalcemia. The QT interval may also be inherently short in some individuals who have no other evidence of heart disease, who are not taking digitalis, and in whom the serum calcium level is normal.[35] These normal subjects have labile T waves; an arrow representing the mean of the electrical forces (vectors) responsible for the T wave changes in direction from time to time. The change may be precipitated by physiologic maneuvers such as assuming the upright position or by a slight increase in heart rate.

Left ventricular hypertrophy

The electrocardiogram of an adult without heart disease shows normal left ventricular dominance. It is difficult to identify an abnormal amount of left ventricular dominance that can be labeled left ventricular hypertrophy.

Left ventricular systolic pressure overload,[36,37] such as occurs with aortic stenosis, systemic hypertension, and idiopathic hypertrophy, causes concentric left ventricular hypertrophy. Left ventricular diastolic pressure overload (due to volume overload of the left ventricle), such as occurs with aortic regurgitation, mitral regurgitation, patent ductus arterosis, or ventricular septal defect, produces left ventricular hypertrophy due to a dilated left ventricle whose wall is also thicker than normal. It is not surprising that these two different types of left ventricular overload would be associated with different types of electrocardiograms. The distinction is not clear-cut, because late in the course of events the electrocardiographic signs of left ventricular diastolic pressure overload shifts to become characteristic of left ventricular systolic pressure overload.

Systolic pressure overload of the left ventricle.[36,37] The duration of the QRS complex may be prolonged slightly from its duration prior to the development of left ventricular hypertrophy; it is usually 0.10 second or less.

An arrow representing the mean of the electrical forces (vectors) produced during the entire QRS complex is usually directed normally. An arrow representing the mean QRS force (vector) associated with left ventricular hypertrophy is usually directed between +80 and −20 degrees. The arrow may shift as much as 30 degrees to the left of its prehypertrophy position, but it should not be directed as far as −30 degrees in the frontal plane. As discussed later in the section on conduction disturbances, when an arrow representing the mean QRS force (vector) for the QRS complex is directed −30 degrees or more to the left, it is likely that left anterosuperior division block is also present. An arrow representing the mean QRS force (vector) associated with systolic pressure overload of the left ventricle tends to be directed more vertically than an arrow representing the direction of the mean QRS force (vector) associated with diastolic pressure overload. This, however, cannot be used to distinguish between the two types of left ventricular hypertrophy.

An arrow representing the direction of the mean QRS force (vector) is always directed posteriorly. It is usually directed 45 to 50 degrees posteriorly but may be directed 60 to 75 degrees posteriorly.

An arrow representing the mean of the electrical forces (vectors) responsible for the initial 0.04 second of the QRS complex may be directed to the right, inferiorly, and anterior to the direction of the arrow representing the mean of the electrical forces (vectors) responsible for the entire QRS complex. This produces a small Q wave in leads I, aV_L, and V_6. The entire QRS loop, which is produced by the change in direction and amplitude of electrical forces (vectors) generated during each millisecond of ventricular depolarization, may be rotated posteriorly, so that no R wave is recorded in leads V_1, V_2, and sometimes V_3. This abnormality can be confused with, and cannot always be separated from, the abnormality caused by a septal myocardial infarction (Fig. 7-75).

An arrow representing the mean of the electrical forces (vectors) responsible for the terminal 0.04 second of the QRS complex is usually directed to the left of, posterior to, and sometimes superior to the arrow representing the mean of the electrical forces (vectors) responsible for the entire QRS complex.

The intrinsicoid deflection may be equal to or greater than 0.05 second in leads V_5 and V_6 when there is left ventricular hypertrophy due to systolic pressure overload of the left ventricle.

The amplitude of the QRS complexes increases when there is left ventricular hypertrophy. As mentioned earlier, the usual cause is either aortic valve stenosis or

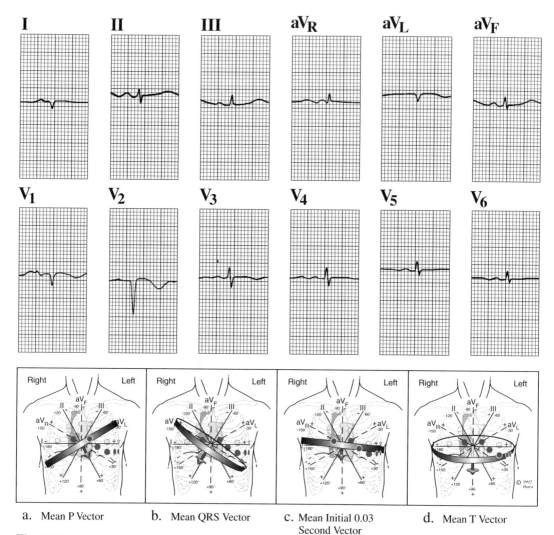

a. Mean P Vector

b. Mean QRS Vector

c. Mean Initial 0.03 Second Vector

d. Mean T Vector

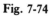

Fig. 7-74

Fig. 7-74. Long QT interval associated with sudden death.

- *Rhythm:* Normal sinus rhythm
  Rate: Undetermined in short strip. There were 85 depolarizations per minute in a longer strip.
  PR interval: 0.17 second
  QT interval: 0.46 second
- *Vector diagrams of electrical forces:* See *a, b, c,* and *d* below the electrocardiogram.
- *Electrophysiologic considerations:*
  The mean P vector is normal.
  The QT interval is markedly prolonged.
  The QRS amplitude is abnormally low. The mean QRS vector is directed +125 degrees to the right; it is directed 5 to 10 degrees posteriorly. This is abnormal. The cause is unknown, but the vector may represent left posteroinferior division block. Leads V_4, V_5, and V_6 are recorded near the transitional pathway. The QRS deflections are resultantly positive, whereas the mean QRS vector shown in *b* would make the QRS deflections negative. This variance may occur when the shape of the patient's chest is significantly different from the diagram of the chest shown in *b*. Also, a slight misplacement of electrodes produces a difference in the deflections when they are recorded from positions that are near the transitional pathway.
  The mean initial 0.03 second QRS vector is directed +95 to 100 degrees to the right; it is parallel with the frontal plane. The mean initial 0.03 second QRS vector is directed too far to the right and posteriorly; it is abnormal. It could be produced by a myocardial dead zone due to one of many causes.
  The mean T vector is directed about +90 degrees to the right and about 40 degrees posteriorly. The ventricular gradient is obviously abnormal, indicating a primary T wave abnormality.
- *Clinical differential diagnosis:* This electrocardiogram could be produced by myocarditis, dilated cardiomyopathy due to one of many causes, or possibly acute pulmonary embolism. The long QT interval could occur with any of the conditions just mentioned. One other possibility exists: the long QT interval could be due to Romano-Ward syndrome. (The remainder of the abnormalities could be the result of the cardiac arrest and resuscitation that occurred in this patient.)
- *Discussion:* This electrocardiogram was recorded from a 32-year-old woman who had recently delivered a baby. She turned over in her bed to check on the baby and had a "convulsion" and cardiac arrest. Her husband resuscitated her with mouth-to-mouth respiration. Her cardiac examination was normal. There was no evidence of pulmonary embolism. The echocardiogram and coronary arteriogram were normal. The electrocardiogram did not change on subsequent tracings.

  This electrocardiogram is presented to point out the seriousness of an abnormally long QT interval. Although the other electrocardiographic abnormalities remain unexplained, there could be some type of myocardial disease. The tracing may, however, represent Romano-Ward syndrome, and the abnormalities (other than the long QT interval) could be a result of cardiac arrest and resuscitation or an unexplained phenomenon.

Electocardiogram courtesy Paul Walter, M.D., Director, Electrophysiologic Laboratory, Emory University Hospital, Alanta, Ga.

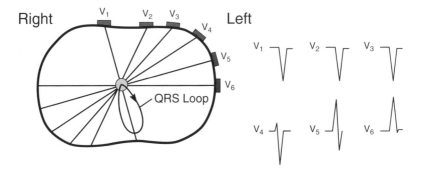

Fig. 7-75. Posterior rotation of the QRS loop (producing absent R waves in leads V_1, V_2, and V_3). This type of electrocardiogram may be recorded from patients with left ventricular hypertrophy due to systolic pressure overload of the left ventricle. Such an electrocardiogram may be erroneously reported as showing "poor R wave progression indicating septal infarction." Although a septal infarction can produce such a finding, it can be caused by left ventricular hypertrophy.

Slightly modified with permission from Hurst JW: *Ventricular electrocardiography*, New York, 1991, Gower, fig 6.8.

hypertension, but cardiomyopathy due to glycogen storage disease, Fabray disease, or idiopathic hypertrophy may produce an enormous increase in QRS voltage. The length of the arrow used to represent the mean of the electrical forces (vectors) responsible for the QRS complex should be drawn longer than normal. Two methods have emerged for use in judging whether or not the amplitude of the QRS complexes is abnormal. They are the Romhilt and Estes system of detecting left ventricular hypertrophy[22,23] (see Table 7-4) and the total QRS amplitude system of Odum et al.[24] (see earlier discussion and Fig. 7-65).

Romhilt and Estes[23] produced a point-score system that uses several abnormalities, in addition to the QRS amplitude, to determine the likelihood of left ventricular hypertrophy being present. They stress that there is no absolute QRS amplitude that has 100% predictive value, and for this reason they use abnormalities of the P waves and ST-T waves, as well as the amplitude of the QRS complexes, to identify the left ventricular hypertrophy (see Table 7-4).

Odum et al.[24] studied the total QRS amplitude of patients who later died of noncardiac causes and established the normal range of the total QRS amplitude. They added the depth of the Q wave to the height of the R wave to the depth of the S wave arithmetically in each of the 12 leads. The total QRS amplitude is determined by adding together the amplitude of the QRS complexes found in all 12 of the leads. They found the normal range to be 85 to 185 mm. When the duration of the QRS complex is 0.09 to 0.10 second and the total QRS amplitude is greater than 185 mm in a patient whose mean QRS vector is directed to the left and posteriorly, left ventricular hypertrophy is highly likely to be present. When the total QRS amplitude is only 160 to 180 mm, left ventricular hypertrophy is still possible, but the predictive value of the measurement is less than when the measurement is greater than 180 mm.

An arrow representing the mean of the electrical forces (vectors) responsible for the T wave may be directed normally when there is left ventricular hypertrophy due to systolic pressure overload of the left ventricle; the QRS-T angle may be 60 degrees or less. The mean T vector will, however, gradually shift, and the QRS-T angle will become abnormally wide. When an arrow representing the mean QRS vector is directed in horizontally and posteriorly, the arrow representing the mean T vector will shift toward the right and anteriorly until it is directed opposite to the direction of the arrow representing the mean QRS vector. When the arrow representing the mean QRS vector is directed inferiorly and posteriorly, the arrow representing the mean T vector will shift anteriorly until it lies superior and anterior to the direction of the arrow representing the mean QRS vector. In either case the QRS-T angle gradually increases until it is 180 degrees.[38] This abnormality was formerly referred to as left ventricular strain, but this term has been discarded. The mean T vector shifts its position because the high systolic pressure load in the left ventricle gradually eliminates the transmyocardial pressure gradient that is normally present; this enables the repolarization process to begin at the endocardium and move toward the epicardium, producing electrical forces (vectors) that are in the opposite direction.[39]

An arrow representing the mean of the electrical forces (vectors) responsible for the ST segment displacement tends to follow the arrow representing the mean T force (vector). The ST segment shift noted with left ventricular hypertrophy due to systolic pressure overload is actually due to early repolarization forces. The angle between the arrows representing the mean T force (vector) and the mean ST force (vector) is usually about 30 degrees or less.

An electrocardiogram illustrating left ventricular systolic pressure overload due to aortic valve stenosis is shown in Fig. 7-76.

Idiopathic hypertrophic cardiomyopathy deserves special emphasis because it is more common than previously appreciated. The diagnosis is commonly missed, especially in the elderly. The amplitude of the QRS complexes is usually increased. An arrow representing the mean of the electrical forces (vectors) responsible for the QRS complex is usually directed as it is in systolic pressure overload of the left ventricle. Arrows representing the mean of the electrical forces (vectors) responsible for the ST and T waves are directed varying degrees away from the arrow representing the mean QRS force (vector). The abnormal T waves are often large, and the electrocardiogram of apical hypertrophy is fairly specific. The arrows representing the mean of the electrical forces (vectors) responsible for the initial 0.04 second of the

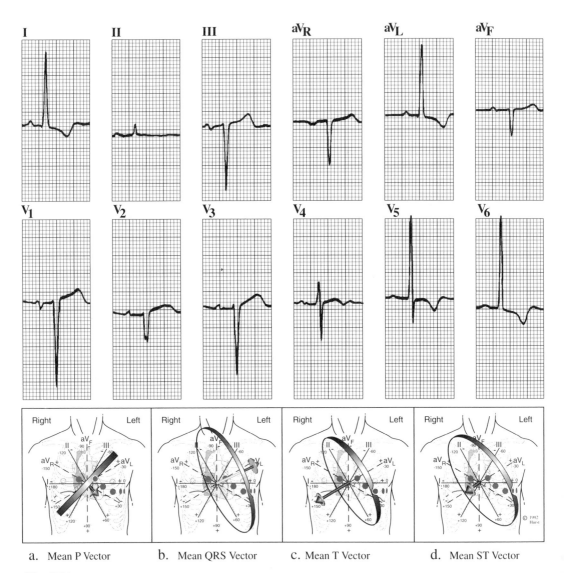

a. Mean P Vector   b. Mean QRS Vector   c. Mean T Vector   d. Mean ST Vector

Fig. 7-76

Fig. 7-76. Left ventricular hypertrophy due to systolic pressure overload of the left ventricle.

- *Rhythm:* Normal sinus rhythm
  Rate: Undetermined in short strip. There were 70 depolarizations per minute in a longer strip.
  PR interval: 0.20 second
  QRS duration: 0.09 second
  QT interval: 0.40 second
- *Vector diagrams of electrical forces:* See *a, b, c,* and *d* below the electrocardiogram.
- *Electrophysiologic considerations:*
  The PR interval is 0.20 second; this is at the upper limit of normal but is more likely to be abnormally long for this patient.
  The mean P vector is directed about +50 degrees inferiorly and is parallel with the frontal plane. The last half of the P wave in lead V_1 measures −0.08 mm/sec. This indicates a definite left atrial abnormality.
  The mean QRS vector is directed about −25 degrees to the left and 50 to 60 degrees posteriorly. The 12-lead QRS amplitude is 202 mm. This indicates left ventricular hypertrophy.
  The mean T vector is directed +150 degrees to the right and 30 to 40 degrees anteriorly. Note that it is directed opposite to the mean QRS vector.
  The mean ST vector is parallel with the mean T vector.
  These abnormalities are characteristic of left ventricular hypertrophy due to systolic pressure overload of the left ventricle.
- *Clinical differential diagnosis:* Systolic pressure overload of the left ventricle may be caused by aortic valve stenosis, systemic hypertension, or primary hypertrophy of the heart, or may occur late in the course of aortic regurgitation.
- *Discussion:* This electrocardiogram was recorded from a 66-year-old man with aortic valve stenosis. The systolic gradient across the aortic valve was 119 mm Hg.

QRS complex, the ST segment displacement, and the T wave may, at times, simulate the abnormalities that are characteristic of myocardial infarction.

Diastolic pressure overload of the left ventricle.[36,37] The duration of the QRS complex may be prolonged only slightly from its duration prior to the development of left ventricular hypertrophy. The duration is usually 0.10 second or slightly less.

An arrow representing the mean of the electrical forces (vectors) produced during the entire QRS complex is directed normally: between +80 and −20 degrees. The arrow may shift as much as 30 degrees to the left of the prehypertrophy position, but it will not be directed to −30 degrees in the frontal plane. As discussed later in the section on conduction disturbances, when the direction of an arrow representing the mean of the electrical forces (vectors) responsible for the QRS complex is directed at −30 degrees or more to the left, it is highly likely that left anterosuperior division block is present. The direction of an arrow representing the mean of the electrical forces (vectors) responsible for the QRS complex associated with diastolic pressure overload of the left ventricle tends to be more horizontal than the direction of an arrow representing the mean of the electrical forces (vectors) responsible for the QRS complex associated with systolic pressure overload of the left ventricle; however, this cannot be used to distinguish between the two types of left ventricular hypertrophy.

An arrow representing the mean of the electrical forces (vectors) responsible for the QRS complex is always directed posteriorly. It is usually directed 45 to 50 degrees posteriorly, but it may be directed 60 to 75 degrees posteriorly.

An arrow representing the mean of the electrical forces (vectors) responsible for the initial 0.04 second of the QRS complex may be directed to the right and inferiorly. It is always directed anterior to the direction of the arrow representing the mean of the electrical forces (vectors) responsible for the entire QRS complex. This often produces a large Q wave in leads I, aV_L, V_5, and V_6 and a larger than usual R wave in lead V_1. These large Q and R waves are produced by the septum, which has probably become thicker, larger, and slightly displaced from its normal position as a result of the remodeling process of the left ventricle, which is produced by diastolic pressure overload of the left ventricle. The large Q waves may be misinterpreted as being due to myocardial infarction.

An arrow representing the mean of the electrical forces (vectors) responsible for the terminal 0.04 second of the QRS complex is usually directed to the left or superior to the arrow representing the mean of the electrical forces (vectors) responsible for the entire QRS complex. It is always directed posteriorly.

The intrinsicoid deflection may be greater than 0.05 second when there is left ventricular hypertrophy due to diastolic pressure overload of the left ventricle.

The amplitude of the QRS complexes is commonly increased when there is diastolic pressure overload of the left ventricle. Two methods are used to distinguish normal from abnormally large QRS complexes. The point score system of Romhilt and Estes[23] is shown in Table 7-4. Note that they use abnormalities of the P waves and ST-T waves, in addition to the QRS abnormalities, to identify left ventricular hypertrophy. Their criteria are more useful in identifying systolic pressure overload and late diastolic pressure overload than in identifying early diastolic pressure overload of the left ventricle. The other method is that described by Odom et al.[24] They recommend the use of the total QRS amplitude, which is determined by adding the depth of the Q wave to the height of the R wave to the depth of the S wave arithmetically in each of the QRS complexes. The total QRS amplitude is then determined by adding together the total amplitude of the QRS complexes found in all 12 of the leads (see Fig. 7-65). They found the normal range to be 80 to 185 mm.

An arrow representing the mean of the electrical forces (vectors) responsible for the T wave in patients with mild diastolic pressure overload should be drawn larger than usual, because the T waves become more prominent than normal; it is directed normally. This occurs because the left ventricle is dilated, as well as hypertrophied, and the transmyocardial pressure gradient is probably not greatly different from normal. With long-standing and severe diastolic pressure overload, the arrow representing the mean of the electrical forces (vectors) responsible for the T waves is directed as it is when there is systolic pressure overload of the left ventricle. This occurs because the diastolic pressure overload may reach a point where systolic pressure overload develops in a patient who initially exhibited electrocardiographic evidence of diastolic pressure overload.

An arrow representing the mean of the electrical forces (vectors) responsible for the ST segment displacement is directed almost parallel with the arrow representing the mean of the electrical forces (vectors) responsible for the T wave. When there is mild diastolic pressure overload of the left ventricle, the arrow representing the electrical forces (vectors) that produce the T wave are directed normally and the arrow representing the mean of the ST forces (vectors) is directed in the same direction. The electrical forces (vectors) responsible for the ST segment displacement are probably due to repolarization forces.

An arrow representing the mean of the electrical forces (vectors) responsible for ST segment displacement due to normal, early, repolarization in normal subjects is directed parallel with an arrow representing the electrical forces (vectors) responsible for the T wave. Although the T wave amplitude is large in these normal subjects, the QRS amplitude is normal. This latter finding may be used to distinguish normal early repolarization from that of diastolic pressure overload of the left ventricle.

An arrow representing the mean of the electrical forces (vectors) responsible for ST segment displacement due to the epicardial injury of pericarditis is usually directed toward the anatomic apex of the left ventricle. Accordingly, the direction of an arrow representing the mean of the electrical forces (vectors) responsible for the ST segment abnormality of pericarditis may be similar to the direction of the arrow representing the mean of the electrical forces (vectors) responsible for the ST segment abnormality related to diastolic pressure overload of the left ventricle. However, the T waves and QRS complexes are not larger than normal in patients with pericarditis, as they are in patients with diastolic pressure overload of the left ventricle. Also, the T waves and ST segments change in size and direction when serial electrocardiograms are recorded from patients with pericarditis.

An electrocardiogram illustrating left ventricular diastolic pressure overload is shown in Fig. 7-77.

Right ventricular hypertrophy

The newborn infant exhibits normal right ventricular dominance. That is, the right ventricular wall is as thick as, or thicker than, the left ventricular wall, and the septum tends to conform to the shape of the right ventricle rather than to the shape of

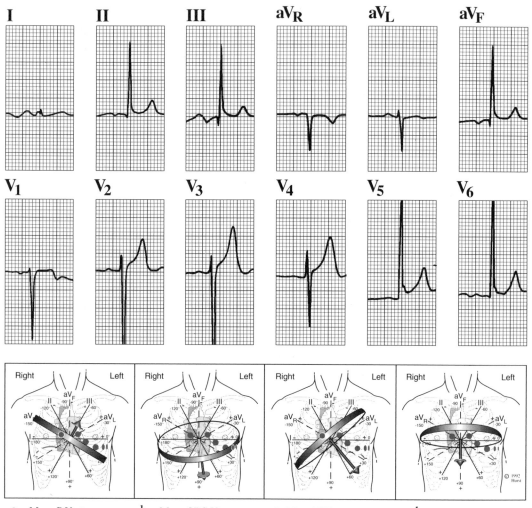

a. Mean P Vector

b. Mean QRS Vector

c. Mean T Vector

d. Mean ST Vector

Fig. 7-77

Fig. 7-77. Left ventricular hypertrophy due to diastolic pressure overload.

- *Rhythm:* Lower atrial rhythm

  Rate: Undetermined in short strip

  PR interval: 0.15 second

  QRS duration: 0.08 second

  QT interval: 0.44 second

- *Vector diagrams of electrical forces:* See *a*, *b*, *c*, and *d* below the electrocardiogram.

- *Electrophysiologic considerations:*

  The mean P vector is directed about −60 degrees superiorly and is parallel with the frontal plane. This indicates retrograde depolarization of the atria. The PR interval is 0.15 second, which eliminates a junctional rhythm. The rhythm originates in an ectopic, lower atrial site.

  The mean QRS vector is directed about +80 degrees inferiorly and at least 60 to 70 degrees posteriorly. The posterior rotation is abnormal. The 12-lead amplitude of the QRS complexes is more than 230 mm; this indicates left ventricular hypertrophy.

  The mean T vector is large and is directed about +50 degrees inferiorly and about 10 degrees anteriorly. The QRS-T angle is abnormal and is about 80 degrees.

  The mean ST vector is relatively parallel with the mean T vector.

  The abnormalities can be caused by diastolic pressure overload of the left ventricle.

- *Clinical differential diagnosis:* The combination of electrocardiographic abnormalities indicates left ventricular hypertrophy. The size of the T waves and ST segment vectors suggests left ventricular hypertrophy due to diastolic pressure overload of the left ventricle. These abnormalities can be caused by aortic valve regurgitation, mitral valve regurgitation, ventricular septal defect, or patent ductus arteriosus.

- *Discussion:* This electrocardiogram was recorded from a 24-year-old man with aortic valve regurgitation due to a bicuspid aortic valve. The echocardiogram and Doppler study revealed aortic regurgitation and a left ventricular diastolic diameter of 60 mm.

Electrocardiogram reproduced with permission from Hurst JW: *Ventricular electrocardiography*, New York, 1991, Gower, fig 9.6.

the left ventricle, as it does in the adult. An arrow representing the mean of the electrical forces (vectors) responsible for the large, wide swinging QRS complex of the newborn is directed to the right and anteriorly, and an arrow representing the mean of the electrical forces (vectors) responsible for the T wave is directed to the left and posteriorly. As months and years pass, the left ventricle begins to be more dominant than the right ventricle, and usually, by the late teenage period, the electrocardiogram attains the configuration that is seen in the normal adult (see Fig. 7-60, *B*).

Just as it is not possible to have rigid criteria distinguishing normal left ventricular dominance from abnormal left ventricular hypertrophy in the adult, it is not possible to develop diagnostic criteria that always distinguishes normal right ventricular dominance from abnormal right ventricular hypertrophy in the infant and young child. Abnormal right ventricular hypertrophy should be suspected in the newborn when an arrow representing the mean QRS vector is directed to the right and anteriorly but an arrow representing the mean T vector is directed anteriorly rather than posteriorly.

Systolic pressure overload and diastolic pressure overload of the right ventricle produce different types of electrocardiograms.

Systolic pressure overload of the right ventricle.[36,37] Systolic pressure overload of the right ventricle can be divided into two subsets: the type seen early in life as a result of congenital heart disease and the type seen later in life as a result of acquired heart disease or congenital heart disease with gradually developing Eisenmenger physiology.

Right ventricular hypertrophy resulting from *systolic pressure overload due to congenital heart disease,* such as occurs with right ventricular outflow tract obstruction (pulmonary valve stenosis or tetralogy of Fallot), has the following characteristics.

The duration of the QRS complex is usually less than 0.10 second. An arrow representing the mean of the electrical forces (vectors) responsible for the QRS complex is directed to the right from +90 to +180 degrees and anteriorly. It is directed toward the hypertrophied right ventricle, which is located anteriorly.

An arrow representing the mean of the electrical forces (vectors) responsible for the initial 0.04 and middle 0.04 second of the QRS complex is directed inferiorly at about +60 degrees and anteriorly.

An arrow representing the mean of the electrical forces (vectors) responsible for the terminal 0.04 second of the QRS complex is directed to the right about +120 degrees or more. It is directed anteriorly, or parallel with the frontal plane.

The amplitude of the QRS complexes is usually greater than normal; however, no absolute measurement in millimeters is necessary, because the direction of the arrow representing the mean of the electrical forces (vectors) responsible for the entire QRS complex in the adult is so different from normal that the exact amplitude need not be determined.

An arrow representing the mean of the electrical forces (vectors) responsible for the T wave is directed to the left and posteriorly. It tends to be directed opposite to the direction of the arrow representing the mean of the electrical forces (vectors) responsible for the QRS complex.

An arrow representing the mean of the electrical forces (vectors) responsible for the T wave tends to be directed away from the right ventricle, because the systolic pressure overload eliminates the right ventricular transmyocardial pressure gradient, so that the repolarization process begins in the endocardium of the thick right ventricle, rather than in the epicardium, and produces electrical forces in an opposite direction.[40]

An arrow representing the mean of the electrical forces (vectors) responsible for the ST segment displacement is directed relatively parallel with the arrow representing the mean of the electrical forces (vectors) responsible for the T wave. The electrical forces (vectors) responsible for the ST segment are, in reality, forces of repolarization.

Right ventricular hypertrophy due to *systolic pressure overload occurs later in life as a result of acquired heart disease,* such as mitral stenosis, pulmonary emboli, or primary pulmonary hypertension. Right ventricular hypertrophy due to systolic pressure overload may also occur later in life in patients with interventricular septal defect, patent ductus arteriosus, or interatrial septal defect who gradually develop Eisenmenger physiology. The sequence of events leading to right ventricular hypertrophy in these patients is different from the sequence of events producing right ventricular hypertrophy in patients with congenital right ventricular outflow tract obstruction or pulmonary valve stenosis. Individuals who develop normal left ventricular dominance before developing a disease that can potentially cause systolic pressure overload of the right ventricle do not initially develop an anterior rotation of the arrow representing the mean of the electrical forces (vectors) responsible for the QRS complex; the arrow may become more vertical but may retain its posterior direction. Later in the course of events the arrow representing the mean of the electrical forces (vectors) responsible for the entire QRS complex becomes directed anteriorly; this always signifies the development of severe right ventricular hypertension. By contrast, patients who are born with pulmonary valve stenosis or tetralogy of Fallot never lose their right ventricular hypertrophy; they never develop left ventricular dominance. Accordingly, an arrow representing right ventricular hypertrophy will, from the beginning, be directed to the right and anteriorly. An exception to this rule may be seen occasionally; an intermediately directed mean QRS vector may be directed anteriorly in an adult with mild pulmonary valve stenosis.

Occasionally an arrow representing right ventricular hypertrophy occurring later in life from acquired heart disease or in relation to Eisenmenger physiology will be directed inferiorly at +60 to +70 degrees, and the R wave in lead V_1 may become greater than 3 mm in such cases. At times in these patients the R wave in V_1 may become equal to, or greater than, the S wave. These abnormalities are caused by an

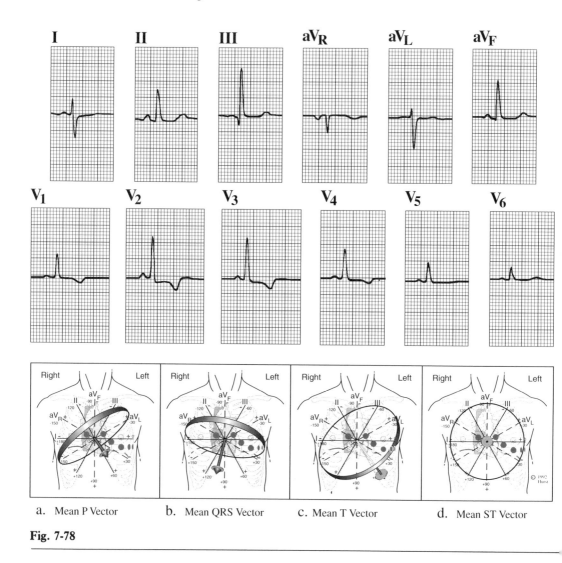

a. Mean P Vector   b. Mean QRS Vector   c. Mean T Vector   d. Mean ST Vector

Fig. 7-78

increase in the size of, and by an anterior rotation of, the initial and middle QRS forces.

The intrinsicoid deflection of the R wave in leads V_1 and V_2 may be prolonged to 0.04 second when right ventricular hypertrophy is present. Normally, the intrinsicoid deflection in leads V_1 and V_2 is 0.02 to 0.03 second.[25]

The arrows representing the mean of the electrical forces (vectors) responsible for the ST segment displacement and T wave in patients with right ventricular hypertrophy due to systolic pressure overload from acquired causes or from the grad-

Fig. 7-78. Right ventricular hypertrophy due to systolic pressure overload of the right ventricle.

- *Rhythm:* Normal sinus rhythm

  Rate: Undetermined in short strip. There were 60 depolarizations per minute in a longer strip.

  PR interval: 0.14 second

  QRS duration: 0.08 second

  QT interval: 0.40 second

- *Vector diagrams of electrical forces:* See *a, b, c,* and *d* below the electrocardiogram.

- *Electrophysiologic considerations:*

  The mean P vector suggests a right atrial abnormality, because it is directed a little more anteriorly than usual.

  The mean QRS vector is directed to the right about +105 degrees. It is directed anteriorly at least 30 degrees (the exact number of degrees cannot be determined without recordings from additional electrode positions). The direction of the mean QRS vector indicates right ventricular hypertrophy.

  The mean T vector is directed about +55 degrees inferiorly and about 80 degrees posteriorly. It is directed away from the right ventricle. The spatial QRS-T angle is at least 110 degrees.

  The mean ST vector is small; it is barely visible in the frontal plane; it is directed 90 degrees posteriorly and is relatively parallel with the mean T vector. The abnormalities are characteristic of systolic pressure overload of the right ventricle such as occurs with congenital pulmonary valve stenosis, congenital subpulmonary valve stenosis, tetralogy of Fallot, and late in the course of primary pulmonary hypertension, repeated pulmonary emboli, Eisenmenger syndrome due to interventricular septal defect, or patent ductus arteriosus. Conceivably, the abnormalities could occur in patients with long-standing, severe mitral stenosis, but this is unlikely.

- *Discussion:* This electrocardiogram was recorded from a 36-year-old woman with congenital subpulmonic infundibular stenosis. The pulmonary artery pressure was 25/17 mm Hg, and the right ventricular pressure was 229/6 mm Hg. The right atrial pressure was 18/10 mm Hg.

---

ual development of Eisenmenger physiology will eventually be directed opposite to the arrow representing the mean of the electrical forces (vectors) responsible for the QRS complex.

An electrocardiogram illustrating systolic pressure overload of the right ventricle due to congenital subpulmonic infundibular stenosis is shown in Fig. 7-78. See Fig. 7-71 for an electrocardiogram showing systolic pressure overload due to mitral stenosis.

Diastolic pressure overload of the right ventricle.[36,37] Theoretically, the same basic pathophysiologic principles should apply to right ventricular diastolic pressure overload of the right ventricle that apply to diastolic pressure overload of the left ventricle. In practice, however, there is only one common cardiac abnormality that produces diastolic pressure overload of the right ventricle: the secundum type of atrial septal defect. When the pulmonary artery pressure is normal, or only slightly elevated, the electrocardiogram reveals right ventricular conduction delay rather than diastolic pressure overload of the right ventricle. Presumably, this occurs because the distal branches of the right bundle become "stretched" and as a result can no longer serve as perfectly normal conduction pathways. Accordingly, the conduction of electrical impulses is delayed in certain portions of the right ventricle. Therefore the right ventricular conduction delay masks, or overshadows, the expected electrocardiographic features of diastolic pressure overload of the right ventricle.

The electrocardiographic characteristics of right ventricular conduction delay are as follows.

The duration of the QRS complex is usually 0.08 to 0.10 second.

An arrow representing the mean of the electrical forces (vectors) responsible for the entire QRS complex is directed to the right at about +100 degrees or more and anteriorly.

An arrow representing the mean of the electrical forces (vectors) responsible for the initial 0.02 second of the QRS complex is directed inferiorly and anteriorly. This produces an initial R wave in lead V_1, but it is not as tall as the R' wave in the same lead.

An arrow representing the mean of the electrical forces (vectors) responsible for the middle 0.03 to 0.04 second of the QRS complex is directed inferiorly and posteriorly. This produces a downward deflection of the middle portion of the QRS complex in lead V_1.

An arrow representing the mean of the electrical forces (vectors) responsible for the terminal 0.02 second of the QRS complex is directed to the right and anteriorly. This produces an R' wave in lead V_1 that is taller than the initial R wave.

Arrows representing the mean of the electrical forces (vectors) responsible for the ST segment displacement and T wave are directed inferiorly and often slightly posteriorly.[41]

When pulmonary hypertension develops in a patient with a secundum atrial septal defect, the QRS complexes begin to resemble those of systolic pressure overload of the right ventricle. Therefore arrows representing the mean of the electrical forces (vectors) responsible for the initial and middle portions of the QRS complex become larger and are directed to the right and anteriorly.

Although the electrocardiogram of an adult with secundum atrial septal defect usually exhibits a right ventricular conduction delay, it may not do so when patients develop acquired heart disease, such as left ventricular hypertrophy due to hypertension or aortic disease, or when the patient has a myocardial infarction.

An electrocardiogram illustrating right ventricular conduction delay is shown in Fig. 7-79.

Biventricular hypertrophy

Biventricular hypertrophy may be a result of aortic and mitral valve disease with pulmonary hypertension or dilated cardiomyopathy including ischemic cardiomyopathy.

Electrocardiograms illustrating biventricular hypertrophy are shown in Figs. 7-80 and 7-81.

P wave abnormality. The P waves may reveal a biatrial abnormality.

Direction of the mean QRS vector. An arrow representing the mean of the electrical forces (vectors) responsible for the QRS complex in patients with biventricular hypertrophy may be directed inferiorly, to the left and slightly anterior to or parallel with the frontal plane, or at more than +90 degrees and posteriorly.

Amplitude of the QRS complexes. The amplitude of the QRS complexes may be greater than normal.

Low-amplitude QRS complexes

Although the amplitude of the QRS complexes *increases* when there is ventricular hypertrophy, the amplitude of the QRS complexes *decreases* when certain conditions are present. The amplitude is considered to be low when it measures 7 mm or less in height in most of the leads. Each measurement has its own predictive value. Accordingly, a QRS complex amplitude of 5 mm in most leads is more likely to indicate an abnormally low amplitude than is a QRS complex amplitude of 10 mm. A QRS complex amplitude of 12 mm in most leads may be abnormal if the amplitude was 15 mm in a previous electrocardiogram.

Odom et al.[24] found the normal total amplitude of the QRS complex to be 80 to 185 mm (see earlier discussion). It is wise to consider conditions that are known to cause a low QRS amplitude whenever the total QRS amplitude is on the low side of normal. Low amplitude of the QRS complexes may be observed in the following conditions:

- Pericardial effusion. The diagnoses can be made with certainty when there is low amplitude of the QRS complexes and electrical alternans of the QRS complexes is also present. Electrical alternans implies that alternate QRS complexes have different amplitudes.
- Constrictive pericarditis.
- Dilated and restrictive cardiomyopathy. Idiopathic cardiomypathy or infiltrative cardiomyopathy such as occurs with amyloid infiltration of the ventricles may produce a low QRS amplitude (Fig. 7-82). The amplitude of the QRS complexes may be abnormally low in patients with progressive systemic sclerosis (scleroderma) because of fibrosis of the myocardium, an increase in skin resistance, or anasarca due to heart failure (Fig. 7-83) or renal failure.

Text continued on p. 304.

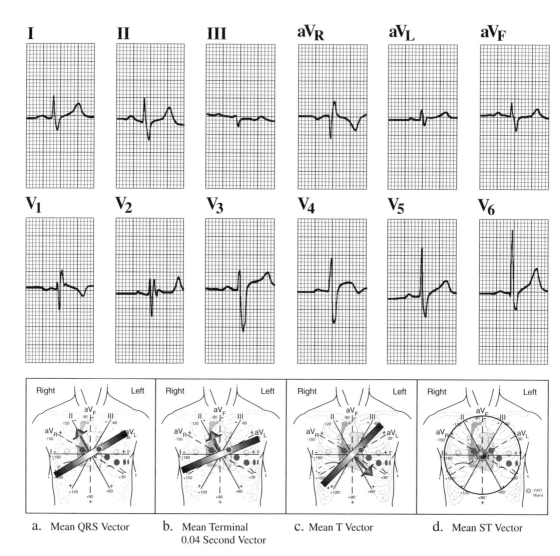

a. Mean QRS Vector

b. Mean Terminal
0.04 Second Vector

c. Mean T Vector

d. Mean ST Vector

Fig. 7-79

Fig. 7-79. Diastolic pressure overload of the right ventricle (right ventricular conduction delay).

- *Rhythm:* Sinus bradycardia
   Rate: Undetermined in short strip. There were 50 depolarizations per minute in a longer strip.
   PR interval: 0.16 second
   QRS duration: 0.10 second
   QT interval: 0.40 second
- *Vector diagrams of electrical forces:* See *a, b, c,* and *d* below the electrocardiogram.
- *Electrophysiologic considerations:*
   The mean QRS vector is directed −120 degrees superiorly and is parallel with the frontal plane. This abnormality is caused by the terminal 0.04 second QRS abnormality.
   The mean terminal 0.04 second QRS vector is directed −115 degrees superiorly and is parallel with the frontal plane. This abnormality is due to right ventricular conduction delay and is commonly associated with diastolic volume overload of the left ventricle. Actually, it masks the theoretic arrangements of vectors that would be predicted to be caused by diastolic pressure overload of the right ventricle.
   The mean T vector is directed about +42 degrees inferiorly and is parallel with the frontal plane.
   The mean ST vector is barely visible in the frontal plane and is directed anteriorly. The cause of the isolated T wave negativity in lead V_4 is not known.
   This type of electrocardiogram occurs in patients with diastolic volume overload of the right ventricle, including secundum atrial septal defect and anomolous drainage of the pulmonary veins into the right atrium. Right ventricular conduction delay can also occur in otherwise normal subjects.
- *Discussion:* This electrocardiogram was recorded from a 26-year-old man with a secundum atrial septal defect. The left-to-right shunt was 1.5 to 1, and the systolic pulmonary artery pressure was 55 mm Hg. This tracing illustrates how right ventricular conduction delay masks, or overshadows, the theoretic arrangements of vectors that could be caused by diastolic volume overload of the right ventricle.

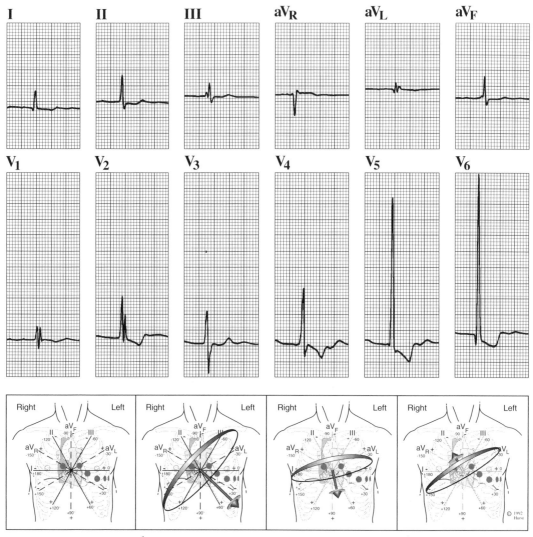

a. Mean P Vector (none)   b. Mean QRS Vector   c. Mean T Vector   d. Mean ST Vector

Fig. 7-80

Fig. 7-80. Biventricular hypertrophy.

- *Rhythm:* Junctional rhythm

  Rate: Undetermined in short strip. There were 74 depolarizations per minute in a longer
   strip.

  PR interval: None

  QRS duration: 0.09 second

  QT interval: 0.36 second

- *Vector diagrams of electrical forces:* See *a*, *b*, *c*, and *d* below the electrocardiogram.

- *Electrophysiologic considerations:*

  No P waves are seen, and the RR interval did not vary in the longer strip. The mean P
  vector cannot be drawn; junctional rhythm is present.

  The mean QRS vector is directed about +43 degrees inferiorly and 10 to 15 degrees anteriorly. The total amplitude of the QRS complexes is more than 235 mm. The direction
  and amplitude of the mean QRS vector indicates right and left ventricular hypertrophy.

  The mean T vector is small (see last hump of ST-T waves; it is directed about +75 degrees
  inferiorly and 15 to 20 degrees anteriorly.

  The mean ST segment vector is directed about −120 degrees superiorly and about 10 degrees posteriorly. The QT interval is 0.36 second. The ST-T wave vector is characteristic
  of digitalis effect.

- *Clinical differential diagnosis:* Several combinations of abnormalities may produce biventricular hypertrophy. The patient might have systemic hypertension and mitral stenosis or aortic valve disease and mitral valve disease with a predominance of mitral stenosis. Hypertrophic cardiomyopathy can also involve both ventricles.

- *Discussion:* The electrocardiogram was recorded from a 64-year-old man with rheumatic aortic stenosis and mitral stenosis. Heart failure was present, and he was receiving digitalis.

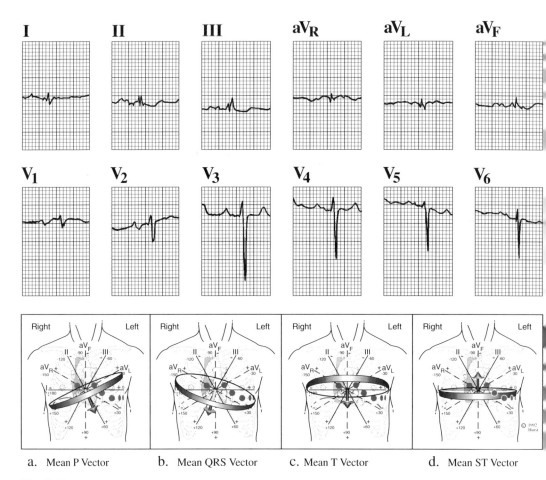

a.   Mean P Vector   b.   Mean QRS Vector   c.   Mean T Vector   d.   Mean ST Vector

Fig. 7-81

Fig. 7-81. Biventricular hypertrophy in another patient.

- *Rhythm:* Normal sinus rhythm

  Rate: Undetermined in short strip. There were 80 depolarizations per minute in a longer strip.

  PR interval: 0.20 second

  QRS duration: 0.08 second

  QT interval: 0.32 second

- *Vector diagrams of electrical forces:* See *a*, *b*, *c*, and *d* below the electrocardiogram.

- *Electrophysiologic considerations:*

  The duration of the P wave is 0.13 second. The P wave amplitude is 2 mm. The P wave is notched at its halfway point. The mean P vector is directed +65 degrees inferiorly and about 15 degrees posteriorly. The second half of the P wave in lead V_1 measures −0.04 mm/sec. The second half of the P wave is also negative in lead V_2. These P wave abnormalities indicate a left atrial abnormality.

  The mean QRS vector is directed about +105 degrees to the right and an undetermined number of degrees posteriorly. Additional precordial leads are needed to determine the exact number of degrees the mean QRS vector is directed posteriorly. The direction of the mean QRS vector suggests right and left ventricular hypertrophy, although the amplitude of the QRS complexes is on the low side of normal.

  The direction of the mean T vector cannot be identified with certainty unless additional precordial leads are acquired. I have used the terminal portion of the ST-T waves to construct the mean T vector. It is directed about +90 degrees inferiorly and 10 degrees anteriorly.

  The mean ST vector is directed −90 degrees superiorly and 10 degrees anteriorly.

  The unusual mean QRS vector could be due to left and right ventricular hypertrophy, because the duration of the QRS complexes is normal and rightward shift (of the QRS vector) is not sufficient to evoke the possibility of left posteroinferior division block. The left atrial abnormality reflects left ventricular disease with or without left atrial enlargement.

- *Clinical differential diagnosis:* The patient could have dilated cardiomyopathy from one of many causes, including aortic or mitral valve disease. The short QT interval and arrangement of the ST and T vectors suggest digitalis effect.

- *Discussion:* This electrocardiogram was recorded from a 67-year-old man with rheumatic heart disease. He had aortic stenosis and regurgitation, mitral stenosis and regurgitation, and tricuspid regurgitation. Heart failure was present, and he was taking digitalis.

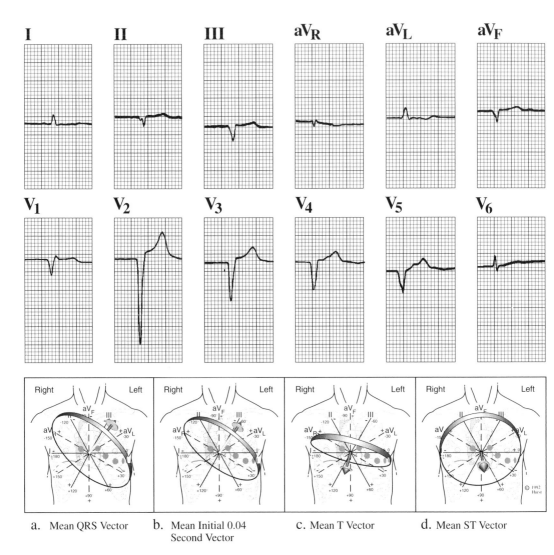

a. Mean QRS Vector

b. Mean Initial 0.04 Second Vector

c. Mean T Vector

d. Mean ST Vector

Fig. 7-82

Fig. 7-82. Low voltage (amplitude) of the QRS complexes.
- *Rhythm:* Accelerated junctional rhythm (no P wave seen)
  Rate: Undetermined in short strip. There were 72 depolarizations per minute in a longer strip.
  PR interval: No P waves seen
  QRS duration: 0.08 second
  QT interval: 0.35 second
- *Vector diagrams of electrical forces:* See *a, b, c,* and *d* below the electrocardiogram.
- *Electrophysiologic considerations:*
  Accelerated junctional rhythm is present.
  The mean QRS vector is directed −55 degrees to the left and posteriorly (the exact amount cannot be determined without additional leads). There is left anterosuperior division block. The total QRS amplitude is about 76 mm, which is abnormally low.
  The mean initial 0.04 second QRS vector is directed −58 degrees to the left and posteriorly (it is directed a few degrees less posteriorly than the mean QRS vector).
  The mean T vector is directed about +110 degrees to the right and anteriorly (the exact amount cannot be determined without additional leads).
  The mean ST vector is directed +85 degrees to the right and 70 to 80 degrees anteriorly.
- *Clinical differential diagnosis:* The QRS amplitude is lower than normal, and the mean 0.04 second QRS vector is directed abnormally leftward and posteriorly. The mean ST and T vectors are directed opposite to the mean QRS vector. This type of electrocardiogram can occur in patients with cardiomyopathy. The cardiomyopathy may be due to atherosclerotic coronary heart disease or to an infiltrative disease, such as amyloid.
- *Discussion:* This electrocardiogram was recorded from a 69-year-old woman with restrictive cardiomyopathy due to amyloid disease. Amyloid cardiomyopathy commonly produces low amplitude of the QRS complexes, and the abnormally directed initial 0.04 second QRS vector may suggest a dead zone simulating myocardial infarction due to atherosclerotic coronary heart disease.

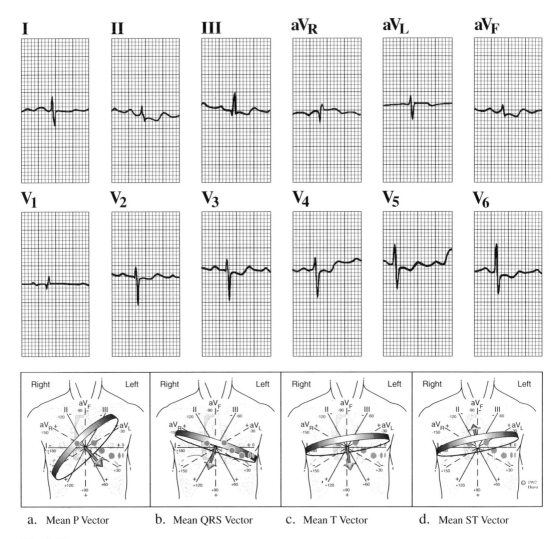

a. Mean P Vector   b. Mean QRS Vector   c. Mean T Vector   d. Mean ST Vector

Fig. 7-83

Fig. 7-83. Low voltage (amplitude) of the QRS complexes in another patient.

- *Rhythm:* Sinus tachycardia

  Rate: Undetermined in short strip. There were 100 depolarizations per minute in a longer strip.

  PR interval: 0.16 second

  QRS duration: 0.08 second

  QT interval: 0.34 second

  Vector diagrams of electrical forces: See *a*, *b*, *c*, and *d* below the electrocardiogram.

- *Electrophysiologic considerations:*

  The mean P vector is normal. The vectors representing the first and second halves of the P wave are normal.

  The mean QRS vector is directed about +115 degrees to the right and slightly anteriorly (note that the deflections shown in leads V_4, V_5, and V_6 are recorded very near the transitional pathway). This indicates right ventricular hypertrophy or right ventricular conduction delay.

  The mean T vector is directed about +80 degrees to the right and about 10 degrees anteriorly.

  The mean ST vector is directed about −95 degrees to the left and about 5 to 10 degrees posteriorly.

- *Clinical differential diagnosis:* The direction of the mean QRS vector suggests right ventricular hypertrophy plus low voltage of the QRS complexes. The short QT interval plus an ST vector that is directed opposite to a small mean T vector suggests digitalis medication. This electrocardiogram could be caused by pulmonary emboli, primary pulmonary hypertension, or Eisenmenger physiology, but the low QRS voltage must be explained. The low voltage could be due to edema or infiltrative myocardial disease.

- *Discussion:* This electrocardiogram was recorded from a 74-year-old woman with progressive systemic sclerosis. She had severe heart failure and a systolic pulmonary artery pressure of 150 mm Hg. She had anasarca. The low QRS amplitude could be due to anasarca due to heart failure plus an increase in skin resistance associated with progressive systemic sclerosis.

Electrocardiogram courtesy Paul Robinson, M.D., Emory University School of Medicine, Atlanta, Ga.

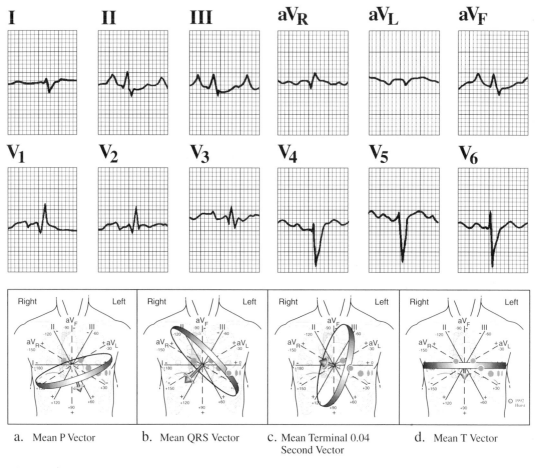

a. Mean P Vector
b. Mean QRS Vector
c. Mean Terminal 0.04 Second Vector
d. Mean T Vector

Fig. 7-84

- Pulmonary emphysema. The inflated lungs and a large chest are responsible for the low amplitude of the QRS complexes (Fig. 7-84).
- Myxedema. The low amplitude of the QRS complexes is due to pericardial effusion, myocardial disease, and high skin resistance. A heart rate below 60 beats per minute in a patient with low voltage of the QRS complexes is an additional clue indicating the presence of myxedema.
- High skin resistance (see Fig. 7-83).
- Anasarca (see Fig. 7-83).
- Improper standardization of the electrocardiograph machine.

When the amplitude of the QRS complexes and T waves is abnormally low in leads V_5 and V_6 but is normal in all other leads, it is wise to consider the presence of a left pleural effusion or a left pneumothorax (Fig. 7-85).

Fig. 7-84. Low QRS voltage due to pulmonary emphysema.

- *Rhythm:* Normal sinus rhythm

  Rate: Undetermined in short strip

  PR interval: 0.14 second

  QRS duration: 0.10 second

  QT interval: 0.48 second

- *Vector diagrams of electrical forces:* See *a*, *b*, *c*, and *d* below the electrocardiogram.

- *Electrophysiologic considerations:*

  The amplitude of the P wave in lead II is 2.5 mm. Note the peaked shape of the P waves in leads II, III, and aV$_F$. The mean P vector is directed +73 degrees inferiorly and 30 degrees posteriorly. There is a right atrial abnormality.

  The mean QRS vector is directed about +135 degrees to the right and about 20 degrees anteriorly. The direction of the mean QRS vector may be due to right ventricular conduction delay or right ventricular hypertrophy (or both). The 12-lead QRS amplitude is about 84 mm, which is on the low side of the normal range.

  The mean terminal 0.04 second QRS vector is directed about −170 degrees to the left and 20 degrees anteriorly because of a right ventricular conduction delay.

  The mean T vector is small and difficult to plot. It seems to be directed +90 degrees inferiorly and parallel with the frontal plane.

  There is a right atrial abnormality, right ventricular conduction delay, and low amplitude of the QRS complexes.

- *Clinical differential diagnosis:* Although the most common cause of this type of electrocardiogram is severe pulmonary emphysema due to obstructive lung disease, other conditions could be responsible for these abnormalities. For example, a patient with secundum atrial septal defect who also had a pericardial effusion might exhibit such an electrocardiogram.

- *Discussion:* This patient had severe pulmonary emphysema and cor pulmonale. The right atrial abnormality, low QRS amplitude, and right ventricular conduction delay strongly suggest emphysema and cor pulmonale.

Electrocardiogram reproduced with permission from Fowler NO, Daniels C, Scott RC et al: The electrocardiogram in cor pulmonale with and without emphysema, *Am J Cardiol* 16:501, 1965.

QRS conduction defects[42,43]

The normal conduction system of the ventricles is discussed earlier in the chapter. Certain ventricular conduction abnormalities may be present when the QRS duration is 0.10 second or less. Other types of ventricular conduction defects may be present when the duration of the QRS complex is 0.12 second, and still other conduction abnormalities may be present when the duration of the QRS complex is greater than 0.12 second. Too often, simple right or left bundle-branch block is said to be present when in reality there is right or left bundle-branch block *plus* an additional QRS conduction abnormality, ST segment abnormality, or primary T wave abnormality.

QRS conduction defects when the QRS duration is less than 0.12 second. There may be an *alteration of the conduction in the first part of the septum.* The direc-

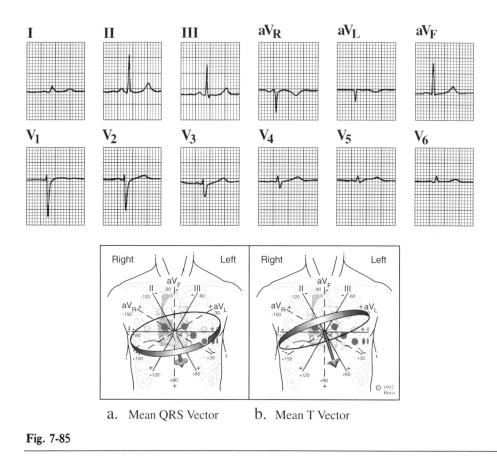

a. Mean QRS Vector   b. Mean T Vector

Fig. 7-85

tion of the electrical forces (vectors) generated by the normal depolarization of the normal septum during the initial 0.01 to 0.02 second is discussed earlier in the chapter. The direction of an arrow representing initial 0.01 to 0.02 second electrical forces (vectors) may be altered when the septum participates in the ventricular remodeling process associated with left or right ventricular hypertrophy, there is septal hypertrophy associated with idiopathic hypertrophy, or there is damage to the septal myocytes and septal conduction system. Such damage may be due to a small anteroseptal infarction resulting from coronary artery disease, fibrosis, myocardial damage from a disease such as amyloid or sarcoid, or from unknown causes. The abnormality may at times be caused by preexcitation of the ventricles or possibly by a congenital alteration of conduction in the septum.

An arrow representing the mean of the electrical forces (vectors) responsible for the abnormal initial 0.01 to 0.02 second of the QRS complex is directed inferiorly and abnormally posteriorly; there is no R wave in leads V_1, V_2, and occasionally lead

Fig. 7-85. Effect of a left pneumothorax on the deflections recorded in the chest leads.

* *Rhythm:* Normal sinus rhythm
  Rate: Undetermined in short strip. There were 80 depolarizations per minute in a longer
    strip.
  PR interval: 0.12 second
  QRS duration: 0.08 second
  QT interval: 0.36 second
* *Vector diagrams of electrical forces:* See *a* and *b* below the electrocardiogram.
* *Electrophysiologic considerations:*
  The P waves are normal.
  The mean QRS vector is directed normally at about +80 degrees in the frontal plane and 45
    degrees posteriorly. Note the low amplitude of the QRS complexes in leads V_3 through
    V_6.
  The mean T vector is directed normally at about +75 degrees and 15 degrees anteriorly.
    The QRS-T angle is normal.
* *Clinical differential diagnosis:* The abnormally low amplitude of the deflections recorded in
  leads V_3 through V_6 can be caused by left pleural fluid or a left pneumothorax.
* *Discussion:* This electrocardiogram was recorded from a 20-year-old woman with a large left
  pneumothorax.

Electrocardiogram courtesy Charles Brown, M.D.

V_3. An arrow representing the mean of the electrical forces (vectors) responsible for the terminal 0.04 second of the QRS complex is directed normally.

Although it is not always possible to identify the exact cause of the alteration of the electrical forces (vectors) generated during the initial 0.01 to 0.02 second of the QRS complex, one must not assume that the abnormality is always due to myocardial infarction; it may have a benign cause.

An example of an isolated, benign alteration of the direction of the initial 0.01 to 0.02 second electrical force (vector) is shown in Fig. 7-86.

The label *left ventricular conduction delay* is used to designate the abnormality of the QRS complex that simulates left bundle-branch block when the QRS duration is 0.10 second or less, rather than 0.12 second, as it is when there is left bundle-branch block.

The direction of an arrow representing the mean of the electrical forces (vectors) responsible for the entire QRS complex is normal.

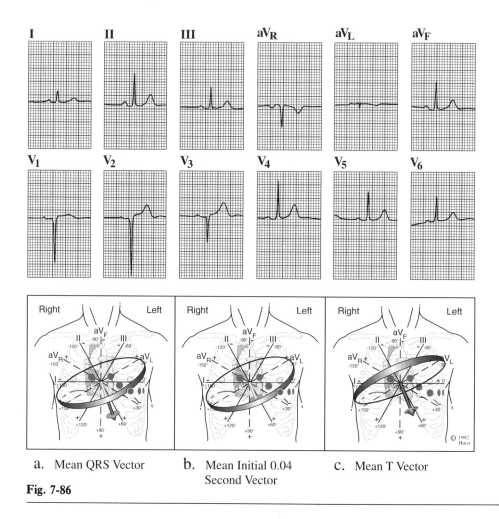

a. Mean QRS Vector b. Mean Initial 0.04 c. Mean T Vector
Second Vector

Fig. 7-86

An arrow representing the direction of the electrical forces (vectors) responsible for the initial 0.01 to 0.02 second of the QRS complex is directed inferiorly and posteriorly, and parallel with or slightly posterior to the frontal plane, so that there is no Q wave in lead I or V_6 and no R wave, or a very small R wave, in leads V_1 and V_2.

An arrow representing the mean of the electrical forces (vectors) responsible for the terminal 0.02 to 0.04 second of the QRS complex is directed to the left and posteriorly. These forces are not, however, sufficiently large to produce an abnormal leftward direction of the arrow representing the mean of the electrical forces responsible for the entire QRS complex.

Fig. 7-86. Alteration of conduction in the first part of the septum.

- *Rhythm:* Sinus bradycardia

  Rate: Undetermined in short strip. There were 56 depolarizations per minute in a longer strip.

  PR interval: 0.16 second

  QRS duration: 0.07 second

  QT interval: 0.36 second

- *Vector diagrams of electrical forces:* See *a, b,* and *c* below the electrocardiogram.

- *Electrophysiologic differential diagnosis:*

  The mean QRS vector is directed about +70 degrees inferiorly and about 40 degrees posteriorly.

  The mean initial 0.04 second QRS vector is directed at about +65 degrees in the frontal plane; it is directed about 40 degrees posteriorly. Normally this vector should be more anteriorly directed than it is in this electrocardiogram. This abnormality may be caused by a conduction defect within the septum or a septal dead zone from some cause.

  The mean T vector is directed about +65 degrees inferiorly and about 15 degrees anteriorly. The mean T vector and the QRS-T angle are normal.

- *Clinical differential diagnosis:* The abnormal initial 0.04 second QRS vector could occur in an otherwise normal patient with a conduction defect located in the first portion of the septum. It could be congenital and unimportant, or it could conceivably be caused by healed myocarditis. The abnormality could also be caused by a dead zone located in the anteroseptal region from atherosclerotic coronary heart disease or from some infiltrative myocardial disease.

- *Discussion:* This electrocardiogram was recorded from a 37-year-old healthy woman. The electrocardiogram has not changed in 14 years. There is no other evidence of heart disease. The abnormality is probably due to a benign conduction defect in the first part of the septum.

This abnormality, illustrated in Fig. 7-87, may be associated with left ventricular hypertrophy, coronary disease, or cardiomyopathy, or the cause may not be identified.

Right ventricular conduction delay is discussed earlier in the context of right ventricular diastolic pressure overload. The abnormality can occur from causes other than diastolic pressure overload and for this reason is discussed again.

The duration of the QRS complex is usually less than 0.10 second.

An arrow representing the mean of the electrical forces (vectors) responsible for the entire QRS complex is usually, but not always, directed vertically or to the right and anteriorly toward the right ventricle.

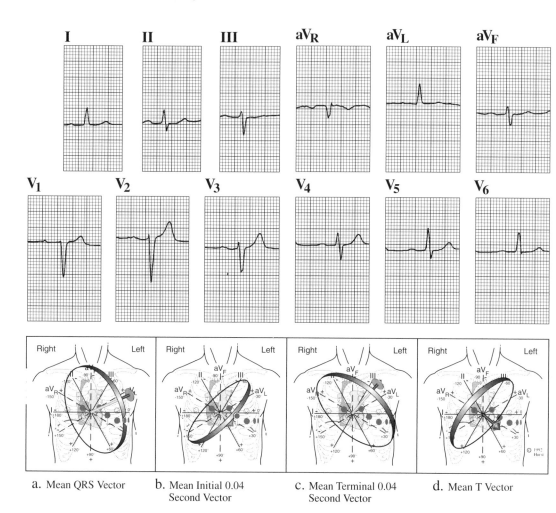

a. Mean QRS Vector   b. Mean Initial 0.04
Second Vector

c. Mean Terminal 0.04
Second Vector

d. Mean T Vector

Fig. 7-87

Fig. 7-87. Left ventricular conduction delay.

- *Rhythm:* Normal sinus rhythm
  Rate: Undetermined in short strip. There were 72 depolarizations per minute in a longer
    strip.
  PR interval: 0.28 second
  QRS duration: 0.09 to 0.10 second
  QT interval: 0.36 second
- *Vector diagrams of electrical forces:* See *a, b, c,* and *d* below the electrocardiogram.
- *Electrophysiologic considerations:*
  The P waves are normal. First-degree atrioventricular block is present.
  The mean QRS vector is directed about −25 degrees to the left and about 60 to 70 degrees
    posteriorly. The mean QRS vector is directed more posteriorly than usual.
  The mean initial 0.04 second QRS vector is directed about +55 degrees inferiorly and about
    20 degrees posteriorly.
  The mean terminal 0.04 second QRS vector is directed about −50 degrees to the left and
    more than 45 degrees posteriorly. This vector is directed farther to the left and more pos-
    teriorly than usual.
  The mean T vector is directed about +40 degrees inferiorly and about 30 degrees anteri-
    orly. This vector is normal.
  The abnormalities noted in this electrocardiogram are similar to those associated with un-
    complicated left bundle-branch block. Note the absence of Q waves in leads I and V_6 and
    a barely visible R wave in lead V_1. It differs from uncomplicated left bundle-branch block
    in that the QRS duration is not 0.12 seconds as it is in left bundle-branch block.
- *Clinical differential diagnosis:* Such an electrocardiogram can be recorded from otherwise normal subjects, patients with atherosclerotic heart disease, dilated cardiomyopathy, or left ventricular hypertrophy due to any cause.
- *Discussion:* This electrocardiogram was recorded from a 67-year-old man with coronary arteriographic evidence of significant obstructive coronary atherosclerosis.

An arrow representing the mean of the electrical forces (vectors) responsible for the initial 0.02 second of the QRS complex is directed normally.

An arrow representing the mean of the electrical forces (vectors) responsible for the terminal 0.02 to 0.04 second of the QRS complex is directed abnormally to the right and anteriorly. This produces an S wave in lead I and an R' wave that is taller than the initial R wave in lead V_1.

This type of conduction defect may occur in otherwise normal subjects. The abnormality occurs commonly in patients with secundum atrial septal defects and in such patients represents diastolic pressure overload of the right ventricle (see earlier discussion and Fig. 7-79). Perhaps the terminal portion of the right ventricular conduction system "stretches" and for this reason conducts more slowly than normally. The delay, however, does not prolong the ventricular conduction sufficiently to produce more than a slight increase in the duration of the QRS complex.

Left anterosuperior division block is a common abnormality and is easy to recognize.[43] Left posteroinferior division block is observed less often and is difficult to identify.[43] Depolarization of the working myocytes of the left ventricle is initiated by the electrical potential delivered to them by the subdivisions of the left bundle branch. The electrical stimulus provided by the left anterosuperior division controls the depolarization sequence of the anterosuperior portion of the left ventricle. This produces electrical forces (vectors) that, when represented as an arrow, are directed at about +60 degrees in the frontal plane and slightly anteriorly. The stimulus provided by the left posteroinferior division controls the depolarization sequence of the posteroinferior portion of the left ventricle. This produces electrical forces (vectors) that, when represented as an arrow, are directed superiorly and posteriorly. These two electrical forces (vectors) occur almost simultaneously, and their vector sum, when represented as an arrow, is usually directed slightly inferiorly or superiorly to the left and posteriorly (see Fig. 7-59).

When the left anterosuperior division of the left bundle branch is damaged (blocked) by some disease process, the depolarization process of the left ventricle is influenced profoundly by the electrical stimulus that travels in the posteroinferior division of the left bundle branch. Therefore the electrical forces (vectors) responsible for the terminal portion of the QRS complex are generated by depolarization of the myocytes that are stimulated by the electrical impulses traveling in the posteroinferior division of the left bundle branch plus the retrograde depolarization of the myocytes normally stimulated by the electrical impulses traveling in the left anterosuperior division of the left bundle branch. An arrow representing the vector sum of these electrical forces (vectors) is directed far to the left and posteriorly (Fig. 7-88).

Left anterosuperior division block is characterized by a QRS duration of about 0.10 second.

An arrow representing the mean of the electrical forces (vectors) occurring dur-

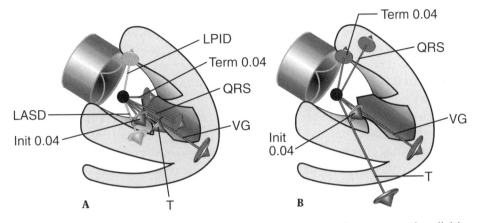

Fig. 7-88. Electrocardiographic abnormalities associated with left anterosuperior division block. **A,** Directions of arrows representing the normal mean initial 0.04 second QRS vector, the normal mean terminal 0.04 second QRS vector, the normal mean QRS vector, and the normal mean T vector. The ventricular gradient *(VG)* is normal. The QRS duration is 0.09 second. Note the direction of electrical forces (vectors) produced by the myocytes stimulated by the left anterosuperior division *(LASD)* of the left bundle branch *(light arrow)* and the direction of the electrical forces (vectors) produced by the myocytes stimulated by the left posteroinferior division *(LPID)* of the left bundle branch *(light arrow)*. The sum of these electrical forces (vectors), which occur almost simultaneously, produces the terminal 0.04 second QRS vector. **B,** Abnormalities. The *QRS duration* is usually 0.10 second. The arrow representing the *mean initial 0.04 second QRS vector* is directed normally. The arrow representing the *mean terminal 0.04 second QRS vector* is directed far to the left and posteriorly, because the left anterosuperior division of the left bundle branch is blocked. In such cases the left posteroinferior branch of the left bundle-branch system stimulates the myocytes. In addition, some of the myocytes ordinarily stimulated by the left anterosuperior division of the left bundle branch undoubtedly depolarize in a manner that is opposite to normal (see text). Accordingly, the electrical forces (vectors) produced by depolarization of the posterobasilar portion of the left ventricle are directed far to the left. The arrow representing the *mean QRS vector* is directed −30 degrees or more to the left and posteriorly, because the arrow representing the mean terminal 0.04 second QRS vector is directed even farther to the left and pulls the mean QRS vector leftward. There may be a *secondary T wave abnormality, as shown in this figure.* The *ventricular gradient* is normal in this illustration.

ing the initial 0.01 to 0.02 second of the QRS complex is directed inferiorly and slightly anteriorly. Its direction is not very different from normal.

An arrow representing the mean of the electrical forces (vectors) responsible for the entire QRS complex is directed −30 degrees or more to the left and posteriorly. The abnormal leftward rotation of this arrow is due, for the most part, to the abnormal leftward rotation of the mean of the electrical forces (vectors) responsible for the terminal 0.04 second portion of the QRS complex.

An arrow representing the mean of the electrical forces (vectors) responsible for the terminal 0.04 second of the QRS complex is directed to the left, superiorly, and posteriorly.

Arrows representing the mean of the electrical forces (vectors) responsible for the ST segment displacement and T wave are directed inferiorly and anterior to the arrow representing the entire QRS complex. The ventricular gradient may or may not be directed normally, depending on the cause of the conduction defect.

A large inferior myocardial infarction can, by removing the electrical forces (vectors) from the inferior portion of the left ventricle, produce a mean QRS vector that is directed far to the left. Other electrocardiographic features associated with inferior infarction serve to distinguish it from left anterosuperior division block. For example, an arrow representing the mean of the electrical forces (vectors) responsible for the initial 0.04 second of the QRS complex in patients with inferior infarction is directed superior to an arrow representing the mean QRS vector. In addition, the ST segment displacement and T wave may be characteristic of inferior infarction.

Left anterosuperior division block may be associated with left ventricular hypertrophy (but is not due to the hypertrophied myocytes); myocardial infarction, myocarditis, or cardiomyopathy (including ischemic cardiomyopathy); Lev disease; Lenegre disease; and elderly patients without other signs of heart disease.

An electrocardiogram illustrating left anterosuperior division block is shown in Fig. 7-89.

When the *left posteroinferior division of the left bundle branch is damaged (blocked),*[43] the duration of the QRS complex remains 0.10 second or less, and an arrow representing the mean of the electrical forces (vectors) produced by the depolarization process responsible for the terminal 0.04 second of the QRS complex is directed to the right and inferiorly. It may be directed slightly anteriorly or posteriorly.

The terminal 0.04 second QRS vector is created by the electrical forces (vectors) produced by the myocytes that are stimulated by electrical impulses transmitted in the left anterosuperior division of the left bundle branch plus the electrical forces (vectors) produced by the retrograde depolarization of the myocytes normally stimulated by electrical impulses transmitted by the left posteroinferior division (Fig. 7-90). This produces an inferiorly directed terminal 0.04 second QRS vector. These electrical forces are probably added to the electrical forces generated by the right ventricle to create electrical forces (vectors) that are directed far to the right.

An arrow representing the mean of the electrical forces (vectors) responsible for the entire QRS complex is directed to the right more than +110 or +120 degrees and slightly posterior to the frontal plane. Remember, the arrow representing the mean of the electrical forces (vectors) may occasionally be normally directed at +110 degrees. Accordingly, it is not always possible to distinguish the rare person without heart disease from the patient with posteroinferior division block, but it is most unusual for the QRS complexes to be directed beyond +120 degrees in the former.

Arrows representing the mean of the electrical forces (vectors) responsible for the ST segment displacement and T wave should be located to the left of, and anterior to, the arrow representing the mean of the electrical forces (vectors) responsible for the entire QRS complex. The ventricular gradient may or may not be directed normally, depending on the cause of the conduction defect.

The electrocardiographic abnormalities caused by left posteroinferior division block occur less often than those due to left anterosuperior division block and are often associated with right bundle-branch block. In fact, posteroinferior division block is more easily recognized when right bundle-branch block is present (see later discussion and Fig. 7–101). Left posteroinferior division block can seldom be recognized without a previous electrocardiogram that does not show the abnormality. The condition must be differentiated from right ventricular hypertrophy or lateral myocardial infarction, although it may actually be caused by the latter. The mean QRS vector associated with right ventricular hypertrophy should not be directed as far to the right as it is with left posteroinferior division block.

Left posteroinferior division block may be caused by myocardial infarction, cardiomyopathy (including ischemic cardiomyopathy), myocarditis, Lev disease, or Lenegre disease.

Pulmonary embolism may produce electrocardiographic abnormalities. A QRS conduction abnormality may occur even though the QRS duration remains normal.[44,45] An arrow representing the mean of the electrical forces (vectors) responsible for the initial 0.04 second of the QRS complex may shift leftward, and an arrow representing the mean of the electrical forces (vectors) responsible for the terminal 0.04 second of the QRS complex may shift to the right and anteriorly (see later discussion).

Preexcitation of the ventricles such as occurs in Wolff-Parkinson-White syndrome produces characteristic electrocardiographic abnormalities.[46] This abnormality, which is a unique variety of conduction defect, is discussed subsequently. It is unique because a bypass tract delivers an electrical stimulus to the ventricle so early that some of the ventricular myocytes are still refractory. The QRS duration may be normal or prolonged; it is usually 0.11 second in duration but may be 0.18 second. The PR interval is short, and a characteristic delta wave is present.

An S_1, S_2, S_3 *type of conduction abnormality* can be identified when there is a terminal S wave in leads I, II, and III.[47] The duration of the QRS complex is usually less than 0.10 second. It is difficult to compute the frontal plane direction of the

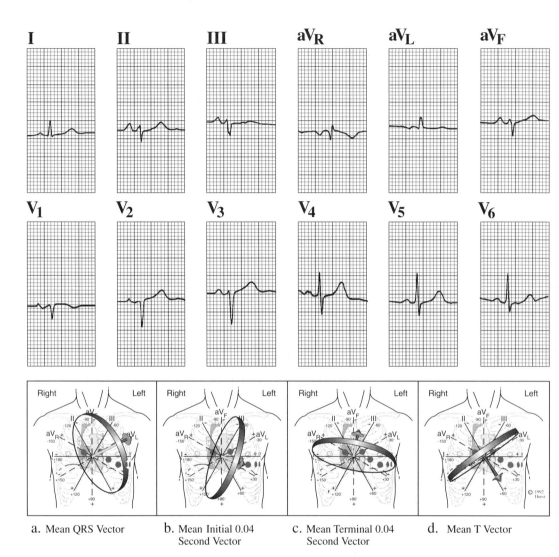

a. Mean QRS Vector

b. Mean Initial 0.04
Second Vector

c. Mean Terminal 0.04
Second Vector

d. Mean T Vector

Fig. 7-89

Fig. 7-89. Left anterosuperior division block.

- *Rhythm:* Normal sinus rhythm
  Rate: Undetermined in short strip. There were 67 depolarizations per minute in a longer strip.
  PR interval: 0.14 second
  QRS duration: 0.08 second
  QT interval: 0.36 second
- *Vector diagrams of electrical forces:* See *a, b, c,* and *d* below the electrocardiogram.
- *Electrophysiologic considerations:*
  The mean QRS vector is directed −28 degrees to the left and about 30 degrees posteriorly. It is directed farther to the left than usual.
  The mean initial 0.04 second QRS vector is directed about +20 degrees inferiorly and about 25 degrees posteriorly. This vector is directed more posteriorly than usual and may represent an alteration of the conduction of the first portion of the septum; it could be misinterpreted as being due to a septal infarction.
  The terminal 0.04 second QRS vector is directed −80 degrees to the left and more than 40 degrees posteriorly. This vector is directed farther to the left than normal and represents left anterosuperior division block.
  The mean T vector is directed +55 degrees to the right and 5 degrees anteriorly.
  The mean initial 0.04 second QRS vector suggests some type of initial conduction defect (see Fig. 7-86). The terminal 0.04 second QRS vector and the mean QRS vector are directed an abnormal degree to the left, suggesting left anterosuperior division block.
- *Clinical differential diagnosis:* Left anterosuperior division block can be associated with left ventricular hypertrophy. It may occur in elderly individuals who have no other clinical evidence of heart disease. It may be caused by cardiomyopathy, atherosclerotic heart disease, or primary disease of the conduction system. Finally, it may occur for unexplained reasons.
- *Discussion:* This electrocardiogram was recorded from a 59-year-old woman who was asymptomatic and had no other evidence of heart disease. The electrocardiogram had not changed in nearly two decades. The cause of the abnormalities is unknown in this case but may be a congenital alteration of the conduction system.

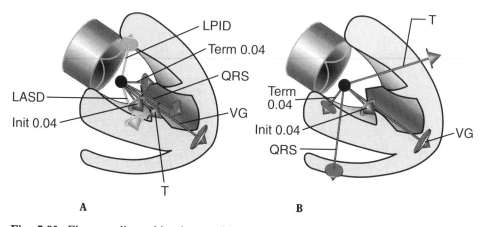

Fig. 7-90. Electrocardiographic abnormalities associated with left posteroinferior division block. **A,** Normal vectors (see legend for Fig. 7-88, *A*). **B,** Abnormalities. The *QRS duration* is usually 0.10 second. The arrow representing the *mean initial 0.04 second QRS* vector is directed normally. The arrow representing the *mean terminal 0.04 second QRS* vector is directed far to the right and posteriorly, because the left posteroinferior division of the left bundle branch is blocked. This alters the direction of the arrow representing the mean of the electrical forces (vectors) that normally produce the leftward and posteriorly directed terminal 0.04 second of the QRS complex. In such cases the left anterosuperior division of the left bundle-branch system stimulates the myocytes. In addition, some of the myocytes ordinarily stimulated by the left posteroinferior division depolarize in a manner opposite to normal (see text). The net result is that the arrow representing the mean terminal 0.04 second QRS vector is directed abnormally to the right; it may be directed posteriorly, parallel with the frontal plane, or slightly anteriorly. The arrow representing the *mean QRS vector* is directed more than +110 degrees to the right. It may be directed posteriorly, parallel with the frontal plane, or slightly anteriorly, because the mean terminal 0.04 second QRS vector is directed far to the right, parallel with the frontal plane, posteriorly, or slightly anteriorly. There may be a *secondary T wave abnormality*. The *ventricular gradient* is normal in this illustration.

electrical forces (vectors) responsible for the QRS complex, because the complexes are equaphasic in most of the extremity leads.

An arrow representing the mean of the electrical forces (vectors) responsible for the terminal 0.04 second of the QRS complex is directed superiorly and posteriorly.

Arrows representing the mean of the electrical forces (vectors) responsible for the ST segment displacement and T wave are large but normally directed.

The abnormality may be seen in patients who have no other evidence of heart disease. It may be due to an anomaly in the Purkinje system within the right ventricle.[47] The defect may also be seen in patients with hypertrophic cardiomyopathy and pulmonary emphysema (Fig. 7-91).

Hypothermia may produce a QRS conduction abnormality (see later discussion).[48] The duration of the QRS complex may be normal or prolonged. The terminal portion of the QRS complex becomes abnormal; this is designated as an Osborn wave.

QRS conduction defects when the QRS duration is 0.12 second. The QRS duration is 0.12 second when there is *uncomplicated* right or left bundle-branch block.[42,43] Furthermore, arrows representing the mean of the electrical forces (vectors) responsible for the entire QRS complex, the initial and terminal 0.04 second of the QRS complex, the ST segment displacement, and the T wave are arranged in a specific manner when there is uncomplicated right or left bundle-branch block. When there is *complicated* bundle-branch block, the duration of the QRS complex may be prolonged beyond 0.12 second, the mean and terminal 0.04 second QRS vectors may be directed farther to the left or right than they are with uncomplicated bundle-branch block, or the initial QRS vector or the ST and T vectors may be directed in a manner different from that of uncomplicated bundle-branch block.

Uncomplicated right bundle-branch block is a common electrocardiographic abnormality (Fig. 7-92).

The duration of the QRS complex is usually 0.12 second but may be 0.11 second. Of course, in children the QRS duration may be 0.09 to 0.10 second.

An arrow representing the mean of the electrical forces (vectors) responsible for the initial 0.01 to 0.02 second of the QRS complex is almost always directed normally.

An arrow representing the mean of the electrical forces (vectors) responsible for the middle portion of the QRS complex is directed inferiorly and parallel with the frontal plane or posteriorly.

An arrow representing the mean of the electrical forces (vectors) responsible for the terminal 0.04 second of the QRS complex is directed to the right and anteriorly (where the right ventricle is located). The direction of these electrical forces (vectors) produces an rS complex in leads I and V_6 and an rsR complex in lead V_1.

An arrow representing the mean of the electrical forces (vectors) responsible for the entire QRS complex may be directed normally at +60 degrees or abnormally at +90 to +110 degrees. It is always directed anteriorly. The direction of this arrow will shift rightward from its preblock direction less than +60 degrees when right bundle-branch block develops. Commonly, the shift will be about +30 rather than +60 degrees. Therefore the direction of the arrow representing the mean of the electrical forces (vectors) responsible for the QRS complex associated with right bundle-branch block is predetermined, to a degree, by the location of the arrow representing the mean of the electrical forces (vectors) responsible for the QRS complex prior to the development of the right bundle-branch block. This explains why it is necessary to consider the addition of some other conduction defect when an arrow representing the mean of the electrical forces (vectors) responsible for the QRS complex

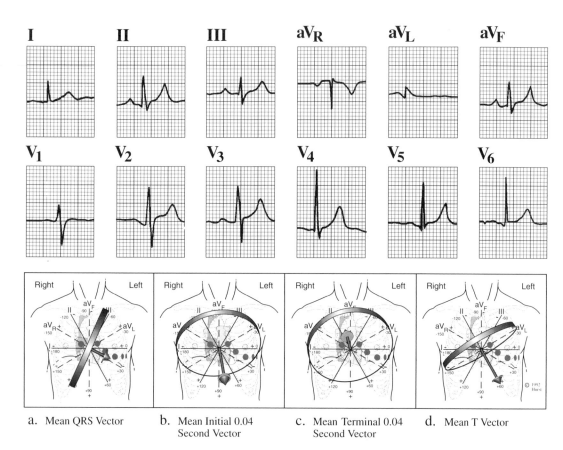

a. Mean QRS Vector

b. Mean Initial 0.04
   Second Vector

c. Mean Terminal 0.04
   Second Vector

d. Mean T Vector

Fig. 7-91

Fig. 7-91. S_1, S_2, S_3 conduction abnormality.

- *Rhythm:* Normal sinus rhythm

  Rate: Undetermined in short strip. There were about 85 depolarizations per minute in a longer strip.

  PR interval: 0.20 second

  QRS duration: 0.08 to 0.09 second

  QT interval: 0.36 second

- *Vector diagrams of electrical forces:* See *a*, *b*, *c*, and *d* below the electrocardiogram.

- *Electrophysiologic considerations:*

  The P waves are normal.

  The mean QRS vector is directed about +30 degrees inferiorly and is parallel with the frontal plane. Note that the QRS complexes are equaphasic in many leads. This is because the initial and terminal QRS electrical forces are directed almost opposite to each other.

  The mean initial 0.04 second QRS vector is directed about +80 degrees inferiorly and almost 90 degrees anteriorly. The mean terminal 0.04 second QRS vector is directed about −100 degrees to the left (superiorly) and almost 90 degrees posteriorly. This arrangement of initial and terminal forces creates the S_1, S_2, and S_3 configuration in the extremity leads.

  Lead I shows a small, broad S wave that is easily overlooked. Even if the terminal electrical forces were isoelectric in lead I, this tracing would still be identified as S_1, S_2, S_3 because the initial QRS electrical forces are opposite to the terminal QRS electrical forces.

  The mean T vector is directed +60 degrees inferiorly and 10 to 15 degrees anteriorly. Note that the T waves are large and the ventricular gradient is normal.

- *Clinical differential diagnosis:* The exact cause of the S_1, S_2, S_3 type of conduction abnormality is not known. It may also occur in otherwise normal individuals. It may occur in patients with pulmonary emphysema and idiopathic hypertrophy.

- *Discussion:* This electrocardiogram was recorded from a normal 35-year-old man.

Electrocardiogram reproduced with permission from Estes EH: Electrocardiography and vectorcardiography. In Hurst JW, Logue RB, editors: *The heart*, ed 1, New York, 1966, McGraw-Hill, p 136.

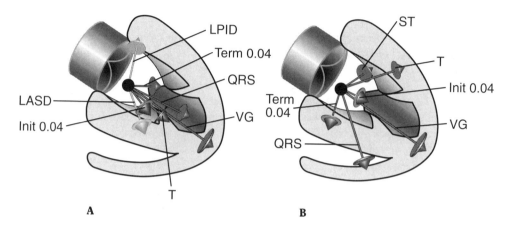

Fig. 7-92. Electrocardiographic abnormalities associated with uncomplicated right bundle-branch block. **A,** Normal vectors (see legend for Fig. 7-88, *A*). **B,** Abnormalities. The *QRS duration* is 0.12 second. The arrow representing the mean *initial 0.04 second QRS vector* is directed normally. The arrow representing the *terminal 0.04 second QRS vector* is directed abnormally to the right and anteriorly, because it is produced later than normal and is unopposed by left ventricular forces. The terminal vector is directed toward the right ventricle. The arrow representing the *mean QRS vector* is usually directed inferiorly and anteriorly. The mean QRS vector associated with right bundle-branch block shifts to the right 60 degrees or less from its preblock direction but is always directed anteriorly. Whenever the arrow representing the mean of the electrical forces (vectors) responsible for the terminal 0.04 second of the QRS complex is directed far to the right and anteriorly, and the arrow representing the mean of the electrical forces (vectors) responsible for the entire QRS complex is directed beyond +120 degrees to the right and anteriorly, one must consider the presence of right bundle-branch block plus left posteroinferior division block (see Fig. 7-100). When there is uncomplicated bundle-branch block, there is a *secondary T wave abnormality;* the arrow representing the mean T vector is directed opposite to the direction of the arrow representing the mean QRS vector. The *ventricular gradient* is normal. The arrow representing the mean vector representing the *ST segment displacement* is directed relatively parallel with the arrow representing the mean T vector.

is directed more than +120 degrees to the right in a patient with a QRS duration of 0.12 second.

Arrows representing the mean of the electrical forces (vectors) responsible for the ST segment displacement and T wave are directed 160 to 180 degrees away from the arrow representing the mean of the electrical forces responsible for the QRS complex. The angle between the arrow representing the mean of the electrical forces (vectors) responsible for the ST segment displacement and the arrow representing the mean of the electrical forces (vectors) responsible for the T wave is usually 60 degrees or less. The T wave configuration, which looks abnormal, is a secondary T wave change. Although it looks abnormal, it is actually normal for the abnormal QRS complex. Whenever the sequence of the repolarization process is altered simply because the depolarization process is altered, it is described as a secondary T wave "abnormality." This occurs in uncomplicated right bundle-branch block. The ventricular gradient is normally directed in such patients.

Right bundle-branch block may occur without any other evidence of heart disease. It may occur in patients with coronary artery disease from any cause, cardiomyopathy, pulmonary embolism, right ventricular hypertrophy from any cause, right ventricular dilatation such as occurs with secundum atrial septal defect, Lenegre disease, Lev disease, or aortic valve disease with calcium impregnation within the septum; or it may occur as a result of drugs or surgical repair of certain types of congenital heart disease.

An example of uncomplicated right bundle-branch block is shown in Fig. 7-93.

Uncomplicated left bundle-branch block is a common electrocardiographic abnormality[42,43] (Fig. 7-94). The sequence of ventricular depolarization is altered initially and terminally when the left bundle branch is damaged (blocked).

The duration of the QRS complex is 0.12 second.

An arrow representing the mean of the electrical forces (vectors) responsible for the initial 0.04 second of the QRS complex is directed inferiorly, to the left, and posteriorly. This is different from normal, because depolarization of the septum is normally directed from left to right rather than from right to left. Therefore, when there is left bundle-branch block, no Q wave is seen in leads I and V_6 as it is in most normal subjects, and there is a very small R wave, or no R wave at all, in lead V_1.

An arrow representing the mean of the electrical forces (vectors) responsible for the middle of the QRS complex is directed to the left and posteriorly.

An arrow representing the mean of the electrical forces (vectors) responsible for the terminal 0.04 second of the QRS complex is directed to the left and posteriorly. It is produced by depolarization of the posterobasilar portion of the left ventricle.

The direction of an arrow representing the mean of the electrical forces (vectors) responsible for the entire QRS complex may be normal; the arrow is never directed more than −30 degrees to the left when there is uncomplicated left bundle-branch block. It is always directed posteriorly. This arrow shifts leftward from its preblock

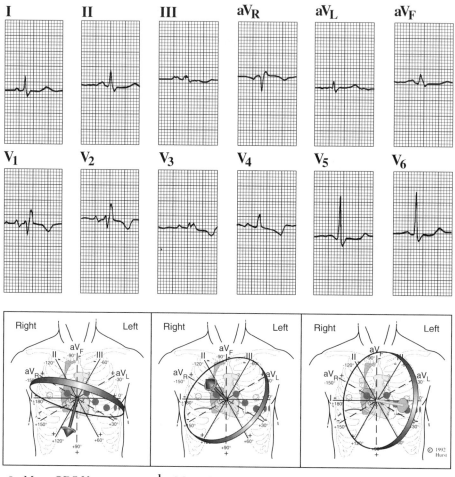

a. Mean QRS Vector

b. Mean Terminal 0.04 Second Vector

c. Mean T Vector

Fig. 7-93

Fig. 7-93. Uncomplicated right bundle-branch block.

- *Rhythm:* Normal sinus rhythm

  Rate: Undetermined in short strip. There were 80 depolarizations per minute in a longer strip.

  PR interval: 0.14 second

  QRS duration: 0.12 second

  QT interval: 0.42 second

- *Vector diagrams of electrical forces:* See *a*, *b*, and *c* below the electrocardiogram.

- *Electrophysiologic considerations:*

  The duration of the QRS complex is 0.12 second. The mean QRS vector is directed about +105 degrees to the right and 15 to 20 degrees anteriorly.

  The mean terminal 0.04 second QRS vector is directed about −135 degrees superiorly and 60 degrees anteriorly. It points toward the right ventricle, signifying right bundle-branch block.

  The mean T vector is directed +10 degrees inferiorly and about 70 degrees posteriorly. The ventricular gradient is normal.

  The abnormalities in this electrocardiogram are characteristic of uncomplicated right bundle-branch block.

- *Clinical differential diagnosis:* Right bundle-branch block may occur when there is no other evidence of heart disease. It may be caused by atherosclerotic coronary heart disease, cardiomyopathy, primary disease of the conduction system, or pulmonary embolism. The abnormal QRS vector associated with right ventricular hypertrophy and dilatation from any cause may progress to right bundle-branch block. For example, the right ventricular delay associated with right ventricular hypertrophy and dilatation associated with a secundum atrial septal defect may gradually change to right bundle-branch block.

- *Discussion:* This electrocardiogram was recorded from a 65-year-old woman with an ostium secundum atrial septal defect. The abnormalities are due to uncomplicated right bundle-branch block. There is a secondary T wave change, and the ventricular gradient is normal.

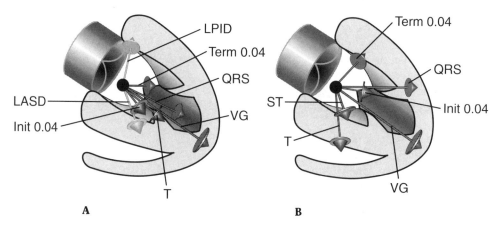

A   **B**

Fig. 7-94. Uncomplicated left bundle-branch block. **A,** Normal vectors (see legend for Fig. 7-88, *A*). **B,** Abnormalities. The *QRS duration* is 0.12 second. The arrow representing the *mean initial 0.04 second QRS vector* is shifted to the left and posteriorly. This eliminates a Q wave in leads I and V_6, and the R wave is either absent or small in lead V_1. The arrow representing the *mean terminal 0.04 second QRS vector* is shifted to the left and posteriorly; it is directed toward the posterobasilar portion of the left ventricle. The arrow representing the *mean QRS vector* is directed to the left and posteriorly. The mean QRS vector will shift less than 60 degrees from its preblock direction. Accordingly, the direction of the mean QRS vector will usually be directed between 0 and +30 degrees; it will never be directed more than −30 degrees to the left. Whenever the arrow representing the mean of the electrical forces (vectors) responsible for the terminal 0.04 second of the QRS complex is directed to the left and posteriorly, and the arrow representing the mean of the electrical forces (vectors) responsible for the entire QRS complex is directed more than −30 degrees to the left and posteriorly, one must consider the presence of left bundle-branch block plus left anterosuperior division block (see Fig. 7-96). When there is uncomplicated left bundle-branch block, there is a *secondary T wave abnormality;* the mean T vector is directed opposite to the mean QRS vector. The *ventricular gradient* is normal. The mean vector representing the *ST segment displacement* is directed relatively parallel with the mean T vector.

direction less than -60 degrees when left bundle-branch block develops. Commonly, the shift would be -30 degrees rather than -60 degrees. Accordingly, the direction of the arrow representing the mean of the electrical forces responsible for the QRS complex is predetermined, to a degree, by its direction before left bundle-branch block developed.

Arrows representing the mean of the electrical forces (vectors) responsible for the ST segment displacement and T wave are directed 160 to 180 degrees away from the arrow representing the mean of the electrical forces (vectors) responsible for the QRS complex. The angle between the arrow representing the mean of the electrical forces (vectors) responsible for the ST segment displacement is usually 60 degrees or less from the arrow representing the mean of the electrical forces (vectors) responsible for the T wave. The T wave alteration is a secondary T wave abnormality; the repolarization sequence is altered because the depolarization sequence is altered. Therefore the ventricular gradient is normally directed.

Left bundle-branch block may be caused by coronary artery disease, myocarditis, cardiomyopathy, Lenegre disease, Lev disease, calcific aortic valve stenosis, extreme left ventricular hypertrophy and dilatation, certain drugs, and cardiac surgery.

An example of uncomplicated left bundle-branch block is shown in Fig. 7-95, *B*. It should be compared with the preblock tracing (Fig. 7-95, *A*).

Preexcitation of the ventricles such as occurs in Wolff-Parkinson-White syndrome is discussed later in the chapter.[46] It is mentioned here because, at times, the QRS duration may be 0.12 second. The electrocardiographic abnormalities due to *hypothermia* are also discussed later in the chapter.[48] They are mentioned here because the QRS duration may be 0.12 second.

Complicated right and left bundle-branch block (QRS duration may be 0.12 second or longer). *Uncomplicated* right or left bundle-branch block is said to be present when the QRS duration is 0.12 second and the mean QRS vector, the initial 0.04 second and terminal 0.04 second vectors, and the mean ST and T vectors are directed in a certain, defined manner (see preceding discussion). *Complicated* right or left bundle-branch block is said to be present when the QRS duration is greater than 0.12 second or the direction of the mean QRS vector, the initial or terminal 0.04 second vector, or the mean ST or T vector is different from that occurring with uncomplicated bundle-branch block. The subsequent discussion deals with the various types of complicated bundle-branch block.

Left bundle-branch block plus left anterosuperior division block[43] (Fig. 7-96). The duration of the QRS complex is 0.12 second or longer. All of the features of left bundle-branch block are present. This abnormality occurs because the left anterosuperior branch of the left bundle, as well as the left bundle itself, is blocked. The depolarization process proceeds from the right side of the septum to the left and enters the left posteroinferior branch of the conduction system. The electrical impulse then continues in the posteroinferior branch and stimulates the myocytes under its

Text continued on p. 332.

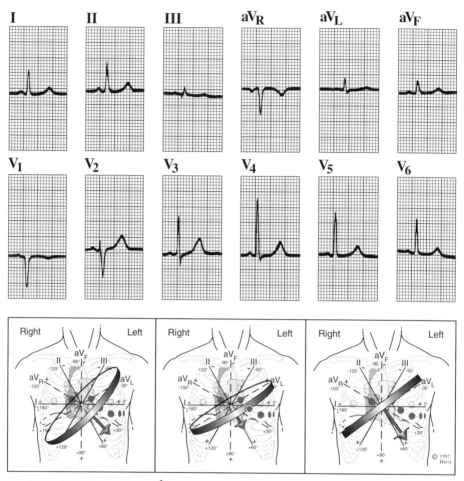

a. Mean QRS Vector   b. Mean Terminal 0.04 Second Vector   c. Mean T Vector

Fig. 7-95, A

Fig. 7-95. A, Normal ventricular electrocardiogram made prior to the development of left bundle-branch block.

- *Rhythm:* Normal sinus rhythm
  Rate: Undetermined in short strip
  PR interval: 0.12 second
  QRS duration: 0.08 second
  QT interval: 0.40 second
- *Vector diagrams of electrical forces:* See *a, b,* and *c* below the electrocardiogram.
- *Electrophysiologic considerations:*

  The P waves are normal. The PR interval is short, suggesting the possibility of Lown-Ganong-Levine syndrome (such patients may have supraventricular tachycardia).

  The mean QRS vector is directed normally, at about +38 degrees inferiorly and about 30 degrees posteriorly. There is no delta wave.

  The mean terminal 0.04 second QRS vector is directed normally, at about +60 degrees inferiorly and about 15 degrees posteriorly.

  The mean T vector is directed about +55 degrees inferiorly and is parallel with the frontal plane.
- *Clinical differential diagnosis:* The electrocardiogram is normal. The heart may be normal, or the patient could have atherosclerotic coronary heart disease, mild valvular disease, a history of arrhythmias, or mild congenital heart disease such as a small interventricular septal defect or patent ductus. Lown-Ganong-Levine syndrome may be present.
- *Discussion:* This normal electrocardiogram is shown as a baseline tracing made prior to the development of uncomplicated left bundle-branch block (see **B**).

Electrocardiogram from Stein E: *Electrocardiographic interpretation: a self-study approach to clinical electro-cardiology,* Philadelphia, 1991, Lea & Febiger, p 432. Reprinted with permission.

Continued.

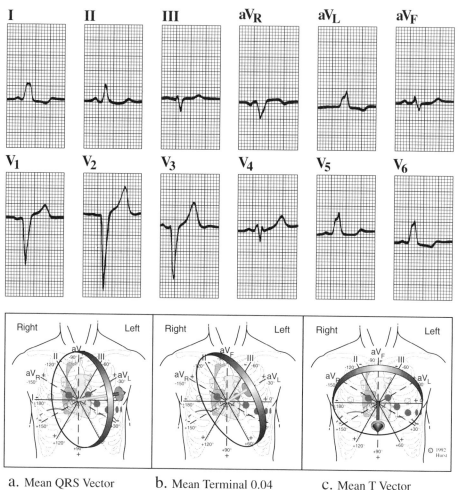

a. Mean QRS Vector

b. Mean Terminal 0.04 Second Vector

c. Mean T Vector

Fig. 7-95, B

Fig. 7-95, cont'd. B, Uncomplicated left bundle-branch block (compare with **A**).

- *Rhythm:* Normal sinus rhythm
  Rate: Undetermined in short strip
  PR interval: 0.14 second
  QRS duration: 0.12 second
  QT interval: 0.42 second
- *Vector diagrams of electrical forces:* See *a, b,* and *c* below the electrocardiogram.
- *Electrophysiologic considerations:*
  The P waves are normal.
  The mean QRS vector is directed about −8 degrees to the left and about 50 degrees poste-
      riorly. Note that it has shifted about 60 degrees to the left of its position prior to the
      development of left bundle-branch block and about 30 degrees posterior to its preblock
      direction.
  The mean terminal 0.04 second QRS vector is directed about −30 degrees to the left and
      about 40 degrees posteriorly. It points toward the basilar portion of the left ventricle and
      is characteristic of left bundle-branch block. Previously (see **A**) it was directed +60 de-
      grees inferiorly and about 70 degrees posteriorly. Note how it has shifted to the left about
      90 degrees.
  The mean T vector is directed about +90 degrees inferiorly and about 85 degrees anteri-
      orly. It is directed about 115 degrees from the QRS vector. The ventricular gradient re-
      mains within the normal range.
  The abnormalities are consistent with the diagnosis of uncomplicated left bundle-branch
      block.
- *Clinical differential diagnosis:* Uncomplicated left bundle-branch block occurs in patients with
  atherosclerotic coronary heart disease, cardiomyopathy, or primary conduction system disease. It also occurs in patients with left ventricular hypertrophy. The QRS gradually wid-
  ens in such patients.
- *Discussion:* The cause of the uncomplicated bundle-branch block in this patient is unknown.
  The tracing is shown in order to compare the changes that occur in the postblock tracing
  with those in the preblock tracing.

Electrocardiogram from Stein E: *Electrocardiographic interpretation: a self-study approach to clinical electro-
cardiology,* Philadelphia, 1991, Lea & Febiger, p 432. Reprinted with permission.

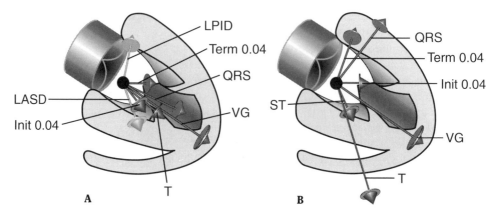

Fig. 7-96. Electrocardiographic abnormalities associated with left bundle-branch block plus left anterosuperior division block (a type of complicated left bundle-branch block). **A,** Normal vectors (see legend for Fig. 7-88, *A*). **B,** Abnormalities. The *QRS duration* is 0.12 second or longer. The arrow representing the *mean initial 0.04 second QRS vector* is directed abnormally to the left and posteriorly, as it is when there is uncomplicated left bundle-branch block. The arrow representing the *mean terminal 0.04 second QRS vector* is directed far to the left and posteriorly. It is directed farther to the left than it is when there is uncomplicated left bundle-branch block, because the electrical forces (vectors) created by the normal sequential stimulation of myocytes by the intact left anterosuperior division of the left bundle branch does not occur. Accordingly, the electrical forces created by the myocytes stimulated by the left posteroinferior division of the left bundle branch plus the electrical forces generated by retrograde depolarization of the myocytes normally stimulated by the left anterosuperior division dominate the electrical field. The arrow representing the *mean QRS vector* is directed more than −30 degrees to the left and posteriorly; it is directed farther to the left than it is when there is uncomplicated left bundle-branch block. Theoretically, this conduction defect should produce a *secondary T wave abnormality* as shown in this figure (the *ventricular gradient* should be normal). In practice, however, this conduction defect is likely to be caused by myocardial damage, and a *primary T wave abnormality* is often present. The mean vector representing the *ST segment displacement* is directed relatively parallel with the mean T vector.

control. The electrical impulse also enters the area of the myocardium normally stimulated by the electrical impulses in the left anterosuperior division branch and stimulates the myocytes in a retrograde manner. The combination of electrical forces (vectors) is directed farther to the left than what occurs with uncomplicated left bundle-branch block.

An arrow representing the mean of the electrical forces (vectors) responsible for the entire QRS complex is directed more than −30 degrees to the left and posteriorly.

An arrow representing the mean of the electrical forces responsible for the terminal 0.4 second of the QRS complex is directed superiorly and posteriorly. This is why the mean QRS vector is directed abnormally to the left (beyond −30 degrees).

Arrows representing the mean of the electrical forces (vectors) responsible for the ST segment displacement and T wave are directed opposite to the mean QRS vector. The ventricular gradient may or may not be directed normally, depending on the cause of the conduction defect.

This conduction defect can be caused by all of the conditions mentioned in the discussion of uncomplicated left bundle-branch block. It is wise, however, to consider more extensive muscular damage when extensive conduction abnormalities are identified.

An electrocardiogram illustrating left bundle-branch block plus left anterosuperior division block is shown in Fig. 7-97.

Right bundle-branch block plus left anterosuperior division block[43] (Fig. 7-98). This common electrocardiographic abnormality occurs because the left anterosuperior division of the left bundle, as well as that of the right bundle, is damaged. Depolarization of the septum is from left to right, because the proximal portion of the left bundle itself is usually intact. Depolarization of the left ventricle is controlled by the left posteroinferior division of the bundle-branch system. Therefore an arrow representing the mean of the electrical forces (vectors) responsible for the terminal 0.04 second of the QRS complexes is directed to the left and superiorly. These electrical forces (vectors) are accompanied by those produced by the retrograde simulation of myocytes ordinarily served by the left anterosuperior division, and they conspire to produce a mean QRS vector that is directed −30 degrees or more to the left. In this condition, however, depolarization of the right ventricle is delayed, and an arrow, which is directed somewhat to the right but markedly anteriorly, representing depolarization of the right ventricle, occurs simultaneously with an arrow representing depolarization of the last portion of the left ventricle. Therefore, when these terminal forces are added together, electrical forces (vectors) are produced that are directed to the left, superiorly, and anteriorly.

Accordingly, the QRS deflections created by this conduction defect produce what appears to be left anterosuperior division block in the extremity leads and right bundle-branch block in the precordial leads.

The duration of the QRS complex is 0.12 second or longer.

Septal depolarization is normal. An arrow representing the mean of the electrical forces (vectors) responsible for the initial 0.04 second of the QRS complex is directed inferiorly and parallel with the frontal plane.

The arrow representing the mean of the electrical forces (vectors) responsible for the terminal 0.04 second of the QRS complex is directed to the left superiorly and anteriorly.

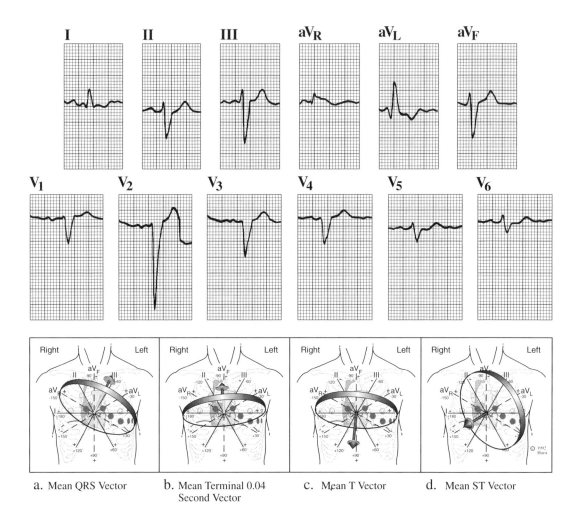

a. Mean QRS Vector

b. Mean Terminal 0.04
   Second Vector

c. Mean T Vector

d. Mean ST Vector

Fig. 7-97

Fig. 7-97. Complicated left bundle-branch block due to additional left anterosuperior division block.

- *Rhythm:* Normal sinus rhythm

  Rate: Undetermined in short strip. There were 73 depolarizations per minute in a longer strip.

  PR interval: 0.18 second

  QRS duration: 0.14 second

  QT interval: 0.42 second

- *Vector diagrams of electrical forces:* See *a*, *b*, *c*, and *d* below the electrocardiogram.

- *Electrophysiologic considerations:*

  The P waves are abnormal. There is a left atrial abnormality; note that the last half of the P wave is negative in leads V_1 and V_2.

  The mean QRS vector is directed −65 degrees to the left and posteriorly; the exact amount of posterior rotation cannot be determined without recordings from additional electrode sample sites.

  The mean terminal 0.04 second QRS vector is directed −95 degrees to the left. It is posteriorly directed; the exact amount of posterior rotation cannot be determined without recordings from additional electrode sample sites. This vector is directed abnormally in that it is directed much farther to the left than normal.

  The mean T vector is directed +95 degrees to the right and anteriorly. The exact amount of anterior rotation cannot be determined without recordings from additional electrode sample sites.

  The mean ST vector is directed about +150 degrees to the right and about 70 degrees anteriorly. It is probably about 60 degrees from the mean T vector.

  The abnormal vectors indicate complicated left bundle branch, because there is additional left anterosuperior division block and the QRS duration is 0.14 second.

- *Clinical differential diagnosis:* Left bundle-branch block plus left anterosuperior division block may occur in patients with dilated cardiomyopathy, severe coronary disease, primary disease of the conduction system (Lenegre disease) Lev disease, or severe aortic valve disease.

- *Discussion:* This electrocardiogram was recorded from a 58-year-old man with severe obstructive triple-vessel coronary atherosclerosis. The left anterior descending coronary artery was totally obstructed. The ejection fraction was 20% of normal, and the large left ventricle contracted poorly. Severe heart failure was present.

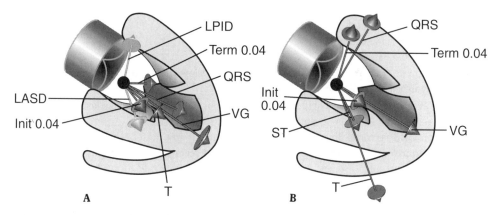

Fig. 7-98. Electrocardiographic abnormalities associated with right bundle-branch block plus left anterosuperior division block (a type of complicated right bundle-branch block). **A,** Normal vectors (see legend for Fig. 7-88, *A*). **B,** Abnormalities. The *QRS duration* is usually 0.12 second or larger. The arrow representing the *mean initial 0.04 second QRS vector* is normal. The arrow representing the *mean terminal 0.04 second QRS vector* is directed far to the left and anteriorly. This, of course, is quite different from the normal direction of this force or the direction when there is left bundle-branch block or right bundle-branch block. This abnormality occurs because the directions of the electrical forces (vectors) produced by the myocytes that are ordinarily stimulated by the left anterosuperior division of the left bundle branch and the myocytes ordinarily stimulated by the right bundle branch are altered because of their blocked pathways. The electrical forces produced by the myocytes stimulated by the intact left posteroinferior division of the left bundle produce a horizontally directed mean vector that, when added to the mean vector created by the myocytes stimulated by the delayed electrical impulses that sweep into the right ventricle from the left ventricle, produce a vector that is directed far to the left and anteriorly. The arrow representing the *mean QRS vector* is directed to the left and anteriorly. It is usually directed more than −30 degrees to the left. This occurs because the arrow representing the mean terminal 0.04 second QRS vector is directed far to the left and anteriorly. Theoretically, this conduction defect should produce a *secondary T wave abnormality* as shown in this figure (the ventricular gradient should be normal). In practice, however, the conduction defect is commonly caused by myocardial damage, and a *primary T wave abnormality* is often present. The mean vector representing the *ST segment displacement* is directed relatively parallel with the mean T vector.

An arrow representing the mean of the electrical forces (vectors) responsible for the entire QRS complex is directed −30 degrees or more to the left and anteriorly.

Arrows representing the mean of the electrical forces (vectors) responsible for the ST segment displacement and T wave are directed opposite to the arrow representing the mean of the electrical forces (vectors) responsible for the QRS complex. The ventricular gradient may or may not be directed normally, depending on the cause of the conduction defect.

Right bundle-branch block plus left anterosuperior division block may be due to myocardial infarction or severe ischemia caused by coronary disease, cardiomyopathy, ostium primum atrial septal defect, myocarditis, calcific aortic valve stenosis, Lenegre disease, Lev disease, or cardiac surgery for valve disease.

Right bundle-branch block plus left anterosuperior division block is illustrated in the electrocardiograms shown in Fig. 7-99.

Right bundle-branch block plus left posteroinferior division block[43] (Fig. 7-100). This electrocardiographic abnormality is uncommon.

The duration of the QRS complex is 0.12 second or longer.

Septal depolarization is normal. An arrow representing the mean of the electrical forces (vectors) responsible for the initial 0.04 second of the QRS complex is directed normally.

An arrow representing the mean of the electrical forces responsible for the terminal 0.04 second of the QRS complex is directed abnormally to the right and anteriorly.

An arrow representing the mean of the electrical forces (vectors) responsible for the entire QRS complex is directed +120 degrees or more to the right and anteriorly. Remember, the arrow representing the mean of the electrical forces (vectors) responsible for the QRS complex commonly shifts to the right only about 30 degrees when uncomplicated right bundle-branch block develops; uncommonly the shift may be as much as +60 degrees. Accordingly, when an arrow representing the mean of the electrical forces (vectors) is directed +120 degrees or more to the right, it is likely that some additional cause is responsible for the markedly rightward direction of the arrow representing the QRS complex.

Left posteroinferior block is more commonly seen in patients who have right bundle-branch block than it is as an isolated conduction defect. For some unexplained reason the left posteroinferior bundle branch is more resistant to damage than is the left anterosuperior division.

It is difficult to identify right posteroinferior division block without a previous electrocardiogram that does not show it.

The direction of an arrow representing the mean of the electrical forces (vectors) responsible for the terminal 0.04 second of the QRS complex is determined by the vector sum of the electrical forces (vectors) responsible for depolarization of the right ventricle during the last 0.04 second of the QRS complex and the electrical forces

Text continued on p. 343.

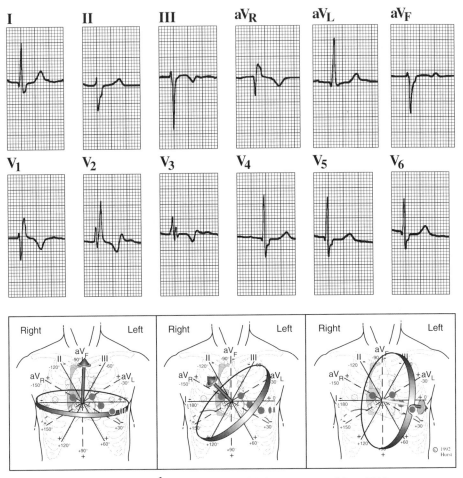

a. Mean QRS Vector

b. Mean Terminal 0.04 Second Vector

c. Mean T Vector

Fig. 7-99, A

Fig. 7-99. A, Complicated right bundle-branch block plus left anterosuperior division block.

- *Rhythm:* Normal sinus rhythm
  Rate: Undetermined in short strip. There were 70 depolarizations per minute in a longer strip.
  PR interval: 0.21 second
  QRS duration: 0.12 second
  QT interval: 0.40 second
- *Vector diagrams of electrical forces:* See *a*, *b*, and *c* below the electrocardiogram.
- *Electrophysiologic considerations:*
  The P waves are normal. First-degree atrioventricular block is present.
  The mean QRS vector is directed about −85 degrees to the left and about 30 degrees anteriorly. This vector is directed farther to the left than is usual for left bundle-branch block. In addition, the vector is directed anteriorly rather than posteriorly, as it is when there is left bundle-branch block.
  The mean terminal 0.04 second QRS vector is directed about −135 degrees to the left and about 40 degrees anteriorly. The anterior direction of this vector indicates that the last portion of the myocardium to be depolarized is the right ventricle.
  The mean T vector is directed about +10 degrees inferiorly and about 40 degrees posteriorly. The ventricular gradient is abnormal.
  This electrocardiogram is abnormal because of right bundle-branch block and left anterosuperior division block. First-degree atrioventricular block is also present.
- *Clinical differential diagnosis:* This type of electrocardiogram can be caused by atherosclerotic coronary heart disease, cardiomyopathy, ostium primum septal defect, primary disease of the conduction system (Lenegre disease), Lev disease, or cardiac surgery for valvular or congenital heart disease.
- *Discussion:* This electrocardiogram was recorded from a 17-year-old woman with an ostium primum septal defect.   *Continued.*

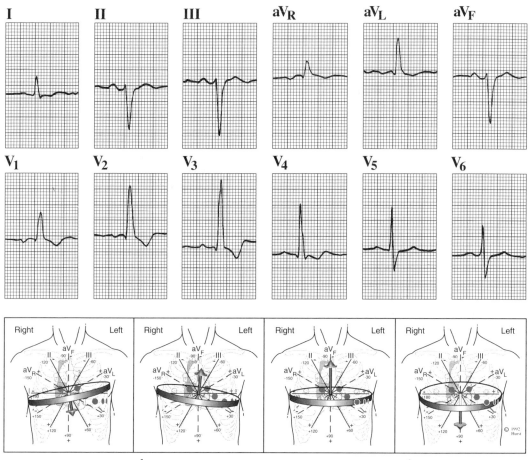

a. Mean Vector for Last
Half of P Wave

b. Mean QRS Vector

c. Mean Terminal 0.04
Second Vector

d. Mean T Vector

Fig. 7-99, B

Fig. 7-99, cont'd. B, Complicated right bundle-branch block plus left anterosuperior division block in another patient.

- *Rhythm:* Normal sinus rhythm
  Rate: Undetermined in short strip. There were 69 depolarizations per minute in a longer strip.
  PR interval: 0.20 second
  QRS duration: 0.13 second
  QT interval: 0.40 second
- *Vector diagrams of electrical forces:* See *a, b, c,* and *d* below the electrocardiogram.
- *Electrophysiologic considerations:*
  There is a left atrial abnormality; note that the second half of the P wave is negative in leads V₁ and V₂.

  The mean QRS vector is directed about -85 degrees to the left and about 20 degrees anteriorly, indicating right bundle-branch block and left anterosuperior division block.

  The mean terminal 0.04 second QRS vector is directed -90 degrees to the left and about 15 degrees anteriorly. This vector is created by the summation of the electrical forces in the myocytes stimulated by the intact left posteroinferior division of the left bundle branch plus the forces generated by the delayed depolarization of the right ventricle caused by the right bundle-branch block.

  The mean T vector is directed about $+90$ degrees to the right and about 50 degrees posteriorly.

  In summary, there is a left atrial abnormality, right bundle-branch block, and left anterosuperior division block.
- *Clinical differential diagnosis:* This type of electrocardiogram may be produced by atherosclerotic coronary heart disease, cardiomyopathy, ostium primum septal defect, primary disease of the conduction system (Lenegre disease), Lev disease, or cardiac surgery for valvular or congenital heart disease.
- *Discussion:* This electrocardiogram was recorded from an 87-year-old man with atherosclerotic coronary heart disease. He had a myocardial infarction 5 weeks before this tracing was made. Coronary arteriography revealed total obstruction of the left anterior descending coronary artery and high-grade obstruction of the circumflex and right coronary arteries.

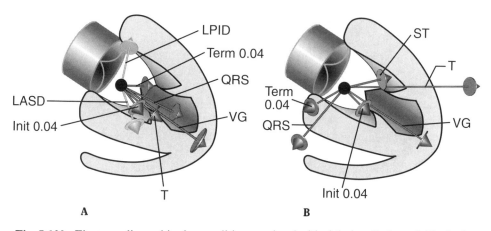

Fig. 7-100. Electrocardiographic abnormalities associated with right bundle-branch block plus left posteroinferior division block (a type of complicated right bundle-branch block). **A,** Normal vectors (see legend for Fig. 7-88, *A*). **B,** Abnormalities. The *QRS duration* is 0.12 second or longer. The arrow representing the *mean initial 0.04 second QRS vector* is normal. The arrow representing the *mean terminal 0.04 second QRS vector* is shifted far to the right and anteriorly. This abnormality occurs because the directions of the electrical forces (vectors) produced by the myocytes that are ordinarily stimulated by the posteroinferior division of the left bundle branch and the myocytes ordinarily stimulated by the right bundle branch are altered because of their blocked pathways. The electrical forces produced by the myocytes stimulated by the intact left anterosuperior division of the left bundle branch produce a vertically directed mean vector that, when added to the mean vector created by the myocytes stimulated by the delayed electrical impulses that sweep into the right ventricle from the left ventricle, produce a vector that is directed far to the right and anteriorly. The *mean QRS vector* is directed farther to the right than is usually seen when there is uncomplicated right bundle-branch block. When right bundle-branch block plus left posteroinferior division block is present, the mean QRS vector is usually directed more than +120 degrees to the right. It is always directed anteriorly. Theoretically, this conduction defect should produce a *secondary T wave abnormality* as shown in this figure (the ventricular gradient should be normal). In practice, however, this conduction abnormality is more likely to be caused by sufficient myocardial damage (see text), and a *primary T wave abnormality* is often present. A mean vector representing the *ST segment displacement* is directed parallel with, or within 30 degrees of, the mean T vector.

(vectors) responsible for depolarization of the left ventricle during the last 0.04 second of the QRS complex. The electrical forces representing the former are altered because of right bundle-branch block and are directed to the right and anteriorly, and the electrical forces representing the latter are altered because of left posteroinferior division block and are directed inferiorly and anteriorly as dictated by the myocytes stimulated by the left anterosuperior division of the left bundle branch. The vector sum of these produces a mean terminal 0.04 second QRS vector that is usually directed far to the right and anteriorly or parallel with the frontal plane.

Arrows representing the mean of the electrical forces (vectors) responsible for the ST segment displacement and T wave are directed opposite to the arrow representing the QRS complex. The ventricular gradient may or may not be normally directed, depending on the cause of the conduction defect.

Right bundle-branch block plus left posteroinferior division block may be caused by myocardial infarction due to coronary disease, cardiomyopathy, myocarditis, Lenegre disease, Lev disease, or cardiac surgery.

An electrocardiogram illustrating right bundle-branch block plus left posteroinferior block, as well as primary T wave and ST segment abnormalities, is shown in Fig. 7-101.

Left or right bundle-branch block plus a primary T wave abnormality representing a type of complicated bundle-branch block. The duration of the QRS complex is 0.12 second or longer.

When an arrow representing the terminal 0.04 second QRS vector is directed to the left and posteriorly, it is typical of uncomplicated left bundle-branch block (Fig. 7-102, *A*). When an arrow representing the terminal 0.04 second QRS vector is directed to the right and anteriorly, it is typical of uncomplicated right bundle-branch block (Fig. 7-103).

Arrows representing the mean of the electrical forces (vectors) responsible for the ST and T waves are directed opposite to the arrow representing the mean of the electrical forces responsible for the QRS complex when there is uncomplicated left or right bundle-branch block. This occurs because the sequence of the repolarization process is predetermined by the sequence of the depolarization process. The T waves in such electrocardiograms are referred to as a *secondary* T wave abnormality. The ventricular gradient is directed normally in such patients. A *primary T* wave abnormality implies that the electrical forces (vectors) produced by repolarization are produced by an abnormality that is unrelated to the depolarization process. An arrow representing the electrical forces (vectors) responsible for a primary T wave abnormality is the vector sum of the normal repolarization forces (vectors) and the abnormal repolarization forces (vectors). Accordingly, the ventricular gradient is abnormally directed.

It is not always possible to determine the presence of a primary T wave abnormality when there is left or right bundle-branch block, because it is not always easy

Text continued on p. 348.

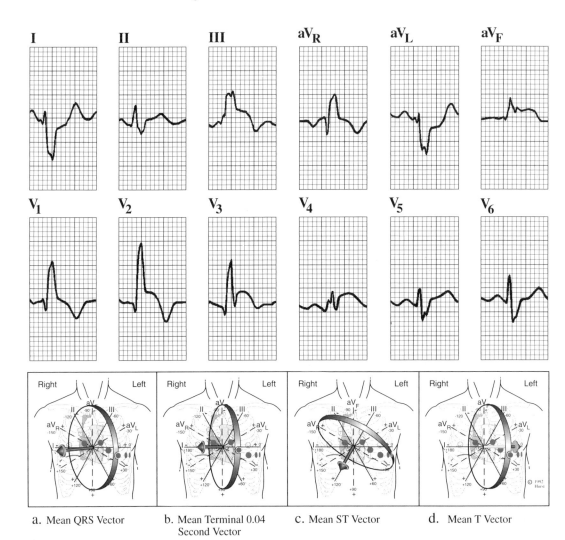

a. Mean QRS Vector

b. Mean Terminal 0.04
Second Vector

c. Mean ST Vector

d. Mean T Vector

Fig. 7-101

Fig. 7-101. Complicated right bundle-branch block plus left posteroinferior division block, primary T wave abnormality, and primary ST segment abnormality.

- *Rhythm:* Sinus tachycardia

  Rate: Undetermined in short strip. There were 104 depolarizations per minute in a longer strip.

  PR interval: 0.15 second

  QRS duration: 0.12 second

  QT interval: 0.36 second

- *Vector diagrams of electrical forces:* See *a*, *b*, *c*, and *d* below the electrocardiogram.

- *Electrophysiologic considerations:*

  The P waves are normal.

  The duration of the QRS complex is 0.12 second. The mean QRS vector is directed about +175 degrees to the right and about 50 degrees anteriorly. This degree of rightward deviation of the mean QRS vector is much more than it should be when there is uncomplicated right bundle-branch block.

  The mean terminal 0.04 second QRS vector is directed +180 degrees to the right and about 25 to 30 degrees anteriorly, signifying the presence of right bundle-branch block. The mean terminal 0.04 second QRS vector is directed farther to the right and more anteriorly than it is when there is uncomplicated right bundle-branch block.

  The extreme rightward deviation of the mean QRS vector and mean terminal 0.04 second QRS vector is probably caused by additional left posteroinferior division block.

  The mean ST vector points toward an area of epicardial injury. It is directed about +120 degrees inferiorly and about 30 degrees anteriorly, and is caused by an inferoanterior myocardial infarction. Note that this is a primary ST segment abnormality because the mean ST vector is not parallel with the mean T vector, as it is when there is a secondary ST segment displacement.

  The mean T vector is directed at ±0 degrees in the frontal plane and about 35 degrees posteriorly. The ventricular gradient is abnormal, suggesting myocardial ischemia.

  This electrocardiogram is abnormal because of right bundle-branch block, left posteroinferior division block, inferoanterior epicardial injury, and myocardial ischemia.

- *Clinical differential diagnosis:* This cluster of electrocardiographic abnormalities is due to an acute myocardial infarction. No other diagnostic option should be considered.

- *Discussion:* This electrocardiogram was recorded from a 56-year-old man with an acute myocardial infarction. Coronary arteriography revealed 80% obstruction of the left anterior descending coronary artery, which wrapped around the cardiac apex, 70% obstruction of the first diagonal, and 60% obstruction of the right coronary artery.

A

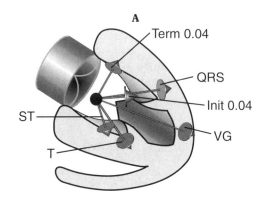

B

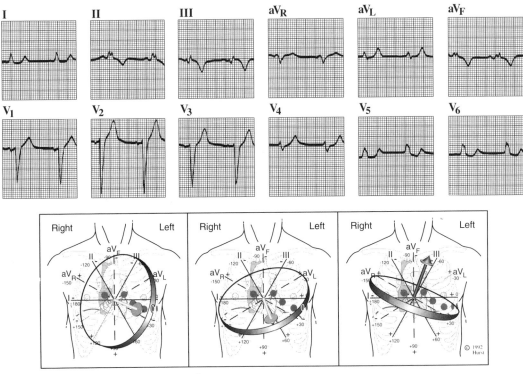

a. Mean QRS Vector

b. Mean Terminal 0.04 Second Vector

c. Mean T Vector

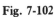

Fig. 7-102

Fig. 7-102. A, Electrocardiographic abnormalities associated with complicated left bundle-branch block plus a primary T wave abnormality. The duration of the QRS complex is 0.12 second or longer. In this example the arrows representing the mean initial 0.04 second QRS vector, the mean terminal 0.04 second QRS vector, and the mean QRS vector are characteristic of uncomplicated left bundle-branch block. The arrow representing the mean T vector, however, is directed posteriorly rather than anteriorly, as it should be when there is a secondary T wave abnormality. This causes the ventricular gradient to be abnormal (it is directed too posteriorly), indicating a primary T wave abnormality. The direction of the ventricular gradient indicates an anterior myocardial repolarization abnormality.

B, Complicated left bundle-branch block due to a primary T wave abnormality.

- *Rhythm:* Normal sinus rhythm

  Rate: 65 depolarizations per minute

  PR interval: 0.18 second

  QRS duration: 0.12 second

  QT interval: 0.40 second

- *Vector diagrams of electrical forces:* See *a, b,* and *c* below the electrocardiogram.

- *Electrophysiologic considerations:*

  The mean P vector is directed about +90 degrees inferiorly and about 40 degrees posteriorly. The second half of the P wave is negative in leads V_1 and V_2. Although the P waves are not large, this probably represents a left atrial abnormality.

  The mean QRS vector is directed about +20 degrees inferiorly and about 65 degrees posteriorly.

  The mean terminal 0.04 second QRS vector is directed about +70 degrees inferiorly and 50 degrees posteriorly.

  The mean T vector is directed −70 degrees to the left and anteriorly. It is not possible to determine the exact number of degrees the mean T vector is directed anteriorly without obtaining recordings from additional electrode sample sites. The ventricular gradient is abnormally directed away from the inferoposterior portion of the left ventricle.

- *Clinical differential diagnosis:* This type of electrocardiogram is usually produced by coronary artery disease with inferoposterior myocardial infarction. Whereas there are many causes of coronary artery disease, the most common cause is coronary atherosclerosis.

- *Discussion:* This electrocardiogram was recorded from a 59-year-old man who had experienced an inferoposterior myocardial infarction.

Electrocardiogram from Hurst JW, Woodson GC Jr: *Spatial vector electrocardiography*, New York, 1952, Blakiston, p 179. The copyright has been transferred from the publisher to me.

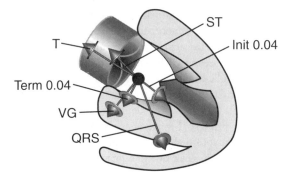

Fig. 7-103. Electrocardiographic abnormalities associated with complicated right bundle-branch block plus a primary T wave abnormality. The duration of the QRS complex is 0.12 second or longer. In this example the arrows representing the mean initial 0.04 second QRS vector, the mean terminal 0.04 second QRS vector, and the mean QRS vector are characteristic of uncomplicated left bundle-branch block. The mean T vector is directed superiorly and to the right, rather than to the left and slightly posteriorly, as it is when there is a secondary T wave abnormality; the ventricular gradient is directed abnormally to the right. This indicates a primary T wave abnormality. The direction of the ventricular gradient indicates an anterolateral myocardial repolarization abnormality.

to compute the direction and size of the ventricular gradient. At times, however, the abnormality can be identified with ease.

The most common cause of a primary T wave abnormality in patients with left or right bundle-branch block is myocardial ischemia due to coronary disease. It can also occur with myocarditis and cardiomyopathy. Pulmonary embolism may be responsible for right bundle-branch block plus a primary T wave abnormality.

An electrocardiogram illustrating left bundle-branch block with a primary T wave abnormality is shown in Fig. 7-102, *B*. Right bundle-branch block plus left posteroinferior division block plus a primary T wave abnormality can be seen in the electrocardiogram in Fig. 7-101.

Left or right bundle-branch block with a primary ST segment abnormality representing a type of complicated bundle-branch block. The duration of the QRS complex is 0.12 second or longer.

The directions of arrows representing the mean of the electrical forces (vectors) responsible for the QRS complex and the mean of the electrical forces (vectors) responsible for the initial and terminal 0.04 second of the QRS complex are typical of uncomplicated left or right bundle-branch block.

An arrow representing the electrical forces responsible for the ST segment displacement should be directed relatively parallel with an arrow representing the mean of the electrical forces (vectors) responsible for the T wave when there is uncomplicated left or right bundle-branch block. The angle between the two arrows is usually 60 degrees or less. This is called a *secondary* ST segment displacement and is due to repolarization forces (vectors). When the arrow representing the mean of the electrical forces (vectors) responsible for the ST segment displacement is directed more than 60 degrees away from the arrow representing the mean of the electrical forces (vectors) responsible for the T wave, or when the ST segment displacement is large compared with the T wave, a *primary* ST segment displacement should be considered. Such an ST segment abnormality is produced by the vector sum of the electrical forces (vectors) responsible for the secondary ST segment displacement plus the electrical forces (vectors) produced by separate epicardial myocardial injury (Figs. 7-104, *A*, and 7-105).

Primary ST segment abnormalities in patients with right or left bundle-branch block are usually caused by epicardial injury due to intense myocardial ischemia due to coronary artery disease.

An electrocardiogram illustrating left bundle-branch block is shown in Fig. 7-104, *B*. It also shows an ST segment abnormality that indicates epicardial injury due to myocardial infarction. The right bundle-branch block shown in the electrocardiogram in Fig. 7-101 also shows an ST segment abnormality that indicates epicardial injury due to myocardial infarction.

Abnormal Q waves due to myocardial infarction in patients with right bundle-branch block. Abnormal Q waves due to myocardial infarction cannot appear when there is left bundle-branch block, because septal depolarization is directed abnormally from right to left rather than from left to right; the spread of the depolarization process is delayed in the endocardium of the left ventricle. This permits the electrical forces (vectors) in the endocardium of the right ventricle to dominate the electrical field during the initial 0.04 second of the QRS complex. Therefore it is not possible for an infarct of the left ventricle to generate abnormal Q waves when there is left bundle-branch block.

Abnormal Q waves due to myocardial infarction *can* be identified in a patient with right bundle-branch block, because the septum is depolarized almost normally (i.e., from left to right) when there is right bundle-branch block; the spread of the depolarization process in the endocardium of the left ventricle occurs normally, whereas the depolarization process in the endocardium of the right ventricle is delayed. The abnormal initial 0.04 second of the QRS complex that occurs in patients with myocardial infarction is discussed later in the chapter.

Abnormal Q waves due to myocardial infarction are commonly due to coronary artery disease. The most common cause of coronary artery disease is obstructive coronary atherosclerosis. Other causes of coronary artery disease include coronary artery thrombosis or spasm with minimal coronary atherosclerosis, dissection of a coronary artery, coronary embolism, Kawasaki disease, and coronary arteritis. Myocar-

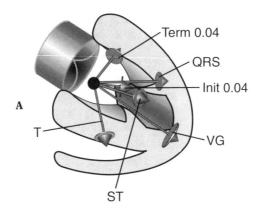

A

| I | II | III | aV$_R$ | aV$_L$ | aV$_F$ |

B

| V$_1$ | V$_2$ | V$_3$ | V$_4$ | V$_5$ | V$_6$ |

a. Mean QRS Vector   b. Mean T Vector   c. Mean ST Vector

© 1992 Hurst

Fig. 7-104

Fig. 7-104. A, Electrocardiographic abnormalities associated with complicated left bundle-branch block due to primary ST segment abnormality. The arrow representing the mean ST segment vector should be relatively parallel with the arrow representing the mean T vector when there is uncomplicated left bundle-branch block. When this occurs, it is labeled as *a secondary ST segment* abnormality and, in reality, is part of the repolarization process. In this example the arrow representing the mean ST vector is directed slightly inferiorly, to the left, and anteriorly; it is not parallel with the arrow representing the mean T vector. This is labeled as a *primary ST segment abnormality* and is usually due to epicardial myocardial injury. The duration of the QRS complex is 0.12 second or longer.

B, Complicated left bundle-branch block due to a primary ST segment abnormality.

- *Rhythm:* Sinus tachycardia

  Rate: Cannot be determined in short strip. There were 125 depolarizations per minute in a longer strip.

  PR interval: 0.14 second

  QRS duration: 0.12 second

  QT interval: 0.30 second

- *Vector diagrams of electrical forces:* See *a, b,* and *c* below the electrocardiogram.

- *Electrophysiologic considerations:*

  The duration of the QRS complex is 0.12 second. It is directed −15 degrees to the left and about 60 degrees posteriorly. The mean terminal 0.04 second QRS vector is directed to the left and posteriorly, indicating left bundle-branch block.

  Ordinarily, when there is left bundle-branch block, the mean initial 0.04 second QRS vector is directed inferiorly or to the left and is commonly parallel with the frontal plane. Accordingly, there will be no Q wave in leads I and V_6 and a small or absent R wave in lead V_1. Accordingly, the Q wave abnormalities of an infarct are usually masked by the left bundle branch. In this example of left bundle-branch block associated with infarction, the abnormal Q waves in leads I and V_6 occurred, I believe, because the infarct did not involve the first portion of the left bundle.

  The mean T vector is directed −170 degrees to the left and 30 to 40 degrees anteriorly. It is directed opposite to the mean QRS vector. The ventricular gradient is abnormal.

  The large mean ST vector is directed −5 degrees to the left and 80 degrees anteriorly. It is not directed parallel with the mean T vector, as it should be with uncomplicated left bundle-branch block. This is a primary ST segment abnormality and represents anterior epicardial injury such as occurs with anterior myocardial infarction.

- *Clinical differential diagnosis:* The abnormal mean initial 0.04 second QRS vector and abnormal primary ST segment vector are diagnostic of anterior myocardial infarction in this patient with left bundle-branch block.

- *Discussion:* This electrocardiogram was recorded from a patient with a characteristic clinical feature of myocardial infarction.

Electrocardiogram from Hurst JW, Woodson GC Jr: *Spatial vector electrocardiography*, New York, 1952, Blakiston, p 183. The copyright has been transferred from the publisher to me.

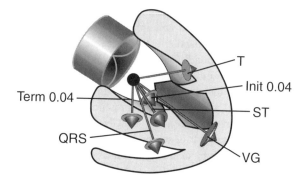

Fig. 7-105. Electrocardiographic abnormalities associated with complicated right bundle-branch block due to primary ST segment abnormality. The duration of the QRS complex is 0.12 second or longer. In this example an arrow representing the mean ST vector is directed inferiorly and anteriorly; it is not parallel with the arrow representing the mean T vector. This is labeled as a primary ST segment abnormality and is usually due to epicardial myocardial injury.

dial diseases such as myocarditis and all types of cardiomyopathy can also produce abnormal Q waves.

An electrocardiogram illustrating right bundle-branch block plus left anterosuperior division block and abnormal Q waves due to myocardial infarction is shown in Fig. 7-106.

Other conditions in which the duration of the QRS complex is 0.12 second or longer. Preexcitation of the ventricles,[46] hypothermia,[48] electrolyte abnormalities, and QRS conduction defects due to drugs are discussed elsewhere in the chapter.

QRS conduction defects in which the QRS duration is 0.14 to 0.20 second. A QRS duration that is greater than 0.12 second is automatically classified as complicated bundle-branch block; it should not be labeled as simple bundle-branch block. Arrows representing the mean of the electrical forces (vectors) responsible for the entire QRS complex, the initial 0.4 second, and the terminal 0.04 second may be typical of left and right bundle-branch block or suggest some ill-defined conduction abnormality. The electrocardiogram, in which the QRS duration may be 0.14 second or more, indicates a Purkinje-myocyte block; the conduction abnormality is located predominantly in the myocardium itself.

Arrows representing the mean of the electrical forces (vectors) responsible for the ST segment displacement and T wave may be those of secondary or primary abnormalities.

Patients with this type of conduction abnormality commonly have myocardial disease. The myocardial disease may be caused by coronary disease, cardiomyopathy, end-stage valve disease, or cardiac surgery.

An electrocardiogram illustrating a QRS duration of 0.16 second is shown in Fig. 7-107.

Myocardial infarction

Myocardial infarction may occur without associated electrocardiographic abnormalities. Also, there is less likelihood that the electrocardiogram will show the new abnormalities of infarction when there are electrocardiographic abnormalities secondary to previous infarctions.

Myocardial infarction may produce abnormal Q waves, primary ST segment abnormalities, and primary T wave abnormalities.

Abnormal Q waves due to myocardial infarction.[49] The initial 0.04 second of the QRS complex of the normal electrocardiogram is produced by the electrical forces (vectors) that result from depolarization of the septum and subendocardium of both ventricles. The direction of the arrows representing these electrical forces (vectors) is discussed earlier in the chapter. When an area of the endocardium of the left ventricle is infarcted, it produces no electrical forces (vectors); the electrical forces (vectors) produced by the myocardium of the opposite "wall" of the left ventricle dominate the electrical field. Accordingly, the mean of the electrical forces (vectors) responsible for the initial 0.04 second of the QRS complex is directed away from the infarct (Fig. 7-108). This vector commonly produces an abnormal Q wave in the electrocardiogram. Note that the area of infarction is larger at the endocardium than at the epicardium.

The normality of a Q wave is determined by identifying the direction of the mean initial 0.04 second QRS vector that produces it and determining its relationship to the mean QRS vector. Normally, an arrow representing the mean of the electrical forces (vectors) responsible for the initial 0.04 second of the QRS complex is directed to the left of a vertically directed mean QRS vector, may be on either side of an intermediately directed mean QRS vector, is directed inferior to a horizontally directed mean QRS vector, and is always anterior to the mean QRS vector. It is usually directed less than 60 degrees away from the mean QRS vector. Commonly, the QRS-T angle is about 30 to 45 degrees. When myocardial infarction occurs, the arrow representing the mean of the electrical forces responsible for the initial 0.04 second of the QRS complex may be directed to the right of a vertical QRS vector, may be more than 60 degrees to the right or left of an intermediate mean QRS vector, may be directed superior to a horizontal or leftward mean QRS vector, and may be directed posterior to the mean QRS vector (Fig. 7-109).

Although it is common for a myocardial infarction to produce an abnormality of the initial 0.04 second of the QRS complex, certain infarcts may alter only the initial 0.02 second of the QRS complex. For example, a small septal infarct may produce electrical forces (vectors) that are directed almost entirely posteriorly. The electrical forces (vectors) may alter the initial portion of the QRS complex very little in the

Text continued on p. 358.

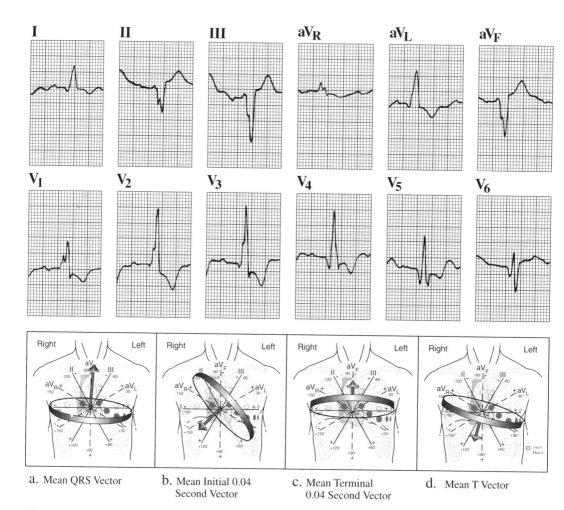

a. Mean QRS Vector

b. Mean Initial 0.04 Second Vector

c. Mean Terminal 0.04 Second Vector

d. Mean T Vector

Fig. 7-106

Fig. 7-106. Complicated right bundle-branch block with left anterosuperior division block and lateral myocardial infarction.

- *Rhythm:* Normal sinus rhythm

  Rate: Undetermined in short strip. There were 76 depolarizations per minute in a longer strip.

  PR interval: 0.23 second

  QRS duration: 0.16 second

  QT interval: 0.44 second

- *Vector diagrams of electrical forces:* See *a, b, c,* and *d* below the electrocardiogram.
- *Electrophysiologic considerations:*

  The P waves are normal. First-degree atrioventricular block is present.

  The mean QRS vector is directed about −85 degrees to the left and about 20 to 30 degrees anteriorly. This is characteristic of right bundle-branch block plus left anterosuperior division block.

  The mean initial 0.04 second QRS vector is directed about +140 degrees to the right and about 20 degrees anteriorly. The direction of this vector is not characteristic of left or right bundle-branch block. It is caused by an endocardial dead zone.

  The mean terminal 0.04 second QRS vector is directed about −90 degrees to the left and about 10 degrees posteriorly. It would be more posterior than this if isolated left bundle-branch block were present.

  The mean T vector is directed +115 degrees to the right and about 20 degrees posteriorly. The ventricular gradient is abnormal, indicating that a primary T wave abnormality is present.

  This electrocardiogram exhibits first-degree atrioventricular block and right bundle-branch block plus left anterosuperior division block. It also shows an initial 0.04 second QRS abnormality that is caused by a dead zone in the endocardium of the lateral portion of the left ventricle. Abnormal Q waves can be produced by myocardial infarction when there is right bundle-branch block. This tracing shows that right bundle-branch block plus left anterosuperior division block does not prevent the development of abnormal Q waves due to infarction.

- *Clinical differential diagnosis:* When all of these abnormalities are present in a single electrocardiogram, the usual cause is coronary artery disease due to atherosclerosis. Other types of coronary artery disease could also cause the abnormalities.
- *Discussion:* This electrocardiogram was recorded from a 69-year-old man with chest pain that was characteristic of myocardial infarction.

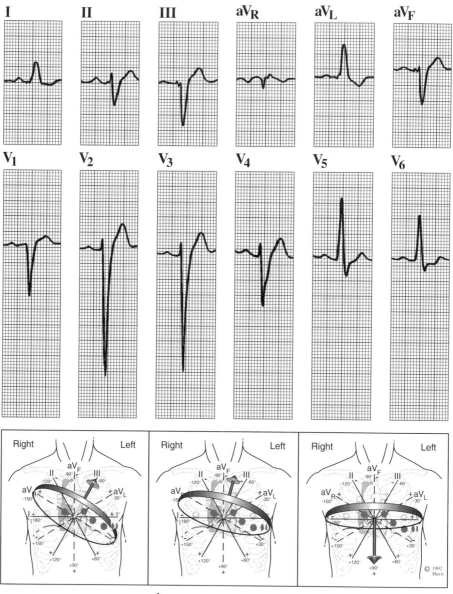

a. Mean QRS Vector

b. Mean Terminal 0.04 Second Vector

c. Mean T Vector

Fig. 7-107

Fig. 7-107. Complicated left bundle-branch block plus left anterosuperior division block with a QRS duration of 0.16 second.

- *Rhythm:* Normal sinus rhythm
  Rate: Undetermined in short strip. There were 78 depolarizations per minute in a longer strip.
  PR interval: 0.20 second
  QRS duration: 0.16 second
  QT interval: 0.40 second
- *Vector diagrams of electrical forces:* See *a*, *b*, and *c* below the electrocardiogram.
- *Electrophysiologic considerations:*
  The P waves are normal.
  The mean QRS vector is directed about −60 degrees to the left and at least 30 degrees posteriorly. The direction of the vector is characteristic of left bundle-branch block plus left anterosuperior division block. Note that the QRS duration is 0.16 second.
  The mean terminal 0.04 second QRS vector is directed more than −75 degrees to the left and at least 30 degrees posteriorly.
  The mean T vector is directed +90 degrees inferiorly and more than 20 degrees anteriorly. The exact number of degrees it is directed anteriorly cannot be determined without recording from additional electrode positions.
  This electrocardiogram is abnormal because of left bundle-branch block, left anterosuperior division block, and a QRS duration of 0.16 second. The greater the QRS duration and the more evidence there is of several ventricular conduction abnormalities, the more likely there is to be myocardial disease. Such abnormalities suggest a generalized Purkinje-myocyte conduction defect.
- *Clinical differential diagnosis:* These abnormalities, indicating a complicated conduction abnormality, may occur with coronary heart disease, cardiomyopathy, primary disease of the conduction system (Lenegre disease), Lev disease, and conditions causing severe and long-standing left ventricular hypertrophy.
- *Discussion:* This electrocardiogram was recorded from a 48-year-old man with acromegaly. The chest x-ray film revealed that the heart was generally enlarged. Such patients have cardiomyopathy, and some of the patients have atherosclerotic coronary heart disease.

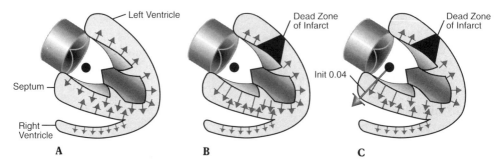

Fig. 7-108. How an abnormal Q wave is produced. **A,** The first portion of the ventricles to undergo depolarization is the left upper portion of the interventricular septum. This occurs because the electrical impulse transmitted by an early twig of the left bundle branch stimulates this area of the heart. The left and right bundles transmit electrical impulses with rapid speed to the endocardial surfaces of the left and right ventricles. Electrical forces are produced as shown by the arrows. Those events occur during the initial 0.04 second of the depolarization of the left and right ventricles. **B,** Suppose a dead zone develops in the superolateral portion of the left ventricle. This removes the electrical forces that are normally produced by this area of the endocardium during the initial 0.03 to 0.04 second of the QRS complex. The electrical forces (vectors) produced by the ventricular muscle that is located opposite the dead zone now dominate the electrical field. **C,** An arrow representing the electrical forces (vectors) responsible for a dead zone is directed away from the dead area. This produces an abnormal Q wave in the electrocardiogram. The location of the abnormal Q wave in the 12-lead electrocardiogram depends on the location and size of the infarct in the left ventricle (and occasionally in the right ventricle).

extremity leads (frontal plane) but will eliminate a small R wave in leads V_1 and V_2. This variation, of course, may be present normally or with systolic pressure overload of the left ventricle. However, when a small Q wave is followed by an R wave, which is followed by an S wave in lead V_3, indicating that the electrical forces (vectors) responsible for the initial 0.01 second of the QRS complex are directed more posteriorly than the subsequent QRS forces, septal infarction is highly likely (Fig. 7-110).

A dead zone due to myocardial infarction can occur in any area of the left ventricle and may occasionally involve the right ventricle. The initial portion of the QRS complex is altered by the dead zone. Accordingly, it is useful to imagine that a dead zone is located in various portions of the endocardium and to predict its effect on the initial electrical forces of the QRS complex (Fig. 7-111).

Abnormal Q waves may not be present in the electrocardiograms of all patients with myocardial infarction for any of the following reasons: the amount of dead tissue may be too small; the dead tissue may be located in the midportion or outer portion of the myocardium; the dead area may shrink in size as time passes; other

Right

Left

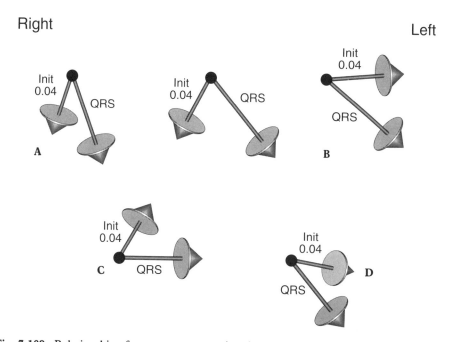

Fig. 7-109. Relationship of an arrow representing the mean initial 0.04 second QRS vector to an arrow representing the mean QRS vector in patients with myocardial infarction. The relationship of an arrow representing the normal mean initial 0.04 second QRS vector to an arrow representing the normal mean QRS vector is shown in Fig. 7-63. **A,** When an arrow representing the mean initial 0.04 second QRS vector is directed to the right of an arrow representing a vertically directed mean QRS vector, it is usually abnormal and often indicates the initial QRS abnormality of an anterolateral myocardial endocardial dead zone. **B,** When an arrow representing the mean initial 0.04 second QRS vector is directed 60 to 90 degrees to the right or left of an arrow representing an intermediately directed mean QRS vector, it often indicates, respectively, a lateral or inferior myocardial dead zone. **C,** When an arrow representing the mean initial 0.04-second QRS vector is directed superior to a horizontally directed arrow representing the mean QRS vector, it usually indicates an inferior myocardial dead zone. **D,** When an arrow representing the mean initial 0.04 second QRS vector is directed posterior to an arrow representing the mean QRS vector, it usually indicates an anterior myocardial dead zone.

Slightly modified with permission from Hurst JW: *Ventricular electrocardiography*, New York, 1991, Gower, fig 6.6.

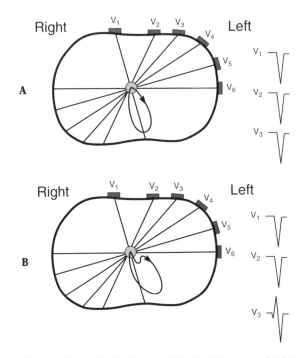

Fig. 7-110. Absent R waves in leads V_1, V_2, and V_3. **A,** When the QRS loop is located posteriorly, the initial portion of the loop may project negatively on leads V_1, V_2, and V_3. This may be produced by left ventricular hypertrophy, septal infarction, or for unknown reasons. In an individual tracing it cannot be declared that it is definitely due to infarction (as is commonly done). **B,** Note the difference in this electrocardiogram as compared with the one shown in **A.** Leads V_1 and V_2 show QRS complexes, and lead V_3 shows a Q wave that is followed by an R wave and S wave. Compare the QRS loop shown here with the QRS loop shown in **A.** Here the initial electrical forces (vectors) are directed posterior to the subsequent electrical forces (vectors). This abnormality usually indicates the presence of a septal dead zone. Only the initial 0.01 to 0.02 second of the electrical forces (vectors) may be altered in this situation. This is an example of an initial QRS abnormality due to a dead zone that does not occupy the initial 0.04 second of the QRS complex. It is usually caused by septal infarction but may be caused by any process that infiltrates the superior portion of the septum.

electrocardiographic abnormalities, such as left bundle-branch block, may mask the effect of the dead zone; and viable myocardium may not be located opposite the area of dead zone, such as occurs when the patient has had previous infarctions, or with an apical infarction, because the atrioventricular valves (and no myocardium) are opposite the apex. On the other hand, there are numerous causes of abnormal Q waves that are not due to myocardial infarction. The abnormalities are referred to as pseudoinfarction and are discussed in the next section.

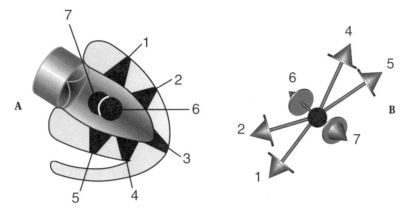

Fig. 7-111. How a dead zone located in the myocardium influences the electrocardiogram. **A,** Cross section of left and right ventricles showing seven dead zones. Most infarcts are located in the left ventricle, but a few also involve the right ventricle. Note that the endocardial portion of the dead zone is larger than the epicardial portion. The usual locations of dead zones are numbered: *1,* anterolateral; *2,* lateral; *3,* apical (note there is no myocardium opposite this dead zone); *4,* inferior; *5,* inferior and sometimes right ventricular; *6,* anteroseptal; *7,* true posterior. **B,** An arrow representing the mean initial 0.03 to 0.04 second QRS vector is directed away from the dead zone. Intact ventricular muscle must be present in an area that is opposite the dead zone for an abnormal initial vector to be produced. The vector is not produced by the dead zone. In fact, electrical forces are removed by the dead zone, permitting electrical forces produced by the intact and opposite myocardium to dominate the electrical field. Note that the vector for dead zone number 3 is omitted, because the atrioventricular valves, rather than myocardium, are located opposite the apex where the dead zone is located. Accordingly, no dead zone vector can be produced by an apical infarct.

The electrocardiographic abnormalities of infarction are currently designated as Q wave infarction or non−Q wave infarction. A non−Q wave infarction is recognized by the typical ST-T wave abnormalities, clinical features, and elevated serum enzyme levels. The terms *transmural* and *nontransmural* are no longer used, because the electrocardiographic abnormalities do not identify accurately whether or not the infarct is transmural. One simply identifies Q wave infarctions and non−Q wave infarctions. In the past the term *subendocardial infarction* was used commonly when no Q waves were present in a patient with infarction; however, this simple approach to the diagnosis of subendocardial infarction proved to be inaccurate. Today subendocardial infarction is diagnosed when an arrow representing the mean of the electrical forces responsible for the ST segment displacement is directed away from the centroid of the endocardial region of the left ventricle and persists for hours. The abnormality may then be followed by electrocardiographic signs of Q wave infarction.

Primary ST segment displacement due to epicardial myocardial injury.[49] An area of injury surrounds the dead zone of myocardial infarction. Usually the area of epicardial injury is larger than the area of subendocardial injury (Fig. 7-112, A), because most of the endocardial portion of the usual infarction is composed of dead tissue rather than injured tissue, whereas the dead area is smaller at the epicardium and the injured area is larger. Therefore the area of epicardial injury is larger because it is not dead.

The electrical forces (vectors) responsible for the ST segment displacement are, for the most part, produced during the TQ interval.[50] The displacement of the baseline of the electrocardiogram is actually opposite to that seen during the ST segment.

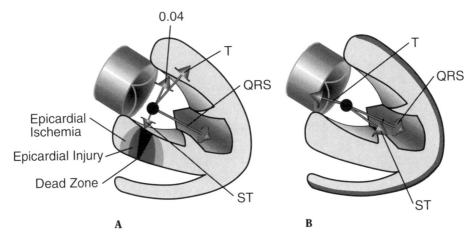

Fig. 7-112. Location of the dead zone, area of injury, and area of ischemia of myocardial infarction as compared with that of epicardial injury and ischemia of acute pericarditis. **A,** The dead zone is located inferiorly. It is largest in the endocardial area and smallest in the epicardial area. The zone of injury surrounds the dead zone and is largest in the epicardial area. The area of ischemia surrounds the area of injury and is largest in the epicardial area. The arrow representing the mean initial 0.03 to 0.04 second QRS vector is directed away from the dead zone. The arrow representing the mean ST vector points toward an area of epicardial injury. The arrow representing the mean T vector points away from the area of epicardial ischemia. **B,** Directions of arrows representing the mean ST and T vectors in a patient with pericarditis. Pericarditis is usually generalized, and the mean ST segment vector points toward the anatomic apex of the left ventricle while the mean T vector points away from the anatomic apex. An apical infarct can produce an ST segment vector that simulates the ST segment vector of pericarditis. No abnormal Q wave of infarction may be produced, because there is no ventricular myocardium located opposite the apex. Pericarditis is usually generalized, as shown in this figure, but it can occasionally be localized. When this occurs, the arrow representing the mean ST vector may simulate the ST segment vector of myocardial infarction. This type of ST segment vector may be associated with pericarditis that follows cardiac surgery, trauma, or myocardial infarction.

The ST segment displacement occurs during electrical diastole of the ventricles and is due to an electrical leak that occurs just after the repolarization process has created the T wave. When the TQ interval is corrected by centering the baseline of the electrocardiogram, it eliminates the displacement noted during the TQ interval. In other words, the machine eliminates the TQ segment displacement by adding an equal and opposite electrical force when the baseline of the tracing is centered on the paper. Following this, ventricular depolarization creates the QRS complex, an act that eliminates most of the electrical forces created by the heart. The machine-induced "artifact" is then unopposed, and this produces the ST segment displacement. There is evidence, too, that a portion of the ST segment displacement is produced by the systolic leak of electrical charges from the injured tissue that occurs just after the depolarization process (QRS complex) is completed.[50]

The mean ST segment vector, representing the mean of the electrical forces (vectors) responsible for *epicardial injury,* is directed toward the injured myocytes. Epicardial injury is localized to segments of the left ventricle when it is due to ischemia associated with coronary disease (Fig. 7-112, *A*), whereas the epicardial injury of pericarditis is usually generalized (Fig. 7-112, *B*). Some years ago it was popular to describe the ST segment displacement of epicardial injury due to infarction as discordant and the ST segment displacement of pericarditis as concordant. This type of designation was a cumbersome way of describing the direction of an arrow representing the mean of the electrical forces (vectors) responsible for the ST segment displacement. Today the arrow representing the mean of the electrical forces (vectors) responsible for the ST segment displacement is visualized and diagrammed.[51]

An arrow representing the mean of the electrical forces (vectors) due to the epicardial injury of infarction is directed toward a segment of the left ventricle, and an arrow representing the mean of the electrical forces (vectors) responsible for epicardial injury due to generalized pericarditis is directed parallel with the anatomic long axis of the heart (see later discussion). The ST segment displacement that is actually part of the normal early repolarization process can be represented by a vector that is directed almost parallel with an arrow representing the mean of the electrical forces (vectors) responsible for the T wave; this ST vector does not change, as does the vector that represents the epicardial injury of myocardial infarction or pericarditis.

ST segment displacement due to epicardial injury may be transient or recurrent in three situations:

- Prinzmetal angina pectoris due to coronary artery spasm usually occurs in patients with coronary atherosclerosis but may occur in its absence. An arrow representing the mean of the electrical forces (vectors) responsible for the ST segment displacement in these cases is directed toward the area of epicardial injury, and the ST segment displacement is transient.[52]
- The syndrome of coronary thrombosis in a patient with coronary atherosclerosis produces a similar ST segment displacement; it, too, may be transient as a result of naturally occurring thrombolysis.

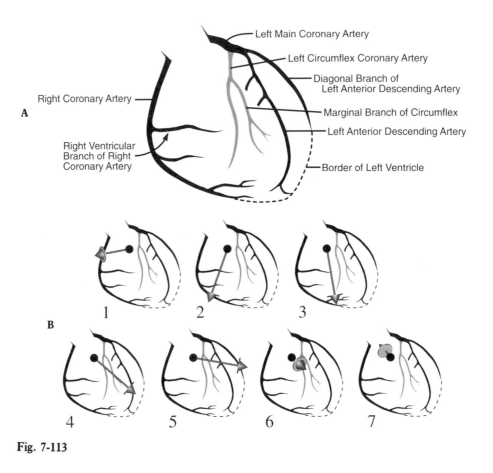

A

Left Main Coronary Artery

Left Circumflex Coronary Artery

Diagonal Branch of
Left Anterior Descending Artery

Right Coronary Artery

Marginal Branch of Circumflex

Left Anterior Descending Artery

Right Ventricular
Branch of Right
Coronary Artery

Border of Left Ventricle

B

1   2   3

4   5   6   7

Fig. 7-113

- An ST segment displacement may vanish when thrombolytic therapy is used for infarction.

An arrow representing the mean of the electrical forces (vectors) responsible for the ST segment displacement due to epicardial injury is often directed toward the obstructed coronary artery that is responsible for it (Fig. 7-113). The direction of the Q wave vector or T wave vector does not indicate the location of the culprit artery as accurately as does the ST segment vector.

An arrow representing the mean of the electrical forces responsible for *endocardial and subendocardial injury* is directed away from the injured myocytes.[53] It is usually directed opposite to the anatomic long axis of the heart (Fig. 7-114). When this injury continues, the entire endocardium of the left ventricle may become infarcted. Later, abnormal Q waves and abnormal T waves may or may not develop.

Fig. 7-113. Identification of the culprit artery believed to be responsible for myocardial infarction. The direction of an arrow representing the mean of the electrical forces (vectors) responsible for the ST segment displacement more accurately identifies the artery responsible for myocardial infarction than does an arrow representing the mean of the electrical forces (vectors) responsible for the initial 0.04 second of the QRS complex or an arrow representing the mean of the electrical forces (vectors) responsible for the T wave. Even so, it is not sufficiently accurate to use for decision-making purposes. Also, this technique gives no information about possible obstructions in the other coronary arteries. **A,** Approximate location of the right coronary artery, the right ventricular branch of the right coronary artery, the left main coronary artery, the left anterior descending coronary artery, a diagonal branch of the left anterior descending artery, and the left circumflex coronary artery. **B,** *Arrow 1* identifies an inferior and right ventricular myocardial infarction. The vector *(arrow)* is pointing toward an obstruction in the proximal portion of the right coronary artery. This obstruction will usually be proximal to the right ventricular branch of the right coronary artery. When the vector (arrow) is directed between the vectors (arrows 1 and 2) and is directed anteriorly, there is a good chance that it is due to an inferior–right ventricular infarction. *Arrow 2* identifies an inferior myocardial infarction. The arrow is pointing toward an obstruction in the distal portion of the right coronary artery. This type of infarction can also be caused by obstruction of the proximal portion of a wraparound left anterior descending artery in which there has been isoembolism to a distal site. *Arrow 3* identifies an inferolateral infarction that may be a result of an obstruction in the distal right coronary artery or in the distal circumflex coronary artery or its marginals. *Arrow 4* identifies an anterolateral myocardial infarction that may be produced by an obstruction in the distal portion of the left anterior descending artery or its diagonals. *Arrow 5* identifies an anteroseptal myocardial infarction that may be produced by an obstruction in the proximal portion of the left anterior descending coronary artery. *Arrow 6* identifies a massive anterior myocardial infarction that may be produced by an obstruction in the left main coronary artery or the initial portion of the left anterior descending artery. *Arrow 7* identifies a true posterior myocardial infarction that may be produced by an obstruction in the proximal portion of the left circumflex coronary artery.

The electrocardiographic abnormalities of most infarcts can be classified as Q wave infarctions or non–Q wave infarctions. Occasionally a subendocardial infarct can be identified (see above). Patients with a hypertrophied left ventricle who have a high diastolic pressure in the left ventricle and obstructive coronary disease may, when there is a fall in systemic blood pressure, develop severe generalized subendocardial injury and generalized endocardial infarction of the left ventricle. The pathophysiology responsible for this sequence of events follows the dictates of LaPlace's law.[54]

Primary T wave abnormalities due to myocardial ischemia.[55] An area of predominant epicardial ischemia surrounds the area of injury due to myocardial infarction (Fig. 7-115, *A*). The area of epicardial ischemia is usually larger than the area of endocardial ischemia. An arrow representing the mean of the electrical forces (vectors) responsible for the T wave is directed away from the area of epicardial ischemia

Text continued on p. 370.

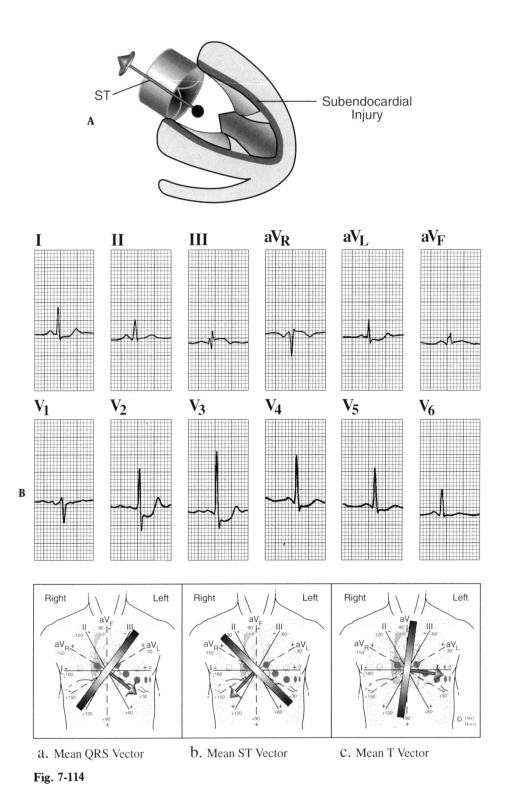

ST

A

Subendocardial
Injury

B

I II III aV_R aV_L aV_F

V₁ V₂ V₃ V₄ V₅ V₆

a. Mean QRS Vector   b. Mean ST Vector   c. Mean T Vector

Fig. 7-114

Fig. 7-114. A, Electrocardiographic abnormalities associated with subendocardial injury or infarction. Subendocardial injury or infarction is commonly due to coronary disease in a patient with left ventricular hypertrophy and elevated left ventricular diastolic pressure. When subendocardial hypoxia lasts a brief period of time, a transient ST segment vector is produced. An arrow representing the mean of the electrical forces (vectors) responsible for the ST segment displacement is directed away from the anatomic apex of the left ventricle. An ST vector persisting for several hours may be due to an infarction of the entire subendocardial area of the left ventricle.

B, Subendocardial injury and infarction or possibly inferior infarction.
- *Rhythm:* Sinus tachycardia
  Rate: Undetermined in short strip. There were 90 depolarizations per minute in a longer strip.
  PR interval: 0.12 second
  QRS duration: 0.08 second
  QT interval: 0.28 second
- *Vector diagrams of electrical forces:* See *a, b,* and *c* below the electrocardiogram.
- *Electrophysiologic considerations:*
  The P waves are normal.
  The mean QRS vector is directed about +38 degrees inferiorly and is parallel with the frontal plane.
  The mean ST segment vector is directed about +140 degrees to the right and is parallel with the frontal plane. Inferior myocardial infarction could also produce this type of ST segment vector.
  The mean T vector is directed at about +10 degrees and is parallel with the frontal plane. The amplitude of the T waves is normal.
  The direction of the mean ST segment vector may indicate subendocardial injury. This is commonly caused by hypoxia of the entire left ventricular endocardium. Whether or not subendocardial infarction develops depends on how long the subendocardium is deprived of an adequate amount of oxygenated blood. Should the ST segment vector persist for several hours, one could conclude that subendocardial infarction has occurred. The ST segment vector could also be caused by inferior myocardial injury.
- *Clinical differential diagnosis:* The usual cause of subendocardial injury is atherosclerotic coronary heart disease. It is commonly observed in patients with coronary artery disease who have left ventricular hypertrophy from some cause plus an increase in left ventricular diastolic pressure. An ST segment vector of this type may be caused by digitalis medication. In such cases the QT interval is short (as it is in this patient). However, the T waves are usually small when the ST segment vector is due to digitalis medication and normal or large when subendocardial injury is responsible for the ST segment vector. The ST segment displacement could be caused by inferior epicardial injury, but subendocardial injury seems more likely, because the mean initial 0.04 second QRS vector and mean T vector do not as yet indicate inferior infarction.
- *Discussion:* This electrocardiogram was recorded from a 60-year-old man with prolonged episodes of chest discomfort believed to be ischemic in origin and considered to be due to atherosclerotic coronary heart disease. Its persistence suggested, but did not prove, subendocardial infarction.

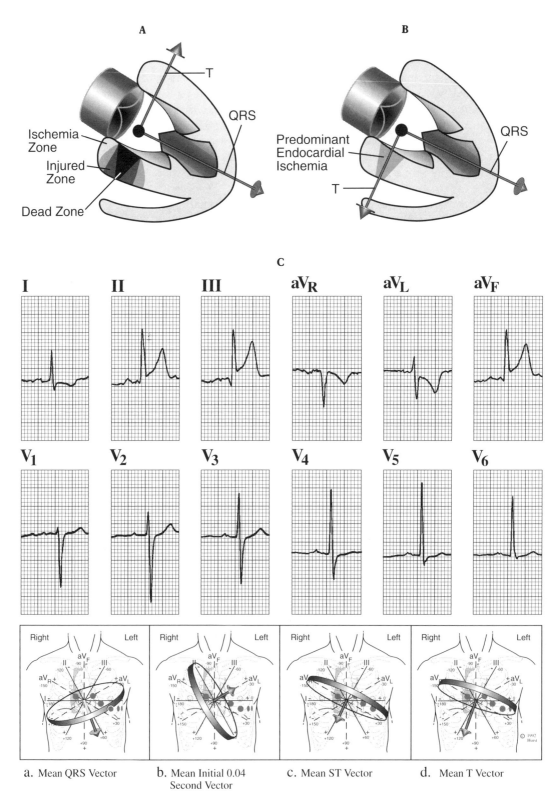

A

T

QRS

Ischemia Zone

Injured Zone

Dead Zone

B

QRS

Predominant Endocardial Ischemia

T

C

I   II   III   aV_R   aV_L   aV_F

V_1   V_2   V_3   V_4   V_5   V_6

a. Mean QRS Vector

b. Mean Initial 0.04 Second Vector

c. Mean ST Vector

d. Mean T Vector

Fig. 7-115

Fig. 7-115. T wave abnormalities due to myocardial ischemia. **A,** The mean T vector is directed away from an area of predominant epicardial ischemia. In myocardial infarction this ischemic area usually surrounds the area of predominant epicardial injury, which surrounds a dead zone whose endocardial base is larger than its epicardial "apex." When no abnormal Q wave is produced and the clinical picture is consistent with infarction, it is called a non–Q wave infarction. When an abnormal Q wave is produced, it is called a Q wave infarction. **B,** The T waves may become "hyperacute" secondary to the acute ischemia that occurs in some patients with fresh myocardial infarction. The T wave vector in such cases points toward the area of predominant localized endocardial ischemia.

C, Hyperacute T waves, inferior epicardial injury, and inferior dead zone.

- *Rhythm:* Normal sinus rhythm
  Rate: Undetermined in short strip. There were 75 depolarizations per minute in a longer
   strip.
  PR interval: 0.16 second
  QRS duration: 0.08 second
  QT interval: 0.36 second
- *Vector diagrams of electrical forces:* See *a, b, c,* and *d* below the electrocardiogram.
- *Electrophysiologic considerations:*
  The P waves are normal.
  The mean QRS vector is normally directed about +68 degrees inferiorly and about 35 to 40
   degrees posteriorly.
  The mean initial 0.04 second QRS vector is directed about −30 degrees to the left and an
   undetermined number of degrees anteriorly (recordings from additional electrode sites
   would be needed to determine exactly how far anteriorly the mean initial 0.04 second
   QRS vector is directed). As drawn, however, the mean initial 0.04 second QRS vector is
   directed abnormally to the left of the mean QRS vector, which suggests an inferior myocardial dead zone.
  The mean ST vector is directed about +118 degrees to the right and about 15 degrees anteriorly. Note how the transitional pathway of the mean ST vector "interdigitates" with
   the precordial electrode position sites; all of the precordial leads are very near the transitional pathway of the mean ST vector. This is why the ST segment shift is so small in the
   lateral precordial leads. The mean ST vector represents inferior epicardial injury.
  The mean T vector is large and is directed about +110 degrees to the right and about 25
   degrees anteriorly. It is due to inferior endocardial ischemia. These large, peaked T waves
   are referred to as hyperacute T waves.
  These abnormalities indicate the presence of a fresh myocardial infarction. There is an inferior endocardial dead zone and the expected inferior epicardial injury. The mean T vector ordinarily would point away from the epicardial area of ischemia that surrounds the
   epicardial injury. In this case, during the early phase of myocardial infarction, the endocardial ischemia is larger than the epicardial ischemia. This produces hyperacute T waves,
   and the mean T vector points toward the area of inferior endocardial ischemia.
- *Clinical differential diagnosis:* This tracing is diagnostic of a fresh myocardial infarction.
  There is likely to be an obstruction of the right coronary artery at its midpoint or just distal
  to the midpoint. The cause of such an obstruction is usually an atherosclerotic plaque and
  its complications.
- *Discussion:* This electrocardiogram was recorded from a 44-year-old man with an acute inferior myocardial infarction due to atherosclerotic coronary heart disease. Coronary arteriography revealed total obstruction of the midportion of the right coronary artery.

that surrounds the zone of injury. The ventricular gradient is commonly abnormal and is directed away from the epicardial area where the repolarization process is delayed.

At times, in the clinical setting of early myocardial infarction, the T waves become large and peaked and are referred to as hyperacute T waves (Fig. 7-115, *B* and *C*). An arrow representing the mean of the electrical forces responsible for these T waves may or may not change in direction. This T wave abnormality may represent predominant endocardial ischemia. This stage of infarction usually gives way to epicardial injury and ischemia.

The electrocardiographic abnormalities that are often, but not always, associated with myocardial infarction may be summarized as follows:

- An arrow representing the mean of the electrical forces (vectors) responsible for the initial 0.04 second of the QRS complex is directed away from a predominantly endocardial dead zone. This is referred to as a Q wave infarction. In some patients there is an abnormality of only the initial 0.01 to 0.02 second of the QRS complex.
- An arrow representing the mean of the electrical forces (vectors) responsible for the primary ST segment displacement is directed toward the area of epicardial injury and away from the area of endocardial injury.
- An arrow representing the mean of the electrical forces (vectors) responsible for the T wave is directed away from the area of epicardial ischemia and toward the area of endocardial ischemia.

An electrocardiogram illustrating inferior myocardial infarction is shown in Fig. 7-116. An electrocardiogram illustrating a true posterior myocardial infarction is shown in Fig. 7-117. An electrocardiogram illustrating right ventricular myocardial infarction is shown in Fig. 7-118. An electrocardiogram illustrating hyperacute ischemic T waves due to obstruction of the left anterior descending artery is shown in Fig. 7-119. An electrocardiogram illustrating an anterolateral myocardial infarction is shown in Fig. 7-120. An electrocardiogram illustrating a non–Q wave myocardial infarction is shown in Fig. 7-121. An electrocardiogram illustrating right bundle-branch block and inferoanterior myocardial infarction is shown in Fig. 7-122. An electrocardiogram illustrating left bundle-branch block and myocardial infarction is shown in Fig. 7-123.

The physician must remember that there are many causes of obstructive coronary disease. The electrocardiogram cannot be used to differentiate among these conditions. For example, myocardial infarction may be caused by coronary atherosclerosis, coronary spasm, coronary thrombosis without identifiable atherosclerosis, coronary artery embolism, dissection of a coronary artery, coronary arteritis, Kawasaki disease, trauma, etc.

Conditions producing electrocardiographic abnormalities of infarction simulating those due to coronary atherosclerotic heart disease. Abnormalities simulat-

ing infarction due to coronary atherosclerotic heart disease may be caused by pulmonary embolism[44,45]; dilated cardiomyopathy from any cause; or myocardial disease
due to amyloid, sarcoid, or neoplastic disease. Fulminating viral myocarditis may
produce abnormal Q waves, ST segments, and T waves. Myocardial necrosis is the
cause, but it is due to infection rather than ischemia. The flood of catecholamines
produced by a pheochromocytoma may produce myocardial necrosis (Fig. 7-124).
Hypertrophic cardiomyopathy may produce abnormal Q waves and ST-T wave abnormalities (Fig. 7-125). Systolic and diastolic pressure overload of the left ventricle
may produce abnormal Q waves that may mimic infarction. Preexcitation of the ventricles, such as may occur with Wolff-Parkinson-White syndrome, may produce abnormal Q waves suggesting infarction.[46] Acute pericarditis commonly produces ST-T
waves that may be misinterpreted as being due to myocardial infarction (see subsequent discussion).

Pericardial disease

Disease of the pericardium is usually generalized. The pericardium produces no electrical forces; the electrocardiographic abnormalities are due to epicardial damage and
pericardial fluid. There are three types of pericardial disease: acute pericarditis, pericardial effusion, and constrictive pericarditis. These are not always separate entities;
there is an overlap of syndromes. For example, acute pericarditis may be relatively
pure or be associated with pericardial effusion, and constrictive pericarditis may be
associated with pericardial effusion.

Acute pericarditis.[56] The rhythm is usually normal, but atrial arrhythmias are
believed to occur more often in patients with acute pericarditis.

The PQ segment may be displaced downward in leads I and V_6 (and I have seen
it in lead V_2 only). It is not always possible to draw an arrow that represents the
mean of the electrical forces (vectors) responsible for this abnormality, because it
may not be seen in all leads. Nor is it possible to consistently distinguish it from the
Ta wave, which is due to atrial repolarization.

During the *first stage* of acute pericarditis an arrow representing the mean of the
electrical forces (vectors) responsible for the ST segment displacement is directed
toward the centroid of epicardial injury; it is usually directed parallel with the anatomic long axis of the heart rather than being precisely parallel with the mean QRS
vector (Fig. 7-126, *A*). It is usually directed anterior to the mean QRS vector. Remember, the mean ST segment vector of epicardial injury due to myocardial infarction is usually directed toward a segment of the left ventricle, whereas the mean ST
segment vector of pericarditis points toward the cardiac apex. This occurs because
the epicardial damage of pericarditis is usually generalized and is not under the control of the conduction system.

Arrows representing the mean of the electrical forces (vectors) responsible for the
abnormal ST and T waves due to pericarditis are somewhat similar to those of early

Text continued on p. 392.

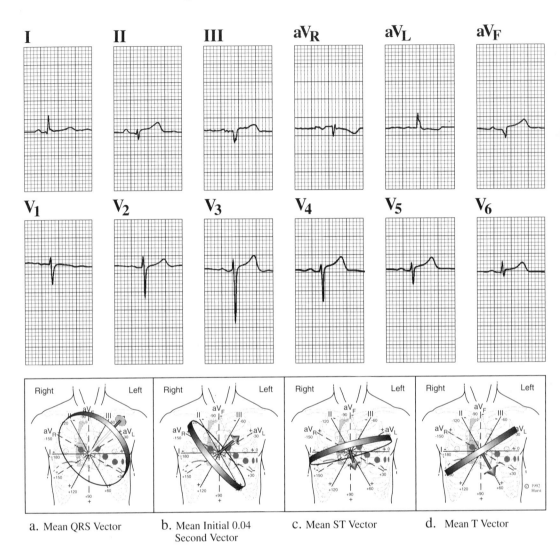

a. Mean QRS Vector

b. Mean Initial 0.04
Second Vector

c. Mean ST Vector

d. Mean T Vector

Fig. 7-116

Fig. 7- 116. Inferior myocardial infarction from thrombotic obstruction of a wraparound left anterior descending coronary artery.

- *Rhythm:* Normal sinus rhythm
  Rate: Undetermined in short strip. There were 71 depolarizations per minute on a longer strip.
  PR interval: 0.14 second
  QRS duration: 0.07 second
  QT interval: 0.32 second
- *Vector diagrams of electrical forces:* See *a, b, c,* and *d* below the electrocardiogram.
- *Electrophysiologic considerations:*
  The P waves are normal.
  The mean QRS vector is directed about −45 degrees to the left and about 60 degrees or more posteriorly. This abnormal degree of leftward deviation of the mean QRS vector is produced by the removal of the electrical forces ordinarily produced by the myocytes that are stimulated by the left anterosuperior division of the left bundle branch. The abnormal direction of the mean QRS vector could also be caused by a large inferior dead zone.
  The mean initial 0.04 second QRS vector is directed about −35 degrees to the left and about 10 degrees anteriorly. Careful scrutiny of leads I and II reveals small 0.01-second Q waves. There is a large Q wave in leads III and aV_F, indicating the presence of an inferior dead zone.
  The mean ST segment vector is directed about +75 degrees to the right and about 10 degrees anteriorly. This represents inferoanterior epicardial injury.
  The mean T vector is directed +60 degrees inferiorly and is parallel with the frontal plane. This is due to endocardial ischemia as discussed in Fig. 7-115, *C.*
- *Clinical differential diagnosis:* These electrocardiographic abnormalities indicate an inferolateral myocardial infarction. The direction of the ST segment vector indicates that the obstructed coronary artery is either the distal right coronary artery, the circumflex coronary artery, or a wraparound left anterior descending artery.
- *Discussion:* This electrocardiogram was recorded from a 24-year-old man who was a heavy smoker. He had severe, prolonged chest pain that was characteristic of myocardial ischemia. Coronary arteriography revealed a clot in the left anterior descending artery with very little atherosclerosis. The left anterior descending artery wrapped around the apex of the heart.

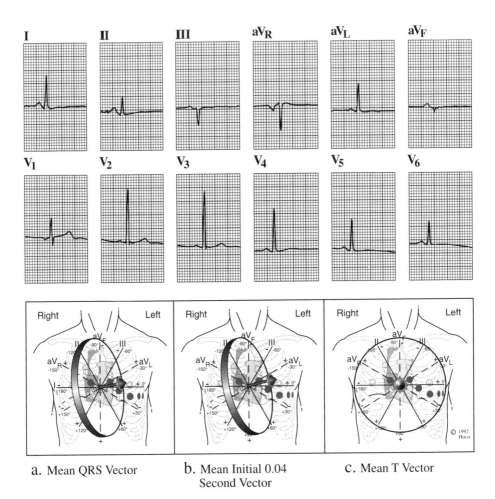

a. Mean QRS Vector

b. Mean Initial 0.04 Second Vector

c. Mean T Vector

Fig. 7-117

Fig. 7-117. True posterior infarction.

- *Rhythm:* Normal sinus rhythm

  Rate: Undetermined in short strip. There were 62 depolarizations per minute in a longer strip.

  PR interval: 0.16 second

  QRS duration: 0.08 second

  QT interval: 0.39 second

- *Vector diagrams of electrical forces:* See *a*, *b*, and *c* below the electrocardiogram.

- *Electrophysiologic considerations:*

  The P waves are normal.

  The mean QRS vector is directed about −10 degrees to the left and about 45 degrees anteriorly (note that the QRS amplitude is approximately the same in leads V_1 and V_6). The direction of the mean QRS vector is abnormal; it is directed too far anteriorly. This could be caused by right ventricular hypertrophy or true posterior infarction. Right ventricular hypertrophy is very unlikely, because the mean QRS vector is directed to the left.

  The mean initial 0.04 second QRS vector is directed about −10 degrees to the left and approximately 45 degrees anteriorly. This abnormality could be caused by right ventricular hypertrophy or a true posterior infarction.

  The mean T vector is directed 90 degrees anteriorly. Note that the T waves are not visible in the extremity leads and that there is a tall T wave in lead V_1 and a flat T wave in lead V_6. It indicates a repolarization abnormality in the posterior epicardial portion of the left ventricle.

- *Clinical differential diagnosis:* The mean QRS vector and the mean initial 0.04-second vector are directed abnormally anteriorly. They are both directed leftward, which makes right ventricular hypertrophy unlikely. The most likely cause of these abnormalities is true posterior infarction from coronary artery disease. The mean T vector points away from an area of true posterior epicardial ischemia surrounding the dead zone.

- *Discussion:* This electrocardiogram shows a true posterior infarction. It was recorded from a man who had coronary bypass surgery 9 years before this tracing was recorded. A coronary arteriogram revealed 40% obstruction of the left main coronary artery, 60% to 70% obstruction of a ramus artery, 70% to 80% obstruction of an obtuse marginal artery, 50% obstruction of the ostium of the right coronary artery, and 90% obstruction of the proximal portion of the right coronary artery.

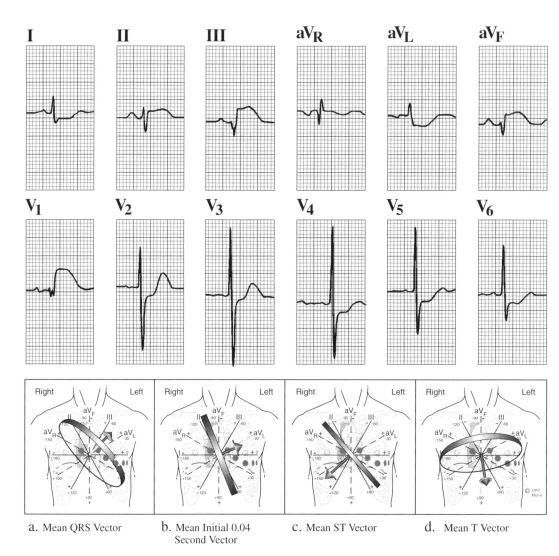

a. Mean QRS Vector

b. Mean Initial 0.04 Second Vector

c. Mean ST Vector

d. Mean T Vector

Fig. 7-118

Fig. 7-118. Right ventricular myocardial infarction.

- *Rhythm:* Normal sinus rhythm
  Rate: Undetermined in short strip. There were 85 depolarizations per minute in a longer
    strip.
  PR interval: 0.16 second
  QRS duration: 0.08 second
  QT interval: 0.40 second
- *Vector diagrams of electrical forces:* See *a*, *b*, *c*, and *d* below the electrocardiogram.
- *Electrophysiologic considerations:*
  The P waves are normal.
  The mean QRS vector is directed about −50 degrees to the left and about 20 degrees pos-
    teriorly. This abnormal direction could be caused by myocardial damage (dead zone) in-
    feriorly or left anterosuperior division block.
  The mean initial 0.04 second QRS vector is directed about −20 degrees to the left and is
    parallel with the frontal plane. Note the small R wave that is 0.02 second in duration in
    lead aV_F. The direction of the mean initial 0.04 second QRS vector could be, but is not
    definitely, due to an inferior myocardial dead zone.
  The mean ST vector is large. It is directed about +120 degrees to the right and is parallel
    with the frontal plane. It is produced by epicardial injury in the inferior portion of the
    septum and lower portion of the right ventricle.
  The mean T vector is directed about +80 degrees to the right and about 30 to 40 degrees
    anteriorly. This is probably a hyperacute ischemic T wave abnormality. As such, it is
    directed toward an area of inferior endocardial ischemia.
  The most easily explained abnormality is the large ST segment vector. It is directed toward
    epicardial injury of the inferior portion of the left ventricle (probably the lowest portion
    of the septum) and the lowest portion of the right ventricle.
- *Clinical differential diagnosis:* The mean ST segment of this electrocardiogram suggests an
  inferior left ventricular infarction that also involves the right ventricle.
- *Discussion:* This electrocardiogram was recorded from a 46-year-old man with an acute inferior–right ventricular myocardial infarction. A coronary arteriogram revealed a 90% obstruction of the right coronary artery proximal to the right ventricular branch of the right
  coronary artery.

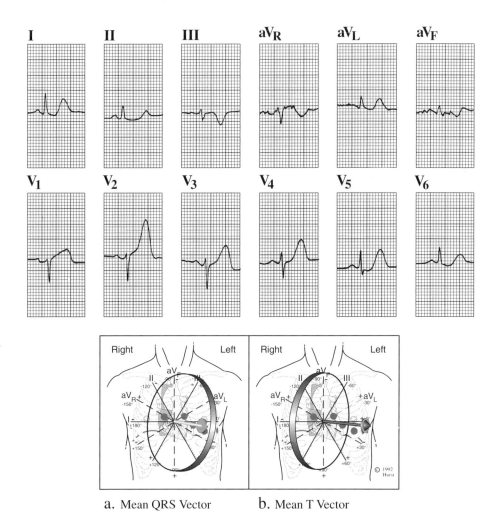

a. Mean QRS Vector   b. Mean T Vector

Fig. 7-119

Fig. 7-119. Hyperacute ischemic T waves due to obstruction of the left anterior descending artery.

- *Rhythm:* Normal sinus rhythm
  Rate: Undetermined in short strip. There were 60 depolarizations per minute in a longer strip.
  PR interval: 0.13 second
  QRS duration: 0.08 second
  QT interval: 0.40 second
- *Vector diagrams of electrical forces:* See *a* and *b* below the electrocardiogram.
- *Electrophysiologic considerations:*
  Note the downward displacement of the PQ segment in leads V_1, V_2, and V_3. This may be due to the repolarization of the atria (T of the P) or represent a left atrial abnormality.
  The mean QRS vector is directed at +10 degrees and about 60 degrees posteriorly.
  The mean T vector is large. It is directed at +10 degrees and about 45 degrees anteriorly.
  The spatial QRS-T angle is abnormally wide. This type of hyperacute T wave abnormality commonly indicates acute endocardial myocardial ischemia.
- *Clinical differential diagnosis:* This type of electrocardiogram may be seen during the hyperacute phase of an acute anterolateral myocardial ischemia. This is usually produced by obstructive atherosclerosis of the coronary arteries. The location of the myocardial ischemia suggests that it is caused by an obstructive lesion in the left anterior descending coronary artery or in the first diagonal.
- *Discussion:* This electrocardiogram was recorded from a 48-year-old woman who was having anterior chest discomfort that was characteristic of myocardial ischemia. Immediate coronary arteriography revealed 90% obstruction of the proximal left anterior descending coronary artery. She was treated with immediate coronary angioplasty.

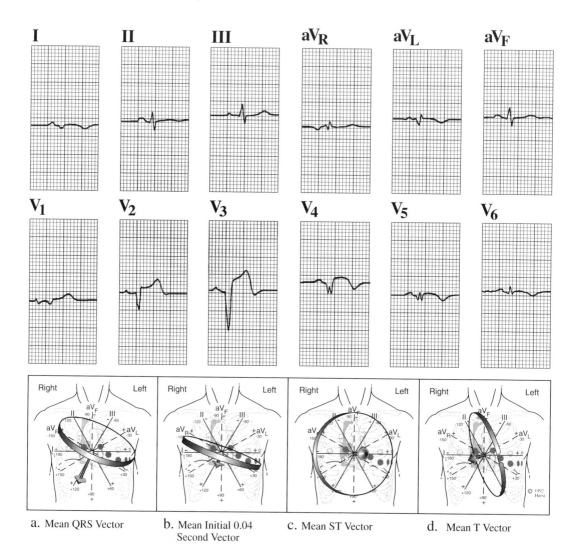

a. Mean QRS Vector

b. Mean Initial 0.04 Second Vector

c. Mean ST Vector

d. Mean T Vector

Fig. 7-120

Fig. 7-120. Anterolateral myocardial infarction.

- *Rhythm:* Normal sinus rhythm

  Rate: Undetermined in short strip. There were 77 depolarizations per minute in a longer strip.

  PR interval: 0.16 second

  QRS duration: 0.08 second

  QT interval: 0.35 second

- *Vector diagrams of electrical forces:* See *a*, *b*, *c*, and *d* below the electrocardiogram.

- *Electrophysiologic considerations:*

  The P waves are normal.

  The mean QRS vector is directed about +125 degrees to the right and about 20 degrees posteriorly. The abnormal direction of the mean QRS vector may be caused by an endocardial dead zone of the lateral portion of the left ventricle, left posteroinferior division block, or both.

  The mean initial 0.04 second QRS vector is directed about +125 degrees to the right and 5 to 10 degrees posteriorly. The direction of this vector is caused by a dead zone in the endocardial region of the anterolateral portion of the left ventricle.

  The mean ST vector is directed at 0 degrees in the frontal plane and 85 to 90 degrees anteriorly. It is produced by extensive anterolateral left ventricular epicardial injury.

  The mean T vector is directed about +170 degrees to the right and about 20 degrees anteriorly. It is produced by lateral epicardial ischemia.

  These abnormalities are caused by an anterolateral myocardial infarction.

- *Clinical differential diagnosis:* These electrocardiographic abnormalities are diagnostic of anterolateral myocardial infarction, which is usually due to obstruction of the proximal portion of the left anterior descending artery or the first diagonal. The obstruction in the artery is usually related to coronary atherosclerosis, but other causes such as coronary embolism may be responsible.

- *Discussion:* This electrocardiogram was recorded from a 59-year-old man with prolonged chest pain that was characteristic of myocardial ischemia. A coronary arteriogram revealed a high-grade obstruction of a long segment of the proximal portion of the left anterior descending coronary artery.

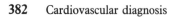

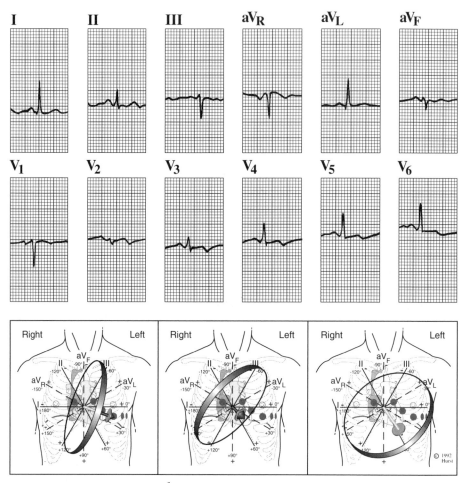

a. Mean QRS Vector

b. Mean Initial 0.04 Second Vector

c. Mean T Vector

Fig. 7-121

Fig. 7-121. Non–Q wave myocardial infarction.

- *Rhythm:* Sinus tachycardia

  Rate: Undetermined in short strip. There were 93 depolarizations per minute in a longer strip.

  PR interval: 0.12 second

  QRS duration: 0.08 second

  QT interval: 0.32 second

- *Vector diagrams of electrical forces:* See *a, b,* and *c* below the electrocardiogram.

- *Electrophysiologic considerations:*

  The P waves are normal.

  The mean QRS vector is normally directed at about +20 degrees inferiorly and 20 degrees posteriorly.

  The mean initial 0.04 second QRS vector is normally directed at +40 degrees inferiorly and about 45 degrees anteriorly. It is directed inferior to and anterior to the mean QRS vector.

  The mean T vector is directed about +58 degrees inferiorly and about 80 degrees posteriorly. It is directed away from the anterolateral surface of the left ventricle and represents a primary repolarization abnormality.

- *Clinical differential diagnosis:* The abnormal mean T vector is most likely due to anterolateral epicardial myocardial ischemia due to obstructive coronary artery disease. The usual cause is coronary arteriosclerosis, but other causes of coronary disease must be remembered and looked for. Pericarditis is unlikely, because the mean T vector is usually directed away from the centroid of generalized epicardial ischemia, whereas in this electrocardiogram the mean T vector is directed away from the anterolateral portion of the left ventricle.

- *Discussion:* This electrocardiogram was recorded from a 67-year-old man with unstable angina pectoris and episodes of prolonged chest discomfort that were characteristic of myocardial ischemia. This electrocardiogram illustrates the electrocardiographic signs of a non–Q wave myocardial infarction.

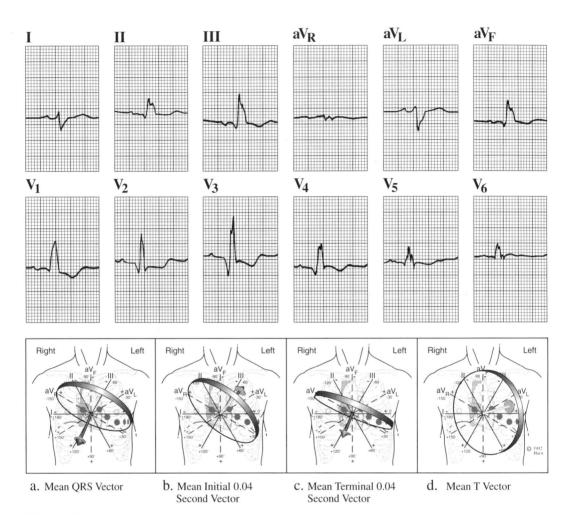

a. Mean QRS Vector

b. Mean Initial 0.04 Second Vector

c. Mean Terminal 0.04 Second Vector

d. Mean T Vector

Fig. 7-122

Fig. 7-122. Complicated right bundle-branch block plus inferoanterior myocardial infarction.

- *Rhythm:* Normal sinus rhythm

    Rate: Undetermined in short strip. There were 67 depolarizations per minute in a longer strip.

    PR interval: 0.19 second

    QRS duration: 0.16 second

    QT interval: 0.42 second

- *Vector diagrams of electrical forces:* See *a, b, c,* and *d* below the electrocardiogram.

- *Electrophysiologic considerations:*

    The mean P vector is directed at −5 degrees and is parallel with the frontal plane. This is probably normal but could represent an abnormal atrial focus.

    The duration of the QRS complex is 0.16 second, which indicates that the bundle-branch block is complicated; this electrocardiogram should not be interpreted as simple, uncomplicated bundle-branch block.

    The mean QRS vector is directed abnormally about +118 degrees to the right and at least 45 degrees anteriorly. Left posteroinferior division block is possible but cannot be diagnosed with certainty.

    The mean initial 0.04 second QRS vector is abnormally directed about −50 degrees to the left and about 45 degrees posteriorly. This abnormality is produced by an inferoanterior endocardial dead zone.

    The mean terminal 0.04 second QRS vector is abnormally directed about +118 degrees to the right and 10 to 20 degrees anteriorly. This abnormally directed terminal force indicates the presence of right bundle-branch block and possibly left posteroinferior division block.

    The mean T vector is directed about −15 degrees to the left and about 80 degrees posteriorly. This abnormality is produced by an abnormality of the repolarization process anteriorly.

    This electrocardiogram is diagnostic of complicated right bundle-branch block plus an inferoanterior myocardial infarction.

- *Clinical differential diagnosis:* As stated above, this electrocardiogram is diagnostic of complicated right bundle-branch block and inferoanterior myocardial infarction. It is complicated for three reasons: the duration of the QRS complex is 0.16 second, the initial 0.04 second QRS abnormality indicates the presence of an inferoanterior myocardial infarction, and left posteroinferior division block may also be present. The usual cause is coronary atherosclerosis, but it is important to remember that there are other causes of obstructive coronary disease.

- *Discussion:* This electrocardiogram was recorded from a 69-year-old man who had coronary bypass surgery 10 years before this tracing was made. He had the clinical features of a recent myocardial infarction.

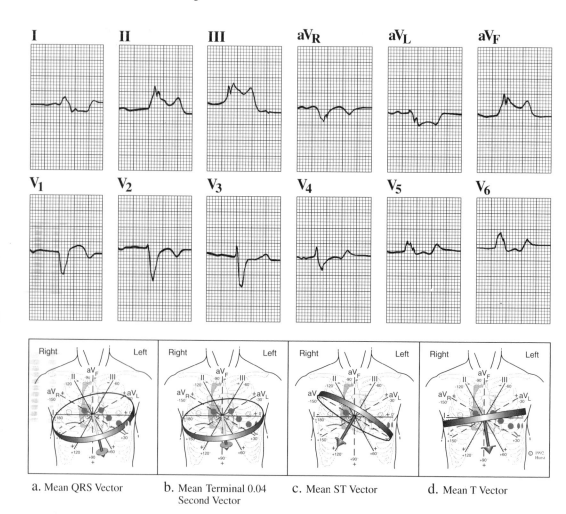

a. Mean QRS Vector

b. Mean Terminal 0.04
Second Vector

c. Mean ST Vector

d. Mean T Vector

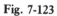

Fig. 7-123

Fig. 7-123. Complicated left bundle-branch block plus right ventricular infarction.

- *Rhythm:* Atrial fibrillation

  Rate: Undetermined in short strip. There were 41 depolarizations per minute in a longer strip.

  PR interval: None

  QRS duration: 0.18 to 0.20 second

  QT interval: 0.48 second

- *Vector diagrams of electrical forces:* See *a*, *b*, *c*, and *d* below the electrocardiogram.

- *Electrophysiologic considerations:*

  Atrial fibrillation is present. The ventricular rate is quite slow.

  The duration of the QRS complex is 0.18 to 0.20 second. The mean QRS vector is directed about +75 degrees inferiorly and about 60 degrees posteriorly. The extremely wide duration of the QRS complex suggests an abnormality at the Purkinje myocyte junction.

  The mean terminal 0.04 second QRS vector is directed about +80 degrees inferiorly and about 60 degrees posteriorly. The posterior direction of the vector indicates that depolarization of the left ventricle is delayed.

  The mean ST vector is directed about +120 degrees to the right and about 20 degrees anteriorly. The direction of this arrow suggests epicardial injury due to inferior myocardial infarction plus a right ventricular infarction.

  The mean T vector is directed about +78 degrees inferiorly and parallel with the frontal plane. It is directed toward an inferior area of subendocardial ischemia.

  The electrocardiogram shows atrial fibrillation, complicated left bundle-branch block, and acute inferior–right ventricular infarction.

- *Clinical differential diagnosis:* The ST segment vector is diagnostic of inferior epicardial injury of the left ventricle plus right ventricular epicardial injury. Myocardial infarction is clearly present. The cause is most likely coronary atherosclerosis, but other causes of obstructive coronary artery disease may be considered.

- *Discussion:* This electrocardiogram was recorded from a 69-year-old man who had a right ventricular infarction. Coronary arteriography revealed high-grade obstruction of the right coronary artery that was proximal to the right ventricular branch of the right coronary artery.

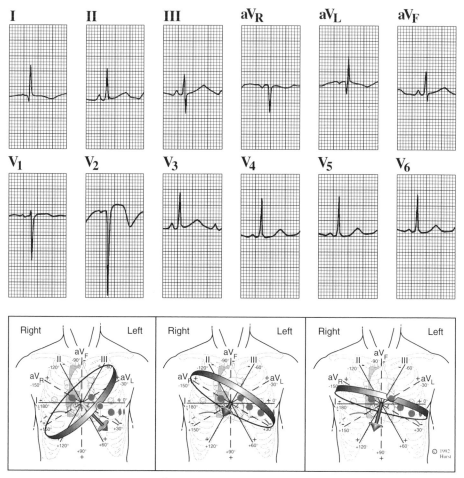

a. Mean QRS Vector   b. Mean ST Vector   c. Mean T Vector

Fig. 7-124

Fig. 7-124. Myocardial infarction due to pheochromocytoma.
- *Rhythm:* Sinus tachycardia
  Rate: Undetermined in short strip. There were 90 depolarizations per minute in a longer strip.
  PR interval: 0.13 second
  QRS duration: 0.7 second
  QT interval: 0.36 second
- *Vector diagrams of electrical forces:* See *a*, *b*, and *c* below the electrocardiogram.
- *Electrophysiologic considerations:*
  The P waves are normal.
  The mean QRS vector is directed about +50 degrees inferiorly and about 25 degrees posteriorly.
  The mean ST vector is barely visible in the frontal plane. It is directed about +120 degrees to the right and about 30 degrees anteriorly. This vector is abnormal and suggests epicardial injury of the anteroseptal portion of the left ventricular muscle and perhaps of the right ventricle.
  The mean T vector is directed about +108 degrees to the right and about 10 degrees anteriorly, suggesting anteroseptal epicardial ischemia.
- *Clinical differential diagnosis:* The ST and T vectors are abnormal and suggest the possibility of anteroseptal and possibly right ventricular infarction. The cause of the abnormalities is most likely an anteroseptal, and possibly right ventricular, myocardial infarction. The cause of the infarction could be the usual one (atherosclerotic coronary heart disease) or an unusual one.
- *Discussion:* This electrocardiogram is presented to remind the reader that many electrocardiographic abnormalities may simulate myocardial infarction due to atherosclerotic coronary heart disease. This electrocardiogram was recorded from a 23-year-old woman with pheochromoctoma who had episodes of hypertension. She developed pulmonary edema and a systolic blood pressure of 320 mm Hg and a diastolic blood pressure of 140 mm Hg. The serum creatine phosphokinase rose to 600 with 10% MB band. This patient undoubtedly had myocardial damage and infarction due to severe catecholenemia. Presumably, the smaller arteries in the myocardium constricted to the point where there was inadequate myocardial perfusion.

Electrocardiogram courtesy Dallas Hall, M.D, Director, Clinical Research Facility, Emory University School of Medicine, Atlanta, Ga.

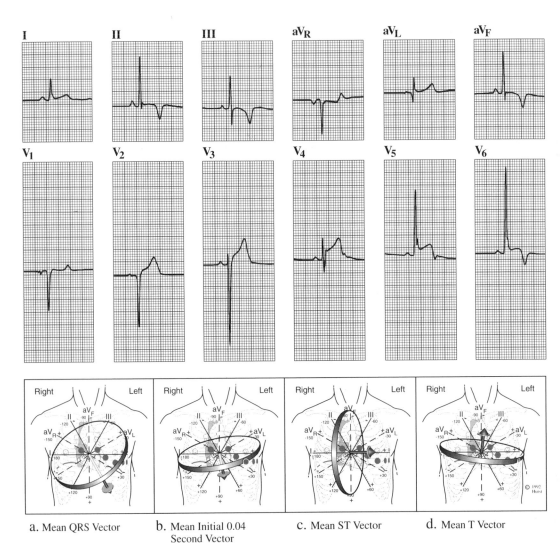

a. Mean QRS Vector

b. Mean Initial 0.04
Second Vector

c. Mean ST Vector

d. Mean T Vector

Fig. 7-125

Fig. 7-125. Pseudomyocardial infarction due to hypertrophic cardiomyopathy.
- *Rhythm:* Sinus bradycardia

  Rate: Undetermined in short strip. There were 53 depolarizations per minute in a longer strip.

  PR interval: 0.16 second

  QRS duration: 0.09 second

  QT interval: 0.40 second
- *Vector diagrams of electrical forces:* See *a, b, c,* and *d* below the electrocardiogram.
- *Electrophysiologic considerations:*

  The P waves are normal.

  The mean QRS vector is directed about +60 degrees inferiorly and about 50 degrees posteriorly. The total amplitude of the QRS complex is about 243 mm, indicating left ventricular hypertrophy.

  The mean initial 0.04 second QRS vector is directed about +80 degrees inferiorly and about 35 degrees posteriorly. This direction is more posterior than usual and could be caused by left ventricular hypertrophy or a dead zone anteriorly.

  The mean ST vector is directed at +0 degrees and 30 degrees anteriorly. It is not parallel with the mean T vector. This abnormal ST vector could be due to acute lateral epicardial injury secondary to myocardial infarction, or, as will become apparent, it may be associated with hypertrophic cardiomyopathy.

  The mean T vector is directed −85 degrees to the left and about 30 degrees anteriorly. The vector in this tracing may be due to left ventricular hypertrophy plus a primary T wave abnormality. The ventricular gradient is obviously abnormal.
- *Clinical differential diagnosis:* The left ventricular hypertrophy, abnormal 0.04 second QRS vector, epicardial injury, and primary T wave abnormality may be caused by myocardial infarction due to coronary atherosclerosis plus some other cause of left ventricular hypertrophy, such as hypertension or aortic valve disease, or it may be due to hypertrophic cardiomyopathy alone. Finally, on rare occasions, patients may have both hypertrophic cardiomyopathy and myocardial infarction due to coronary atherosclerosis.
- *Discussion:* This electrocardiogram was recorded from a 37-year-old man with nonobstructive hypertrophic cardiomyopathy. He gave a history of cardiac arrhythmia and syncope.

normal repolarization, with the exception that the T waves are usually smaller in patients with pericarditis than they are in patients with early normal repolarization.

An arrow representing the mean of the electrical forces (vectors) responsible for the ST segment displacement is directed toward the anatomic apex when there is an apical infarction. Fortunately, this condition is rare, because the electrocardiographic abnormality is similar to that of pericarditis. Abnormal Q waves may not develop with apical infarction, because there is no ventricular myocardium opposite the apex. One must rely on other electrocardiographic and clinical data to identify apical infarction.

The amplitude and configuration of the QRS complexes do not change as a result of acute pericarditis unless there is pericardial effusion.

During the *second stage* of pericarditis the ST segment displacement diminishes and an arrow representing the mean of the electrical forces responsible for the T wave may be directed opposite to the anatomic apex (Fig. 7-126, *B*).

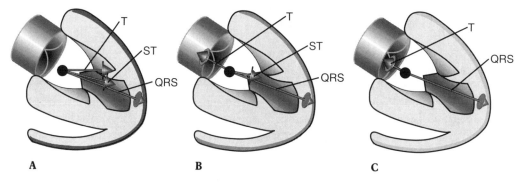

A   **B**   **C**

Fig. 7-126. Electrocardiographic abnormalities produced by acute pericarditis. **A,** Pericarditis usually produces generalized epicardial myocardial injury (see dark area). Initially, during the early stage of pericarditis, an arrow representing the mean of the electrical forces (vectors) responsible for the ST segment is directed toward the anatomic apex of the left ventricle. It is produced by generalized epicardial injury. The PQ segment may become displaced downward in leads where the P waves are upright. It cannot be represented by an arrow, because it is rarely seen in all leads. **B,** During the second stage of acute pericarditis the arrow representing the ST segment vector becomes smaller than it was in **A,** and an arrow representing the mean of the electrical forces (vectors) responsible for the T wave is directed somewhat opposite to the anatomic apex of the left ventricle; it is due to generalized epicardial ischemia. **C,** During the third stage of acute pericarditis an arrow representing the mean of the electrical forces (vectors) responsible for the ST segment decreases markedly, and the arrow representing the mean of the electrical forces (vectors) responsible for the T wave may become larger than it was in **B.** The T waves may then decrease in size, as shown here. When pericardial fluid develops, the amplitude of the QRS complexes and T waves decreases, and electrical alternans of the QRS complexes and T waves may appear.

Finally, in the *third stage* of pericarditis the ST segment displacement may disappear, leaving the T wave abnormality (Fig. 7-126, *C*). An arrow representing the mean of the electrical forces (vectors) responsible for the T wave may shift in direction, producing a QRS-T angle of 90 degrees or less. The T waves may become small. Pericarditis is often unrecognized, and it is likely that some unexplained T wave abnormalities are due to old, undiagnosed pericarditis.

The electrocardiographic abnormalities of acute pericarditis are illustrated in the electrocardiogram shown in Fig. 7-127.

The epicardial myocardial damage associated with pericarditis is usually generalized. Acute pericarditis may be due to viral or bacterial infection, collagen disease, or neoplastic disease. Although uremia may cause pericarditis, the electrocardiographic changes may not be as pronounced as they are with viral pericarditis. The conditions just mentioned produce generalized epicardial damage and the electrocardiographic abnormalities described above. More localized pericarditis can occur with myocardial infarction or trauma, and especially after cardiac surgery. In such cases the ST segment displacement, when represented as a vector, may be directed toward a segment of the left ventricle; and the T wave, when represented as a vector, may be directed away from a segment of the left ventricle. When this occurs, the abnormalities are difficult to distinguish from non–Q wave myocardial infarction.

Pericardial effusion. Although there may be lingering electrocardiographic signs of acute pericarditis, the hallmark of pericardial effusion is a decrease in amplitude of the QRS complexes and T waves. Although the electrocardiogram may reveal a QRS complex amplitude of 5 to 7 mm, no absolute figure should be used to designate low amplitude of the QRS complexes. The normal total QRS complex amplitude ranges from 80 to 185 mm[24] (see earlier discussion). Pericardial effusion should be considered, along with other causes of low QRS complex amplitude, whenever the total QRS amplitude is on the low side of normal. When pericardial effusion develops, the total QRS amplitude may be lowered but still be within the normal range, but the decrease in size may not be appreciated unless a previously recorded electrocardiogram is available.

Electrical alternans may occur in patients with pericardial effusion. The amplitude of the QRS complexes alternates with every other ventricular depolarization. The T waves may also alternate in size, because the heart swings back and forth like a pendulum when there is a large pericardial effusion. This phenomenon was called "cardiac nystagmas" by Lipmann and is often seen in the echocardiogram. The "swinging" of the heart produces a different electrical field every other beat. Electrical alternans has no relationship to pulsus alternans.

The amplitude of the QRS complexes may be diminished in patients with dilated cardiomyopathy, pulmonary emphysema, or anasarca, and in patients with an increased skin resistance. The low amplitude of the QRS complexes in patients with myxedema is due to pericardial effusion, increased skin resistance, and possibly myocardial disease.

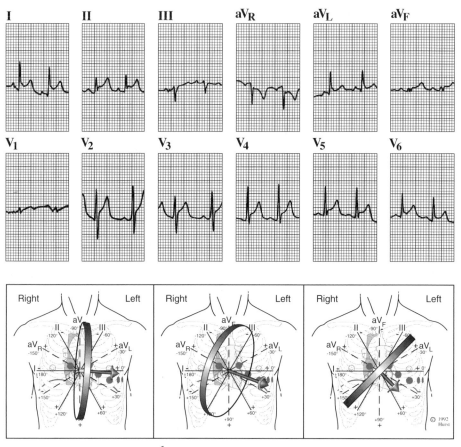

a. Mean QRS Vector   b. Mean ST Vector   c. Mean T Vector

Fig. 7-127

Fig. 7-127. Acute pericarditis.

- *Rhythm:* Sinus tachycardia
  Rate: 130 depolarizations per minute
  PR interval: 0.14 second
  QRS duration: 0.08 second
  QT interval: 0.28 second
- *Vector diagrams of electrical forces:* See *a, b,* and *c* below the electrocardiogram.
- *Electrophysiologic considerations:*

  The P waves are normal. The PQ segment in lead II may be displaced downward, but one cannot be certain of this observation.

  The mean QRS vector is directed about +5 degrees inferiorly and about 5 to 10 degrees posteriorly.

  The mean ST vector is directed about +20 degrees inferiorly and about 20 to 30 degrees anteriorly. The ST segment vector indicates the presence of generalized epicardial injury.

  The mean T vector is directed about +45 degrees inferiorly and is parallel with the frontal plane.

- *Clinical differential diagnosis: Generalized epicardial injury* is a clue to generalized pericarditis. This electrocardiographic abnormality occurs early; it precedes the T wave abnormality, which tends to occur as the ST segment vector decreases in size. When the abnormal T wave vector appears, it can be represented by a vector that is directed opposite to the mean ST vector. An *apical myocardial infarction* can produce such an ST segment vector, but such an infarct is unusual. An abnormal Q wave may not appear with apical infarction, because there is no myocardium opposite the apex; the aortic and mitral valves are opposite the cardiac apex. *Segmental pericarditis* may cause the ST segment vector to be directed toward the epicardium of a segment of myocardium, as it does with infarction. For example, postoperative pericarditis, traumatic pericarditis, and the pericarditis of infarction may be segmental rather than generalized, as it is with viral pericarditis.

- *Discussion:* This electrocardiogram was recorded from a 68-year-old man with acute pericarditis. He had rheumatoid arthritis and clinical clues suggesting lupus erythematosis.

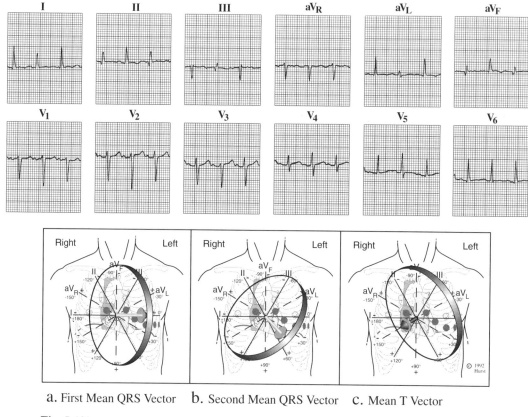

a. First Mean QRS Vector   b. Second Mean QRS Vector   c. Mean T Vector

Fig. 7-128

An electrocardiogram illustrating the abnormalities due to pericardial effusion is shown in Fig. 7-128.

Constrictive pericarditis. Atrial arrhythmias may be present. In addition, the amplitude of the QRS complexes may be low. Years ago, when calcific pericardial disease was more common, it was not unusual to observe QRS abnormalities, because the calcium commonly impregnated the ventricular muscle.

T wave abnormalities are common. An arrow representing the mean of the electrical forces (vectors) responsible for the T wave may be directed 60 to 180 degrees away from an arrow representing the mean of the electrical forces (vectors) responsible for the QRS complex.

An electrocardiogram illustrating the electrocardiographic abnormalities due to constrictive pericarditis is shown in Fig. 7-129.

Fig. 7-128. Pericardial effusion.

- *Rhythm:* Sinus bradycardia
  Rate: 140 depolarizations per minute
  PR interval: 0.13 second
  QRS duration: 0.08 second
  QT interval: 0.28 second
- *Vector diagrams of electrical forces:* See *a, b,* and *c* below the electrocardiogram.
- *Electrophysiologic considerations:*
  Sinus tachycardia is present.
  The direction and amplitude of the mean QRS vector alternates with every other depolarization. This is called electrical alternans. The total QRS amplitude (97 mm) is on the low side of the normal range.
  The T waves are small. The mean T vector is directed +150 degrees to the right and about 85 to 90 degrees anteriorly. This is a primary T wave abnormality.
- *Clinical differential diagnosis:* Electrical alternans, QRS voltage on the low side of normal, low-amplitude T waves, and a primary T wave abnormality indicate the presence of pericardial effusion. Electrical alternans may also be associated with atrial tachycardia.
- *Discussion:* This electrocardiogram was recorded from a 40-year-old man with a pericardial effusion caused by what was presumed to be a sarcoma of the thymus with involvement of the pericardium.

Cor pulmonale due to pulmonary emphysema[57]

When the electrocardiogram reveals the characteristic features of cor pulmonale, the disease has usually advanced to the degree that heart failure is present; hypoxia and mild to moderate pulmonary hypertension are also present. Atrial arrhythmias such as atrial fibrillation may be present.

Direction of the mean P wave vector. When the rhythm is normal, a right atrial abnormality is commonly present; an arrow representing the mean of the electrical forces (vectors) responsible for the P wave may be directed +80 to +90 degrees in the frontal plane; it is commonly directed more anteriorly than normal. The amplitude of the P waves may be 2.5 mm or more. An arrow representing the first half of the P wave may be directed vertically and anteriorly; the first half of the P wave in lead V_1 becomes more prominent than normal. As stated above, the amplitude of

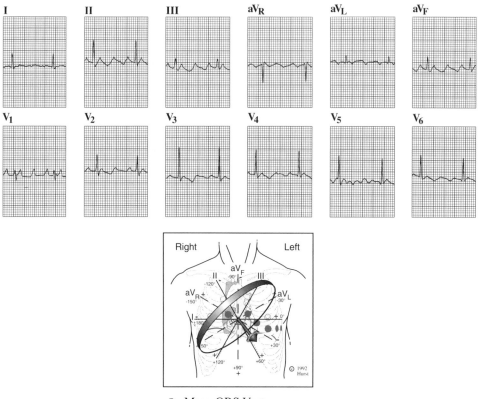

a. Mean QRS Vector

Fig. 7-129

the P waves may be increased, but in some patients the P waves are of low amplitude, as are the QRS complexes.

Duration and amplitude of the QRS complex. The duration of the QRS complex may remain normal or become slightly prolonged as a result of right ventricular conduction delay. Right bundle-branch block occurs when the duration of the QRS complex is prolonged to 0.12 second. The amplitude of the QRS complexes is usually on the low side of the normal range as a result of emphysematous lungs.

Direction of the mean QRS vector. An arrow representing the mean of the electrical forces (vectors) responsible for the QRS complex may be directed inferiorly, to the right, and anteriorly; the R wave in lead V_1 may become taller than the S wave is deep.

Direction of the mean T vector. An arrow representing the mean of the electrical forces (vectors) responsible for the T wave is directed to the left and posteri-

Fig. 7-129. Constrictive pericarditis.
- *Rhythm:* Atrial flutter with 3:1 atrioventricular block
  Rate: 77 ventricular depolarizations per minute
  PR interval: Not applicable because of atrial flutter
  QRS duration: 0.08 second
  QT interval: Undetermined (obscured by F waves)
- *Vector diagrams of electrical forces:* See *a* below the electrocardiogram (only the QRS vector is shown; the T waves are obscured by the F waves).
- *Electrophysiologic considerations:*
  The rhythm is abnormal because of atrial flutter with 3:1 atrioventricular block.
  The mean QRS vector is directed +50 degrees inferiorly and about 10 degrees anteriorly.
  The total QRS amplitude is about 78 mm. This is low QRS voltage.
  The mean T wave vector cannot be computed, because the large F waves obscure them.
  This tracing shows atrial flutter and low amplitude of the QRS vector, as well as slight anterior rotation of the mean QRS vector.
- *Clinical differential diagnosis:* The atrial flutter and decreased QRS amplitude could be caused by infiltrative cardiomyopathy or constrictive pericarditis. The anterior rotation of the mean QRS vector could be caused by right ventricular preponderance, which in turn could be due to a condition that causes the right ventricle to be larger than the left ventricle, or to a condition that decreases the electrical potential transmitted from the left ventricle but does not alter the transmission of the electrical potential transmitted from the right ventricle. Constrictive pericarditis involving predominantly the left ventricle could produce such an electrocardiogram.
- *Discussion:* This electrocardiogram was recorded from a 24-year-old woman with calcific constrictive pericarditis.

Electrocardiogram courtesy Paul Walter, M.D., Director, Electrophysiologic Laboratory, Emory University Hospital, Atlanta, Ga.

---

orly away from the right ventricle. The amplitude of the T waves may be diminished.

An electrocardiogram illustrating the abnormalities due to cor pulmonale secondary to emphysema is shown in Fig. 7-130.

Acute pulmonary embolism[44,45]

Most pulmonary emboli produce no electrocardiographic abnormalities. When an embolus is large, or when the lungs are already congested at the time the embolus occurs, the electrocardiogram may change. Sinus tachycardia may develop, and an atrial arrhythmia may occur.

Duration of the QRS complex. The QRS duration may remain normal or become slightly prolonged. The duration of the QRS complex may become 0.12 second when right bundle-branch block develops.

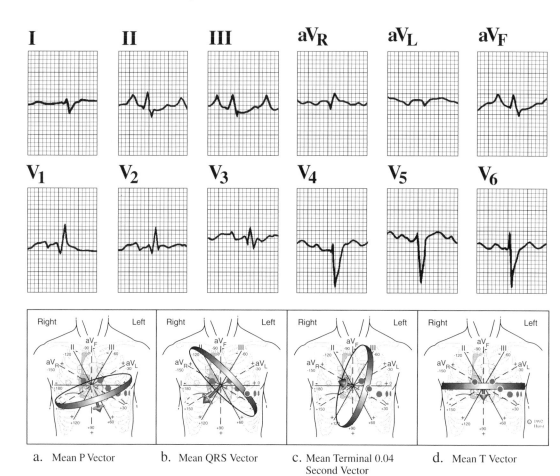

a. Mean P Vector

b. Mean QRS Vector

c. Mean Terminal 0.04 Second Vector

d. Mean T Vector

Fig. 7-130

Fig. 7-130. Pulmonary emphysema.

- *Rhythm:* Normal sinus rhythm
  Rate: Undetermined in short strip
  PR interval: 0.14 second
  QRS duration: 0.09 second
  QT interval: 0.48 second
- *Vector diagrams of electrical forces:* See *a, b, c,* and *d* below the electrocardiogram.
- *Electrophysiologic considerations:*

  The amplitude of the P wave in lead II is 2.5 mm. Note the peaked shape of the P waves in leads II, III, and aV$_F$. The mean P vector is directed +73 degrees inferiorly and 30 degrees posteriorly. There is a right atrial abnormality.

  The mean QRS vector is directed about +135 degrees to the right and about 20 degrees anteriorly. This abnormality is due to right ventricular conduction delay or right ventricular hypertrophy (or both). The 12-lead QRS amplitude is about 84 mm, which is on the low side of the normal range.

  The mean terminal 0.04 second QRS vector is directed at −170 degrees and 20 degrees anteriorly as a result of right ventricular conduction delay.

  The mean T vector is small and difficult to plot. It seems to be directed +90 degrees inferiorly and parallel with the frontal plane.

  There is a right atrial abnormality, right ventricular conduction delay, and low amplitude of the QRS complexes.

- *Clinical differential diagnosis:* The most common cause of this type of electrocardiogram is extensive pulmonary emphysema due to obstructive lung disease. Other conditions could be responsible for these abnormalities. For example, a patient with secundum atrial septal defect who also had a pericardial effusion might exhibit such an electrocardiogram.
- *Discussion:* This patient had severe pulmonary emphysema and cor pulmonale. The right atrial abnormality, low QRS amplitude, and right ventricular conduction delay should strongly suggest emphysema and cor pulmonale.

Electrocardiogram reproduced with permission from Fowler NO, Daniels C, Scott RC et al: The electrocardiogram in cor pulmonale with and without emphysema, *Am J Cardiol* 16:501, 1965.

Direction of the mean QRS vector and the initial and terminal 0.04 second QRS vectors. An arrow representing the mean of the electrical forces (vectors) responsible for the QRS complex may be directed at +80 to +105 degrees. An arrow representing the mean of the electrical forces (vectors) responsible for the initial 0.04 second of the QRS complex may be directed -20 degrees or more to the left and parallel with the frontal plane. An arrow representing the mean of the electrical forces (vectors) responsible for the terminal 0.04 second of the QRS complex may be directed to the right and anteriorly. This arrangement of electrical forces (vectors) may simulate those due to inferior infarction; it is due to asynchronous ventricular depolarization with right ventricular conduction delay. Right bundle-branch block may develop.

Direction of the mean ST vector. Occasionally the ST segment displacement may be characteristic of subendocardial injury. In such cases an arrow representing the mean of the electrical forces (vectors) produced by subendocardial injury is directed away from the anatomic cardiac apex.

Direction of the mean T vector. An arrow representing the mean of the electrical forces (vectors) responsible for the T wave may be directed to the left and posteriorly away from the right ventricle.

Multiple pulmonary emboli may produce electrocardiographic signs of right ventricular hypertrophy or persistent right bundle-branch block. In the proper clinical setting, especially in patients with coronary heart disease, an acute pulmonary embolus may produce electrocardiographic evidence of subendocardial injury or myocardial infarction.

An electrocardiogram illustrating the signs of an acute pulmonary embolus is shown in Fig. 7-131.

Preexcitation (Wolff-Parkinson-White syndrome)[46]

Patients with Wolff-Parkinson-White syndrome may have episodes of supraventricular tachycardia or atrial fibrillation. Because the QRS duration is commonly wider than normal, this electrocardiographic abnormality may be misinterpreted as being due to ventricular tachycardia. When atrial fibrillation is present, the ventricular rate may be 250 depolarizations per minute or more, because the atrioventricular node is bypassed by the accessory bundle. The PR interval is shorter than normal; the P waves abut the QRS complexes.

Duration of the QRS complex. The duration of the QRS complex may be slightly prolonged to 0.10 second or as wide as 0.18 second.

Direction of the mean initial 0.04 second QRS vector. The initial portion of the QRS complex is slurred and is referred to as a delta wave. An arrow representing the mean of the electrical forces (vectors) responsible for the initial 0.4 second of the QRS complex is directed abnormally; its direction may simulate that of inferior infarction or anterior infarction.

Direction of the mean ST and T vectors. There may be a secondary T wave abnormality. An arrow representing the mean of the electrical forces (vectors) responsible for the ST segment displacement is directed relatively parallel with an arrow representing the mean of the electrical forces (vectors) responsible for the T wave.

Preexcitation of the ventricles occurs more often than is generally appreciated. We formerly believed that there were two basic types of preexcitation: type A and type B. Then other types were discovered. Now it seems that there are numerous types, and there may be more than one anomalous tract in the same heart. It is not possible to identify the exact location of the bypass tract from the routine surface electrocardiogram.

When the episodes of tachycardia occur frequently and are not controlled with appropriate medication, it may be necessary to have the bypass tract(s) ablated or severed at surgery. Accordingly, under such circumstances, the precise location of the bypass tract can be identified by electrophysiologic testing, although body surface mapping is proving to be useful. When atrial fibrillation complicates preexcitation of the ventricles, the ventricular rate is usually 250 depolarizations or more per minute. Digitalis must not be used in an attempt to slow the ventricular rate.

Preexcitation of the ventricles may occur with no evidence of other cardiac abnormalities. The condition occurs with greater frequency in patients with idiopathic cardiac hypertrophy, Ebstein anomaly, or atrial septal defect. The abnormality is commonly misdiagnosed as being due to myocardial infarction.

An electrocardiogram illustrating the abnormalities that are characteristic of preexcitation of the ventricles is shown in Fig. 7-132.

Hypothermia[48]

Patients exposed to cold weather may develop a characteristic electrocardiogram. The baseline of the electrocardiogram shows considerable motion as a result of muscular shivers. Atrial fibrillation may be noted, but the ventricular rate may be slower than usual.

The duration of the QRS complex may be longer than normal because of an unusual abnormality of the terminal portion of the QRS complex. Called an Osborne wave, this terminal QRS abnormality may be due to extreme cooling of the posterobasilar portion of the left ventricle.

The T waves may be broad and grossly abnormal; there is a primary T wave abnormality.

An electrocardiogram illustrating the abnormalities that are characteristic of hypothermia is shown in Fig. 7-133.

Text continued on p. 410.

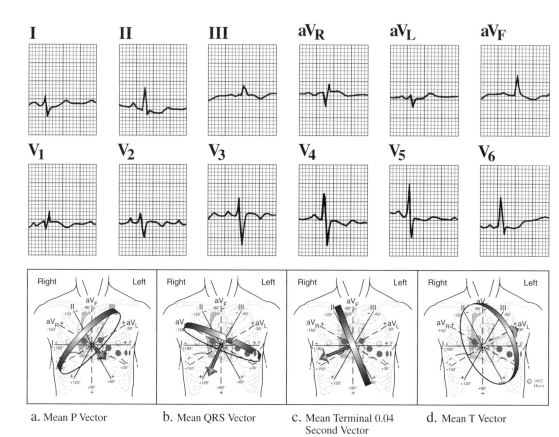

| I | II | III | aV_R | aV_L | aV_F |

a. Mean P Vector   b. Mean QRS Vector   c. Mean Terminal 0.04 Second Vector   d. Mean T Vector

Fig. 7-131

Fig. 7-131. Acute pulmonary embolus.

- *Rhythm:* Normal sinus rhythm
  Rate: Undetermined in short strip
  PR interval: 0.16 second
  QRS duration: 0.08 second
  QT interval: 0.32 second
- *Vector diagrams of electrical forces:* See *a*, *b*, *c*, and *d* below the electrocardiogram.
- *Electrophysiologic considerations:*

  The mean P vector is directed +45 degrees inferiorly and about 20 degrees anteriorly. The anterior rotation suggests a right atrial abnormality, but this is not definite.

  The mean QRS vector is directed +110 degrees to the right and about 10 degrees anteriorly. Note that the QRS complexes in leads V_5 and V_6 are resultantly positive, whereas the transitional pathway of the mean QRS that is shown in *b* would cause the QRS complexes in leads V_5 and V_6 to be resultantly zero. This discrepancy occurs because the electrode positions for leads V_5 and V_6 are near the transitional pathway of the mean QRS vector. Accordingly, a small electrode placement error could cause such a variance.

  The mean terminal 0.04 second QRS vector is directed +160 degrees to the right and is parallel with the frontal plane. This is characteristic of right ventricular conduction delay.

  The mean T vector is directed almost −30 degrees to the left and 70 degrees posteriorly. The mean T vector points away from a repolarization abnormality of the right ventricle.

  The possible right atrial abnormality, right ventricular conduction defect, and anterior repolarization abnormality strongly indicate an acute pulmonary embolism. Such patients may have right bundle-branch block. Also, the mean initial 0.04 second QRS vector may shift to the left, producing a Q wave in leads III and AV_F, suggesting an inferior myocardial infarction.

- *Clinical differential diagnosis:* When these electrocardiographic abnormalities appear in a patient with syncope, acute dyspnea, or acute pleuritic pain and a previous electrocardiogram is normal (or does not show the same abnormalities), the clinician should diagnose acute pulmonary embolism.
- *Discussion:* This electrocardiogram was recorded from a 54-year-old patient with an acute pulmonary embolism.

Electrocardiogram from Hurst JW, Woodson GC Jr: *Atlas of spatial vector electrocardiography*, New York, 1952, Blakiston, p 203. The copyright has been transferred from the publisher to me.

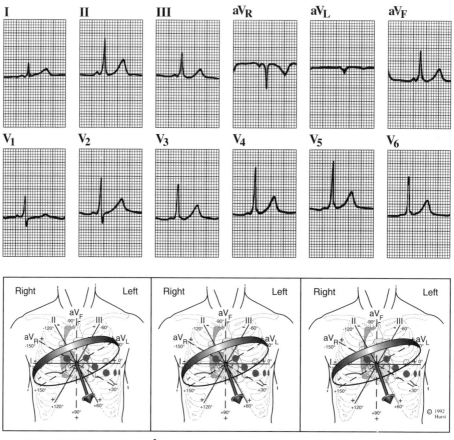

a. Mean QRS Vector

b. Mean Initial 0.04
   Second Vector

c. Mean T Vector

Fig. 7-132

Fig. 7-132. Preexcitation of the ventricle responsible for the Wolff-Parkinson-White syndrome.

- *Rhythm:* Normal sinus rhythm
  Rate: Undetermined in a short strip. There were 74 depolarizations per minute in a longer
      strip.
  PR interval: 0.08 to 0.09 second
  QRS duration: 0.09 second
  QT interval: 0.42 second
- *Vector diagrams of electrical forces:* See *a, b,* and *c* below the electrocardiogram.
- *Electrophysiologic considerations:*
  The PR interval is abnormally short. This finding alone should lead one to consider the
      possibility of a bypass tract that circumvents the atrioventricular node, causing early elec-
      trical activation of the ventricles.
  The mean QRS vector is directed about +70 degrees inferiorly and anteriorly (the exact
      number of degrees cannot be determined without recording from additional electrode sam-
      ple sites). There are two unusual features of the QRS complex:
  The slur of the first portion of the QRS complex, called a delta wave.
  The mean initial 0.04 second QRS vector is directed +70 degrees inferiorly and ante-
      riorly, producing a tall R wave in leads V_1 and V_2. This is abnormal and could be
      produced by a true posterior myocardial infarction.
  The mean T vector is directed +70 degrees inferiorly and anteriorly. It is probably directed
      about 20 degrees anteriorly, because the T wave in lead V_1 is much smaller than the T
      wave in lead V_6.
- *Clinical differential diagnosis:* The short PR interval and delta wave are diagnostic of preexcitation of the ventricles caused by a bypass tract that circumvents the atrioventricular node.
  This type of electrocardiogram is usually seen in patients who have episodes of supraventricular tachycardia (including atrial fibrillation) and who have no other evidence of heart
  disease. The clinician should, however, search for idiopathic hypertrophic cardiomyopathy,
  an ostium secundum atrial septal defect, or Ebstein anomaly, because the abnormality is
  more common in patients with these conditions as compared with a population of individuals without such diseases.
- *Discussion:* This electrocardiogram was recorded from a 22-year-old woman who had experienced episodes of rapid heartbeat since the age of 6. The electrocardiographic abnormalities plus the episodes of rapid heartbeat qualify her as having Wolff-Parkinson-White syndrome. Abnormal Q waves are commonly seen in the electrocardiograms of patients who
  have preexcitation of the ventricles. Because of this, clinicians must be alert to the characteristics of preexcitation so that an erroneous diagnosis of myocardial infarction is not made.
  Once this is learned, the clinician must then be alert to the fact that patients whose electrocardiograms show preexcitation of the ventricles may also have myocardial infarction. Preexcitation does not prevent coronary atherosclerosis.

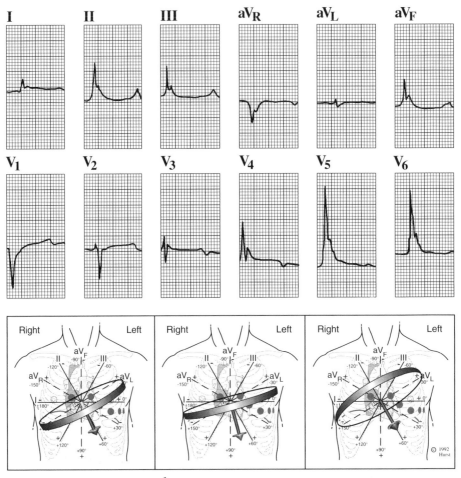

a. Mean QRS Vector

b. Mean Terminal 0.04
   Second Vector

c. Mean T Vector
   (an estimation)

Fig. 7-133

Fig. 7-133. Electrocardiographic effects of environmental hypothermia.

- *Rhythm:* Atrial fibrillation

  Rate: Undetermined in short strip. There were 40 ventricular depolarizations per minute in a longer strip.

  PR interval: None

  QRS duration: 0.16 second

  QT interval: 0.72 second

- *Vector diagrams of electrical forces:* See *a*, *b*, and *c* below the electrocardiogram.

- *Electrophysiologic considerations:*

  Atrial fibrillation is present with a slow ventricular rate.

  The mean QRS vector is directed about +65 degrees inferiorly and about 20 degrees posteriorly.

  The terminal 0.04 second QRS vector is directed about +75 degrees inferiorly and about +20 degrees posteriorly. Note the unusual configuration of the QRS complex. The slur of the last half of the QRS complex is diagnostic of an Osborn wave, which in turn is diagnostic of hypothermia.

  The mean T vector is directed +60 degrees inferiorly. It is difficult to determine the anteroposterior rotation of the vector, because the T waves are upright in V_1 and V_2, inverted in V_3 and V_4, and upright (but low) in V_4 and V_5. The inverted T waves in V_3 and V_4 do not fit the spatial orientation concept in that there is an area of isolated T wave inversion located within an area of T wave positivity. The cause of this is unknown, but it is not unique to hypothermia. Perhaps a body surface map might show why T waves in leads V_3 and V_4 are negative.

  The atrial fibrillation, slow ventricular rate, wide QRS complex, and peculiar and unique slur of the last half of the QRS complex are characteristic of the electrocardiographic abnormalities produced by hypothermia.

- *Clinical differential diagnosis:* These electrocardiographic abnormalities are typical of those produced by hypothermia.

- *Discussion:* This electrocardiogram was recorded from a 58-year-old man with chronic obstructed lung disease, pylonephritis, and previous myocardial infarction. His rectal temperature was 75° F. He had been exposed to a low environmental temperature in a nursing home.

Electrocardiogram reproduced with permission from Clements SD, Hurst JW: Diagnostic value of electrocardiographic abnormalities observed in subjects accidentally exposed to cold, *Am J Cardiol* 29:729, 1972.

Hypokalemia and hyperkalemia

Hypokalemia.[58] Hypokalemia makes the heart more susceptible to the development of atrial tachycardia or atrial fibrillation, especially when the patient is receiving digitalis. Other arrhythmias may occur, such as premature atrial and ventricular depolarizations. The QRS complex is not altered unless there is a ventricular arrhythmia.

The T wave becomes smaller than normal, and the U wave becomes larger. The U wave abuts the T wave, and they eventually blend together to produce the QU interval. The QU interval may then be erroneously perceived to be a prolonged QT interval.

An electrocardiogram illustrating the abnormalities of hypokalemia and hypocalcemia is shown in Fig. 7-134.

Hyperkalemia.[58] Hyperkalemia may profoundly affect atrial depolarization, and the P waves may vanish. All types of ventricular conduction defects may occur. The QT interval becomes prolonged, and the T wave becomes abnormal. The T wave becomes tall and peaked; the first and second halves of the T wave become symmetric. They are commonly called tentlike in appearance. A primary T wave abnormality may be present.

An electrocardiogram illustrating the abnormalities due to hyperkalemia is shown in Fig. 7-135.

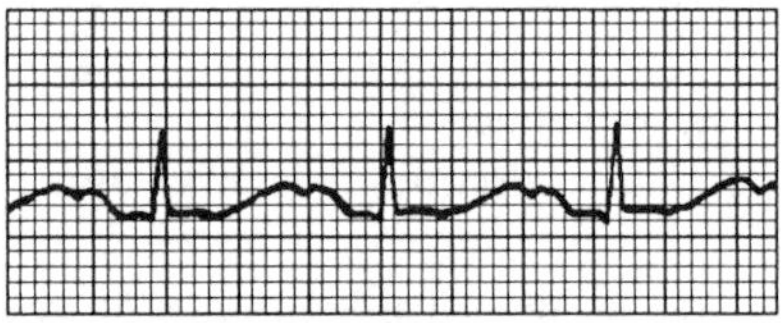

Fig. 7-134. Electrocardiographic effects of hypokalemia and hypocalcemia.
- *Rhythm:* Sinus tachycardia
    Rate: Undetermined in short strip. There were about 100 depolarizations per minute in a longer strip.
    PR interval: Approximately 0.20 second
    QRS duration: 0.06 second
    QT interval: 0.44 second
- *Electrophysiologic considerations:* The long QT interval is abnormal, and the amplitude of the T waves is low. In this tracing the T waves abut the P waves, and it is not possible to identify U waves.
- *Clinical differential diagnosis:* The long QT interval and low-amplitude T waves suggest the possibility of hypokalemia. The QT segment seems a little long, suggesting hypocalcemia.
- *Discussion:* This electrocardiogram was recorded from a 57-year-old woman with cirrhosis of the liver. The serum potassium level was 2.7 mEq/L, and the serum calcium level was 4.4 mg%.

Effect of digitalis on the electrocardiogram[59,60]

Digitalis produces a characteristic effect on the electrocardiogram. The PR interval may be prolonged, and the QT interval becomes shorter as a result of digitalis medication.

All types of arrhythmias may be produced by digitalis medication, but an excess of digitalis commonly produces premature ventricular depolarizations, Wenckebach phenomenon, 2:1 atrioventricular block, atrial tachycardia with 2:1 atrioventricular block when hypokalemia is also present, ventricular tachycardia, and ventricular fibrillation. Complete heart block can occur but is rare.

Digitalis medication does not alter the depolarization sequence of the ventricles unless there is a ventricular rhythm disturbance.

The repolarization process is profoundly altered. The myocytes repolarize so rapidly as a result of digitalis medication that the repolarization process is already underway before the last part of the ventricles depolarize. The QT interval may become 0.32 second or less. Accordingly, the repolarization sequence is not influenced by the transmyocardial pressure gradient, as it is when repolarization occurs at the end of mechanical systole. In fact, digitalis medication enables the myocytes to repolarize during the early phase of mechanical systole rather than waiting until the late phase. This occurs as the QT interval becomes shorter.

Duration of the QRS complex. The duration of the QRS complex does not change.

Duration of the QT interval. The duration of the QT interval becomes shorter than it was before digitalis was taken. The QT interval may be 0.32 second or less.

Direction of the mean QRS vector. An arrow representing the mean of the electrical forces (vectors) responsible for the QRS complex does not change.

Direction of the mean ST segment vector. As the effect of digitalis increases, an ST segment displacement develops. An arrow representing the mean of the electrical forces (vectors) responsible for the ST segment displacement is directed opposite to an arrow representing the mean of the electrical forces (vectors) responsible for the T wave. The ST segment displacement is due to extremely early repolarization (Fig. 7-136, C).

Direction of the mean T vector. The direction of the mean T vector does not change when digitalis is given. The T waves become smaller and may disappear, but the direction of the vector (arrow) representing them does not change (Fig. 7-136, A and B).

The electrocardiographic abnormalities due to digitalis medication must be differentiated from those due to generalized subendocardial injury. The latter abnormality is not associated with a short QT interval, and the T waves may not become smaller, as they commonly do with digitalis medication.

The clinician must always appreciate that the patient who is taking digitalis, but who shows little evidence of it in the electrocardiogram, may develop all of the elec-

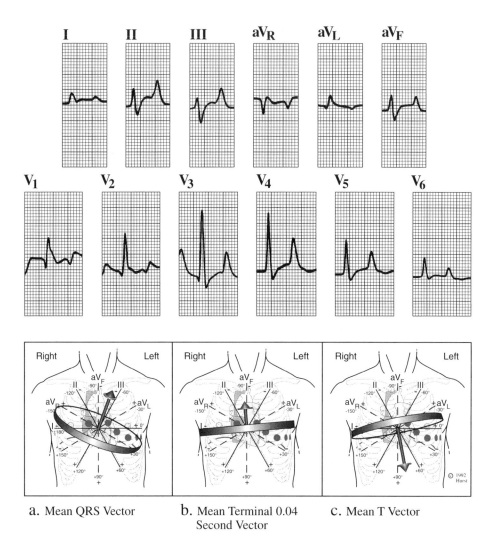

a. Mean QRS Vector

b. Mean Terminal 0.04
Second Vector

c. Mean T Vector

Fig. 7-135

Fig. 7-135. Electrocardiographic effects of hyperkalemia.

- *Rhythm:* Junctional rhythm

  Rate: Undetermined in short strip. There were 90 depolarizations per minute in a longer strip.

  PR interval: None

  QRS duration: 0.12 second

  QT interval: 0.44 second

- *Vector diagrams of electrical forces:* See *a, b,* and *c* below the electrocardiogram.

- *Electrophysiologic considerations:*

  P waves cannot be identified.

  The mean QRS vector is directed about −70 degrees to the left and about 20 degrees anteriorly. The direction of the mean QRS vector is characteristic of right bundle-branch block plus left anterosuperior division block.

  The mean terminal 0.04 second QRS vector is directed −95 degrees to the left and is parallel with the frontal plane. This, too, is typical of right bundle-branch block plus left anterosuperior division block.

  The mean T vector is directed about +80 degrees to the right and 5 to 10 degrees anteriorly. Note the shape of the T waves. They are tall and narrow, and the ascending and descending limbs are sloped to the same degree. Such T waves are referred to as being tent shaped.

  The long QT interval, abnormal rhythm, right bundle-branch block plus left anterosuperior division block, and tent-shaped T waves are characteristic of hyperkalemia.

- *Clinical differential diagnosis:* This cluster of abnormalities is almost diagnostic of hyperkalemia.

- *Discussion:* This electrocardiogram was recorded from an 85-year-old man with diabetic ketoacidosis. His serum potassium level was 9.1 mEq/L.

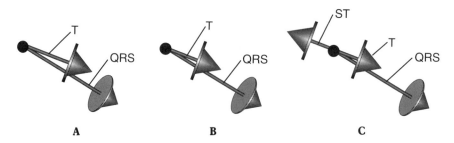

Fig. 7-136. Electrocardiographic effects of digitalis. **A,** The direction and magnitude of arrows representing the mean of the electrical forces (vectors) responsible for the normal QRS complex and normal T wave prior to digitalis medication are illustrated. The QT interval is 0.36 second. **B,** Early signs of digitalis medication may be recognized as a decrease in the amplitude of the T wave. Note in this illustration that the arrow representing the T wave becomes shorter than in **A** but the direction of the arrow has not changed. The QT interval is now 0.30 second. The direction and magnitude of the arrow representing the mean of the electrical forces (vectors) responsible for the QRS complex show no change from the direction and magnitude of the arrow shown in **A**. **C,** More advanced electrocardiographic changes of digitalis medication are shown here. An arrow representing the mean of the electrical forces (vectors) responsible for the T waves is shorter, but its direction has not changed from that shown in **A** and **B**. An arrow representing the mean of the electrical forces (vectors) responsible for the ST segment displacement is shown; it is actually due to the early forces of repolarization (see text) and is directed opposite to the arrow representing the mean T vector. The QT interval is 0.28 second. The direction and magnitude of the arrow representing the QRS vector show no change from the direction and magnitude of the arrows shown in **A** and **B**.

trocardiographic signs of digitalis medication when the heart rate is accelerated. Accordingly, a patient who is receiving digitalis may exhibit a false positive exercise stress test.

Hypercalcemia may produce the same electrocardiographic abnormalities as those produced by digitalis medication.

An electrocardiogram illustrating the abnormalities characteristic of digitalis medication is shown in Fig. 7-137.

Neuromuscular disease and the heart

Friedrich ataxia, as well as most other neuromuscular diseases, is associated with ventricular conduction abnormalities and cardiomyopathy. Perhaps this is true because the genetic abnormality responsible for neuromuscular disease produces abnormalities in other tissue, such as the heart, that is composed of nerve (conduction system) and muscle (myocytes).

The x-linked humeroperoneal disease (Emery-Dreifuss syndrome) deserves special emphasis, because such patients may have atrial paralysis, cardiac arrhythmias requiring a pacemaker, and sudden death.[61,62]

An electrocardiogram illustrating the abnormalities of the Emery-Dreifuss syndrome is shown in Fig. 7-138.

Acute cerebral disease.[33] Head trauma may produce primary T wave abnormalities and large U waves. Unique electrocardiographic abnormalities may develop as a result of cerebral tumor, cerebral hemorrhage, cerebral thrombosis, or subarachnoid hemorrhage.[33] Sinus bradycardia may occur as a result of an increase in intracranial pressure. The QT interval becomes prolonged, and the T waves become grossly abnormal in that they become broad and deeply inverted. An arrow representing the mean of the electrical forces responsible for the grotesque Niagara Falls–type T wave may be directed far to the right. The area encompassed by the T waves is 5 to 10 times the area encompassed by the QRS complexes. The cause of this abnormality is far from clear. One theory holds that cerebral disease alters the influence of the sympathetic nervous system on the right and left ventricles.

The only other electrocardiographic abnormality that simulates "cerebral" T waves is the repolarization abnormality associated with apical hypertrophic cardiomyopathy.

An electrocardiogram illustrating the abnormalities associated with a cerebral hemorrhage is shown in Fig. 7-139.

Athlete's electrocardiogram.[63] The electrocardiogram of a trained athlete is often abnormal. Sinus bradycardia is usually present, and the P waves may become slightly taller than usual. Arrhythmias, including premature atrial depolarizations, and junctional and ventricular depolarizations may occur. Conduction abnormalities, including first- and second-degree atrioventricular block and the Wenckebach phenomenon, may also appear.

The amplitude of the QRS complexes may increase as the left ventricular thickness increases. An ST segment displacement due to early repolarization is common. An arrow representing the mean of the electrical forces (vectors) responsible for the T wave may be directed to the right and anteriorly as a result of left ventricular hypertrophy.

These abnormalities decrease or vanish after the individual discontinues his or her exercise program.

It may be impossible to distinguish the QRS and T wave abnormalities described above from the abnormalities occurring with hypertrophic cardiomyopathy. Echocardiographic examination will assist in this differentiation.

Abnormal initial QRS electrical forces (vectors) and QRS conduction abnormalities are not produced by exercise training.

An electrocardiogram of an athlete is shown in Fig. 7-140.

Effect of drugs on the electrocardiogram.[64] The effect of digitalis on the electrocardiogram is discussed earlier in the chapter. Several other cardiac drugs and cer-

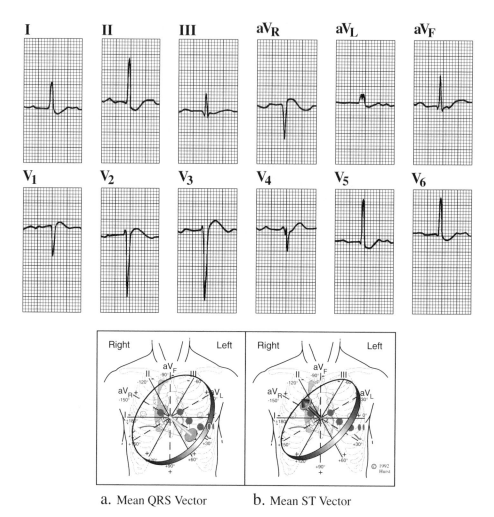

a. Mean QRS Vector   b. Mean ST Vector

Fig. 7-137

Fig. 7-137. Electrocardiographic effects of digitalis and a high serum calcium level.

- *Rhythm:* Sinus tachycardia
  Rate: Undetermined in short strip. There were 96 depolarizations per minute in a longer strip.
  PR interval: 0.28 second
  QRS duration: 0.08 second
  QT interval: 0.29 second
- *Vector diagrams of electrical forces:* See *a* and *b* below the electrocardiogram.
- *Electrophysiologic considerations:*
  The PR interval is prolonged, indicating first-degree atrioventricular block.
  The QT interval is shorter than normal.
  The mean QRS vector is directed +40 degrees inferiorly and 70 degrees posteriorly. It is more posteriorly directed than usual.
  The mean ST segment vector is large. It is directed at −140 degrees and 30 to 40 degrees anteriorly.
  The T waves are not seen in all leads. Therefore a mean vector for the T waves cannot be drawn. The T waves are small and upright in leads aV_L, V_5, and V_6.
  The longer than normal PR interval, the shorter than normal QT interval, and an ST segment vector that is opposite in direction to the mean QRS vector are characteristic of the effect of digitalis on the electrocardiogram (see text). The same effect occurs with hypercalcemia.
- *Clinical differential diagnosis:* There are two causes of these abnormalities: the digitalis effect and hypercalcemia. Subendocardial injury can produce an ST segment displacement of this magnitude, but the QT interval is usually prolonged and the T waves are usually more obvious than what are shown here.
- *Discussion:* This electrocardiogram was recorded from a 66-year-old woman with *Staphlococcus aureus* and *Streptococcus viridans* endocarditis of the aortic valve, a history of hypertension, severe heart failure, a digoxin blood level of 3.2 ng/ml, and a serum calcium level of 12.2 mg%. The patient also had hyperparathyroidism.

  The ST segment and T wave abnormalities in this electrocardiogram are undoubtedly due to digitalis plus hypercalcemia.

tain noncardiac drugs can produce electrocardiographic abnormalities. For example, phenothiazine and tricyclic antidepressant drugs can produce sinus arrest, sinoatrial block, and atrioventricular block. The QT interval may be prolonged, which may precipitate ventricular tachycardia or ventricular fibrillation. The duration of the QRS complex may become longer than normal, and bundle-branch block may develop. Primary T wave abnormalities may develop.

Quindine, procainamide, and disopyramide may produce sinus arrest, atrioventricular block, ventricular conduction defects, prolongation of the QT interval, and repolarization abnormalities.

Lidocaine produces few abnormalities in the electrocardiogram, but sinus arrest and atrioventricular block may occur. Mexiletine and tocainide may produce repolarization abnormalities.

Verapamil may produce sinus bradycardia and varying degrees of atrioventricular block. Diltiazem may slow the heart rate slightly and may have a small effect on atrioventricular conduction but not to the degree noted with verapamil. Nifedipine produces no significant changes in the electrocardiogram.

The beta-blocking drugs may slow the heart rate and prolong atrioventricular conduction.

It is not uncommon for a beta blocker, digitalis, and a calcium antagonist to be used in the same patient. The clinician should be aware that the combination of drugs, especially if the calcium antagonist is verapamil, may precipitate high-grade atrioventricular block.

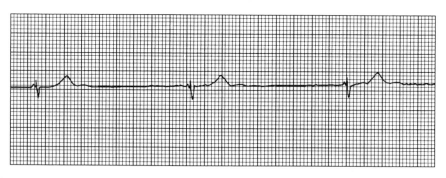

Fig. 7-138. Atrial standstill associated with Emery-Driefuss syndrome. This electrocardiogram was recorded from a 37-year-old man with Emery-Driefuss syndrome. No P waves are seen, and the ventricular rate is about 30 depolarizations per minute. Such patients have atrial paralysis, conduction disturbances, and sudden death. Despite the installation of a pacemaker, this patient died suddenly while mowing the lawn.

Electrocardiogram courtesy Linton Hopkins, M.D., Professor of Neurology, Emory University School of Medicine, Atlanta, Ga.

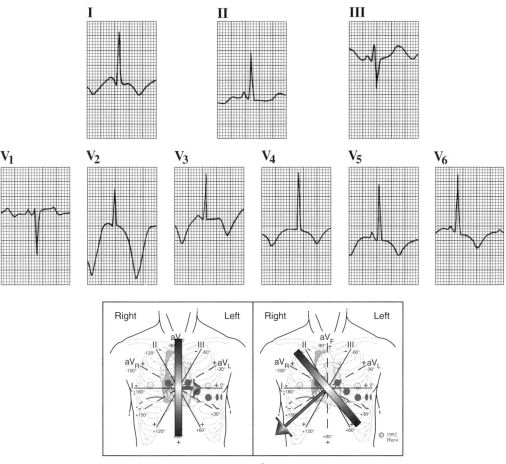

a. Mean QRS Vector   b. Mean T Vector

Fig. 7-139. Huge, abnormal T waves associated with cerebral hemorrhage, cerebral thrombosis, or subarachnoid hemorrhage. The heart rate may be slow because of an increase in intracerebral pressure. The T waves may become huge and may be directed abnormally. The cause of these "cerebral" T waves is not known.

Electrocardiogram from Burch GE, Meyers R, Abildskov JA: A new electrocardiographic pattern observed in cerebrovascular accidents, *Circulation* 9:720, 1954. Reproduced by permission of the American Heart Association, Inc.

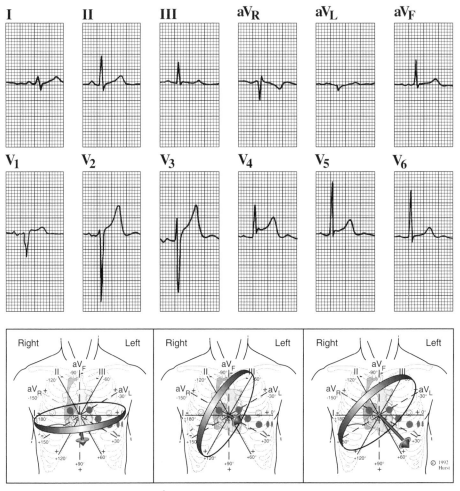

a. Mean QRS Vector   b. Mean ST Vector   c. Mean T Vector

Fig. 7-140

Fig. 7-140. Normal early repolarization in a young athlete.

- *Rhythm:* Sinus bradycardia
    Rate: Undetermined in short strip. There were 46 depolarizations per minute in a longer strip.
    PR interval: 0.16 second
    QRS duration: 0.08 second
    QT interval: 0.36 second
- *Vector diagrams of electrical forces:* See *a, b,* and *c* below the electrocardiogram.
- *Electrophysiologic considerations:*
    The P waves are normal.
    The mean QRS vector is directed normally. It is directed about +80 degrees inferiorly and 25 to 30 degrees posteriorly.
    The mean ST vector is directed about 30 degrees inferiorly and about 30 degrees anteriorly. It is directed parallel with the large mean T vector. The ST vector in this case is due to the repolarization process.
    The mean T vector is large. It is directed about +50 degrees inferiorly and about 30 degrees anteriorly.
    The ST vector could be due to generalized epicardial injury, possibly as a result of pericarditis or apical myocardial ischemia. Subsequent tracings would, however, show a change. The ST segment displacement would decrease in size, the mean T vector would become smaller, and, finally, the mean T vector would be directed opposite to the mean QRS vector (see Fig. 7-127).
    Hyperkalemia can produce a large T wave with symmetric sides. Note that the ascending limb of the T wave in this tracing is more slanted than the descending limb of the T wave.
    Finally, this could be a normal varient such as occurs with normal early repolarization.
- *Clinical differential diagnosis:* This electrocardiogram could be normal or be due to pericarditis. It is not characteristic of hyperkalemia.
- *Discussion:* This electrocardiogram was recorded from a normal 27-year-old athlete. An electrophysiologic study was normal.

Electrocardiogram reproduced with permission from Hurst JW: *Ventricular electrocardiography*, New York, 1991, Gower, fig 13.6.

Key Points

- Electrocardiography commonly reveals diagnostic clues that, when added to the clues gleaned from the history, physical examination, chest roentgenogram, and routine laboratory tests, enable the physician to make a cardiac diagnosis. At times the electrocardiogram reveals important diagnostic clues and the remainder of the initial examination may be normal. At other times a patient may have serious cardiac disease, as determined by other methods, and the electrocardiogram may be normal.

- It is necessary for the physician to appreciate the appropriate cardiac anatomy, the depolarization and repolarization sequences of the atria and ventricles, and the spatial vector concept in order to interpret electrocardiograms. It is not wise to memorize "patterns" without an understanding as to their origin. The Grant method of analysis is attractive because it requires the interpreter to use basic principles to interpret each electrocardiogram he or she inspects. This is far better than memorizing some basic principles and then ignoring them as one proceeds to memorize the patterns of deflections. When pattern recognizition is used, the interpreter soon forgets basic mechanisms and has no tools to work with when a new pattern is encountered.

- Electrocardiography is needed to identify accurately most cardiac arrhythmias.

- Careful analysis of P waves gives important information about the ventricles of the heart.

- Electrocardiographic abnormalities may be caused by diseases of the coronary arteries, heart valves, heart muscle, and pericardium, as well as by systemic and pulmonary hypertension.

- Abnormal levels of serum electrolytes and certain drugs may produce alterations of the electrocardiogram.

- The physician should always use a four-step approach to interpret electrocardiograms:

  Determine the heart rhythm and heart rate. Measure all intervals. Create a clinical differential cardiac diagnosis to explain these abnormalities.

  Diagram the spatial vectors for the first and last halves of the P wave. Diagram the mean spatial vectors for the initial and terminal 0.04 second of the QRS complex, the entire QRS complex, the ST segment displacement, and the T wave. Determine how the vectors of the patient differ from normal.

  Create an electrical differential cardiac diagnosis to explain the abnormalities.

  Finally, to reach the goal, create a clinical differential cardiac diagnosis that might cause the electrical abnormalities.

- The electrocardiographic data should then be correlated with the data collected from the history, physical examination, chest roentgenogram, and routine laboratory tests.

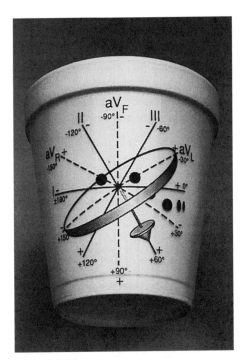

Fig. 7-141. Use of a styrofoam cup as a model for visualizing the spatial orientation of electrical forces (vectors). The beginning, as well as the seasoned, clinician may profit from the use of a model for visualizing the electrical forces in three-dimensional space. Whereas very sophisticated models can be (and have been) created, a styrofoam cup is inexpensive and readily available. The top of the cup should be visualized as the shoulders of the patient, and the base of the cup should be visualized as the waist of the patient. The origin of electrical activity should be imagined to be in the center of the cup, and the hexaxial lead system and chest lead electrode positions can be drawn on the front of the cup (the chest). The fact that the cup is circular enables the clinician to appreciate the effect a curved surface has on one's perception of the location of the transitional pathway and the direction of various vectors.

● The beginner may find it beneficial to use a model to visualize the arrows that symbolize the electrical forces. A styrofoam cup may be used for this purpose (Fig. 7-141).

COMMENTS

The statements made in this chapter on electrocardiography represent a clinically useful approach to the subject. Most of the statements are supported by the scientific studies of Frank Wilson and Robert Grant. At times statements are made that are not supported by scientific data. Such statements are based on many years of experience, which included the correlation of electrocardiographic data with other clinical data.

At times electrocardiographic interpretation is based on logic rather than scientific data. It is like watching the wind blow the leaves of a tree. If you are standing in a closed-in space watching the leaves on a tree move in a certain direction, you deduce that the wind is blowing the leaves in that direction. How do you know it is true? You know because of your previous experience with wind and leaves. You do not feel the wind, because you are in a closed-in space, but logic dictates that the wind is blowing the leaves. It would be ridiculous, based on your past experience, to suggest that something is sucking the leaves.

REFERENCES

1. Wilson FN: Foreword. In Barker JM: *The unipolar electrocardiogram: a clinical interpretation*, New York, 1952, Appleton-Century-Crofts, pp xi-xii.
2. Grant RP, Estes EH: *Spatial vector electrocardiography*, Philadelphia, 1951, Blakiston.
3. Hurst JW: The hypothetical myocardial cell. In Hurst JW: *Ventricular electrocardiography*, New York, 1991, Gower, pp 3.2-3.12.
4. Becker AE: Personal communication, May 20, 1988.
5. Katz LN: *Electrocardiography: including an atlas of electrocardiograms*, Philadelphia, 1941, Lea & Febiger, pp 62-63.
6. Lewis T, Rothschild MA: The excitatory process in the dog's heart. II. The ventricles, *Philos Trans R Soc Lond (Biol)* 206:181, 1915.
7. Lazzara R: Cellular basis for the U wave and its translation to the surface ECG, *J Electrocardiol* 24(suppl):44-45, 1992.
8. Durrer E: Electrical aspects of human cardiac activity: a clinical physiological approach to excitation and stimulation, *Cardiovasc Res* 2:5, 1968.
9. Katz LN, Hellerstein HK: Electrocardiography. In Fishman AP, Richards DW, editors: *Circulation of the blood*, New York, 1944, Oxford University Press, pp 265-351.
10. Einthoven W: The galvanometric registration of the human electrocardiogram, likewise a review of the use of the capillary-electrometer in physiology. In Willius FA, Keys E, editors: *Cardiac classics*, translated by Willius FW, St Louis, 1941, Mosby.
11. Bayley R: *Electrocardiographic analysis*, vol 1, *Biophysical principles*, New York, 1958, Paul Hoeber, p 41.
12. Wilson FN, Johnston FD, MacLeod AG, Barker PS: Electrocardiograms that represent potential variations of single electrode, *Am Heart J* 9:477, 1934.
13. Goldberger E: Simple indifferent, electrocardiographic electrode of zero potential and a technique of obtaining augmented, unipolar, extremity leads, *Am Heart J* 23:483, 1942.
14. Mirvis DM: *Body surface electrocardiographic mapping*, Boston, 1988, Kluwer, pp 1-204.
15. Hayes JJ, Stewart RB, Greene, Bardy GH: Narrow QRS complex ventricular tachycardia, *Ann Intern Med* 114:460, 1991.
16. Romano C, Gemme G, Pongiglione R: Aritmie cardiache rare dell' eta' pediatrica. II. Accessi sincopali per fibrillazione ventricolane passossistica, *Clin Pediatr* 45:656, 1963.
17. Ward OC: A new familial cardiac syndrome in children, *J Irish Med Assoc* 54:103, 1964.
18. Jervell A, Lange-Nielsen F: Congenital deaf-mutism, functional heart disease with prolongation of the QR interval, and sudden death, *Am Heart J* 54(1):59, 1957.
19. Morris JJ, Estes EH Jr, Whalen RE et al: P wave analysis in valvular heart disease, *Circulation* 29:242, 1964.
20. Jin L, Weisse AB, Hernandez F et al: Significance of electrocardiographic isolated abnormal terminal P wave force (left atrial abnormality): an echocardiographic and clinical correlation, *Arch Intern Med* 148(7):1545, 1988.
21. Horan LG, Sridharan MR, Hand RC et al: Variation in the precordial QRS transition zone in normal subjects, *J Electrocardiol* 21(1):25, 1988.
22. Romhilt DW, Bove KE, Norris RJ et al: A critical appraisal of the electrocardiographic criteria for the diagnosis of left ventricular hypertrophy, *Circulation* 40:185, 1969.
23. Romhilt DW, Estes EH Jr: A point-score system for the ECG diagnosis of left ventricular hypertrophy, *Am Heart J* 75(6):752, 1968.
24. Odom H II, Davis JL, Dinh HA et al: QRS voltage measurements in autopsied men free of cardiopulmonary disease: a basis for evaluating total QRS voltage as an index of left ventricular hypertrophy, *Am J Cardiol* 58:801, 1986.
25. Goldberger E: *Unipolar lead electrocardiography*, ed 2, Philadelphia, 1949, Lea & Febiger, pp 128, 129.
26. Wilson FN, MacLeod AG, Barker PS: The T deflection of the electrocardiogram, *Trans Assoc Am Physicians* 46:29, 1931.
27. Burch G, Winsor T: *A primer of electrocardiography*, Philadelphia, 1945, Lea & Febiger.

28. Hurst JW: The hypothetical myocardial cell. In Hurst JW: *Ventricular electrocardiography*, New York, 1991, Gower, fig 3.4.
29. Hurst JW: *Ventricular electrocardiography*, New York, 1991, Gower, p 5.19, fig 5.16.
30. Hurst JW: *Ventricular electrocardiography*, New York, 1991, Gower, p 5.22.
31. Wilson FN, MacLeod AG, Barker PS, Johnston FD: The determination and the significance of the areas of the ventricular deflections of the electrocardiogram, *Am Heart J* 10:46, 1934.
32. Wilson F: Foreword. In Lepeschkin E, editor: *Modern electrocardiography*, Baltimore, 1978, Little, Brown.
33. Burch GE, Meyers R, Abildskov JA: A new electrocardiographic pattern observed in cerebrovascular accidents, *Circulation* 9:719, 1954.
34. Hersch C: Electrocardiographic changes in head injuries, *Circulation* 23:853, 1961.
35. Personal observation.
36. Cabrera E, Monroy JR: Systolic and diastolic loading of the heart. I. Physiologic and clinical data, *Am Heart J* 43:661, 1952.
37. Cabrera E, Monroy JR: Systolic and diastolic loading of the heart. II. Electrocardiographic data, *Am Heart J* 43:669, 1952.
38. Hurst JW: *Ventricular electrocardiography*, New York, 1991, Gower, fig 6.20.
39. Hurst JW: *Ventricular electrocardiography*, New York, 1991, Gower, fig 6.21.
40. Hurst JW: *Ventricular electrocardiography*, New York, 1991, Gower, fig 6.23.
41. Hurst JW: *Ventricular electrocardiography*, New York, 1991, Gower, p 6.25.
42. Wilson FN: Concerning the form of the QRS deflections of the electrocardiogram in bundle branch block, *J Mt Sinai Hosp* 8:1110, 1942.
43. Rosenbaum MB, Elizari MV, Lazzari JO et al: The differential electrocardiographic manifestations of hemiblocks, bilateral bundle branch block, and trifascicular blocks. In Schlant RC, Hurst JW, editors: *Advances in electrocardiography*, vol 1, New York, 1972, Grune & Stratton, p 145.
44. McGinn S, White PD: Acute cor pulmonale resulting from pulmonary embolism, *JAMA* 104:1473, 1935.
45. Stein PD, Dalen JE, McIntyre KM et al: The electrocardiogram in acute pulmonary embolism, *Prog Cardiovasc Dis* 27(4):247, 1975.
46. Wolff L, Parkinson J, White PD: Bundle branch block with short PR interval in healthy young people prone to paroxysmal tachycardia, *Am Heart J* 5:685, 1930.
47. de Luna AB, Carrio I, Subirana MT et al: Electrophysiological mechanisms of the S1 SII SIII electrocardiographic morphology, *J Electrocardiol* 20(1):38, 1987.
48. Clements SD Jr, Hurst JW: Diagnostic value of electrocardiographic abnormalities observed in subjects accidentally exposed to cold, *Am J Cardiol* 29:889, 1972.
49. Wilson FN, MacLeod AG, Barker PS et al: The electrocardiogram in myocardial infarction with particular reference to the initial deflections of the ventricular complex, *Heart* 16:155, 1933.
50. Holland RP, Brooks H: TQ-ST segment mapping: critical review and analysis of current concepts, *Am J Cardiol* 40:110, 1977.
51. Hurst JW: *Ventricular electrocardiography*, New York, 1991, Gower, p 6.20.
52. Prinzmetal M, Kennamer R, Merlis R et al: Angina pectoris. I. A variant form of angina pectoris, *Am J Med* 27:375, 1959.
53. Hurst JW: *Ventricular electrocardiography*, New York, 1991, Gower, p 6.21, fig 6.18.
54. Hurst JW, editor-in-chief: *Atlas of the heart*, New York, 1988, McGraw-Hill and Gower, figs 2.7, 2.11, 2.12.
55. Antaloczy Z, Barcsak J, Magyar E: Correlation of electrocardiologic and pathologic findings in 100 cases of Q wave and non–Q wave myocardial infarction, *J Electrocardiol* 21(4):331, 1988.
56. Hurst JW: *Ventricular electrocardiography*, New York, 1991, Gower, p 10.2.
57. Fowler NO, Daniels C, Scott RC et al: The electrocardiogram in cor pulmonale with and without emphysema, *Am J Cardiol* 16:500, 1965.
58. Fisch C: Electrolytes and the heart. In Hurst JW, editor: *The heart*, ed 6, New York, 1986, McGraw-Hill, p 1473.
59. Grant RP: *Clinical electrocardiography*, New York, 1957, McGraw-Hill, pp 96-100.
60. Hurst JW: *Ventricular electrocardiography*, New York, 1991, Gower, p 6.33, fig 6.24.
61. Emery AEH, Dreifuss FF: Unusual type of benign X-linked muscular dystrophy, *J Neurol Neurosurg Psychiatry* 29:338, 1966.
62. Waters DD, Nutter DO, Hopkins LC, Dorney ER: Cardiac features of an unusual X-linked humeroperoneal neuromuscular disease, *N Engl J Med* 293:1017, 1975.
63. Zeppilli P, Venerando A: Sudden death and physical exertion, *J Sports Med Phys Fitness* 21:299, 1981.
64. Hurst JW: *Ventricular electrocardiography*, New York, 1991, Gower, p 12.2.

ADDITIONAL READINGS

Hayes JJ et al: Narrow QRS complex ventricular tachycardia, *Ann Intern Med* 114:460, 1991.
Wellens HJJ et al: The value of the electrocardiogram in the differential diagnosis of a tachycardia with a widened QRS complex, *Am J Med* 64:27, 1978.

CHAPTER 8

Interpretation of the chest roentgenogram

Roentgenology (Roentgen, the discoverer, and aoyos, knowledge) or radiology (Latin, radius, ray, and aoyos, knowledge) has been sufficiently developed in technique and application to allow us to judge something of its real clinical value (Roentgen, 1895). It is not superfluous to examine fluoroscopically every individual with cardiovascular symptoms or signs when such roentgenological examination is readily available, even though no measurements are made.* Sometimes surprising and frequently useful and interesting information results from such routine study. Only by this method may the size and shape of the heart be determined with certainty during life, and occasionally aortic aneurysms and cardiovascular malformations are revealed in routine roentgen study when they had not even been suspected previously. It must be admitted, however, that serious heart disease may be present, as discovered in other ways, when no clew is given to its presence by roentgenology. Also, early and slight cardiovascular lesions usually escape notice in the application of this method, as happens frequently in the case of other methods, because the heart and vessels may show no definite abnormalities of size, shape, or action. For the most part, therefore, roentgenology merely reveals evidence of well established or advanced disease which is difficult or impossible to eradicate. Although this mainly affords only "interesting" data for the student of pathology, it does help the practitioner of medicine appreciably in the establishment of exact diagnoses which are so essential to accuracy of prognosis and to the handling of patients with chronic heart disease.

The chief difficulty in the routine application of roentgenology to the circulation lies not in the technique, which can be mastered without great difficulty, but in the interpretation of the normal limits of heart size, shape, and action, and therefore in the diagnosis of slight abnormalities. There are so many factors, for example, age, size, build,

---

*Routine fluoroscopic examination of the heart was discontinued in the 1950s because of the danger of excessive exposure to radiation in uncontrolled physicians' offices. This technique enabled the clinician to more readily identify abnormalities of ventricular contractility, calcification of the heart valves, the size of the heart chambers and great vessels, and pulmonary blood flow than was possible using routine chest roentgenograms.[1] The cost of the examination in 1950 was $3. The necessary discontinuation of this valuable technique has been viewed as a step backward. Surely, a safe fluroscope could be developed. The echocardiogram has replaced fluoroscopic examination of the heart; however, the cost of performing an echocardiogram prohibits its routine use in every patient. The cost of a transthoracic echocardiogram in 1992 was $553, and the cost of an esophageal echocardiogram was $723.

respiration, and nervousness resulting in individual variations within the normal, that it is at present impossible to recognize them all, or at least to take them all into consideration in the establishment of any satisfactory tables of measurement of size, or rules about shape or action. Not only are the normal limits difficult or impossible to define accurately, but in a given individual important changes may occur in heart size or shape insufficient to produce definite roentgenological abnormalities at the time of examination, but which would have been noted if such study had been previously made. For example, a heart showing a roentgen ray shadow area of 80 square centimetres at the lower limit of the normal figures may increase in area 38 per cent before it equals even the average normal measurement (110 square centimetres) and as much as 75 per cent before it equals the upper normal limit of 140 square centimetres (Smith and Bloedorn, 1922).[2] Successive records of heart size and shape in the same individual carefully made under varying conditions of health should be more useful than a single comparison of this individual case with a table of normal averages or a set of rules; it is, however, usually impossible to possess information about the roentgen ray findings prior to the onset of trouble in a given case. In spite of these difficulties some rules are necessary and normal standards for measurements of size are useful if we realize their inaccuracy in application to individual patients, and do not lull ourselves into a false sense of security which tends to develop from the use of figures and formulas.

PAUL DUDLEY WHITE 1931[3]*

Careful inspection of the chest roentgenogram is extremely valuable in the detection of heart disease, diseases of the aorta and pulmonary vessels, and heart failure.[3,4] Abnormalities identified in the x-ray film of the chest must be correlated with abnormalities discovered through the history, physical examination, electrocardiogram, and routine laboratory data.

VIEWS OF THE HEART

Clinicians should personally view the chest roentgenograms of the patients they examine. Posteroanterior (PA) and left lateral views of the chest are sufficient and should be obtained routinely.

OVERALL HEART SIZE

The size of the heart must be determined, because an enlarged heart is definitely abnormal. When the heart silhouette is enlarged, it is necessary to determine if the enlargement is due to enlargement of the heart itself or to pericardial effusion. How-

---

ever, a normal heart size does not rule out abnormalities; the patient may have coronary heart disease, slight aortic or mitral valve disease, severe aortic valve stenosis, acute rupture of a chordae tendineae of the mitral valve, hypertrophic cardiomyopathy, cardiac arrhythmias, or mild to moderate hypertension.

The experienced clinician is able to inspect a chest film and determine if the heart size is normal, whereas the beginner should make certain measurements (Fig. 8-1). The intrathoracic diameter of the chest should be determined by measuring the inside of the rib cage at the level of the superior portion of the dome of the right leaf of the diaphragm. A vertical line is then drawn down the middle of the spine (this line is referred to as the midline). Horizontal lines are then extended from the midline to the right and left cardiac borders. The sum of these two lines constitutes the transverse diameter of the heart, which should not normally exceed one half of the intrathoracic diameter of the chest. The measurements are made in centimeters.

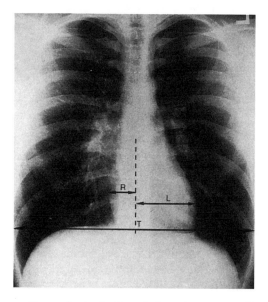

Fig. 8-1. Measurement of heart size in the frontal view. A transverse line is drawn at the level of the upper portion of the right leaf of the diaphragm and extended to reach the internal margins of the ribs on the right and left. This line represents the transverse diameter of the chest *(T)*. A vertical line is drawn down the middle of the thoracic vertebra. A horizontal line is drawn from the vertical line to the outer border of the right cardiac margin *(R)*. Another horizontal line is drawn from the vertical line to the outer border of the left cardiac margin *(L)*. The length of the lines labeled *T, R,* and *L* are measured in centimeters. The cardiothoracic ratio is computed as follows: normally, R + L is equal to or less than one half of T.

Reproduced with permission from Rubens MB: Chest x-ray in adult heart disease. In Julian DG, Camm AJ, Fox KM, Hall RJC, Poole-Wilson PA, editors: *Diseases of the heart,* London, 1989, Baillière Tindall, p 260.

The range of normal for heart size is large, and it is possible for the heart to be on the small side of the normal range at one point in time and then become larger but still remain within the normal range. The change in heart size, however, is abnormal. This illustrates the value of having a baseline roentgenogram made when the patient is in good health.

When the cardiac silhouette is large, there are three possible causes: pericardial effusion alone, cardiac chamber enlargement alone, or cardiac enlargement combined with pericardial effusion. When the correct cause cannot be determined by inspection of the chest roentgenogram, it is necessary to seek other clues from the physical examination and electrocardiogram.

PERICARDIAL EFFUSION

The overall size of the heart silhouette may increase very little when a small pericardial effusion accumulates rapidly. When the fluid accumulates gradually, the cardiac silhouette may become huge.

There are several clues to the recognition of pericardial effusion. The usual concavity that is present in the region of the main pulmonary artery in the PA view, including the contour of the main pulmonary artery itself, is obscured by the peri-

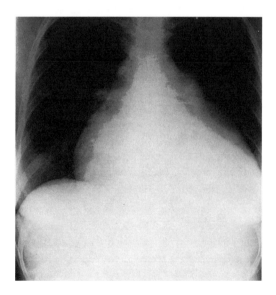

Fig. 8-2. Pericardial effusion. The cardiac silhouette is enlarged without specific chamber enlargement. Note that the contour produced by the main pulmonary artery is "ironed out." The pulmonary vascularity is normal or diminished in size.
Courtesy Wade Shuford, M.D., Professor of Radiology, Emory University School of Medicine, and the Radiology Service at Grady Memorial Hospital, Atlanta, Ga.

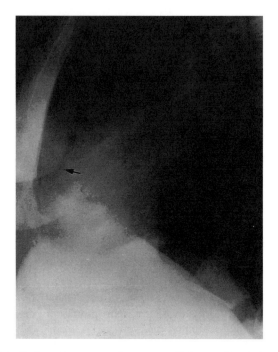

Fig. 8-3. Pericardial effusion. An arrow points to a radiolucent line (epicardial fat stripe) that is displaced inward by fluid in the pericardial sac.

Courtesy Wade Shuford, M.D., Professor of Radiology, Emory University School of Medicine, and the Radiology Service at Grady Memorial Hospital, Atlanta, Ga.

cardial fluid. This occurs because the pericardium attaches to the aorta at a level that is higher than the main pulmonary artery. Accordingly, fluid can collect and "iron out" the outer border of the main pulmonary artery. The lung fields are clear when there is isolated pericardial fluid without heart failure (Fig. 8-2). An epicardial fat stripe may be seen in the lateral view. The stripe is displaced posteriorly by fluid in the intervening pericardial sac (Fig. 8-3).

Causes of pericardial effusion

Pericardial effusion may be caused by pericarditis of any type, including viral pericarditis, collagen disease, neoplasia, trauma, myxedema, uremia, or heart failure.

INDIVIDUAL CARDIAC CHAMBER ENLARGEMENT

The names of the individual cardiac chambers are misleading. Normally, the *left atrium* is not located on the left; it is located in a central position posteriorly. It lies below the carina of the trachea and the mainstem bronchi on the PA view and abuts the esophagus posteriorly on the lateral view (Figs. 8-4 and 8-5). The *left ventricle* is

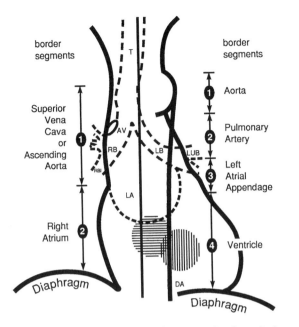

Fig. 8-4. Diagram of the normal adult heart as shown on the frontal chest roentgenogram. The left border of the mediastinum is divided into four segments: *1*, distal aortic arch segment; *2*, main pulmonary artery segment; *3*, left atrial appendage segment; *4*, ventricular segment. The right border is divided into two segments: *1*, superior vena cava or ascending aortic segment; *2*, right atrial segment. *LA*, Right margin of left atrium (often seen in this region in the normal heart); *T*, trachea; *AV*, azygous vein; *RB*, right main bronchus; *RBI*, right intermediate bronchus; *LB*, left main bronchus; *LUB*, left upper lobe bronchus; *DA*, left margin of descending aorta. The horizontally lined area represents the usual position of the aortic valve, and the vertically lined area represents the usual position of the mitral valve. The dashed lines represent the tracheal and main bronchial outlines.

Modified with permission from the Criteria Committee of the New York Heart Association: *Nomenclature and criteria for diagnosis of diseases of the heart and great vessels,* ed 8, Boston, 1979, Little, Brown and Company, p 294.

not simply on the left. The long anatomic axis of the normal left ventricle is directed inferiorly, to the left, and slightly anteriorly. The left lower heart border is produced by the left ventricle in the PA view. The left ventricle extends posteriorly and toward the observer in the left lateral view. The normal *right atrium* makes up the lower right heart border in the PA view. The normal *right ventricle* is not located on the right; it is an anterior structure, and its size cannot be determined by inspecting the PA radiographic view of the chest. The normal right ventricle forms the anterior surface of the lower cardiac silhouette on the lateral view.

Enlargement of the individual heart chambers is illustrated in Figs. 8-6 through 8-11.   *Text continued on p. 437.*

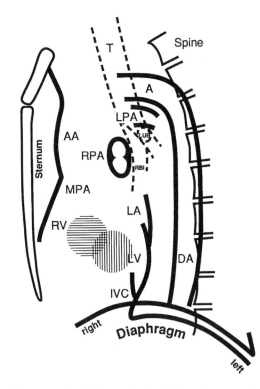

Fig. 8-5. Diagram of the normal adult heart in the left lateral projection. *A,* Aorta; *LPA,* left pulmonary artery at left hilus arching over *LUB* (circular image of left upper lobe bronchus); *RPA,* right pulmonary artery at right hilus; *RBI,* right intermediate bronchus; *LA,* dorsal margin of left atrium; *LV,* dorsal margin of left ventricle; *DA,* descending aorta; *IVC,* dorsal margin of intrathoracic inferior vena cava; *RV,* ventral margin of right ventricular outflow tract; *MPA,* ventral margin of main pulmonary artery; *AA,* ventral margin of ascending aorta; *T,* trachea. The horizontally lined area represents the usual position of the aortic valve, and the vertically lined area represents the usual position of the mitral valve.

Reproduced with permission from the Criteria Committee of the New York Heart Association: *Nomenclature and criteria for diagnosis of diseases of the heart and great vessels,* ed 8, Boston, 1979, Little, Brown and Company, p 295.

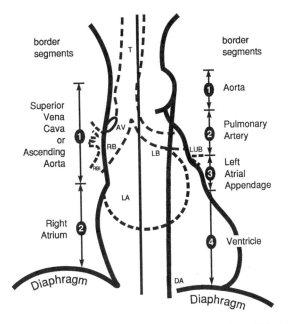

Fig. 8-6. Enlargement of the left atrium as seen in the frontal view of the chest. Compare its size with that of the normal left atrium shown in Fig. 8-4. Note that the large left atrium produces elevation of the left main bronchus. On the PA chest x-ray film the left atrium forms a larger than normal double contour, and the left atrial appendage may become prominent. The main pulmonary artery may be larger than normal, because left atrial pressure is often higher than normal. The so-called four-bump heart is produced when the left border of the heart is composed of the aortic knob, main pulmonary artery, left atrial appendage, and border of the left ventricle. See Fig. 8-4 for an explanation of numbers and abbreviations.

Modified with permission from the Criteria Committee of the New York Heart Association: *Nomenclature and criteria for diagnosis of diseases of the heart and great vessels,* ed 8, Boston, 1979, Little, Brown and Company, p 294.

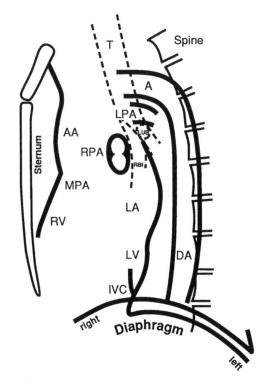

Fig. 8-7. Enlargement of the left atrium as seen in the left lateral view of the chest. Note that the large left atrium extends from the left main bronchus inferiorly and posteriorly. Compare its size with that of the normal left atrium shown in Fig. 8-5. The left lateral roentgenogram will reveal compression of the barium-filled esophagus. See Fig. 8-5 for an explanation of abbreviations.

Modified with permission from the Criteria Committee of the New York Heart Association: *Nomenclature and criteria for diagnosis of diseases of the heart and great vessels*, ed 8, Boston, 1979, Little, Brown and Company, p 295.

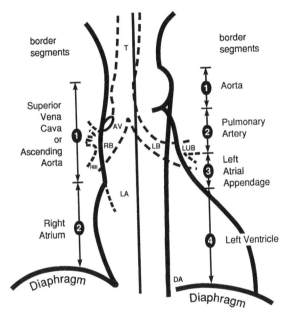

Fig. 8-8. Enlargement of the left ventricle as seen in the frontal view of the chest. Note that the left lower border of the large left ventricle extends more to the left and inferiorly than does the normal left ventricle. Compare the size of the large left ventricle with the size of the normal left ventricle shown in Fig. 8-4. See Fig. 8-4 for an explanation of numbers and abbreviations.

Modified with permission from the Criteria Committee of the New York Heart Association: *Nomenclature and criteria for diagnosis of diseases of the heart and great vessels,* ed 8, Boston, 1979, Little, Brown and Company, p 294.

Fig. 8-9. Enlargement of the left ventricle as seen in the left lateral view. Compare the size of the large left ventricle with the size of the normal left ventricle shown in Fig. 8-5. See Fig. 8-5 for an explanation of abbreviations.

Modified with permission from the Criteria Committee of the New York Heart Association: *Nomenclature and criteria for diagnosis of diseases of the heart and great vessels*, ed 8, Boston, 1979, Little, Brown and Company, p 295.

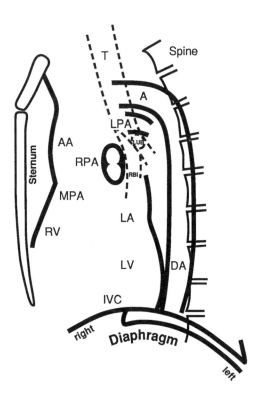

Fig. 8-10. Enlargement of the right atrium as seen in the frontal view of the chest. Compare the size of the large left atrium with the size of the normal left atrium shown in Fig. 8-4. See Fig. 8-4 for an explanation of numbers and abbreviations.

Modified with permission from the Criteria Committee of the New York Heart Association: *Nomenclature and criteria for diagnosis of diseases of the heart and great vessels*, ed 8, Boston, 1979, Little, Brown and Company, p 294.

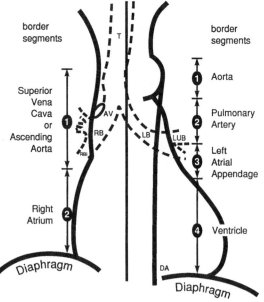

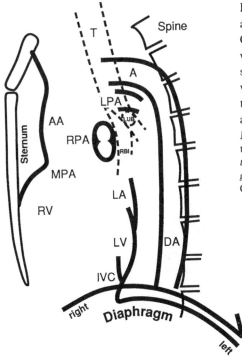

Fig. 8-11. Enlargement of the right ventricle as seen in the left lateral view of the chest. Compare the size of the large right ventricle with the size of the normal right ventricle shown in Fig. 8-5. Note that the large right ventricle occupies a larger than normal portion of the retrosternal space. See Fig. 8-5 for an explanation of abbreviations.

Modified with permission from the Criteria Committee of the New York Heart Association: *Nomenclature and criteria for diagnosis of diseases of the heart and great vessels,* ed 8, Boston, 1979, Little, Brown and Company, p 295.

Left atrial enlargement

When the left atrium enlarges, it may elevate and displace posteriorly the left main bronchus. Normally, in the PA view there may be three contour shadows along the left border of the heart: the aortic knob, the main pulmonary artery, and the left ventricle (see Fig. 8-4). With left atrial enlargement the pulmonary artery may become larger than normal, because the left atrial pressure is often higher than normal, and the left atrial appendage may dilate and become border forming along the mid–left cardiac contour, resulting in the so-called four-bump heart (Figs. 8-12 and 8-13, *A*). Also, a double density may be seen on the PA view. The barium-filled esophagus may be displaced to the right on the PA view and posteriorly on the lateral view (Fig. 8-13, *B*).

When the left atrium becomes greatly enlarged, it may be noted on the right side of the heart (Fig. 8-14); a giant left atrium may touch the rib cage on the right.

Causes of left atrial enlargement. The left atrium may become larger than normal when there is mitral stenosis or mitral regurgitation. It may also become larger than normal when there is long-standing atrial fibrillation without other evidence of heart disease. A giant left atrium is usually due to a combination of long-standing mitral regurgitation, atrial disease due to a past episode of rheumatic fever, and atrial fibrillation. The left atrium may be slightly enlarged as a result of aortic valve disease, especially when there is secondary mitral regurgitation and poor left ventricular compliance. Left atrial enlargement is a common participant in generalized cardiac enlargement such as occurs in patients with cardiomyopathy, in which all heart chambers are enlarged. A large left atrial appendage is usually caused by mitral valve stenosis or regurgitation.

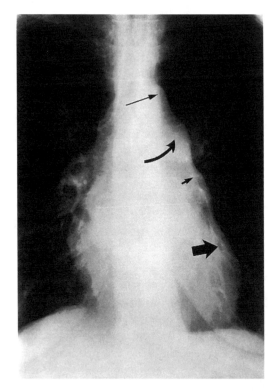

Fig. 8-12. Left atrial enlargement in a patient with mitral stenosis. A large double contour can be seen in the central portion of the heart. This is a so-called four-bump heart. The four "bumps" are produced on the left border of the heart by the aortic knob *(long narrow arrow)*, main pulmonary artery *(curved arrow)*, left atrial appendage *(short arrow)*, and left ventricle *(broad arrow)*. The right pulmonary artery is larger than normal and tapers promptly, suggesting pulmonary hypertension. The right atrium is large.

Courtesy Wade Shuford, M.D., Professor of Radiology, Emory University School of Medicine, and the Radiology Service at Grady Memorial Hospital, Atlanta, Ga.

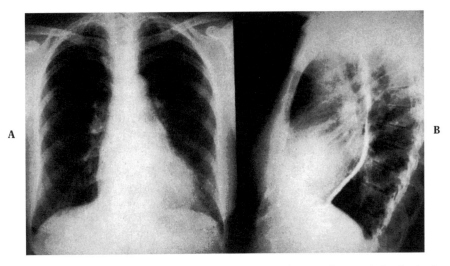

Fig. 8-13. Mitral valve stenosis. **A,** Note the four bumps that are characteristic of mitral stenosis. **B,** Posterior deviation of the barium-filled esophagus due to a large left atrium.

Reproduced with permission from Cobbs BW Jr: Clinical recognition and medical management of rheumatic fever and valvular heart disease. In Hurst JW, Logue RB, editors: *The heart*, ed 1, New York, 1966, McGraw-Hill, p 540.

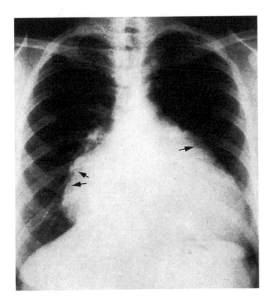

Fig. 8-14. Gross enlargement of the left atrium due to mitral valve disease. The left atrium forms the right border of the heart (*double arrows*), and the left atrial appendage is prominent (*single arrow*). The left ventricle and right atrium are enlarged.

Reproduced with permission from Rubens MB: Chest x-ray in adult heart disease. In Julian DG, Camm AJ, Fox KM, Hall RJC, Poole-Wilson PA, editors: *Diseases of the heart*, London, 1989, Baillière Tindall, p 277.

Left ventricular hypertrophy and enlargement

Concentric hypertrophy of the left ventricle may be present while the overall heart size remains within the normal range. Accordingly, patients with concentric left ventricular hypertrophy due to valvular aortic stenosis or patients with idiopathic cardiac hypertrophy may have signs of left ventricular hypertrophy that are apparent on the electrocardiogram but not on the chest x-ray film. When left ventricular dilatation plus left ventricular hypertrophy is present, the left lower region of the cardiac silhouette extends farther to the left and below the diaphragm in the PA view (see Fig. 8-8). The large left ventricle extends more posteriorly than normal in the lateral view (see Fig. 8-9). A roentgenogram illustrating left ventricular hypertrophy and enlargement is shown in Fig. 8-15.

Causes of left ventricular enlargement. The left ventricle may become enlarged as a result of hypertension, aortic stenosis and regurgitation, mitral regurgitation, dilated cardiomyopathy, a patent ductus arteriosus, or a ventricular septal defect. Volume overload of the left ventricle is likely to produce a larger left ventricle than that produced by pressure overload. The left ventricle may not appear enlarged until late in the course of primary hypertrophy of the heart or aortic valve stenosis.

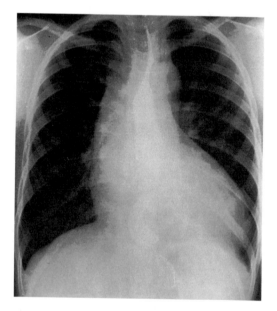

Fig. 8-15. Aortic valvular regurgitation. The left ventricle is dilated. There is downward and lateral displacement of the cardiac apex. The proximal portion of the aorta is dilated, and the pulmonary artery vasculature is normal.

Courtesy Wade Shuford, M.D., Professor of Radiology, Emory University School of Medicine, and the Radiology Service at Grady Memorial Hospital, Atlanta, Ga.

Right atrial enlargement

The lower right region of the heart extends farther to the right than normal when the right atrium is enlarged (see Fig. 8-10). However, the right atrium must be moderately enlarged for the increased size to be detected. A roentgenogram illustrating right atrial enlargement in a patient with Ebstein anomaly is shown in Fig. 8-16.

Causes of right atrial enlargement. The right atrium may be enlarged when the other three chambers of the heart are enlarged. It may also be larger than normal when there is primary pulmonary hypertension, pulmonary valve stenosis, tetralogy of Fallot, tricuspid stenosis, Eisenmenger syndrome, or Ebstein anomaly.

Right ventricular hypertrophy and enlargement

The right ventricle is an anterior structure. Accordingly, enlargement of the right ventricle does not alter the PA x-ray view of the chest. When the right ventricle enlarges, it may obliterate the retrosternal space. An x-ray film illustrating right ventricular enlargement is shown in Fig. 8-17.

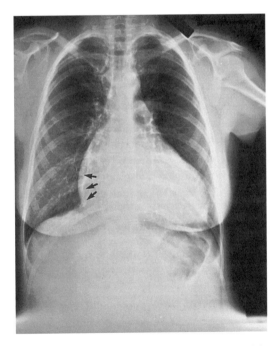

Fig. 8-16. Enlargement of the right atrium *(arrows)* in a 50-year-old woman with Ebstein anomaly. Compare the size of the large right atrium with the size of the normal right atrium shown in Fig. 8-4.

Courtesy Paul Robinson, M.D., Professor of Medicine (Cardiology); William Casarella, M.D., Professor and Chairman of the Department of Radiology of Emory University School of Medicine; and the Radiology Service of Emory University Hospital, Atlanta, Ga.

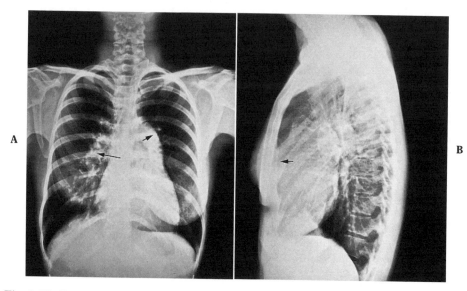

Fig. 8-17. Enlargement of the right ventricle, main pulmonary artery, and right pulmonary artery. **A,** The PA view of the chest shows a large main pulmonary artery (*short arrow*). The left branch of the pulmonary artery is not seen. The right branch of the pulmonary artery is large and tapers abruptly, suggesting severe pulmonary artery hypertension (*long arrow*). **B,** The left lateral view reveals right ventricular enlargement. Note how the right ventricle crowds out the retrosternal space (*arrow*). Compare the size of the right ventricle with the size of the normal right ventricle illustrated in Fig. 8-5. The patient had surgical repair of an ostium secundum atrial septal defect as a child; she is shown here at age 39 with severe pulmonary hypertension, which is probably primary pulmonary hypertension, because the pulmonary artery pressure was only slightly elevated at the time of the surgical repair of the atrial septal defect. She has since had a successful lung transplant.

Courtesy William Casarella, M.D., Professor and Chairman of the Department of Radiology of Emory University School of Medicine, and the Radiology Service of Emory University Hospital, Atlanta, Ga.

Causes of right ventricular enlargement. The right ventricle may be larger than normal when there is enlargement of the other three chambers of the heart. It may also be larger than normal when there is primary pulmonary hypertension, severe lung disease, Eisenmenger syndrome, tetralogy of Fallot, or pulmonary valve stenosis.

LOCATION, SHAPE, AND SIZE OF THE AORTA

The first part of the normal aorta is not seen on the PA chest x-ray film. The root of the aorta courses upward from the aortic valve, arching to the left of the trachea and esophagus to descend down the left side of the spine (see Fig. 8-4).

The root and ascending aorta

An example of dilatation of the first portion of the aorta due to congenital aortic valve stenosis is shown in Fig. 8-18.

Causes of dilatation of the first portion of the aorta. The root and ascending portion of the aorta may be increased in size by an atherosclerotic aneurysm, dissection of the aorta, medial disease associated with Marfan syndrome, annuloaortic ectasia, syphilis, poststenotic dilatation of the aorta due to congenital or acquired aortic valve stenosis, or aortic regurgitation from congenital or acquired disease.

The arch and descending portion of the aorta

The arch and the descending (thoracic) portion of the aorta may be abnormal as a result of the *figure 3 sign of coarctation* of the aorta (Fig. 8-19), dissection of the aorta, or an atherosclerotic or traumatic aneurysm of the aorta. The aorta may become elongated and tortuous as a result of sclerosis of its media.

A *right aortic arch* is present in approximately 25% of patients with tetralogy of Fallot (Fig. 8-20) and in 50% of patients with truncus arteriosus. This anomaly may occur as an incidental finding when there are no other cardiovascular anomalies.

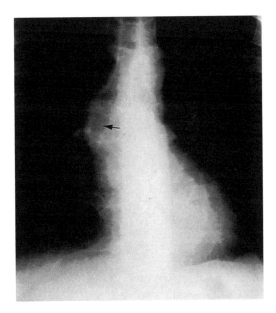

Fig. 8-18. Dilatation of the proximal portion of the aorta *(arrow)* due to severe aortic valve stenosis (congenital bicuspid aortic valve). The enlargement of the proximal aorta in this example is almost aneurysmal in contour; the enlargement is usually more subtle. The left ventricle is large.

Courtesy Wade Shuford, M.D., Professor of Radiology, Emory University School of Medicine, and the Radiology Service at Grady Memorial Hospital, Atlanta, Ga.

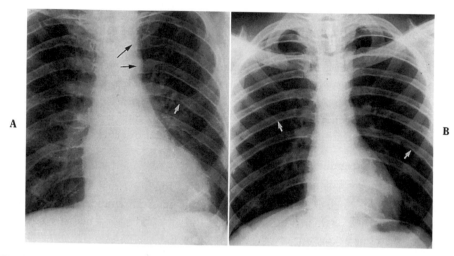

Fig. 8-19. A, Coarctation of the aorta. There is notching of the inferior rib margins (*white arrow*). Note the figure 3 sign (*black arrows*). The upper segment is composed of dilated left subclavian artery (*long black arrow*). The lower segment is produced by poststenotic dilatation of the descending aorta (*short black arrow*). **B,** Coarctation of the aorta. Note the slight notching of the inferior margins of the ribs (*arrows*). There is moderate cardiac enlargement as a result of left ventricular enlargement.

Courtesy Wade Shuford, M.D., Professor of Radiology, Emory University School of Medicine, and the Radiology Service at Grady Memorial Hospital, Atlanta, Ga.

Calcification of the intima of the ascending portion of the aorta, the arch of the aorta, and the descending portion of the aorta is due to atherosclerosis, but other disease processes may encourage its predilection for the aortic root just distal to the aortic valve. For example, syphilis of the aorta or giant cell arteritis should be suspected when flecks of calcium are noted in the initial portion of the aortic root (Fig. 8-21).

LOCATION, SHAPE, AND SIZE OF THE PULMONARY ARTERIES

The main pulmonary artery can be identified in the frontal roentgenogram. It is normally smaller than the aorta, forming the left upper cardiac border immediately below the aortic knob. The left branch of the pulmonary artery appears as a direct extension of the main pulmonary artery, coursing posteriorly behind the left mainstem bronchus. Accordingly, it may not be as visible as the right branch of the pulmonary artery, which emerges as an easily visible structure in the right hilum.

The size of the main pulmonary artery and its branches should be studied carefully, because normal pulmonary blood flow, increased pulmonary blood flow, de-

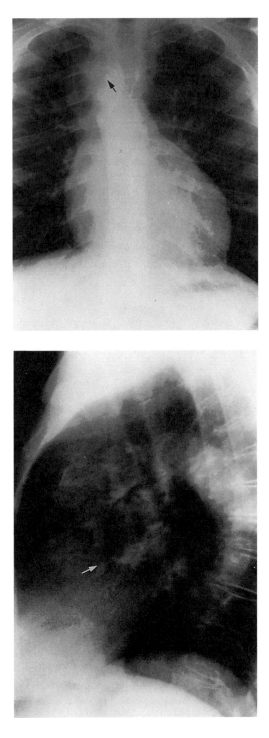

Fig. 8-20. Tetralogy of Fallot. The right aortic arch *(arrow)* indents the tracheal air column. The main pulmonary artery segment is flat. The right and left pulmonary arteries are small, indicating a decrease in pulmonary artery blood flow.

Courtesy Wade Shuford, M.D., Professor of Radiology, Emory University School of Medicine, and the Radiology Service at Grady Memorial Hospital, Atlanta, Ga.

Fig. 8-21. Syphilitic aortitis. Note the calcification of the intima of the first portion of the aorta *(arrow)* in the left lateral roentgenogram.

Courtesy Wade Shuford, M.D., Professor of Radiology, Emory University School of Medicine, and the Radiology Service at Grady Memorial Hospital, Atlanta, Ga.

creased pulmonary blood flow, and increased pulmonary artery pressure can be suspected from their size and shape.

Normal pulmonary blood flow

The pulmonary blood flow is considered normal when the main pulmonary artery and its right and left branches are normal in size and distribution (Fig. 8-22).

Decreased pulmonary blood flow

The main pulmonary artery and its left and right branches are smaller than normal when there is decreased pulmonary blood flow. The small size of the pulmonary arteries makes the lung fields appear radiolucent. A roentgenogram illustrating a decrease in pulmonary blood flow is shown in Fig. 8-23.

Causes of decreased pulmonary blood flow. Patients with tetralogy of Fallot have decreased pulmonary blood flow. Other conditions associated with a decrease in pulmonary blood flow are tricuspid atresia, type 4 truncus arteriosus, and pulmonary artery atresia.

Increased pulmonary blood flow

When the pulmonary blood flow is increased, the main pulmonary artery and hilar branches may appear larger than normal on the chest roentgenogram. The periph-

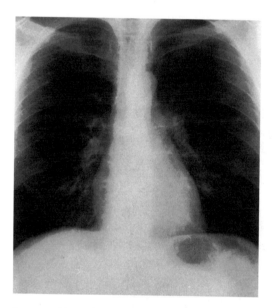

Fig. 8-22. Normal pulmonary blood flow. Note the size and shape of the pulmonary arteries. Courtesy Wade Shuford, M.D., Professor of Radiology, Emory University School of Medicine, and the Radiology Service at Grady Memorial Hospital, Atlanta, Ga.

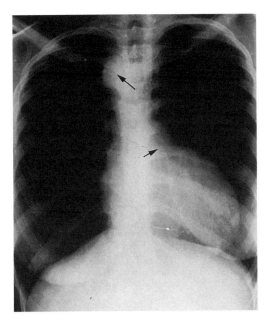

Fig. 8-23. Decreased pulmonary blood flow in a patient with tetralogy of Fallot. Note the right aortic arch *(long arrow)*. The main pulmonary artery is not visible *(short arrow)*. The shadows of the pulmonary arteries and veins are barely visible. The cardiac apex is elevated. These findings are characteristic of marked right ventricular hypertrophy rather than left ventricular hypertrophy.

Courtesy Wade Shuford, M.D., Professor of Radiology, Emory University School of Medicine, and the Radiology Service at Grady Memorial Hospital, Atlanta, Ga.

eral branches of the pulmonary artery dilate, giving the lungs a plethoric appearance. An example of this abnormality is shown in Fig. 8-24.

Causes of increased pulmonary blood flow. An increase in pulmonary blood flow is seen in patients with patent ductus arteriosus and an interventricular septal defect, in which cases the aortic knob is normal or larger than normal; in patients with secundum atrial septal defect, in which cases the aortic knob is small; in patients with transposition of the great vessels; and in patients with type 1, 2, or 3 truncus arteriosus. In types 1, 2, and 3 truncus arteriosus the pulmonary arteries arise from the common trunk.

Increased pulmonary artery pressure

Patients with an increase in pulmonary artery pressure may exhibit a larger than normal main pulmonary artery. The hilar branches also enlarge and taper abruptly (Fig. 8-25; see also Fig. 18-17).

Fig. 8-24. Increased pulmonary blood flow in a patient with an ostium secundum atrial septal defect. Note the large main pulmonary artery *(long arrow)*, large right pulmonary artery *(curved arrow)*, large pulmonary veins *(broad arrows)*, and small aortic knob *(short arrow)*. The heart is slightly enlarged as a result of right ventricular and right atrial enlargement.

Courtesy Wade Shuford, M.D., Professor of Radiology, Emory University School of Medicine, and the Radiology Service at Grady Memorial Hospital, Atlanta, Ga.

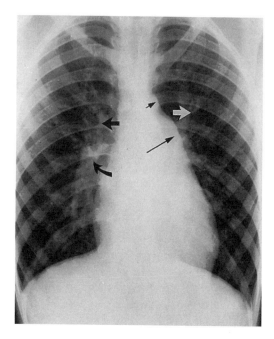

Fig. 8-25. Pulmonary artery hypertension. The main pulmonary artery is large *(long arrow)*. The left pulmonary artery is not seen, because it courses posteriorly. The right pulmonary artery is large *(short arrow)*; it tapers *(broad arrow)* abruptly, signifying pulmonary artery hypertension. The patient had primary pulmonary hypertension.

Reproduced with permission from Weens HS, Gay BB Jr: Radiologic examination of the heart. In Hurst JW, Logue RB, editors: *The heart,* ed 1, New York, 1966, McGraw-Hill, p 162.

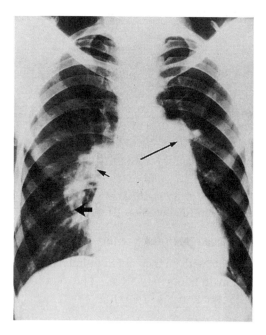

Causes of pulmonary artery hypertension

Pulmonary artery hypertension occurs in patients with primary pulmonary hypertension; in patients with Eisenmenger physiology associated with interventricular septal defect, patent ductus arteriosus, or ostium secundum atrial septal defect; in patients with repeated pulmonary emboli; in patients with mitral stenosis; and, to a lesser degree, in patients with left ventricular heart failure.

The main pulmonary artery may become larger than normal when there is pulmonary valve stenosis. This abnormality may be similar to the large pulmonary artery that accompanies pulmonary hypertension. The size of the right and left branches of the pulmonary artery are different in the two conditions. The left branch may be large and the right branch is normal size in patients with pulmonary valve stenosis, whereas the right branch is large in patients with pulmonary hypertension.

PULMONARY VEINS

The pulmonary veins, which course from their superior position in the lungs toward the left atrium, are barely seen in the normal PA chest roentgenogram (see Fig. 8-22).

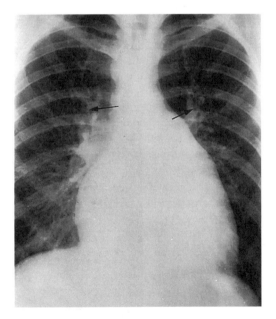

Fig. 8-26. Prominent pulmonary veins *(arrows)* in the upper lobes of the lungs in a patient with mitral valve stenosis and regurgitation. This abnormal redistribution of blood flow from the lungs is associated with an elevated left atrial pressure. Note the four bumps of the left lateral heart border. There is left atrial and left ventricular enlargement.

Courtesy Wade Shuford, M.D., Professor of Radiology, Emory University School of Medicine, and the Radiology Service at Grady Memorial Hospital, Atlanta, Ga.

The pulmonary veins become more prominent when the left atrial pressure is higher than normal from any cause, including mitral stenosis (Fig. 8-26); mitral regurgitation; and heart failure due to aortic valve disease, hypertension, coronary artery disease, or cardiomyopathy. The pulmonary veins may also be prominent when there is an increase in pulmonary blood flow, such as occurs with a large ostium secundum septal defect (see Fig. 8-24).

CALCIFICATION OF CARDIOVASCULAR STRUCTURES

Intracardiac calcification

Calcification of the aortic valve. The aortic valve may become calcified in patients with aortic valve stenosis due to rheumatic heart disease, congenital aortic valve stenosis, or calcific aortic valve disease of the elderly. The location of the aortic valve itself is illustrated in Figs. 8-4 and 8-5. Aortic valve calcification is seen best in the left lateral x-ray film of the chest (it is difficult to visualize in the PA x-ray film of the chest, because the sternum and vertebral column mask its visibility). When a line is drawn from the carina to the anterior costophrenic angle, the aortic valve calcification lies superior to the line or straddles it (Fig. 8-27).

Calcification of the mitral valve. The mitral valve leaflets may become calcified in patients with rheumatic mitral valve stenosis or regurgitation. The calcification can be identified best in the lateral chest roentgenogram; it is located posterior to a line drawn from the carina to the anterior costophrenic angle (Fig. 8-28).

Calcification of the mitral valve annulus. Calcification of the mitral valve annulus produces a large, smooth, curved intracardiac structure (Fig. 8-29). Calcification

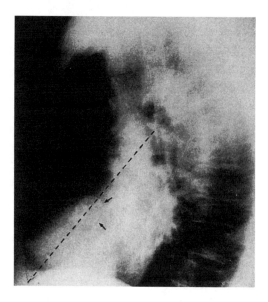

Fig. 8-27. Calcific aortic valve stenosis (*arrows*). Note in the lateral view of the chest that the calcification straddles a line drawn from the carina to the anterior costophrenic angle.

Reproduced with permission from Rubens MB: Chest x-ray in adult heart disease. In Julian DG, Camm AJ, Fox KM, Hall RJC, Poole-Wilson PA, editors: *Diseases of the heart*, London, 1989, Baillière Tindall, p 284.

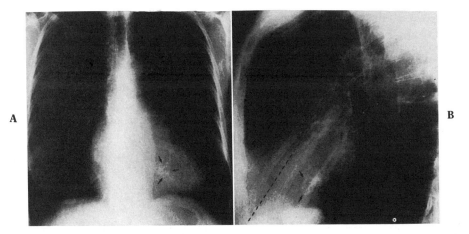

Fig. 8-28. Mitral valve calcification. **A,** On the frontal view the calcified valve *(arrows)* is lateral to the spine. **B,** On the lateral view the calcification *(arrows)* is posterior to a line drawn from the carina to the anterior costophrenic angle.

Reproduced with permission from Rubens MB: Chest x-ray in adult heart disease. In Julian DG, Camm AJ, Fox KM, Hall RJC, Poole-Wilson PA, editors: *Diseases of the heart*, London, 1989, Baillière Tindall, p 285.

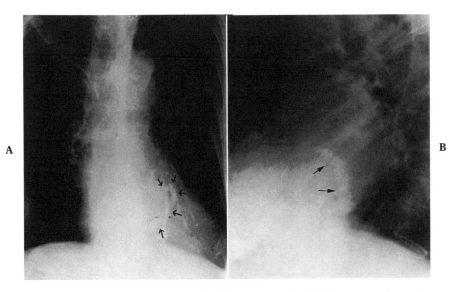

Fig. 8-29. Calcified mitral valve annulus. **A,** A large curved calcified structure *(arrows)* is seen in the PA view of the heart. **B,** A large curved calcified structure *(arrows)* is seen in the left lateral view of the heart.

Courtesy Wade Shuford, M.D., Professor of Radiology, Emory University School of Medicine, and the Radiology Service at Grady Memorial Hospital, Atlanta, Ga.

of the mitral valve annulus is caused by a degenerative process that is poorly understood.

Calcification of an atrial myxoma. Calcification of an atrial myxoma may be seen within the left atrium (Fig. 8-30).

Calcification within the atrial and ventricular myocardium

Curvilinear calcification of the myocardium may occur at the site of an old myocardial infarction (Fig. 8-31).

Calcification of the atrial wall is illustrated in Fig. 8-32. It is rarely seen but may follow myocarditis resulting from rheumatic fever.

Calcification of the coronary arteries

Calcification of atherosclerotic lesions may be seen in the larger coronary arteries (Fig. 8-33). This signifies advanced coronary atherosclerosis.

Calcification of the pericardium

Calcification of the pericardium is identified best in the lateral chest x-ray film (Fig. 8-34). It does not in itself indicate constrictive pericarditis; the appropriate physiologic derangements must be present before cardiac constriction can be diagnosed.

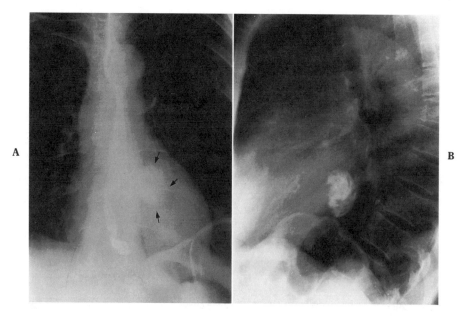

Fig. 8-30. A, Calcification of a left atrial myxoma (*arrows*) as seen in the PA view. **B,** Calcification of a left atrial myxoma as seen in the lateral roentgenogram of the heart.

Courtesy Wade Shuford, M.D., Professor of Radiology, Emory University School of Medicine, and the Radiology Service at Grady Memorial Hospital, Atlanta, Ga.

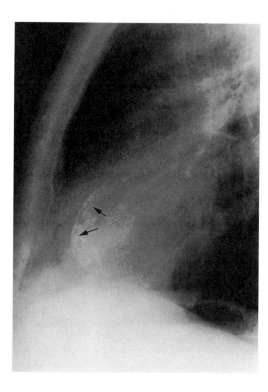

Fig. 8-31. Calcification at the site of an anteroseptal myocardial infarction (*arrows*).

Courtesy Wade Shuford, M.D., Professor of Radiology, Emory University School of Medicine, and the Radiology Service at Grady Memorial Hospital, Atlanta, Ga.

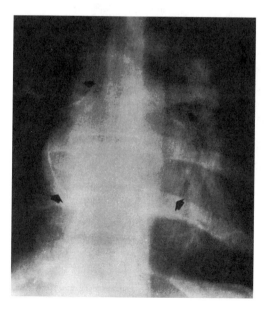

Fig. 8-32. Extensive curvilinear calcification of the left atrial wall (*arrows*).

Reproduced with permission from Weens HS, Gay BB Jr: Radiologic examination of the heart. In Hurst JW, Logue RB, editors: *The heart*, ed 1, New York, 1966, McGraw-Hill, p 156.

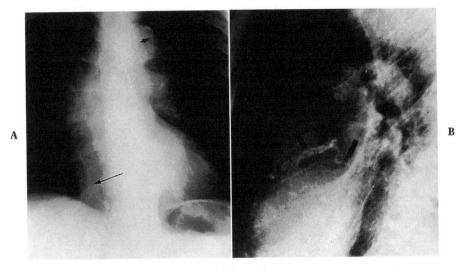

Fig. 8-33. A, PA view of the chest showing a calcified right coronary artery *(long arrow)*. The aorta is dilated and tortuous. Note calcification of the interior of the aorta in the region of the aortic knob *(short arrow)*. **B,** Calcification of the left anterior descending and circumflex coronary arteries *(arrows)*.

A courtesy Wade Shuford, M.D., Professor of Radiology, Emory University School of Medicine, and the Radiology Service at Grady Memorial Hospital, Atlanta, Ga. **B** reproduced with permission from Weens HS, Gay BB Jr: Radiologic examination of the heart. In Hurst JW, Logue RB, editors: *The heart*, ed 1, New York, 1966, McGraw-Hill, p 156.

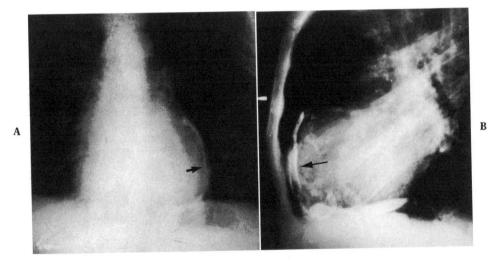

Fig. 8-34. Calcification of the pericardium. Calcification of the pericardium is usually seen more easily in the left lateral view; in this patient it is seen in the PA, **A,** and left lateral, **B,** views *(arrows)*.

Reproduced with permission from Weens HS, Gay BB Jr. Radiologic examination of the heart. In Hurst JW, Logue RB, editors: *The heart*, ed 1, New York, 1966, McGraw-Hill, p 157.

Calcification of the intima of the aortic root and ascending, transverse, and descending portions of the aorta

See earlier discussion and Fig. 8-21.

ABNORMAL BULGE OF THE LEFT VENTRICLE

A left ventricular aneurysm may follow myocardial infarction (Fig. 8-35).

ABNORMALITIES OF THE LUNGS

Pulmonary disease such as pulmonary emphysema due to obstructive lung disease, pneumoconiosis such as silicosis, interstitial fibrosis, and granulomatous disease such as sarcoidosis may be detected in the frontal chest x-ray film. These diseases may be responsible for cor pulmonale.

A *pneumothorax* may be identified on the PA chest x-ray film. This, at times, explains a patient's chest discomfort and dyspnea.

A *pulmonary infarct* is suspected when there is a wedgelike shadow adjacent to a pleural surface, elevation of one of the leaflets of the diaphragm, and pleural fluid.

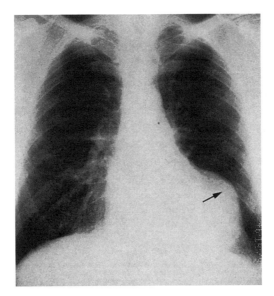

Fig. 8-35. Left ventricular aneurysm. Note the bulge in the middle of the left cardiac border (*arrow*).

Reproduced with permission from Rubens MB: Chest x-ray in adult heart disease. In Julian DG, Camm AJ, Fox KM, Hall RJC, Poole-Wilson PA, editors: *Diseases of the heart*, London, 1989, Baillière Tindall, p 280.

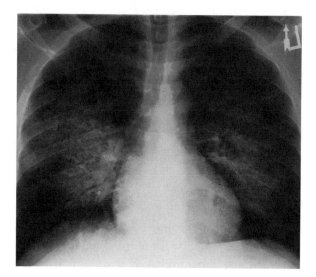

Fig. 8-36. Acute alveolar pulmonary edema as seen in the PA view of the chest. Diffuse alveolar bilateral infiltrates are noted in the central and posterior aspects of the lungs, forming a pattern of distribution that simulates butterfly wings. This type of pulmonary edema is caused by abrupt dysfunction of the left ventricle. It can also be caused by noncardiac conditions (see Fig. 8-38).

Courtesy Wade Shuford, M.D., Professor of Radiology, Emory University School of Medicine, and the Radiology Service at Grady Memorial Hospital, Atlanta, Ga.

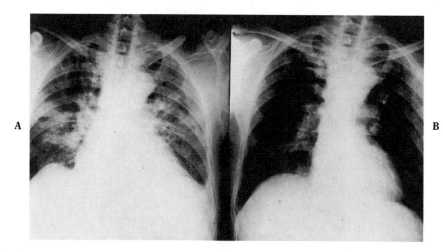

Fig. 8-37. Alveolar pulmonary edema due to acute heart failure in a 64-year-old man with atherosclerotic heart disease and aortic regurgitation. **A,** Alveolar pulmonary edema of the lobular type that may be mistaken for pulmonary infection, pulmonary infarction, or pulmonary neoplasm. **B,** Clearing after 4 days of heart failure.

Reproduced with permission from Logue RB, Hurst JW: Etiology and clinical recognition of heart failure. In Hurst JW, Logue RB, editors: *The heart,* ed 1, New York, 1966, McGraw-Hill, p 263.

HEART FAILURE

The PA chest x-ray film may reveal numerous signs of congestive heart failure.

Acute *alveolar pulmonary edema* can be identified by a great increase in haziness occurring near the hilum of each lung and extending like butterfly wings into the lung tissue (Figs. 8-36 and 8-37). This pattern of haziness is caused by an excess of fluid in the alveolar spaces. The area of increased density may be patchy, especially when previous lung disease has produced pulmonary scar tissue. Acute pulmonary edema may be precipitated by an acute myocardial infarction, acute rupture of a chordae tendineae of the mitral valve, uncontrolled atrial fibrillation in a patient with tight mitral stenosis, or a cardiac arrhythmia with a rapid rate in a patient with poor left ventricular function from any cause. When acute pulmonary edema occurs as the result of acute myocardial infarction or ruptured chordae tendineae, the heart size is normal. There are, however, some noncardiac causes of acute alveolar pulmonary edema, including smoke inhalation, toxic nephritis from carbon tetrachloride (Fig. 8-38), drowning, extreme hypervolemia, and extensive viral pneumonia. High-altitude pulmonary edema may occur in patients with normal hearts, but it is actually caused by an alteration in cardiovascular physiology.

Interstitial pulmonary edema may also occur acutely, although its radiographic characteristics are discussed on p. 458 with the abnormalities identifying chronic heart failure. It is caused by the appearance of fluid in the interstitial spaces between the

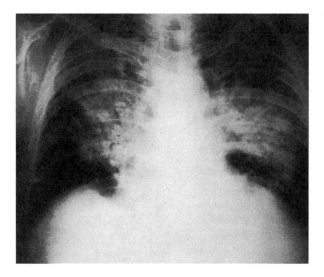

Fig. 8-38. Alveolar pulmonary edema in a 53-year-old man following ingestion of carbon tetrachloride.

Reproduced with permission from Logue RB, Hurst JW: Etiology and clinical recognition of heart failure. In Hurst JW, Logue RB, editors: *The heart*, ed 1, New York, 1966, McGraw-Hill, p 265.

alveoli rather than by the entrance of fluid into the alveolar spaces. It may be caused by the same conditions mentioned in relation to alveolar pulmonary edema.

Chronic heart failure can be identified in the PA chest x-ray film by identifying one or more of the following abnormalities:

- The superior pulmonary veins become more prominent when there is an increase in left atrial pressure (see Fig. 8-26).
- Kerley B lines may become visible when the left atrial pressure becomes elevated (Fig. 8-39). These lines, which are due to edematous intralobular septa, occur more commonly in patients with mitral stenosis than in patients with heart failure from other causes.
- Interstitial pulmonary edema is due to the accumulation of excess fluid in the interstitial tissues of the lungs (Fig. 8-40, *B*). It is also seen around the branches of the pulmonary arteries (referred to as periarterial cuffing). The margins of the pulmonary artery branches seem to be out of focus, because the periarterial fluid blurs their margins (Fig. 8-41).
- Pleural fluid, as well as subpulmonary fluid, due to heart failure may be seen in both costophrenic angles but is greater on the right than on the left (Figs. 8-42 and 8-43). Pleural fluid due to heart failure is rarely seen on the left side only. With a large right pleural effusion due to heart failure the mediastinum may not shift, because the lungs are stiffer than normal as a result of reduced lung compliance.

A "phantom tumor" is due to encapsulated pleural effusion that is trapped in the right major interlobar fissure. The "tumor" clears with the treatment of heart failure (Fig. 8-44).

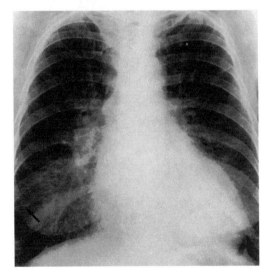

Fig. 8-39. Kerley B lines are noted in the lower lung fields (*arrow*). There is also perivascular cuffing, and the pulmonary veins are prominent. These abnormalities are all due to left ventricular dysfunction. The heart is enlarged. Courtesy Wade Shuford, M.D., Professor of Radiology, Emory University School of Medicine, and the Radiology Service at Grady Memorial Hospital, Atlanta, Ga.

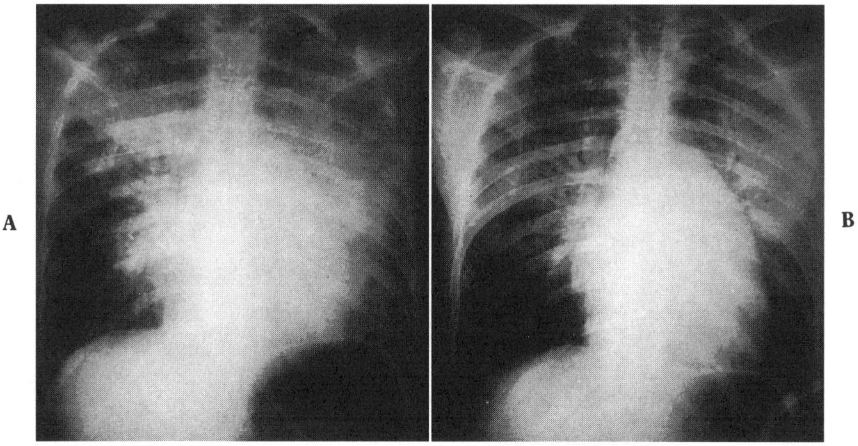

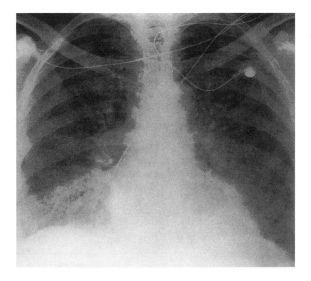

Fig. 8-40. Roentgenogram of a 24-year-old man with tight mitral stenosis. **A,** PA view of the chest showing alveolar pulmonary edema. **B,** PA view of the chest showing partial clearing on the right and interstitial pulmonary edema on the left.

Reproduced with permission from Logue RB, Hurst JW: Etiology and clinical recognition of heart failure. In Hurst JW, Logue RB, editors: *The heart*, ed 1, New York, 1966, McGraw-Hill, p 265.

Fig. 8-41. Interstitial edema of the lungs due to left ventricular dysfunction. Note the haziness and clouding of the lungs. The borders of the pulmonary arteries are indistinct (periarterial cuffing), and the pulmonary veins are prominent. The heart is enlarged.

Courtesy Wade Shuford, M.D., Professor of Radiology, Emory University School of Medicine, and the Radiology Service at Grady Memorial Hospital, Atlanta, Ga.

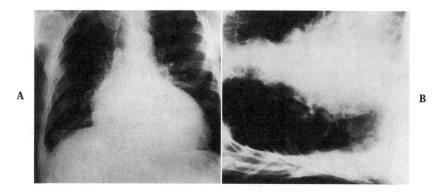

Fig. 8-42. Subpulmonary fluid on the right in a patient with congestive heart failure. **A,** PA view with the patient upright. The right leaf of the diaphragm appears to be elevated. **B,** Film made in the decubitus position (right side down) showing that the subpulmonary fluid has gravitated to the dependent portion of the chest.

Reproduced with permission from Fowler NO: Radiologic clues to cardiac diagnosis. In Fowler NO, editor: *Cardiac diagnosis*, New York, 1968, Harper & Row, p 59.

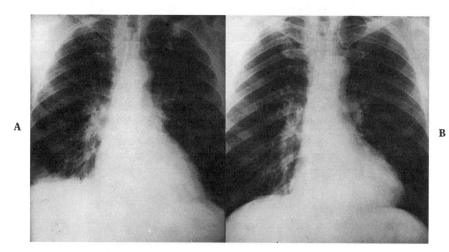

Fig. 8-43. Roentgenograms of a 57-year-old man with atherosclerotic coronary heart disease and heart failure. **A,** Subpulmonary fluid is noted on the right; there is also slight interstitial pulmonary edema. **B,** Clearing of the subpulmonary fluid and interstitial pulmonary edema after 4 days of treatment for heart failure.

Reproduced with permission from Logue RB, Hurst JW: Etiology and clinical recognition of heart failure. In Hurst JW, Logue RB, editors: *The heart*, ed 1, New York, 1966, McGraw-Hill, p 264.

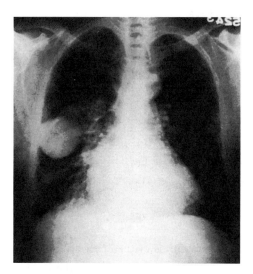

Fig. 8-44. "Phantom tumor." Pleural fluid due to heart failure may accumulate in the major interlobar fissure on the right, giving the appearance of a tumor. The fluid disappears after treatment for heart failure.

Reproduced with permission from Fowler NO: Radiologic clues to cardiac diagnosis. In Fowler NO, editor: *Cardiac diagnosis*, New York, 1968, Harper & Row, p 58.

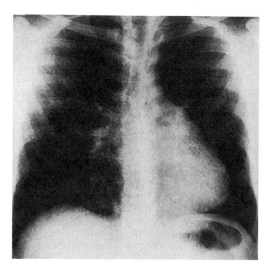

Fig. 8-45. Depression of the sternum causing apparent cardiac enlargement. Note leftward displacement of the heart in the PA view.

Reproduced with permission from Rubens MB: Chest x-ray in adult heart disease. In Julian DG, Camm AJ, Fox KM, Hall RJC, Poole-Wilson PA, editors: *Diseases of the heart*, London, 1989, Baillière Tindall, p 262.

ABNORMALITIES OF THE BONES

Rib notching occurs in patients with coarctation of the aorta (see Fig. 8-19). The scalloping of the inferior surface of the posterior ribs is rarely seen in patients under the age of 8 but is commonly seen in adults. It is due to tortuous, dilated intercostal arteries.

The PA and left lateral chest x-ray films of patients with *ankylosing spondylitis* are diagnostic. Patients with this condition may have aortic regurgitation and complete heart block.

A *depressed sternum* may force the heart toward the left, and this appearance on the x-ray film may be mistaken for cardiac enlargement (Fig. 8-45).

Key Points

- The PA and left lateral x-ray films of the chest are excellent diagnostic tools.
- The overall heart size, as well as enlargement of the individual cardiac chambers, can be detected through use of the chest x-ray film.
- The x-ray film of the chest may reveal evidence of pericardial effusion. The size and location of the aortic arch and the size and shape of the pulmonary arteries can be identified, and an increase or decrease in pulmonary artery blood flow can be detected.
- Pulmonary artery hypertension and an elevation of pulmonary venous pressure can be detected through use of the chest x-ray film.
- Calcification of the pericardium, myocardium, left atrium, coronary arteries, aortic and mitral valves, and aortic root, as well as an intracardiac tumor, can be seen on the chest x-ray film.
- Signs of heart failure may be seen on the chest x-ray film even when few clues are detected in the history or physical examination.
- A chest x-ray film may reveal evidence of lung disease and bone disease that may cause or be associated with heart disease.
- Despite the abnormalities that may be observed on the chest x-ray film, serious heart disease can be present and the chest x-ray film may be normal. Thus the technique of chest roentgenography does have limitations.

REFERENCES

1. Chen JTT: Technique of cardiac fluoroscopy. In Hurst JW, editor-in-chief: *The heart*, ed 7, New York, 1990, McGraw-Hill, p 1853.
2. Smith HW, Bloedorn WA: The size of the normal heart, a teleroentgen study, *US Naval Med Bull* 16:219, 1922.
3. White PD: *Heart disease*, New York, 1931, Macmillan, pp 143-144.
4. Weens HS, Gay BB Jr: Radiologic examination of the heart. In Hurst JW, Logue RB, editors: *The heart*, ed 1, New York, 1966, McGraw-Hill, p 148.

CHAPTER 9

Routine examination of the urine and blood

We need some imaginative stimulus, some not impossible ideal such as may shape vague hope, and transform it into effective desire, to carry us year after year, without disgust, through the routine work which is so large a part of life.

WALTER PATER 1885*

There is little information about the diagnostic value of routine examination of the urine and blood in textbooks on medicine[1] and cardiology.[2] This is proper, because routine examination of the urine and blood rarely yields diagnostic clues indicating the presence of cardiovascular disease. This will not always be the case, because the biochemical, molecular biologic, and genetic era of cardiology is just beginning; in the future it is likely that the early markers of many cardiovascular problems will be discovered by testing the urine and blood. When such tests are devised, new routine testing will be done.

EXAMINATION OF THE URINE

Routine urine examination may yield information in the following areas. *Albuminuria* may occur in patients with hypertension and renal disease. *Red blood cells* may appear in the urine of patients with acute glomerular disease or renal emboli from infective endocarditis. *Glycosuria* and *microproteinuria* occur in patients with diabetes mellitus and indicate that the patient is at risk for the future development of coronary and peripheral arterial atherosclerosis.

EXAMINATION OF THE BLOOD

Anemia from many causes may be recognized by a hematocrit value that is less than 40 vol% in men and 37 vol% in women.

Anemia may contribute to the development, or worsening, of angina pectoris and

*Pater W: *Marius the epicurean*, 1885.

heart failure. Severe anemia alone may cause high-output cardiac failure, and sickle cell anemia may cause myocardial disease and painful joints.

Patients who are hypoxic as a result of congenital heart disease with a right-to-left shunt may have *erythrocytosis* and an *elevated hematocrit value*. Such patients may develop cerebral thrombosis.

Leukocytosis may occur in patients with infective endocarditis. The total white blood cell count is usually only slightly elevated, and counts in the range of 15,000/dl^3 to 20,000/dl^3 may signal the presence of myocardial abscess, including a valve ring abscess, in a patient with infective endocarditis. *Leukemia* may also be detected by an elevation of the leukocyte or lymphocyte count; this disease may affect the myocardium.

Eosinophilia may occur in patients with "blue toe" syndrome, which is due to cholesterol emboli to the toes from proximal atherosclerotic plaques in the arteries to the legs. Eosinophilia may also occur in Fiedler myocarditis; in eosinophilic myalgia syndrome, which may be associated with myocarditis; and in toxic oil syndrome, which causes pulmonary hypertension.

Elevated blood urea nitrogen and *creatinine levels* may occur in patients with renal disease and are a common finding in patients with long-standing hypertension. Renal failure, of course, may contribute to heart failure and should always be considered when a physician prescribes digitalis, potassium supplements, and any drug that is eliminated by the kidneys.

A repeated *elevation of the blood glucose level* to 140 mg/dl or more in the fasting patient is strong evidence of diabetes mellitus. Accordingly, when the level of the initial blood glucose measurement is above 140 mg/dl, it is necessary to repeat the measurement. Diabetes, of course, puts the patient at risk for developing atherosclerotic arterial disease.

The *total plasma cholesterol* should be measured initially and routinely in all patients above the age of 20. A total plasma cholesterol value of 199 mg/dl or below is considered desirable; testing in patients with a cholesterol level in this range need not be repeated for several years. These patients should, however, follow the American Heart Association's recommendation regarding their diet in an effort to prevent atherosclerotic coronary heart disease. When the total plasma cholesterol value is above 199 mg/dl, additional lipid studies are recommended (see Chapter 10).[3] More specific treatment may be needed in these patients in order to reduce the likelihood of atherosclerotic coronary heart disease. The total plasma cholesterol should be measured initially in children who are above age 2 when there is a family history of atherosclerotic coronary heart disease or hypercholesterolemia.[3]

It is likely that other lipids will be measured routinely in the future. For example, some experts on atherosclerosis suggest that the total cholesterol, high- and low-density lipoproteins, and triglycerides be measured routinely in all adults.

Routine measurement of the *serum electrolytes* can be justified in patients who are ill and do not have simple, self-limiting diseases and in all hospitalized patients. Although the yield of abnormalities revealed through such testing is low, there is no other way to ensure that there is no electrolyte abnormality. A *serum calcium level that is low or high* may explain an abnormality in the electrocardiogram and assist one in the search for hypoparathyroidism or hyperparathyroidism, renal disease, etc. A *low serum potassium level* may occur in patients receiving diuretics or in patients with hyperaldosteronism and may explain a patient's electrocardiographic abnormality, hypertension, or weakness. The alert physician will be cautious in the use of digitalis in such a patient. A surprisingly *high serum potassium level* may occur secondary to renal failure or the use of potassium-sparing diuretics and may also explain certain abnormalities in the electrocardiogram. The *serum sodium level may be alarmingly low* as a result of dilutional hyponatremia in a patient with heart failure or in a patient who has been diuresed excessively.

The level of *lactic dehydrogenase (LDH)*, which is measured when the SMA panel of tests is ordered, may be elevated in a patient who is taking lovastatin (Mevacor) for hyperlipidemia.

CAVEAT

It is not easy to define the tests that should be performed on the urine and blood of every patient. Practically, one would require that the yield of abnormalities be sufficiently high to justify the time, effort, and cost of performing the test. However, such testing reveals abnormalities in only a small percentage of patients. The problem is compounded, because an SMA panel of tests is as easy, and as inexpensive, to order as a single specific test.

It appears that practicing physicians have determined, on the basis of their day-to-day experience, that it is diagnostically useful and cost-effective to order routine urine and blood examination and an SMA for every patient. It is clearly the best way to diagnose early diabetes mellitus and the only way to detect abnormal lipid metabolism and early renal failure. A primary care physician is profoundly influenced by his or her recent experiences with patients. If the physician missed a diagnosis of diabetes mellitus in a patient he or she saw recently, the physician is likely to order a routine blood glucose determination for all patients, even if a scientific study shows that the yield of abnormal test results is small.

The discussion in this brief chapter is not complete, because the behavioral patterns and beliefs of thousands of physicians cannot be summated. This problem is highlighted by the following examples.

Suppose, on routine testing, that a certain test is positive in 1% of the population tested. Suppose, too, that the test costs $100 and, when positive, implies that the patient has a certain benign disease for which there is no current treatment. Would you, the reader, order this test for every patient?

Suppose, on routine testing, that a certain test is positive in 0.1% of the population tested. Suppose, too, that the test costs $1 and, when positive, implies that the patient has a certain malignant disease for which a cure is available. Would you, the reader, order this test for every patient?

These two examples emphasize the difficulty encountered in trying to establish the tests that one can justify ordering in the so-called routine examination of the blood and urine. Accordingly, this chapter has dealt with only a small part of the problem. Furthermore, the discussion is limited to the value of routine testing of the urine and blood in one's quest for the diagnosis of the presence of, or the future development of, cardiovascular disease.

REFERENCES

1. Hurst JW, editor-in-chief: *Medicine for the practicing physician,* ed 3, Boston, 1992, Butterworth.
2. Hurst JW, editor-in-chief: *The heart,* ed 7, New York, 1990, McGraw-Hill.
3. Brown WV: Lipoproteins: what, when, and how often to measure, *Heart Dis Stroke* 1(1):20, 1992.

CHAPTER 10

Use of high technology for diagnostic purposes

Be not the first by whom the new are tried nor yet the last to lay the old aside.

ALEXANDER POPE 1711*

The quotation attributed to Alexander Pope has always intrigued me. If his admonition were believed by everyone, there would be no research. This, of course, would be catastrophic, because without research there would be no improvement in medicine. On the other hand, wise clinicians perceive a great deal of truth in Pope's statement. Clinicians, whose primary mission is to care for their patients, soon learn that the value of a new procedure or treatment may not be determined until the procedure or treatment has been used in the field for several years after the research has been completed.

Chapters 5 through 9 of this book deal with use of the medical history, the physical examination, analysis of the electrocardiogram, interpretation of the chest x-ray film, and interpretation of the results of "routine" examination of the blood and urine. These techniques are referred to as being part of low technology. Proficiency in these techniques enables clinicians to either make a specific cardiovascular diagnosis or create a differential cardiovascular diagnosis in virtually every patient they examine. Having done so, clinicians must ask the questions presented here.

If a single, specific cardiovascular diagnosis has been formulated after a review of the abnormalities discovered by the use of low technology, the clinician should ask if the diagnosis *could be* further refined and, just as important, if it *should be* further refined. Two case studies are presented to serve as examples for further discussion:

PATIENT 1

A 75-year-old woman with long-standing diabetes mellitus has dyspnea on effort, a pulsus alternans, a cardiac apex that is easily seen in the midaxillary line, a deep systolic jugular venous pulse, no heart murmurs, left bundle-branch block in the electrocardiogram, evidence of generalized cardiac enlargement and heart failure in the chest x-ray film, a blood glucose level of 180 mg/dl, and 1+ glycosuria. The complete cardiac diagnosis is as follows:

---

*Pope A: *An essay on criticism,* 1711, L 135.

Problem 1: Organic heart disease
 Etiology: *Dilated cardiomyopathy (etiology unknown)*
 Anatomy: *All heart chambers enlarged*
 Physiology: *Severe heart failure, normal sinus rhythm, left bundle-branch block*
 Cardiac status: *Severely compromised*
 Prognosis: *Poor with medical therapy*
Problem 2: Diabetes mellitus

What, if any, additional testing is needed in the above example? Some physicians would obtain an echocardiogram in order to measure the exact size of the cardiac chambers and determine the ejection fraction, whereas others would feel secure that there was ample evidence that all heart chambers were quite large and that the pulsus alternans found in this setting indicated that the ejection fraction was below 30% and was probably 15% to 20%. Some physicians would order catheterization of both sides of the heart and coronary arteriography in order to state the physiologic derangement with more precision and to determine if the dilated heart was caused by atherosclerotic coronary heart disease. Others would think that if coronary disease were found, it would not matter, because the heart muscle had been destroyed and neither bypass surgery nor angioplasty could be used. Some would order a myocardial biopsy when, in fact, the results would not alter the treatment of the patient. Some astute clinician might suggest that this diabetic woman might have hemochromatosis, and results of the myocardial biopsy might reveal it. A specific treatment might be available should this be the correct diagnosis. An even more astute physician might respond that it would be simpler to measure the serum ferritin and transferrin levels.

The above example serves to emphasize that, at times, although many diagnostic procedures could be ordered, because the diagnosis is obvious and the cardiac status is so severely compromised, further diagnostic testing should not be ordered.

PATIENT 2

A tall 22-year-old asymptomatic woman plans to apply for a life insurance policy. The entire examination is normal except for a midsystolic click at the cardiac apex followed by a grade 1 late systolic murmur. The cardiac diagnosis is as follows:
Problem 1: Organic heart disease
 Etiology: *Mitral valve prolapse*
 Anatomy: *Unknown*
 Physiology: *Slight mitral regurgitation*
 Cardiac status: *Not compromised*
 Prognosis: *Good with medical treatment (bacterial endocarditis prophylaxis)*

In this example it would be appropriate to obtain an echocardiogram. The procedure is not needed for diagnostic purposes, because the auscultatory findings are definite. The echocardiogram is needed to determine if the mitral valve leaflets are normal or reveal evidence of myxomatous degeneration and to study the size of the aortic root. Aortic root dilatation is difficult to detect on the routine chest x-ray film, and because mitral valve prolapse may occur in patients with Marfan syndrome, it would be prudent to order an echocardiogram to determine the size of the aortic root even though there are no physical signs of arachnodactyly. If the echocardiogram reveals a normal aortic root and the mitral valve leaflets are normal size, the echocardiogram should not be repeated for several years, and the patient should be encouraged to live a normal life but take antibiotics to prevent bacterial endocarditis.

If a specific cardiovascular diagnosis cannot be made after a review of the abnormalities discovered with the use of low technology, a differential diagnosis must be created. The following case report should serve as an example of this type of diagnostic problem:

PATIENT 3

A 30-year-old woman has intermittent attacks of severe dyspnea. In between attacks she has normal exercise tolerance. A chest x-ray film made during an attack of dyspnea reveals pulmonary edema. Auscultation of the heart reveals a low-pitched diastolic rumbling murmur at the cardiac apex. The electrocardiogram and "routine" examination of the blood and urine are normal. She is asymptomatic at the time of the examination.

The complete cardiac diagnosis at this point is as follows:

Problem 1: Organic heart disease

Etiology: *Unknown*

Anatomy: *Obstruction of the mitral valve*

Physiology: *Diastolic rumble at the apex, intermittent pulmonary edema, normal rhythm*

Cardiac status: *Severely compromised*

Prognosis: *Unknown until the exact cause is identified*

The initial plans for this patient should be written as follows:

Problem 1: Organic heart disease

Diagnostic:

   Rheumatic mitral valve stenosis—to obtain an echocardiogram.

   Left atrial myxoma—to obtain an echocardiogram.

Therapeutic: *No treatment until the echocardiogram has been reviewed.*

Educational: *The patient should be informed that there seems to be a blockage of the mitral valve. The echocardiogram should clarify the problem. The usual causes of mitral valve blockage can be successfully corrected by surgery.*

IMPORTANT CONSIDERATIONS

Low-technology procedures should be perfected until the clinician can either make a specific cardiovascular diagnosis or create a differential diagnosis.

High-technology procedures should be used to further clarify the specific diagnosis or to permit the selection of the specific diagnosis from a list of possible diagnoses (differential diagnosis).

High-technology procedures should not be used unless the answers they provide will improve the decision making, treatment, and outcome of the patient. They should not be done because the images created by the high-technology procedures are pretty or even because the measurements they yield are more accurate than those derived from the use of low-technology procedures.

The examples cited on the preceding pages serve to illustrate some of the indications for and contraindications to the use of high-technology procedures. Note that in each example the proper use of high-technology procedures was determined by the perception the clinician had of the patient's problem as determined by the use of low-technology procedures:

- The first patient, the 75-year-old diabetic woman with dilated cardiomyopathy, needed *no* high-technology procedures, although such procedures are often obtained. The condition, dilated cardiomyopathy, was so severe that little could be done other than to provide medical treatment for heart failure. Although high-technology procedures could more accurately measure the size of the heart chambers, the ejection fraction, etc., such measurements would add nothing to the evaluation of the patient.

  A metaphor might be as follows. It is equally as serious to fall out of a window located on the ninetieth floor of a building as it is to fall out of a window located on the one-hundredth floor of the building. An accurate measurement of the distance one falls when he or she falls such a great distance is of no value in estimating the outcome of the fall.

- The second patient, the 22-year-old woman with a midsystolic click and grade 1 systolic murmur at the apex, has mitral valve prolapse. An echocardiogram might be indicated to study the shape of the mitral valve leaflets and to determine the size of the aortic root. Because this was done and the aortic root was found to be normal, the echocardiogram need not be repeated for several years unless the murmur changes on auscultation.

  A metaphor might be as follows. A photographer does not continue to take photographs of the same building. He or she might make a new photograph when the scene changes (different shadows, etc.).

- The third patient, the 30-year-old woman with a diastolic rumble at the apex, needed an echocardiogram to determine if the mitral valve obstruction was caused by rheumatic mitral valve stenosis or a left atrial myxoma. The echocardiogram was diagnostic—the mitral valve blockage was due to a left atrial myxoma. It was not necessary to obtain magnetic resonance imaging (MRI) (which was obtained in this patient). Those who ordered it undoubtedly believed that it was a chance to learn how the tumor would look on an MRI scan. I always remind house officers that they have no contract with the patient that obligates the patient or taxpayer to pay for their education. I ask if they have reviewed the numerous videotapes available that show the cardiac abnormalities that can be identified with MRI.

A metaphor for this misadventure might be as follows. A gold-headed stethoscope may be prettier than the usual stethoscope, but it does not add to one's ability to listen to the heart.

- The example of the first patient indicates the overuse of high technology. The examples of the last two patients indicate the great value of appropriately used high technology. These examples serve to emphasize that this book is not a diatribe against the use of high technology. Rather, it strongly supports the idea that high technology may be misused unless it is used to clarify problems that should be clarified and that have been identified with the use of low technology. It follows that the more skilled clinicians are in the use of low technology, the more likely they are to use high technology properly.

• • •

The discussions of the following procedures and tests, except for most of the discussion on echocardiography, represent my own view and use of the techniques. I recognize that others may have different views. In each case, however, high technology should be used to answer questions raised by low technology.

The approximate cost of each procedure or test is listed. The cost undoubtedly varies with the locale. The cost listed represents the cost of the procedure or test at Emory University Hospital and Clinic in January 1993.

ECHOCARDIOGRAPHY

Echocardiography is a commonly used diagnostic procedure. At times the echocardiogram can clarify a diagnostic problem, and such clarification will assist in the decision making regarding the treatment of the patient. For example, a patient who has chest pain and a simultaneous neurologic deficit usually has dissection of the aorta. An esophageal echocardiogram may not only prove the diagnosis, but may also give the cardiovascular surgeon insight regarding the surgical procedure that may be needed. Also, and most important, an echocardiogram may be the best method to identify a cardiovascular source of an embolic stroke. At other times the echocardiogram is used for improper reasons and merely signifies the user's misunderstanding of its use. For example, one does not obtain an echocardiogram "to determine if a murmur is present." Such an action is simply a cover-up for inadequate auscultatory ability. Also, when a diagnosis has been clarified by an echocardiogram, it may not be necessary to repeat the procedure each time the patient visits the physician. A decision should be made regarding the need for repeat echocardiograms. For example, the echocardiogram need not be repeated when the problem is mild mitral valve prolapse unless a change is detected in auscultation, whereas the echocardiogram should be repeated perhaps twice a year when a dilated aortic root is being followed in a patient with Marfan syndrome.

Clinical application

The American College of Cardiology and the American Heart Association appointed a task force to produce guidelines for the clinical application of echocardiography. The document created by the task force is reproduced in the Appendix.

Cost

The cost of a transthoracic echocardiogram, including the technical and professional fee, is approximately $553. The cost of a transesophageal echocardiogram, including the technical and professional fee, is approximately $723. When a transthoracic echocardiogram is followed by a transesophageal echocardiogram the total charge is that of a transesophageal echocardiogram.

EXERCISE ELECTROCARDIOGRAPHY

Exercise electrocardiography, usually referred to as stress electrocardiography, is the most commonly performed procedure for the detection and evaluation of patients with atherosclerotic coronary heart disease.

Indications

General indications. General indications for exercise electrocardiography include the following:

- An exercise electrocardiogram may be obtained in asymptomatic men and women over the age of 40 years whose occupation involves serving the general public. This includes school bus drivers, airplane pilots, firemen, policemen, etc. (A positive test result is more likely to be a false positive response in young women than it is in young men. A negative test result is more likely to be a true negative response in young women than it is in young men.)
- An exercise electrocardiogram may be obtained in asymptomatic men and women who are 35 years old or older and who plan a vigorous exercise program.
- An exercise electrocardiogram may be obtained in men and women over the age of 35 who have chest discomfort and the physician determines that the pretest probability of coronary heart disease is 30% to 70% (see Chapter 5). (A positive test result is more likely to be a false positive response in women than it is in men. A negative test result is more likely to be a true-negative response in young women than it is in men.)
- An exercise electrocardiogram may be obtained in asymptomatic men and women with several risk factors for coronary atherosclerosis.

Exercise electrocardiography for prognostic purposes. An exercise electrocardiogram may be used to determine the functional capacity of patients with known coronary heart disease.

A submaximal exercise electrocardiogram may be used to assist in the risk stratification of patients following an uncomplicated myocardial infarction. This test is usually performed toward the end of hospitalization. (Some physicians prefer a thallium scan for this purpose, and others prefer a coronary arteriogram.)

Exercise electrocardiography to determine the effects of therapy. An exercise electrocardiogram may be used to determine the success or failure of medical treatment, coronary angioplasty, or coronary bypass surgery. The stress test may be repeated once a year in asymptomatic patients who fall into these categories.

Contraindications

Contraindications to exercise electrocardiography include the following:

- The test should not be performed in patients during the early, acute phase of myocardial infarction or to study a patient with a recent clinical syndrome suggesting infarction (i.e., chest discomfort thought to possibly be due to prolonged myocardial ischemia).
- The procedure should not be performed in patients with unstable angina pectoris or what is thought to possibly be unstable angina pectoris (i.e., recent onset of chest discomfort that has some, but not all, of the features characteristic of angina pectoris).
- The stress test should not be used for diagnostic purposes when stable angina pectoris has been diagnosed with a predictive value of 90% (see Chapter 5). Under these circumstances a positive test result adds nothing to the diagnosis, and a negative response should not negate the conclusion drawn by the analysis of the symptoms.
- An exercise stress test should not be performed in patients with heart failure.
- An exercise stress test should not be performed when the patient is known to have serious arrhythmias. There are times, however, when the test is performed to determine if an arrhythmia is exercise induced. These are special situations, and the operator must be prepared to treat the arrhythmia, including using a defibrillator.
- An exercise stress test should not be performed to assist in the evaluation of a patient with chest discomfort when aortic valve disease is present.
- An exercise stress test should not be performed in patients with severe systemic hypertension (systolic pressure over 200 mm Hg and diastolic pressure over 120 mm Hg.
- An exercise stress test should not be performed when there is evidence of dilated or hypertrophic cardiomyopathy.
- An exercise stress test should not be performed in a patient with right or left bundle-branch block, because it is usually difficult to interpret the ST segment displacement.

- An exercise stress test should not be performed in a patient who is receiving digitalis medication, because the drug causes a false positive response.
- An exercise stress test should not be performed in patients with hypokalemia, because the electrolyte abnormality causes a false positive response.
- An exercise stress test should not be performed in patients with noncardiac debilitating diseases.

Comment

My use of stress electrocardiography differs somewhat from that of most published texts on the subject. This is because I perceive that the prevalence of coronary atherosclerosis is increasing in the female population. Furthermore, the disease may occur at an earlier age in women today than it did in the past. Accordingly, I have dealt with women as I have dealt with men, although I have emphasized that false positive responses are still more common in young women than in young men.

The reader is referred to the literature for the technique of actually performing the test[1] and for the interpretation of the stress electrocardiogram itself.[2] The physician who uses the test must understand Bayes' theorem, how to determine pretest probability, sensitivity, specificity, predictive value, a false positive response, a false negative response, and, above all, the hazards associated with the test.

Cost

The cost of exercise electrocardiography, including the technical and professional fee, is approximately $249.

AMBULATORY RECORDING OF THE ELECTROCARDIOGRAM (HOLTER MONITORING)

Indications

Ambulatory (24-hour) recording of the electrocardiogram is commonly used to identify the cause of a patient's complaint of palpitation or syncope. The cause of the palpitation or syncope may be discovered to be due to supraventricular tachycardia, ventricular tachycardia, sick-sinus syndrome, or multiple premature atrial or ventricular depolarizations.

Ambulatory (24-hour) recording of the electrocardiogram (Holter monitoring) has also been used to determine the efficacy of the drug treatment of ventricular tachycardia. In certain patients Holter-guided antiarrhythmic therapy is as accurate in predicting the efficacy of treatment as is antiarrhythmic treatment selected by the results of electrophysiologic studies.

Ambulatory (24-hour) recording of the electrocardiogram may be used to identify "painless" myocardial ischemia. This condition is identified when ST segment displacement develops in the electrocardiogram. How reliable is such a finding as compared with exercise electrocardiography? I do not believe that the technique of ambulatory (24-hour) monitoring with a Holter monitor is as accurate as 12-lead exercise electrocardiography in the detection of "painless" myocardial ischemia. Sharp et al.[3] have studied this problem and have written the following summary of their work:

> Data from previous studies are debatable regarding whether Holter monitors are a reliable electrocardiographic indicator of ischemia, for which the 12-lead electrocardiogram (ECG) is the standard. Simultaneous 12-lead and Holter ECGs were performed on 30 patients with typical angina pectoris during coronary angiography or exercise testing. ST depression recorded by both methods was directly compared, using the 12-lead ECG as the reference. The Holter tapes were also scanned by two automated ST analysis programs and the results were compared to 12-lead ECGs. Only 66 of the 178 12-lead ECG ST depression events were also present on the Holter recordings (37.1% Holter sensitivity). ST depression was underestimated by the Holter recordings compared to the 12-lead ECGs (p < 0.0001). The majority (67.0%) of ST depression events identified by one computer program were false positive events. The degree of ST depression was overestimated compared to 12-lead ECGs by the second program (p = 0.0033). Holter-detected ST depression may not be a reliable ECG indicator for myocardial ischemia.*

Cost

The cost of continuous electrocardiographic (Holter) monitoring, including the technical and professional fee, is approximately $298.

SIGNAL-AVERAGED ELECTROCARDIOGRAPHY

Special equipment has been designed to isolate, if present, the delayed and fragmented spread of electrical activity that occurs, usually in a region of infarcted myocardium, during depolarization of the heart. Areas of the myocardium that have such conduction characteristics are thought to represent potential sites for certain ventricular arrhythmias. The equipment attempts to eliminate the baseline "noise" and artifact and reveal, at the end of the QRS complex, the underlying very low amplitude voltage "late potential" arising from these small areas. A "positive" recording, meaning that a late potential is present, is rarely seen in normal subjects, whereas about 80% of patients with prior myocardial infarction who have ventricular tachycardia have positive recordings.

The hope, with signal-averaged electrocardiography, is to use it alone or in combination with other tests to assist in the risk stratification and accurate selection of

---

*Reproduced with permission from Sharp SD, Mason JW, Bray B: Comparison of ST depression recorded by Holter monitors and 12-lead ECGs during coronary angiography and exercise testing, *J Electrocardiol* 25(4):323, 1992.

patients at high risk for future ventricular tachyarrhythmias. The three clinical situations specifically indicating the signal-averaging technique are (1) after myocardial infarction, a condition that is prone to serious arrhythmic events, (2) patients with nonsustained ventricular tachycardia, and (3) patients with syncope. For example, about one third of patients with recent myocardial infarction who have a positive recording and an ejection fraction of less than 40% will have ventricular tachycardia or sudden death in the subsequent 12 months. Also, a positive recording is found in the majority of patients with syncope who are induced into ventricular tachycardia during electrophysiologic testing. Currently the negative predictive accuracy of signal-averaged electrocardiography seems to be higher than its positive predictive accuracy. More research is needed to improve its clinical significance.

Cost

The cost of a signal-averaged electrocardiogram, including the technical and professional fee, is approximately $229.

ELECTROPHYSIOLOGIC STUDIES

Electrophysiologic studies are commonly used to (1) diagnose the type of cardiac arrhythmia in those patients who are suspected of having arrhythmia-related symptoms, (2) determine the cause of syncope, (3) evaluate patients who have been resuscitated from sudden cardiac death, (4) determine the appropriate medical treatment of certain arrhythmias (especially ventricular tachycardia), and (5) map and localize a suitable site for catheter ablation or ablation treatment of various cardiac arrhythmias.[4]

This technique is complex and lengthy as compared with many other procedures. It should not be used until an expert in arrhythmias has reviewed the history, physical examination, electrocardiogram (including, at times, the record produced by a 24-hour recording using a Holter monitor), and chest x-ray film. Also, at times, a signal-averaged electrocardiogram, an exercise stress test, or upright tilt-table testing may be needed before electrophysiologic testing is performed. The technique of electrophysiologic testing will surely be modified and simplified as time passes.

Indications

The indications for electrophysiologic testing are listed in Box 10-1.[4]

Complications

The risks associated with electrophysiologic testing are low. Significant complications include perforation of the heart (0.5% of procedures),[5] arterial damage (0.2%), venous thrombosis (0.5%), pulmonary embolism (0.3%), and thrombophlebitis (0.6%). The mortality associated with electrophysiologic studies is about 0.12%.[5]

Box 10-1   Guidelines for the use of electrophysiologic studies in patients with symptoms due to heart disease

Symptomatic patients who have suspected sinus node dysfunction (SND):

In whom SND is suspected to cause symptoms but causal relationship cannot be shown by other means.

Symptomatic patients with acquired atrioventricular block:

In whom His-Purkinje block is suspected to cause symptoms but cannot be documented by ECGs, or

Who are being treated with pacemakers yet remain symptomatic, and in whom VT is suspected to cause symptoms.

Symptomatic patients with chronic intraventricular conduction delay:

In whom a ventricular arrhythmia is suspected as a cause.

Patients who have narrow QRS complex tachycardias:

In whom the tachycardias are frequent or poorly tolerated, drug refractory, and in whom detailed information about the tachycardia is essential, or

Who prefer ablative therapy to antiarrhythmic drugs.

Patients with wide QRS complex tachycardias:

In whom the tachycardias are sustained, symptomatic, or both, when correct diagnosis is unclear.

Patients who have Wolff-Parkinson-White syndrome:

And are being considered for nondrug therapy because of drug intolerance or arrhythmias that are life-threatening or incapacitating.

Patients who have unexplained syncope:

And known or suspected structural heart disease.

Survivors of cardiac arrest:

Without acute Q wave myocardial infarction, and

In whom cardiac arrest occurred 48 hours or more after acute myocardial infarction.

Patients who have unexplained palpitations:

Whose pulse rates are inappropriately fast (e.g., >150 beats/min), and

In whom ECG recordings fail to document the cause of symptoms.

Reproduced with permission from An interview with Mark E. Josephson, M.D.: The role of the electrophysiologist in the diagnosis of tachyarrhythmias, *Medtronic News* 21(1):14, 1992. Based on data from Zipes DP, Akhtar M, Denes P et al: Guidelines for clinical intracardiac electrophysiologic studies: a report of the American College of Cardiology/American Heart Association Task Force on Assessment of Diagnostic and Therapeutic Cardiovascular Procedures (Subcommittee to Assess Clinical Intracardiac Electrophysiologic Studies), *J Am Coll Cardiol* 14:1827, 1989.

Cost

The cost of an electrophysiologic study, including the technical and professional fee, is approximately $5000 dollars.

EXERCISE THALLIUM-201 SCAN

Radionuclear techniques are commonly used to evaluate patients with coronary artery disease or patients with possible coronary artery disease. Thallium-201 imaging is used more often than any other nuclear test for this purpose.

A thallium-201 scan is obtained after exercise when an area of decreased myocardial perfusion is more likely to be seen. The area of decreased myocardial perfusion is detected by comparing the scan made after injection during exercise with the resting scan made 4 hours later. A false negative thallium scan may be obtained when the exercise is inadequate or when cardiac therapy, such as the use of a beta-blocker, prevents an increase in heart rate. A false positive thallium scan may be obtained in patients with bundle-branch block or in women with large breasts or breast implants.

Indications

A discussion of the use of thallium-201 for the diagnosis of atheroscleratic coronary heart disease can be divided into two parts: the use of thallium-201 for symptomatic patients and its use for asymptomatic patients.

Use of thallium-201 for symptomatic patients. Symptomatic patients may be divided into five groups:

- Symptomatic patients who have stable angina pectoris in which the predictive value is 90% (see Chapter 5) should not have a thallium scan or an exercise electrocardiogram. I believe the diagnostic procedure of choice is a coronary arteriogram. A thallium scan is sometimes needed if the coronary arteriogram reveals coronary lesions that are of borderline significance (i.e., less than 50% luminal diameter). The result of the scan assists in determining the significance of borderline coronary lesions.
- Symptomatic patients with what is believed to be unstable angina pectoris should not have an exercise electrocardiogram or an exercise thallium scan. This rule holds even if the predictive value of the symptoms for unstable angina is as low as 50%. Such a patient should have a coronary arteriogram. Here again, a thallium scan may be indicated after the coronary arteriogram reveals that the coronary artery lesions are of borderline significance (i.e., less than 50% luminal diameter).
- A thallium scan may be performed in symptomatic patients in whom the predictive value of the symptoms indicating myocardial ischemia (stable angina pec-

toris) is 30% to 70% (see Chapter 5). When the thallium scan is positive, a coronary arteriogram should be performed.

- Women who are under 50 years of age should have a thallium scan if they have chest discomfort suggesting stable angina pectoris with a predictive value of 30% to 70%. An exercise electrocardiogram may be performed, but there is considerable likelihood that a positive response for myocardial ischemia is a false positive response. A negative response is, of course, useful. If the breasts are large or if breast implants are present, it may be wise to obtain a positron emission tomography (PET) scan or proceed directly with coronary arteriography.
- A thallium scan can be performed on patients recuperating from an uncomplicated myocardial infarction in an effort to determine if there are remaining areas of myocardial ischemia. Only submaximal exercise should be used in such patients. The test is performed before the patient is discharged from the hospital. If the thallium scan is positive for myocardial ischemia, a coronary arteriogram should be performed. Some physicians, including myself, prefer to omit the thallium scan and proceed with coronary arteriography before the patient is discharged from the hospital.
- Patients with angina pectoris following a myocardial infarction should have a coronary arteriogram rather than a thallium scan.

Use of thallium-201 for asymptomatic patients. Asymptomatic patients who have a positive exercise electrocardiogram may have a thallium scan in an effort to determine if the ST segment displacement represents myocardial ischemia or is a false positive response. Some physicians, including myself, may obtain a coronary arteriogram rather than a thallium scan in an effort to clarify the situation. It is uncommon for a thallium scan to be used initially to screen asymptomatic patients for silent myocardial ischemia. An exception to this rule is the middle-aged man with risk factors for coronary disease who cannot exercise for some reason (such as severe intermittent claudication of the legs) but who can have a thallium scan using dipyridamole as a stress agent. If such a patient has a positive thallium scan, a coronary arteriogram should be performed.

Comment

This discussion describes the thallium scan as I have used it. I have found it to be very useful in the decision-making process regarding my patients. I do wish to point out that many physicians use it differently and that some use it more frequently than I have suggested.

Cost

The cost of a thallium scan, including the technical and professional fee, is approximately $1350. When a dipyridamole test is performed, the cost is about $1500.

POSITRON EMISSION TOMOGRAPHY

Positron emission tomography (PET), which uses rubidium-82, is more accurate than thallium-201 scanning. In addition, a PET scan takes only 1½ hours, whereas a thallium scan requires 5 hours.

The PET camera is able to correct the cardiac images for attenuation by different body builds. Accordingly, a PET scan is much more accurate in women and in large individuals. While this is true, there are no satisfactory data to suggest that the improved accuracy allows physicians to make decisions that improve their patients' outcome as compared with decisions based on thallium-201 images.

A PET scan can be used to determine if a nonperfused area of myocardium is stunned, hibernating, or dead. This is accomplished by using the glucose analogue FDG. How much the data obtained using this technique will alter decision making and patient outcome has not yet been determined. Theoretically, the study of myocardial metabolism should eventually lead to useful information.

Because exercise PET scans are not usually available, dipyridamole testing is used. Exercise PET can be performed using the cyclotron-produced isotope nitrogen-13 ammonia for myocardial perfusion and FDG for metabolism.

Cost

The cost of a PET scan, including the use of dipyridamole, is approximately $1750. This figure includes the technical and professional fee.

COMPUTED TOMOGRAPHY

Computed tomography (including contrast-enhanced scans) is only occasionally needed to diagnose cardiovascular disease. The indications for, and limitations of, the technique are discussed below. The technique can be used to determine the volume of the ventricles, myocardial mass, ejection fraction, presence of pulmonary congestion, and amount of blood flow in an artery. However, the technique is seldom used for these purposes.

Congenital heart disease is rarely clarified with computed tomography. Echocardiography and cardiac catheterization are used to answer questions raised by the results of low-technology procedures.

A *pericardial effusion* can be identified by computed tomography. This technique is rarely needed, because an echocardiogram usually identifies the presence of pericardial fluid. Rarely, computed tomography may be needed to clarify a false positive echocardiogram that suggests pericardial fluid.

Constrictive pericarditis may be identified with computed tomography when the pericardium is greater than 4 mm thick and the inferior vena cava is abnormally dilated as it enters the right atrium. Constrictive pericarditis is usually recognized using low-technology procedures, echocardiography, and cardiac catheterization. These techniques, however, may not always enable the physician to differentiate restrictive cardiomyopathy from constrictive pericarditis. Computed tomography may be useful under such circumstances. Computed tomography may reveal a thicker than normal pericardium, which indicates the presence of constrictive pericarditis, whereas the pericardium appears to be normal in patients with restrictive cardiomyopathy.

A *pericardial cyst* is usually suspected on the chest x-ray film. Computed tomography may enable the physician to make a definite diagnosis and differentiate the abnormality from a lipoma or large lymph node due to neoplastic disease.

Although *myocardial infarction* can be identified with this technique, there are two reasons why it is not used:

- Low-technology procedures usually detect the condition, and other high-technology procedures are superior to computed tomography when additional studies are needed.
- It is not wise to place patients with a recent infarction in the machine for a prolonged period of time and give hypertonic iodinated fluid, which is needed to identify a myocardial infarction when computed tomography is used.

A *ventricular aneurysm* due to myocardial infarction can be identified with computed tomography. It is doubtful, however, whether computed tomography is superior to left ventricular angiography or echocardiography, which are commonly used for other reasons in such patients.

Masses within the heart may be detected by computed tomography. Echocardiography usually detects tumors and thrombi, but there is still a place for the occasional use of computed tomography in the identification of intracardiac masses. Computed tomography may identify neoplastic processes that have infiltrated the myocardium and conform to the ventricular wall rather than projecting into the chamber cavity. Also, computed tomography may rarely identify thrombi in the left ventricle, atrium, or atrial appendage that are not detected by echocardiography. Accordingly, if the clinician is searching for a source of a cerebral embolus and the echocardiogram is negative, computed tomography may be indicated. Apparently, clots that adhere to the curve of the left ventricle or left atrial wall are more easily seen with contrast-enhanced computed tomography than they are with echocardiography. It may well be that, as echocardiography improves (especially with esophageal echocardiography), computed tomography will be totally discarded for this purpose.

A *dissecting aneurysm* and other abnormalities of the aorta may be identified with contrast-enhanced computed tomography. Esophageal echocardiography has virtually replaced computed tomography and aortography for the diagnosis of dissection of the aorta.

Other important anomalies of the aorta may be identified by computed tomography. The procedure is usually ordered when an unexplained shadow is seen on the chest x-ray film.

Venous grafts used in coronary bypass surgery can be visualized with computed tomography. This technique has not replaced angiographic examination of the grafts. Internal mammary artery grafts cannot be detected with computed tomography.

Ultrafast computed tomography can be used to detect calcification in the coronary arteries. This technique is now being investigated by several groups, and the results of their initial investigation are quite promising. Current investigators believe the following. When ultrafast computed tomography reveals calcium in the coronary arteries, it is a marker for intimal atherosclerosis. When no calcium is seen, there is little liklihood that the patient will develop significant coronary atherosclerosis. Additional research is needed before the sensitivity and specificity of the results of the technique are known. It may become the best screening procedure for the presence of coronary atherosclerosis.

Cost

The cost of computed tomography of the chest with use contrast media, including the technical and professional fee, is approximately $705.

MAGNETIC RESONANCE IMAGING

The development of magnetic resonance imaging (MRI) has been a great advance in diagnostic cardiology. Further development of the technology will make it possible to diagnose coronary disease and assess its consequences without invading the body.[6]

Magnetic resonance images are beautiful and clear. No one can remain unimpressed by the images the machine creates. Despite the magnificence of the images, several factors have inhibited the wide use of the technique:

- The MRI machines are not portable, and the first-generation systems have limited physical access and require that most electronic monitors and defibrillators be several feet away in order to operate. Accordingly, the use of MRI in acutely ill patients, particularly those who are hemodynamically unstable, is restricted.
- While the information MRI can provide about cardiac structure and left ventricular function is precise, detailed, and quantitatively accurate, much of this information needed for routine patient management can be obtained adequately by simpler techniques.
- Uniform reimbursement by insurance companies has been slow to come, and MRI is incorrectly perceived as being considerably more expensive than other tests (MRI costs about the same as SPECT thallium at Emory University Hospital).
- Many cardiologists and other referring physicians have limited familiarity with the practical capabilities and relative strengths and weaknesses of the technique.
- The technical ability currently required for performing and analyzing a thorough study is relatively great.

To restate for emphasis: it is highly likely that these negative factors will change as the technique is further improved.

Types of information obtained

Pettigrew[7] has divided the types of information obtained by MRI into three groups: (1) visualization of cardiovascular structure in three dimensions; (2) characterization of cardiac and pericardiac tissues by means of evaluation of relaxation times; and (3) determination of global and local functions, including myocardial contractility, determination of the degree of valvular regurgitation and shunts, and determination of the ejection fraction, stroke volume, and cardiac output.

The cardiovascular applications of MRI are summarized in Table 10-1.

Table 10-1   Cardiovascular applications of MRI

Disorder	MRI information
Congenital heart disease	Three-dimensional structure Biventricular function, pre- and postoperative Shunt identification Valve areas Severity of valvular insufficiency
Aortic aneurysm, dissection, coarctation	Cross-sectional area Site of dissection/intimal flap Thrombus identification Location of important branches Flow quantification
Ischemic heart disease	Site and extent of infarction and sequelae Viable myocardium vs. scar Ventricular aneurysms, thrombi Segmental wall motion and systolic thickening Global function and indexes, eg, RVEF, LVEF, CO
Cardiac masses	Lesions, site, and extent Resectability Functional consequence Limited tissue characterization
Cardiomyopathies	Myocardial function/dysfunction Hypertrophic site and distribution Myopathic vs. reaction hypertrophy
Valvular heart disease	Ventricular mass Visualization of regurgitant jets Regurgitant fractions/volumes Valve area Chamber volumes
Pericardial disease	Thickened pericardium Intrapericardial adhesions Effusion volume Transudative vs. exudative Functional consequence

Reproduced with permission from Pettigrew RI: Magnetic resonance imaging of the heart and great vessels. In Hurst JW, editor-in-chief: *The heart*, ed 7, New York, 1990, McGraw-Hill, p 1977.

Limitations

In day-to-day diagnostic work it seems that echocardiography provides adequate information about left ventricular function and many cardiac masses, so that the higher detail and three-dimensional completeness of MRI is frequently not required. However, in instances where echocardiography is nondefinitive, MRI may be a useful adjunctive technique.[8] Today, many physicians use transesophageal echocardiography to identify the presence and extent of dissection of the aorta in acutely ill patients. Although esophageal echocardiography is modestly invasive, it is usually preferred to the use of MRI, because hemodynamic instability in acute dissection limits the use of MRI.

As stated earlier, the nonportability of the MRI system is a limitation, and some patients are too unstable to be placed in the machine. Other notable limitations with current MRI systems include inability to image during physical stress and lack of routine imaging of myocardial perfusion so that ischemia is not detected. Patients with cardiac pacemakers are an absolute contraindication, as are patients with pre-6000 Starr Edwards valves.

The procedure is somewhat expensive but is comparable in cost to other noninvasive cardiac tests and considerably less costly than cardiac catheterization.

Indications

At present, MRI is primarily indicated for nonacute aortic disease and complex congenital heart disease. At our institutions the surgeons prefer MRI of the aorta with three-dimensional reconstruction over angiography as the preoperative procedure of choice in patients with aortic aneurysms. MRI also is superb, relative to other techniques, in evaluating pericardial disease and right ventricular function—the latter being particularly difficult to assess accurately by other noninvasive techniques. MRI also has an adjunctive role in assessing masses when echocardiography is not definitive. One additional indication is in distinguishing regions of viable myocardial tissue from scar tissue in the setting of remote infarction. Viability is established if systolic thickening is observed, whereas scar tissue has a combination of segmental diastolic thinning and absence of thickening.

Future use

Innovations on the horizon promise a significant role for MRI in the diagnosis and assessment of coronary artery and ischemic heart disease. Developments that are currently in progress include MRI angiography of the coronaries, imaging of myocardial perfusion using magnetic contrast media, and pharmacologic stress MRI, all of which have been demonstrated at various research centers.[6,9,10]

Cost

The cost of MRI, including the technical and professional fee, is approximately $1000.

CARDIAC CATHETERIZATION AND ANGIOGRAPHY

Catheterization of the human heart remains the greatest technologic advance in cardiovascular medicine. It stimulated the development of all other diagnostic procedures and encouraged the eventual surgical and medical advances that are commonly used today.

In the beginning (see Chapter 1), cardiac catheterization was used as an investigative tool in an effort to understand normal and abnormal cardiac physiology. Later, the procedure was used as a diagnostic tool, and recently it has been used as a therapeutic tool (e.g., dilatation of coarctation of the aorta).

Diagnostic use

Right- and left-sided cardiac catheterization can be used to identify and quantify left-to-right and right-to-left shunts due to congenital heart disease. The technique can be used to identify the presence and severity of valve disease by identifying pressure gradients across obstructed valves. Aortic and mitral valve regurgitation can be identified and quantified. Valve areas can be computed. Left and right ventricular systolic and diastolic pressure and pulmonary artery pressure can be measured. Contrast material is usually injected into the right and left ventricles. This enables one to identify intracardiac shunts, hypertrophic cardiomyopathy, and cardiac tumors and thrombi, and to estimate the left ventricular ejection fraction.

Readers who wish to know more about this time-tested, commonly used technique are referred to entire books that are written on the subject.[11]

The technique may be used less frequently in infants and children than it was in the past, because echocardiography has been developed to the point where in many instances a complete diagnosis can be made without cardiac catheterization. Cardiac surgeons are now accepting echocardiographic diagnoses and in many instances do not demand cardiac catheterization prior to cardiac surgery. Echocardiography is also used in the follow-up of adult patients with valve disease, and this has decreased the need for repeated cardiac catheterization. Cardiac catheterization and coronary arteriography are commonly performed in adults who have valve disease, because echocardiography does not identify the anatomic features of the coronary arteries.

Complications

Cardiac catheterization and angiography are relatively safe procedures.[12] Considering how sick many of the patients are, it is remarkable that complications are so rare. Death due to catheterization of the right side of the heart is very rare. Death due to catheterization of the left side of the heart, including coronary arteriography, is less than 0.02%, and the risk of stroke or excessive blood loss is less than 0.5%. A few patients will have dissection of the coronary artery (see section on coronary arteriography), and a small percentage of patients will have retroperitoneal bleeding. An arteriovenous fistula in the region of the femoral artery may occur in a small percentage of patients.

Comment

Cardiac catheterization and angiography are safe and reliable methods of studying valvular heart disease, congenital heart disease, cardiomyopathy, and coronary artery disease. Echocardiography has developed to the point where it is replacing cardiac catheterization for the study of many conditions. Echocardiography has not, however, replaced coronary arteriography in the study of coronary artery disease. Ultrafast computed tomography and MRI may be used in the future to identify the absence or presence of coronary atherosclerosis.

Cost

The cost of left-sided cardiac catheterization and coronary arteriography, including the technical and professional fee, is approximately $2407. The cost of right-sided and left-sided cardiac catheterization and coronary arteriography, including the technical and professional fee, is approximately $3395.

CORONARY ARTERIOGRAPHY

Coronary arteriography remains the gold standard for identifying the presence of obstructive and nonobstructive coronary atherosclerosis.[13] No one doubts, however, that the genesis of coronary events is far more complex and complicated than the degree of obstruction noted in the coronary arteriogram. Also, no one doubts that in the future similar information may be obtained by using a simpler technique.

Coronary arteriography is indicated for two reasons: (1) as a diagnostic procedure to identify atherosclerotic coronary artery disease (or some other coronary disease, including congenital anomalies) or (2) to determine the exact coronary anatomy in patients with known atherosclerotic coronary heart disease in order to determine the need and feasibility for coronary angioplasty, coronary bypass surgery, or medical therapy. A left ventriculogram, performed at the same sitting, will reveal the left ventricular ejection fraction and left ventricular wall motion abnormalities.

Indications

The discussion of the indications for coronary arteriography can be divided into two parts.

Indications for patients without symptoms of myocardial ischemia. A coronary arteriogram is indicated when the exercise electrocardiogram shows a positive response, suggesting the possibility of painless myocardial ischemia (silent ischemia). Most often, a coronary arteriogram is performed, rather than a thallium scan, in an effort to determine if the positive response in the exercise electrocardiogram is a true-positive or a false positive response. At times an exercise thallium scan is performed, along with an exercise electrocardiogram, as the initial screening procedure. When the thallium scan is positive, a coronary arteriogram should be performed.

The usual reasons for performing an exercise electrocardiogram or thallium scan in a patient without symptoms or signs of myocardial ischemia are as follows:

- Patients with peripheral vascular disease due to atherosclerosis may have severe claudication of the leg muscles and may be unable to exercise. Such patients commonly have severe coronary atherosclerosis. A thallium scan, using dipyridamole rather than exercise, may be performed, especially if surgery is planned for the peripheral vascular disease. When the thallium scan is positive, a coronary arteriogram is performed because, at times, coronary angioplasty or coronary bypass surgery is indicated prior to surgery for peripheral vascular disease.

- Older patients without symptoms of myocardial ischemia who are to have aortic or mitral valve surgery should have a coronary arteriogram performed prior to valve surgery. Atherosclerotic coronary heart disease is common in older patients with aortic valve stenosis and occurs sufficiently often in older patients with aortic regurgitation or mitral valve disease to warrant the performance of a coronary arteriogram. When the surgeon is armed with such information, he or she will usually perform bypass surgery on the coronary arteries that are obstructed more than 50% of the luminal diameter at the time the valve surgery is performed.

- An exercise electrocardiogram or thallium scan may be indicated in airline pilots, school bus drivers, policemen, firemen, etc. These tests are also performed when a middle-aged asymptomatic individual decides to become an avid runner. When the noninvasive test is positive, it should be followed with a coronary arteriogram.

Indications for patients with symptoms that might be due to myocardial ischemia. Chest discomfort is common. At times it may be characteristic of angina pectoris due to coronary atherosclerotic heart disease with a predictive value of 90% (see Chapter 5). At other times, however, the chest discomfort may suggest the possibility of angina pectoris, and the predictive value of the symptoms may be only 50% (see Chapter 5). Some patients have what is believed to be chronic stable angina, and other patients have what is believed to be unstable angina. Patients with prolonged chest discomfort, suggesting prolonged myocardial ischemia, may have additional clinical signs of myocardial infarction, so that a definitive diagnosis of myocardial infarction can be made. At times, however, there may be no other signs of infarction. Patients with the following symptoms are potential candidates for coronary arteriography:

- Patients with chest discomfort in which chronic stable angina pectoris is thought to be present with a predictive value of 90% (see Chapter 5). An exercise electrocardiogram or a thallium scan is not needed (see discussions of exercise electrocardiography and exercise thallium-201 scan).

The chronic stable angina should be graded according to the Canadian Cardiovascular Society Classification (see Chapter 4). The physician uses the grade of symptoms (Class 1 to 4), the coronary anatomy, the ejection fraction, the age of the patient, and the presence of coexistent disease to make a decision regarding the need for bypass surgery, angioplasty, or medical treatment.

Some patients who are 75 to 80 years of age or older who have Class 1 to 2 chronic stable angina (predictive value of 90%) and who are satisfied with their lifestyle may be managed as if they have coronary disease and may not require a coronary arteriogram to eliminate the 10% of patients who do not have coronary disease. Many of these patients may be treated medically. My own rule is to be aggressive in young patients and more conservative in older patients, because the operative risk and chance of postoperative stroke are increased in patients beyond the age of 75.

- Patients with possible unstable angina pectoris should have a coronary arteriogram performed. I believe that an exercise electrocardiogram or a thallium scan is contraindicated for the following reasons.

The molecular biology and pathophysiology of coronary artery lesions causing unstable angina are different from the molecular biology and pathophysiology of lesions responsible for stable angina; the lesions are far more "active" than those associated with stable angina. Accordingly, the response to exercise is unpredictable and is more often associated with complications, including death. In addition, patients with a recent onset of chest discomfort may not be able to describe the relationship of the discomfort to effort or emotional disturbances or to recognize the reproducibility of the chest discomfort. Knowledge of all of these features is needed to determine the likelihood (predictive value) that the discomfort is due to myocardial ischemia. If such features are present and the predictive value of the symptoms is 90%, an exercise electrocardiogram or thallium scan is not needed and, being more dangerous than when it is performed for stable angina pectoris, should not be performed. A coronary arteriogram is needed. If sufficient symptoms are not present (because so little time has elapsed to make the observations) and an accurate assessment cannot be made, it is not wise to obtain additional information by exercising the patient. Under such circumstances a coronary arteriogram may be associated with less risk than an exercise electrocardiogram or exercise thallium scan.

To summarize, I favor a coronary arteriogram as the diagnostic procedure of choice for patients with possible unstable angina pectoris even when the predictive value of the symptoms is 50%.

- Patients with chest discomfort in whom the symptoms indicate the presence of chronic stable angina pectoris with a predictive value of 30% to 70% may be studied further with an exercise electrocardiogram or exercise thallium scan. If the noninvasive test is positive for myocardial ischemia, a coronary arteriogram should be performed.

- Patients with angina pectoris following a myocardial infarction should have a coronary arteriogram performed. Patients who have a complicated course with arrhythmias, angina, or heart failure following a myocardial infarction should have a coronary arteriogram performed rather than a submaximal exercise electrocardiogram or thallium scan.
- Patients with myocardial infarction who have received thrombolytic therapy should have a coronary arteriogram performed several days after the therapy. A decision is then made as to whether angioplasty, bypass surgery, or medical therapy is needed.
- There is a move afoot to have coronary arteriography performed immediately in patients with a recent myocardial infarction in preference to the use of thrombolytic therapy. If appropriate coronary lesions are found, coronary angioplasty is used. At times bypass surgery may be used, or medical treatment will be implemented.
- Patients with angina pectoris who are to have valve surgery should have cardiac catheterization performed, because the cardiac surgeon will often perform valve surgery and coronary bypass surgery at the same operation.

Contraindications

The relative contraindications to coronary arteriography include a history of reaction to contrast material, concurrent infection, gastrointestinal bleeding, severe anemia, recent stroke, and advanced noncardiac disease.

The patient must understand that the diagnostic procedure is being used to determine if coronary atherosclerosis is truly present and, if it is present, to delineate the coronary anatomy and determine the contractile ability of the left ventricle so that a decision can be made regarding the need for angioplasty, bypass surgery, or medical treatment. Simply stated, the patient needs to understand that when a coronary arteriogram is performed, the findings may lead to another procedure. If the patient does not wish to have bypass surgery or angioplasty performed, a coronary arteriogram should not be done when the diagnosis of angina pectoris has a predictive value of 90%.

Complications

Coronary arteriography carries a low complication rate. Death occurs in less than 0.02% of patients, and the risk of myocardial infarction, stroke, or excessive blood loss is less than 0.5%.[12] Coronary artery dissection and retroperitoneal bleeding from trauma to an atheromatous plaque in the abdominal aorta may occur as rare complications.

Comment

Coronary arteriography has revolutionized the diagnosis and treatment of atherosclerotic coronary heart disease. It remains the gold standard against which all other procedures are compared. I have expressed here my own use of the technique with full knowledge that others may have a different view. A final caveat: remember that the genesis of coronary events is more complex and complicated than the obstruction produced by the atheromatous plaque itself.

Cost

The cost of coronary arteriography, including the technical and professional fee, is approximately $2407.

MYOCARDIAL BIOPSY

Indications and limitations

Myocardial biopsy is routinely used at specified intervals to detect *cardiac allograft rejection.*

Myocardial biopsy has been used to diagnose *acute myocarditis.* The value of this procedure has been brought into question because of the recent clinical study that revealed that therapy could not be determined by the results of the biopsy.[14] Also, the study revealed that the biopsy of one half of patients with unexplained heart failure showed no evidence of myocarditis.

Myocardial biopsy is sometimes performed in patients with *unexplained chronic congestive heart failure (cardiomyopathy)* in an effort to discover the etiology of this universally serious problem. Myocardial biopsy may enable the clinician to diagnose amyloid deposits, sarcoidosis, carcinoid syndrome, hemochromatosis, anthracycline toxicity, endocardial fibrosis, antineoplastic drug toxicity, radiation fibrosis, glycogen storage disease, Fabry disease, and neoplastic disease of the heart. Although myocardial biopsy is capable of revealing the cause of the cardiomyopathy, the question arises as to *why* the procedure is done. In the first place, the etiology of the cardiomyopathy can be determined by simpler means in patients with carcinoid syndrome, hemochromatosis, Fabry disease, or glycogen storage disease. Second, there is no specific treatment available for myocardial disease with the exception of hemochromatosis, which can be diagnosed without a biopsy, and alcoholic cardiomyopathy, a common cause of cardiomyopathy, which can be treated (with poor results) by asking the patient to abstain from the use of alcohol.

Because of the above problems, I have rarely recommended a myocardial biopsy for presumed myocarditis or chronic heart failure due to cardiomyopathy. I have been able to manage these patients despite my ignorance of the exact etiology of the cardiomyopathy until the time arrives when cardiac transplantation should be performed. At that time a myocardial biopsy might be used to exclude a systemic disease that would contraindicate cardiac transplantation.

Medical centers that are engaged in the research of myocarditis or cardiomyopathy may perform myocardial biopsies as part of a research protocol that is designed to discover an improved treatment for the serious problems of acute and chronic myocardial disease. For example, some progress has been made in the treatment of amyloid heart disease, but this treatment is still experimental. To restate for emphasis, a myocardial biopsy that is performed routinely and not in relation to a carefully designed research effort is rarely useful, whereas one can justify the procedure when it is performed within the setting of an excellent research protocol.

Complications

Complications are rare. Cardiac tamponade occurs in 0.1% to 0.2% of patients with atrial fibrillation, pneumothorax, air embolism, transient laryngeal paresis, and Horner syndrome.[15] Death was reported to occur in 0.03% of the patients in whom the procedure was performed.[16]

Cost

The cost of myocardial biopsy, including the technical fee, professional fee of the operator, and professional and technical fee of the pathologist, is approximately $2632.

OTHER IMPORTANT DIAGNOSTIC TESTS AND PROCEDURES

No attempt has been made to list and discuss all of the tests and procedures that may be needed to answer questions raised by the initial examination. The following are the tests and procedures that I have used most often in my own work. They are only used when the initial examination raises questions that might be answered by such testing.

Additional noninvasive and invasive procedures

Pulmonary function tests may be indicated when the patient has diagnostic clues suggesting cor pulmonale. The diagnostic workup of a patient with cor pulmonale, defined as heart disease due to respiratory system disease, may, at times, also include the workup of sleep-apnea syndrome. The cost of pulmonary function tests, including the technical and professional fee, varies according to the tests that are ordered. The cost of partial spirometry, including the technical and professional fee, is approximately $64. If a bronchodilator is given, the cost is approximately $113. As other tests are added, the total may reach approximately $450.

Whenever the clinician suspects that the abdominal aorta is enlarged, it is wise to obtain an *ultrasound examination of the aorta*. If the abdominal aorta is only slightly enlarged, the ultrasound should be repeated at about 6-month intervals in order to determine whether or not the aneurysm is increasing in size. The cost of an ultrasound of the aorta, including the technical and professional fee, is approximately $342.

Patients with transient ischemic attacks should have an *echo-Doppler study of the carotid arteries* performed. If this study is abnormal, a *carotid arteriogram* may be needed prior to carotid artery surgery. The cost of an echo-Doppler study of the carotid arteries, including the technical and professional fee, is approximately $476. The cost of a bilateral carotid arteriogram, including the technical and professional fee, is approximately $2507.

An *esophageal echocardiogram* may be needed to identify the cardiac origin of an embolic stroke. The embolus (1) may have originated in the left atrium or left atrial appendage in a patient with atrial fibrillation, with or without mitral stenosis; (2) may have originated from a left ventricular mural thrombus following a myocardial infarction; (3) may have originated from a mural thrombus in a dilated left ventricle; (4) may have originated in the leg veins and enter the left side of the heart through a patent foramen ovale; (5) may be from a left atrial tumor; (6) may be related to mitral valve annulus calcification; or (7) may be caused by endocarditis of the aortic or mitral valve.

An esophageal echocardiogram is also indicated in patients in whom the "shaggy" aorta syndrome may be responsible for stroke or in patients with the "blue toe" syndrome that occurs with eosinophilia. See earlier discussion on echocardiography for the cost of an esophageal echocardiogram.

A *pulmonary scan* may be indicated in patients with signs and symptoms suggesting pulmonary embolism. The cost of a pulmonary scan, including the technical and professional fee, is approximately $709.

An *aortogram* may be indicated in patients with signs and symptoms of dissection of the aorta; however, surgeons are beginning to accept the results of an esophageal echocardiogram. When the condition is not acute, MRI may be preferable. An aortogram may also be indicated when an abdominal aortic aneurysm is detected by ultrasound examination. The ultrasound is usually ordered when the examiner palpates a larger than normal pulsation in the abdomen or identifies calcification in the wall of the dilated aorta in an x-ray film made of the abdomen for some other reason. The cost of an aortogram, including the technical and professional fee, is approximately $1490.

An *angiographic study of the renal arteries* is indicated in patients who have signs of renovascular hypertension that has been proved by an increase in the renal vein blood level of renin. The information provided by angiography will assist in decision making regarding the feasibility of using renal artery angioplasty or surgical intervention in an effort to relieve the renal artery obstruction. The cost of an angiographic study of the renal arteries, including the technical and professional fee, is approximately $2080.

Deep vein thrombosis of the veins of the legs may be studied with *Doppler techniques*. Other studies of deep veins of the legs, including plethysmographic studies, are used less often today. *Phlebography* is sometimes used, but the test is painful, which limits its use. The cost of phlebography, including the technical and professional fee, is approximately $619. The cost of a Doppler study of the leg veins, including the technical and professional fee, is approximately $170. The cost of a duplex Doppler study of the venous system, including the technical and professional fee, is approximately $334.

Angiographic studies of the arteries of the legs are needed when the clinical signs suggest that surgery should be performed on the peripheral arteries. An angiographic study of the arteries of the legs, including the technical and professional fee, is approximately $2111.

When obstruction of a renal artery has been identified, it is useful to *measure the renin level in each renal vein* in order to establish the functional significance of the obstruction. The cost of determing the level of renin in the renal veins, including the technical and professional fee, is approximately $48.

Swann-Ganz catheterization of the right side of the heart and pulmonary artery may be needed to access the physiologic competence of the cardiovascular system in patients who are seriously ill with cardiogenic shock or severe heart failure, or to identify the presence of acute mitral regurgitation due to a ruptured papillary muscle or rupture of the interventricular septum. The cost of Swann-Ganz catheterization, including the technical and professional fee, ranges from approximately $931 to $1267.

Blood and urine tests

The costs of the tests listed here are for outpatients who visit our clinic. As in most medical centers, the cost is often higher for patients who are hospitalized.

Blood tests. Abnormalities noted on routine examination of the blood and their relevance to disease of the cardiovascular system are discussed in Chapter 9. The following blood tests may be needed depending on the questions raised by the initial examination of the patient (using low-technology procedures):

- Sickle cell anemia may be the cause of cardiomyopathy and a syndrome suggesting rheumatic fever. The cost of a special sickle cell preparation is approximately $11. Hemoglobin electrophoresis is used to identify the phenotype of the condition. The cost of this test is approximately $27.
- Patients who have diabetes mellitus or cirrhosis and who also have cardiomyopathy may have hemochromatosis. A determination of the level of serum ferritin and serum transferrin is indicated. The costs of these tests are approximately $43 and $36, respectively.
- Blood cultures are obtained in an effort to diagnose bacterial endocarditis. Blood cultures are indicated when a patient with a heart murmur due to valvular or congenital heart disease has fever without an obvious cause. Blood cultures

should also be obtained when a patient with a heart murmur has fever and there is an apparent cause, such as an obvious bacterial infection. The cost of these blood cultures is approximately $49.

- Arterial blood gases are obtained in order to identify arterial oxygen desaturation that may be due to congenital heart disease or cor pulmonale. The arterial P_{O_2} and P_{CO_2} may be abnormally low secondary to pulmonary embolism. The cost of blood gas determination, including the technical and professional fee and electrolyte determination, is approximately $64.

- Hypothyroidism and hyperthyroidism can usually be diagnosed by obtaining a T_4 and thyroid-stimulating hormone (TSH) determination of the serum. The costs of these tests are approximately $46 and $52, respectively.

- Acromegaly may cause cardiomyopathy and coronary artery disease. Acromegaly can be diagnosed by measuring the level of growth hormone in the serum 1 hour after ingestion of 100 g of oral glucose solution. The cost of this test is approximately $43.

- The level of the antistreptolysin titer should be measured in the serum, and throat cultures should be obtained in patients whose initial examination suggests the possibility of acute rheumatic fever. The cost of a serum antistreptolysin titer determination is approximately $24.

- A serologic test for syphilis is indicated when the initial examination reveals a cardiovascular condition that could be produced by syphilis. The cost of this test is approximately $14.

- The serologic test for Lyme disease should be performed when the initial examination reveals fever, rash, atrioventricular block, and cardiomyopathy. The cost of this test is approximately $88.

- Lupus erythematosus may cause pericarditis, coronary arteritis, aortic regurgitation, and Libman-Sacks disease. Lupus erythematosus can usually be diagnosed by obtaining a serum antinuclear antibody profile. The cost of this test is approximately $46.

- Rheumatoid arthritis may be associated with pericarditis, constrictive pericarditis, coronary arteritis, aortic valve disease, and myocardial disease. The rheumatoid factor is usually positive. The cost of this test is approximately $22.

- Gout may be associated with coronary artery disease. The serum uric acid level is usually elevated. The cost of this test is approximately $16.

- Certain electrolyte abnormalities affect the heart. Although hyperkalemia, hypokalemia, hypercalcemia, and hypocalcemia are usually identified on "routine" blood work, hypomagnesemia, which can also affect the heart and circulation, can only be detected by ordering its determination specifically. The cost of this test is approximately $20.

- It is uncommon that the cause of sporadically occurring acute pericarditis or myocarditis, which is usually viral in origin, can be identified by blood tests.

When an epidemic of acute pericarditis or myocarditis occurs, it may be possible to identify the exact viral cause of the epidemic. The cost of blood cultures for viruses is approximately $22.

- The blood test for pheochromocytoma consists of measuring the blood catecholamines (epinephrine plus norepinephrine). The test, of course, is only performed if the initial examination suggests the possible presence of pheochromocytoma. The cost of the test is approximately $85.
- At times, when the clinician suspects cardiac drug toxicity as the cause of a clinical problem or wishes to determine if there is an adequate blood level of the drug, it is useful to measure the level of the drug in the blood. Accordingly, the blood levels of digoxin and antiarrhythmic drugs such as quinidine and procainamide may be measured. The cost of determining the level of digoxin in the blood is approximately $46. The cost of determining the level of quinidine in the blood is approximately $34. The cost of determining the level of procainamide in the blood is approximately $48.

Urine tests. The following urine tests may be ordered:

- Patients with symptoms and signs of carcinoid heart disease should have their urine tested for 5-hyroxyindoleacetic acid. The cost of this test is approximately $48.
- Primary aldosteronism may be the cause of hypertension. The condition is usually diagnosed by identifying an elevation of serum or urinary levels of aldosterone that fail to be suppressed by volume expansion. The cost of the test on the serum is approximately $49. The cost of the test on the urine is approximately $89.
- Cushing disease may be the cause of systemic hypertension. The 24-hour free cortisol excretion test is an excellent screening test. The cost of this test is approximately $55.

FINAL COMMENT

The procedures and tests listed here are not performed routinely, because they are either expensive, hazardous, or time consuming, or their diagnostic usefulness is small when applied to every patient who is seen by a physician. These procedures and tests are used when the results of the initial examination of the patient suggest conditions that can be diagnosed or further refined with their use.

REFERENCES

1. DeBusk RF: Techniques of exercise testing. In Hurst JW, editor-in-chief: *The heart*, ed 7, New York, 1990, McGraw-Hill, pp 1825-1834.
2. Reeves TJ: Use of stress electrocardiography in practice, *Heart Dis Stroke* 1(1):13, 1992.
3. Sharp SD, Mason JW, Bray B: Comparison of ST depression recorded by Holter monitors and 12-lead ECGs during coronary angiography and exercise testing, *J Electrocardiol* 25(4):323, 1992.
4. Zipes DP, Akhtar M, Denes P et al: Guidelines for clinical intracardiac electrophysiologic studies: a report of the

American College of Cardiology/American Heart Association Task Force on Assessment of Diagnostic and Therapeutic Cardiovascular Procedures (Subcommittee to Assess Clinical Intracardiac Electrophysiologic Studies), *J Am Coll Cardiol* 14:1827, 1989.

5. Horowitz LN: Safety of electrophysiologic studies, *Circulation* 73:11, 1986.
6. Edelman RR, Manning WJ, Burstein D, Paulin S: Coronary arteries breath-hold MR angiography, *Radiology* 181:641, 1991.
7. Pettigrew RI: Magnetic resonance imaging of the heart and great vessels. In Hurst JW, editor-in-chief: *The heart*, ed 7, New York, 1990, McGraw-Hill pp 1975-1989.
8. Lund JT, Ehman RL, Julsrud PR et al: Cardiac masses: assessment by MR imaging, *AJR* 152:469, 1989.
9. Manning WJ, Atkinson DJ, Grossman W et al: First-pass MRI using Gd-DTPA in patients with coronary artery disease, *J Am Coll Cardiol* 18:959, 1991.
10. Pettigrew RI, Martin S, Eisner R et al: Quantitative catecholamine stress MR imaging to evaluate ischemic heart disease, *Radiology* 177:278, 1990 (abstract).
11. Grossman W: *Cardiac catheterization, angiography and intervention*, ed 4, Philadelphia, 1991, Lea & Febiger.
12. Kennedy JW: Registry Committee of the Society for Cardiac Angiography: complications associated with cardiac catheterization and angiography, *Cathet Cardiovasc Diagn* 8:5, 1982.
13. Ross J, Brandenburg RO, Dinsmore RE et al: Guidelines for coronary angiography: a report of the American College of Cardiology/American Heart Association Task Force on Assessment of Diagnostic and Therapeutic Cardiovascular Procedures (Subcommittee on Coronary Angiography), *Circulation* 76(4):963A, 1987.
14. Mason J: Personal communication, December 1992.
15. Fowles RE, Mason JW: Endomyocardial biopsy, *Ann Intern Med* 97:885, 1982.
16. Sekiguchi M, Take M: World survey of catheter biopsy of the heart. In Sekiguchi M, Olson EGJ, editors: *Cardiomyopathy: clinical, pathological and theoretical aspects*, Baltimore, 1980, University Park Press/University of Tokyo Press, pp 217-225.

ADDITIONAL READINGS
Exercise electrocardiography

Mark DB, Shaw L, Harrell FE Jr et al: Prognostic value of a treadmill exercise score in outpatients with suspected coronary artery disease, *N Engl J Med* 325:849, 1991.
McNeer JF, Margolis JR, Lee KL et al: The role of the exercise test in the evaluation of patients for ischemic heart disease, *Circulation* 57:64, 1978.
Schlant RC, Friesinger GC II, Leonard JJ: Clinical competence in exercise testing: a statement for physicians from the ACP/ACC/AHA Task Force on Clinical Privileges in Cardiology, *Am J Cardiol* 16:1061, 1990.

Holter monitoring

Hammill SC: Evaluation of a Holter system to record ST-segment changes, *J Electrocardiol* 20(suppl):12, 1987.
Nademanee K, Christenson PD, Intarachot V et al: Variability of indexes for myocardial ischemia: a comparison of treadmill tests, ambulatory electrocardiographic monitoring and symptoms of myocardial ischemia, *J Am Coll Cardiol* 13:574, 1989.
Stern S, Tzivoni D, Stern Z: Diagnostic accuracy of ambulatory ECG monitoring in ischemic heart disease, *Circulation* 52:1045, 1975.
Tzivoni D, Benhorin J, Gavish A, Stern S: Holter recordings during treadmill testing in assessing myocardial ischemia changes, *Am J Cardiol* 55:1200, 1985.
Wolf E, Tzivoni D, Stern S: Comparison of exercise test and 24-hour ambulatory electrocardiographic monitoring in detection of ST-T changes, *Br Heart J* 36:90, 1974.

Signal-averaged electrocardiography

Breithardt G, Borggrefe M: Recent advances in the identification of patients at risk of ventricular tachyarrhythmias: role of ventricular late potentials, *Circulation* 75:1091, 1987.
Denniss AR, Richards DA, Cody DV et al: Prognostic significance of ventricular tachycardia and fibrillation induced at programmed stimulation and delayed potentials detected on the signal-averaged electrocardiograms of survivors of acute myocardial infarction, *Circulation* 74:731, 1986.
Gomes JA, Winters SL, Stewart D: A new noninvasive index to predict sustained ventricular tachycardia and sudden death in the first year after myocardial infarction: based on signal-averaged electrocardiogram, radionuclide ejection fraction and Holter monitoring, *J Am Coll Cardiol* 10:349, 1987.
Kuchar DL, Thorburn CW, Sammel NL: Late potentials detected after myocardial infarction: natural history and prognostic significance, *Circulation* 74:1280, 1986.
Walter PF: Technique of electrophysiological testing. In Hurst JW, editor-in-chief: *The heart*, ed 7, New York, 1990, McGraw-Hill, pp 1847-1848.

Electrophysiologic studies

Dimarco JP, Garan H, Ruskin JN: Complications in patients undergoing cardiac electrophysiologic procedures, *Ann Intern Med* 97:490, 1982.

Exercise thallium-201 scan/positron emission tomography

O'Rourke RA, Chatterjee K, Dodge HT et al: Guidelines for clinical use of cardiac radionuclide imaging, December 1986: a report of the American College of Cardiology/American Heart Association Task Force on Assessment of Cardiovascular Procedures (Subcommittee on Nuclear Imaging), *Circulation* 74(4):1469A, 1986.

Computed tomography

Baron MG: Computed tomography of the heart. In Hurst JW, editor-in-chief: *The heart*, ed 7, New York, 1990, McGraw-Hill, pp 1950-1962.

Cipriano P, Nassi M, Brody WR: Clinically applicable gated cardiac computed tomography, *AJR* 140:604, 1983.

Daniel WG, Dohring W, Stender HS et al: Value and limitations of computed tomography in assessing aortocoronary bypass graft patency, *Circulation* 67:983, 1983.

Doppman JL, Rienmuller R, Lissner J et al: Computed tomography in constrictive pericardial disease, *J Comput Assist Tomogr* 5:1, 1981.

Godwin JD, Korobkin M: Acute disease of the aorta: diagnosis by computed tomography and ultrasonography, *Radiol Clin North Am* 21:551, 1983.

Modic MT, Janicki PC: Computed tomography of mass lesions of the right cardiophrenic angle, *J Comput Assist Tomogr* 4:521, 1980.

Niehues B, Heuser L, Jansen W et al: Noninvasive detection of intracardiac tumors by ultrasound and computed tomography, *Cardiovasc Intervent Radiol* 6:30, 1983.

Silverman PM, Harell GS, Korobkin M: Computed tomography of the abnormal pericardium, *AJR* 140:1125, 1983.

Tomoda H, Hoshai M, Furuya H et al: Evaluation of pericardial effusion with computed tomography, *Am Heart J* 99:701, 1980.

Magnetic resonance imaging

Amparo EG, Higgins CB, Hricak H et al: Aortic dissection: magnetic resonance imaging, *Radiology* 155:399, 1985.

Go RT, O'Donnell JK, Underwood DA et al: Comparison of gated cardiac MRI and 2D echocardiography of intracardiac neoplasms, *AJR* 145:21, 1985.

Soulen RL, Stark DD, Higgins CB: Magnetic resonance imaging of constrictive pericardial disease, *Am J Cardiol* 55:480, 1985.

ACC/AHA guidelines for the clinical application of echocardiography

A report of the American College of Cardiology/American Heart Association Task Force on Assessment of Diagnostic and Therapeutic Cardiovascular Procedures (Subcommittee to Develop Guidelines for the Clinical Application of Echocardiography)

Subcommittee members
Gordon A. Ewy, M.D., F.A.C.C., *Chairman*
Christopher P. Appleton, M.D., F.A.C.C.; Anthony N. DeMaria, M.D., F.A.C.C.;
Harvey Feigenbaum, M.D., F.A.C.C.; Edwin W. Rogers, Jr., M.D., F.A.C.C.;
James A. Ronan, Jr., M.D., F.A.C.C.; David J. Skorton, M.D., F.A.C.C.;
Abdul J. Tajik, M.D., F.A.C.C.; and Roberta G. Williams, M.D., F.A.C.C.

Task force members
Charles Fisch, M.D., F.A.C.C., *Chairman*
George A. Beller, M.D., F.A.C.C.; Roman W. DeSanctis, M.D., F.A.C.C.;
Harold T. Dodge, M.D., F.A.C.C.; J. Ward Kennedy, M.D., F.A.C.C.;
T. Joseph Reeves, M.D., F.A.C.C.; and Sylvan Lee Weinberg, M.D., F.A.C.C.

Reproduced with permission. ACC/AHA guidelines for the clinical application of echocardiography,
Circulation 82(6):2323, 1990. Copyright American Heart Association. Also reprinted with permission from
the American College of Cardiology (*Journal of the American College of Cardiology* 16[7]:1505, 1990).
"Guidelines for the Clinical Application of Echocardiography" were approved by the American College of
Cardiology Board of Trustees on March 17, 1990, and by the American Heart Association Steering Com-
mittee on May 18, 1990.

PREAMBLE

It is becoming more apparent each day that despite a strong national commitment to excellence in health care, the resources and personnel are finite. It is, therefore, appropriate that the medical profession examine the impact of developing technology on the practice and cost of medical care. Such analysis, carefully conducted, could potentially have an impact on the cost of medical care without diminishing the effectiveness of that care.

To this end, the American College of Cardiology and the American Heart Association in 1980 established a Task Force on Assessment of Diagnostic and Therapeutic Cardiovascular Procedures with the following charge:

The Task Force of the American College of Cardiology and the American Heart Association shall define the role of specific noninvasive and invasive procedures in the diagnosis and management of cardiovascular disease.

The Task Force shall address, when appropriate, the contribution, uniqueness, sensitivity, specificity, indications, contraindications, and cost-effectiveness of such specific procedures.

The Task Force shall include a Chairman and six members, three representatives from the American Heart Association and three representatives from the American College of Cardiology. The Task Force may select ad hoc members as needed upon the approval of the Presidents of both organizations. Recommendations of the Task Force are forwarded to the President of each organization.

The members of the Task Force are: George A. Beller, M.D., Roman W. DeSanctis, M.D., Harold T. Dodge, M.D., J. Ward Kennedy, M.D., T. Joseph Reeves, M.D., Sylvan Lee Weinberg, M.D., and Charles Fisch, M.D., Chairman.

This document was reviewed by the officers and other responsible individuals of the two organizations and received final approval in May 1990. It is being published simultaneously in *Circulation* and the *Journal of the American College of Cardiology*. The potential impact of this document on the practice of cardiology and some of its unavoidable shortcomings are clearly set out in the introduction.

CHARLES FISCH, M.D., F.A.C.C.

GENERAL CONSIDERATIONS AND SCOPE

Echocardiography is an examination technique that provides images of cardiac and great vessel anatomy and blood flow by ultrasound. Although ultrasound may be applied in different forms (M-mode, two-dimensional, spectral, and color flow Doppler imaging) and by different techniques (transthoracic, transesophageal), all are encompassed in the term echocardiography. When applied by the customary transthoracic approach, the examination involves little, if any, patient discomfort and has not been associated with patient risk. The ability of echocardiography to provide unique information regarding cardiac structure and function, the lack of ionizing radiation, the portability of the instrument, and the potential for repeated studies have led to the widespread utilization of echocardiography for virtually all categories of known and suspected cardiovascular disease.

When the role of echocardiography is discussed, it is assumed that the patients who are given the test have undergone a complete physical examination with medical history and that the usefulness and likely diagnostic yield have been carefully considered. The decision to perform an echocardiogram and interpret the results should not be done without consideration of other factors relevant to the individual patient.

In discussing the optimal use of echocardiography, it is important to consider the relation between the information derived and the ability to establish a definitive diagnosis or make a therapeutic decision. In some cases, echocardiography will definitively establish the etiology of a symptom complex (such as acquired ventricular septal defect after myocardial infarction). Echocardiography may establish the need for interventional therapy (as in patients with left atrial myxoma or cardiac tamponade, for example). Commonly, echocardiography will indicate the need for corrective therapy or specific follow-up (as in mitral or aortic stenosis). Often, it provides data that are confirmatory in nature, that have prognostic significance, or that aid in the overall evaluation of a disease state. The primary reason not to perform echocardiography in many cases is economic. The cost-effectiveness of echocardiography in these settings is related to the individual case. Societal resources must be considered by the physician. In addressing instances where echocardiography provides neither definitive diagnosis nor data on which therapeutic decisions may be based, this report attempts to indicate those situations in which the performance of echocardiography is not generally cost-effective.

The report is based on the assumption that the echocardiogram is performed and interpreted in accordance with the guidelines for optimal training set forth by the American Society of Echocardiography, the American College of Cardiology,[1,2] and the Society of Pediatric Echocardiography.[3]

This report is divided into two parts, the adult and the pediatric guidelines. In classifying the usefulness of echocardiography in clinical cardiovascular practice, each part is divided into two major sections. In the first, the usefulness of echocardiography in *specific cardiovascular disorders* is considered. In the second, the usefulness of echocardiography in evaluating general *symptoms and signs* is considered. The latter method of categorizing the appropriateness of echocardiography corresponds to the frequent use of the technique in the evaluation of the significance and mechanism of such common presenting complaints as dyspnea, chest discomfort, and cardiac murmur. It is hoped that this symptom- and sign-based classification will provide guidance to physicians regarding the utility of echocardiography in the evaluation of common clinical problems. The pediatric guidelines include those for fetal echocardiography.

Throughout this report, we have used the following classification system:

Class I: Conditions for which or patients for whom there is general agreement that echocardiography is appropriate

Class II: Conditions for which or patients for whom echocardiography is frequently used but there is a divergence of opinion with respect to its appropriateness

Class III: Conditions for which or patients for whom there is general agreement that echocardiography is not appropriate

VALVULAR HEART DISEASE

In evaluating the patient with valvular heart disease, the clinician seeks information about valvular structure and function, as well as about the effect of the valvular abnormality on cardiac anatomy and physiology. Assessment of the cardiac consequences of stenotic valve lesions requires estimation of the transvalvular pressure gradient and valve area and assessment of the cardiovascular consequences. In the case of regurgitant valves, assessment requires determination of not only the degree of regurgitation but also the anatomy of the receiving chamber and ventricular function. Thus, complete evaluation of the patient with acquired valvular heart disease requires attention not only to the valve lesion as such but also to its integrated role in overall cardiac function.

Echocardiography has become the noninvasive diagnostic method of choice for the evaluation of valvular heart disease. Because of the precision and accuracy of modern echocardiographic data, selected patients may undergo definitive surgical therapy without the need for cardiac catheterization.[4-6] In general, echocardiographic methods are more precise in defining the severity of valvular stenosis than of valvular regurgitation; however, this is also true of the alternative methods.

Native valve disease

Echocardiography is extremely useful in the diagnosis of stenosis and regurgitation of all four native cardiac valves. The largest clinical experience and most definitive validation studies have been reported in mitral and aortic valve disease, with less experience in the study of tricuspid and pulmonary valve disease.[7-9]

A particular strength of echocardiography is its ability to help identify the etiology of specific valvular abnormalities. Thus, calcification and fibrosis (due to degenerative and rheumatic diseases), prolapse (either idiopathic or related to specific connective tissue disorders), endocarditis, and other pathophysiologic mechanisms of valve dysfunction may be characterized using ultrasound examination techniques. Special mention should be made of mitral valve prolapse. Although of undisputed value in the diagnosis of mitral prolapse, some controversy continues as to the optimal echocardiographic criteria for this diagnosis.[10,11]

The degree of valvular fibrosis, calcification, and immobility bears an approximate relation to the degree of valvular stenosis. The severity of mitral stenosis may be accurately quantified in most patients by planimetric measurement of the valve area.[25] In all other valvular stenoses, hemodynamic measurement with Doppler echocardiography gives more accurate assessment of severity. Doppler echocardiographic techniques can accurately estimate instantaneous and mean transvalvular pressure gradient across stenotic mitral,[12] aortic,[12-14] and pulmonary[8] valves. In the evaluation of semilunar valvular stenosis, peak instantaneous and mean pressure gradient, as well as estimates of aortic valve orifice area based on the "continuity" principle,[6,14] have been successfully used to assess severity. In studies of stenotic atrioventricular (AV) valves, measurement of mean pressure gradient as well as estimation of orifice area by the continuity principle or by the pressure half-time method[15-19] have been employed.

Doppler echocardiographic methods are by far the most sensitive means of identifying the presence of valvular regurgitation. In fact, Doppler techniques are so sensitive that care must be taken not to interpret a physiologic phenomenon as indicating pathologic regurgitation. Studies[20,21] have indicated that mild apparent retrograde flow disturbances are frequently detected in Doppler echocardiograms of normal subjects by both pulsed and color flow Doppler methods.

Precise assessment of the severity of regurgitant valvular lesions is difficult using any invasive or noninvasive imaging technique. Pulsed Doppler and Doppler color flow mapping techniques yield only semiquantitative estimates of the severity of mitral and aortic regurgitation.[22-25] Due in part to difficulties in defining an appropriate independent standard, studies validating echocardiographic grading of the severity of tricuspid and pulmonary valve regurgitation are few. Echocardiography is the most sensitive noninvasive method of identifying valvular annular calcification.

Infective endocarditis

Transthoracic two-dimensional echocardiography has been utilized for the diagnosis and characterization of these valvular masses. However, the sensitivity of transthoracic examination in visualization of valvular vegetations ($\geq$4 to 5 mm in size) has ranged from 50% with M-mode echocardiography to 70% with two-dimensional echocardiography. Transesophageal echocardiography promises to improve the sensitivity of visualization of vegetations to nearly 90%.[26] Because of the possibility of false negative examination results, echocardiography should not be used as the sole means of excluding the presence of endocarditis. Echocardiography may be of use in identifying vegetations in patients with culture-negative endocarditis.[27]

In addition to identifying the presence of valvular vegetations, echocardiography offers important information about the complication of endocarditis, including not only the valvular sequelae (such as ruptured chordae tendineae), abscesses, and shunt lesions, but also the hemodynamic and pathologic consequences.

Prosthetic valve dysfunction

Echocardiographic imaging can be used to define abnormalities of prosthetic disk or ball motion; however, this usefulness is limited. Thrombus on struts, stents, or disks is difficult to appreciate because of reverberations and shadowing from the prosthetic valve structure. This is especially true of mitral prosthetic valves. In this situation the addition of transesophageal echocardiography is helpful since the combination of techniques allows a view of the valves from several angles.

Evaluation of the severity of prosthetic valvular dysfunction is best performed by Doppler techniques. The pressure gradient across aortic and mitral prostheses may be estimated accurately utilizing Doppler techniques in the majority of prosthetic valves.[28,29] Special care must be taken in the identification of the highest velocity jets, particularly in valves that produce eccentric flow, such as tilting disk and ball valve prostheses. The transvalvular pressure gradient expected across normally functioning prosthetic valves will vary with valve type and size. However, sufficient data are available concerning in vivo and in vitro flow behavior of these valves to interpret the velocities measured in the clinical setting.[30] Assessment of prosthetic valve effective orifice areas, particularly AV valve areas by pressure half-time methods, may be less accurate than the assessment of mean and peak pressure gradients.[31] Diagnosis of mild prosthetic obstruction may be difficult because of the variable transvalvular pressure gradients expected in valves of differing designs and sizes.

Echocardiography can identify bioprosthetic valve regurgitation. When employing Doppler techniques to identify abnormal mechanical prosthetic valve insufficiency, the normal occurrence of small amounts of regurgitation through these devices should be kept in mind.[32] Doppler color flow mapping appears capable of discriminating between central regurgitant flow jets and eccentric jets due to paravalvular leaks, although this differentiation is not perfect.[33,34]

The strengths and limitations of assessing severity of prosthetic regurgitation are in general similar to those noted for native valves. However, reverberations and attenuation (shadowing) associated with prostheses complicate the process of mapping regurgitant tricuspid and mitral jets. Transesophageal imaging methods avoid some of these problems, [35] especially when imaging the prosthetic mitral valve. Insufficient data are available to classify the usefulness of echocardiographic assessment of the severity of dysfunction of regurgitant pulmonary valve prostheses.

Prosthetic valve infective endocarditis

Diagnosis of prosthetic valve endocarditis by the transthoracic technique is more difficult than the diagnosis of endocarditis of native valves because of the reverberations, attenuation, and other image artifacts related to both mechanical valves and bioprostheses. Particularly in the case of mechanical valves, echocardiography is probably helpful only when there is a large or mobile vegetation. Thus, the technique cannot be used to exclude the presence of vegetations. These limitations are diminished with the use of transesophageal recording techniques because of the superior imaging quality. Transesophageal techniques have enhanced echocardiographic assessment of prosthetic valve infective endocarditis, especially of the mitral valve and of both mitral and aortic annular areas for abscesses.

Doppler techniques offer important information about the functional consequences of endocarditis of prosthetic valves, such as the existence of paravalvular leaks. It should be noted, however, that paravalvular leaks are not specific for endocarditis. Importantly, echocardiography may identify vegetations on native valves in patients with suspected prosthetic endocarditis.

Indications for echocardiography

Class I
  1. Native cardiac valve disease
  2. Prosthetic cardiac valve disease
  3. Suspected or proved infective endocarditis

Class II
  None

Class III
  None

ISCHEMIC HEART DISEASE

Because atherosclerosis still represents the major health threat to adults in Western societies, there has been tremendous effort expended on the development of noninvasive techniques for the diagnosis of coronary artery disease and its consequences. As a result, echocardiography has evolved to become a powerful tool in the assessment of patients at all stages of the ischemic disease process. It is useful to consider its application in the following circumstances:

Diagnosis

Acute myocardial infarction. Segmental ventricular wall motion abnormalities are characteristic of myocardial infarction in all but the smallest of infarctions and correlate with specific coronary artery distribution and pathology.[36-45] However, the loss of systolic contraction, the loss of wall thickening during systole, and even frank systolic bulging of a ventricular segment may also occur in acute and chronic ischemia or myocardial scar and therefore are not pathognomonic for infarction.[37-45] Segmental wall motion abnormalities may also occur in myocarditis and other conditions not associated with coronary occlusion, but the lack of systolic wall thickening is more specific for ischemia.[46] In patients with acute myocardial infarction, the ventricular wall motion abnormalities include not only the acutely infarcted segment but also previously infarcted segments as well as ischemic, "stunned," and "hibernating" myocardium in adjacent zones.[39,41,42,45,47] Together these represent the functional infarct size, which may be an overestimation of the true anatomic infarct size in some patients. Nevertheless, echocardiography-derived infarct size[42] correlates with thallium-201 perfusion defects,[40] peak creatine kinase levels,[41] hemodynamic changes,[42] results of catheterization ventriculography,[43] and coronary angiography,[44] early[48] and late[49] complications, mortality,[42,50] and pathologic findings.[45]

In acute myocardial infarction, clinical status and ventricular function may not be static, especially after reperfusion therapy. Serial echocardiography is a noninvasive method for monitoring the changes that occur.

Evaluation of myocardial segments uninvolved by the acute infarction is also important. The lack of the expected compensatory hyperkinesia can indicate multivessel disease,[47] and, therefore, the presence of asynergy in a remote segment carries an increased risk of postinfarction angina, progression in Killip classification, shock, and death.[41]

The right ventricle is involved to some degree in one third of inferior myocardial infarctions,[51] and an associated right ventricular infarction can have significant hemodynamic implications for patient management. Although somewhat more difficult to image, echocardiography is useful in the diagnosis of biventricular infarction.[52]

Complications of acute myocardial infarction

In addition to revealing and allowing quantitation of wall motion abnormalities, the echocardiogram can be used to detect five major early complications of acute myocardial infarction:

1. *Thrombus.* Echocardiography is the definitive test for intracardiac thrombi.[53-58] The true frequency of postinfarction thrombus was not appreciated until echocardiographic studies were done. Thrombi are more common in anterior and apical than in inferior infarctions.[56-58] Patients developing a mural thrombus are at increased risk of mortality.[54] The therapeutic implications of left ventricular thrombi are evolving and therefore the need for serial imaging is controversial.

2. *Acute mitral regurgitation.* The importance of new onset of mitral regurgitation is demonstrated by its correlation with prognosis.[59] Acute mitral regurgitation can occur from several mechanisms. One of the heads of the papillary muscle may acutely rupture.[60]

Alternatively, the papillary muscle and associated free wall may be acutely ischemic or may develop late fibrosis and foreshorten, rendering the valve regurgitant.[61] Both are evident echocardiographically. Doppler ultrasonography can be used to locate the regurgitant jet, and color flow mapping can help in its quantitation.[62]

3. *Ventricular septal rupture.* Two-dimensional echocardiography can be used to visualize the typical interventricular septal defect [63] and Doppler ultrasonography can be used to locate the left-to-right shunt[64] and differentiate it from mitral valve regurgitation[65] or from tricuspid valve regurgitation resulting from right ventricular infarction. This information is essential when surgical intervention is being considered.

4. *Free wall rupture.* Patients who survive free wall rupture develop a pseudoaneurysm that has a characteristic echocardiographic appearance.[66] Echocardiography also provides information regarding the presence or absence of associated cardiac tamponade[67] and can prove helpful in determining the timing of surgical intervention.

5. *Infarct expansion.* Infarct expansion may occur after myocardial infarction. When this occurs, the patient's prognosis has been shown to be worse.[68] Echocardiography has been shown to be excellent at making this diagnosis[69] and at differentiating expansion from infarct extension.

Therefore, in patients with acute myocardial infarction, echocardiography can be used to make a rapid diagnosis, to stratify patients into high- or low-risk categories, to monitor serial changes, to look for associated injury such as right ventricular infarction, and to diagnose the complications of infarction.

Chronic ischemic heart disease

Echocardiography is frequently useful in assessing patients with chronic ischemic heart disease for both prognostic and therapeutic reasons. Quantitative global and regional systolic function indexes include fractional shortening, fractional area change, and ejection fraction.

A left ventricular aneurysm is a finding of chronic ischemic heart disease, and echocardiography is a helpful test for this condition.[70,71] Assessment of function of residual cardiac segments is one of the key factors in selecting medical or surgical therapy in these patients. Doppler echocardiographic evaluation of the tricuspid valve usually detects sufficient tricuspid regurgitation to allow an estimation of right ventricular and pulmonary artery systolic pressure.[72] Doppler echocardiography is also helpful in assessing diastolic dysfunction (see below).

Echocardiography is most helpful in patients with chronic ischemic heart disease at initial evaluation of the patient for risk stratification and to assess the changes produced by therapeutic interventions or unexpected clinical deterioration. Little additional information is added, however, by serial imaging at predetermined intervals during routine follow-up.

Detection of myocardial ischemia

Echocardiography in coronary artery disease does not image the primary lesion but only its consequences. Segmental wall motion abnormalities with lack of normal systolic thickening are therefore highly specific but not sensitive for latent underlying coronary artery disease.

Stress echocardiography, including exercise and pharmacologic stress, is more informative than studies at rest for the detection of myocardial ischemia.[73-75] Stress echocardiography is discussed in more detail in the section on chest pain. Exercise examination may be warranted in patients with clinical evidence of coronary artery disease in those circumstances in which the standard graded exercise tests may prove nondiagnostic. Examples include conditions that produce abnormal rest echocardiographic results and others likely to produce false positive stress echocardiographic results.

Indications for echocardiography

Rest echocardiography
Class I
   1. Myocardial infarction (acute and chronic) when there is a specific question that can be resolved by echocardiography
Class II
   1. Clinical evidence of coronary artery disease
Class III
   1. Screening test for coronary disease in the general population
Stress echocardiography
Class I
   None
Class II
   1. Whenever there is a high pretest probability that an indicated standard exercise stress test would be inadequate, nondiagnostic, or produce false positive results
Class III
   1. Routine screening of the general population without significant coronary risk factors

DISEASE OF THE HEART MUSCLE

Cardiomyopathies are heart muscle disorders of unknown etiology and are classified into three broad categories: dilated, hypertrophic, and restrictive forms.[76] Echocardiography provides comprehensive morphologic assessment as well as characterization of the hemodynamics.

Dilated cardiomyopathy

Echocardiography demonstrates dilation of ventricles, usually with normal wall thickness and reduced systolic function.[76,77] Intracardiac thrombi may be detected. Doppler echocardiography is used to determine valvular regurgitation, pulmonary pressures, and diastolic dysfunction.[77] Echocardiography is useful for serial follow-up as well as for assessment of the effectiveness of therapeutic interventions. It is useful in assessing and monitoring patients at risk of developing toxic cardiomyopathy, such as adriamycin cardiomyopathy.

Hypertrophic cardiomyopathy

Echocardiography not only establishes the diagnosis of hypertrophic cardiomyopathy by revealing diffuse or localized areas of ventricular hypertrophy but also permits comprehensive morphologic assessment, specifically in patients with unusual areas of ventricular hypertro-

---

phy.[78] Doppler techniques are utilized to assess severity of intraventricular obstruction at rest and with provocative maneuvers and to assess associated mitral regurgitation and diastolic filling abnormalities.[78] In many patients, cardiac catheterization is no longer necessary to establish the diagnosis or for hemodynamic assessment. Echocardiography is useful for serial follow-up and for assessment of the effectiveness of therapeutic interventions.

Restrictive cardiomyopathy

The two-dimensional echocardiographic features of restrictive cardiomyopathy are distinctive in that the ventricular chambers are usually normal in dimension and wall thickness and that frequently there is normal systolic function. However, the atria are markedly dilated, reflecting abnormal diastolic compliance of the ventricles. Doppler studies have shown characteristic ventricular inflow velocity profiles consisting of increased peak early flow velocity, reduced peak late flow velocity, and shortened deceleration time.[79-81] Combined two-dimensional and Doppler echocardiographic examination may be helpful in patients with restrictive cardiomyopathy and may allow differentiation from constrictive pericarditis.

Indications for echocardiography

Class I
1. Establishment of the morphologic diagnosis and assessment of hemodynamic status of patients with cardiomyopathies
2. Systemic illness associated with cardiac involvement, with clinical symptoms
3. Exposure to cardiotoxic agents

Class II
1. Systemic illness with high incidence of cardiac involvement but no clinical evidence of cardiac involvement
2. Clinical evidence suggesting cardiomyopathy
3. Family history of genetically transmitted cardiac disease

Class III
1. Systemic illness with low incidence of cardiac involvement and no clinical evidence of cardiac involvement

PERICARDIAL DISEASE

One of the earliest applications of echocardiography was in the detection of pericardial effusion,[82] and it remains the procedure of choice for evaluating this clinical problem. The pericardium usually responds to disease or injury by inflammation that may result in pericardial thickening, the formation of an exudate, or both, which in turn is manifested in the clinical picture of pericardial effusion, with or without tamponade or constriction. The anatomic evidence of pericardial disease and its effects on cardiovascular physiology can often be seen on M-mode, two-dimensional, and Doppler echocardiograms.

Pericardial effusion

Pericardial effusions as small as 15 ml in volume can be detected by echocardiography, their location and configuration determined, and their size estimated in a semiquantitative fashion. Differentiation among types of pericardial fluid (blood, exudate, transudate, and others) cannot be made, but fibrous strands, tumor masses, and blood clots can often be distinguished. It should be remembered that all "echo-free" spaces adjacent to the heart are not the result of pericardial effusion.[83]

Most pericardial effusions that require pericardiocentesis are located both anteriorly and posteriorly, but loculated effusions may occur, particularly after cardiac surgery. In such cases, echocardiography can define the distribution of the fluid so that the safest and most effective approach (subcostal, apical, or parasternal) can be planned for the pericardiocentesis.[84]

Cardiac tamponade

Enlarging pericardial effusions may cause cardiac tamponade. Although the diagnosis of cardiac tamponade can usually be made on the basis of the clinical evidence, when two-dimensional or Doppler echocardiography, alone or in combination, is combined with those clinical findings, the diagnosis is more certain, even in difficult cases. The elevated intrapericardial pressure in tamponade decreases the transmural pressure gradient between the pericardium and the right atrium and ventricle and increases the distending force necessary for ventricular filling. Echocardiographic evidence of right atrial invagination (collapse) at end-diastole and right ventricular collapse in early diastole are signs of hemodynamic compromise.[85-87] Right atrial collapse is a sensitive sign of tamponade but is not specific; diastolic right ventricular compression is more specific. Distension of the inferior vena cava that does not diminish on deep inspiration may also be seen and indicates an elevation of central venous pressure.[88] Doppler flow studies have shown marked respiratory variation in transvalvular flow velocities, left ventricular ejection, and left ventricular isovolumetric times in patients with pericardial tamponade.[89,90]

Increased pericardial thickness

Increased echo density behind the posterior wall suggests pericardial thickening, but echocardiographic measurement of the precise pericardial thickness may be inaccurate.[91] The causes of such thickening include fibrosis, calcification, and neoplasms, and it is usually not possible to differentiate the specific cause by echocardiography.

Pericardial tumors and cysts

Tumor in the pericardium is usually metastatic from the breast or lung, but other types occasionally occur.[92] The clinical findings are typically a sizable pericardial effusion, at times leading to tamponade, but tumor may also present as single or multiple epicardial tumor nodules, as effusive-constrictive pericarditis, or even as constrictive pericarditis. The effects of radiation therapy on the tumor may further affect the pericardium, resulting in inflammation, effusion, or fibrosis.

Pericardial cysts are rare and are usually located at the right costophrenic angle. They are readily visualized by echocardiography and their cystic nature can be differentiated from that of a solid mass.[93]

Constrictive pericarditis

In constrictive pericarditis there are such prominent pathologic and physiologic changes that echocardiographic abnormalities are always present, and in most cases there are multiple abnormalities. However, there is no single echocardiographic sign, or combination of signs, that is absolutely diagnostic of constrictive pericarditis. Some frequently seen findings are pericardial thickening, mild atrial enlargement with a normal-sized left ventricle, dilation of the vena cava, flattening of left ventricular endocardial motion in mid and late diastole, various abnormalities of septal motion, and premature opening of the pulmonary valve. Although these findings are nonspecific,[94-98] when they are considered in the clinical context they can usually confirm the diagnosis of constrictive pericarditis. Doppler flow studies show marked changes in early mitral and tricuspid flow velocity at the onset of inspiration and expiration, and they provide useful information about physiology that can be combined with anatomic information from two-dimensional echocardiography.[79,80] These Doppler findings are helpful in differentiating restrictive cardiomyopathy from constrictive pericarditis.

Congenital absence of the pericardium

In both total and partial absence of the pericardium, there are echocardiographic findings that are helpful in establishing the diagnosis.[99,100]

Indications for echocardiography

Class I
Patients with clinical manifestations of or suspected pericardial disease.
Class II
Follow-up studies. The precise timing of follow-up studies is highly individualized, but they are usually done when there is other clinical evidence that the clinical status of the patient has changed or when further information is needed for guiding treatment.
Class III
None

CARDIAC MASSES

Echocardiography is a well-established technique for diagnosis of various types of intracardiac masses.[53,54,58,101] Cardiac masses include tumors, thrombi, and vegetations. The most common primary cardiac tumor is a myxoma, and echocardiography has proved to be the diagnostic technique of choice for characterization of this tumor (location, attachment, size, appearance, and mobility). Echocardiography similarly is highly sensitive and specific for diagnosis of rhabdomyoma in patients with tuberous sclerosis. It also is useful for diagnosis of suspected cardiac metastases.

Intracardiac thrombi can be present in any of the cardiac chambers, and echocardiography is also the diagnostic technique of choice for localization and characterization of various intracardiac thrombi. With transesophageal echocardiography, thrombi in the left atrial appendage can be readily visualized. Echocardiography not only detects thrombus but also provides information pertaining to its size and shape and on whether it is sessile, pedunculated, or freefloating. Such characterization has important clinical and therapeutic implications.

Indications for echocardiography

Class I
1. Evaluation of patients with suspected cardiac masses

Class II
None

Class III
None

DISEASES OF THE GREAT VESSELS

Echocardiography can be effectively utilized to visualize the entire thoracic aorta in most adults. Complete aortic visualization by combined transthoracic (left and right parasternal windows), suprasternal, supraclavicular, and subcostal windows can be often achieved in 80% to 85% of patients. Good visualization of the main pulmonary artery segment and the proximal right and left pulmonary arteries can also be achieved in 85% of adults. The proximal portion of the innominate veins along with superior vena cava visualization can be achieved in nearly all patients with use of the right supraclavicular fossa and suprasternal notch approaches. Similarly, the proximal inferior vena cava and hepatic (subcostal) and pulmonary veins (apical and transesophageal) can be visualized in most patients.

Aortic dissection

Acute aortic dissection is a life-threatening emergency, and an early and prompt diagnosis is mandatory for appropriate patient care. The feasibility of using transthoracic echocardiography to visualize the intimal flap has been demonstrated by various investigators.[102,103] Transesophageal echocardiography is currently regarded as a sensitive diagnostic procedure.[26] In cooperative European studies the sensitivity and predictive accuracy of transesophageal echocardiography in aortic dissection were 98% and 99%, respectively. Limitations of single-plane transesophageal echocardiography include the "blind spot" of the ascending aorta because of the interposition of the trachea and the difficulty of detecting branch vessel involvement. In addition to establishing the diagnosis and the extent of aortic dissection, echocardiography is extremely useful in delineating any associated complications, such as pericardial effusion, with or without tamponade, and aortic regurgitation, as well as in evaluating left ventricular size and function. Transesophageal echocardiography is also suited for serial follow-up of postoperative patients with aortic dissection.[104]

Aortic aneurysm

Aneurysms of the ascending aorta can be characterized by transthoracic echocardiography. The aneurysm may be localized to one of the sinuses of Valsalva. With Doppler color flow imaging, rupture of an aneurysm in the sinus of Valsalva can be diagnosed and its communication with the receiving cardiac chamber can be documented. Annuloaortic ectasia as well as localized atherosclerotic aneurysms of the ascending aorta can be well visualized with use of the left as well as the right parasternal windows. Echocardiography is particularly well suited for serial follow-up of patients with ascending aortic aneurysms (especially in patients with Marfan's syndrome) for determination of increase in the size of the aneurysm in a serial manner. Descending thoracic aortic aneurysms are difficult to visualize with the transthoracic approach. Transesophageal echocardiography is particularly suited for complete characterization of these aneurysms.

The great veins

Echocardiography is a useful technique for visualizing the superior vena cava and for diagnosing various congenital and acquired abnormalities. A persistent left superior vena cava often can be imaged directly from the left supraclavicular fossa. Its connection, which is frequently to the coronary sinus, can be seen from a parasternal window as dilation. In some cases the connection to the coronary sinus can be better delineated with the use of contrast echocardiography with injection into the left arm. Other abnormalities, such as vena caval thrombosis, can also be diagnosed with combined use of echocardiographic and Doppler techniques. The proximal inferior vena cava can be readily visualized in nearly all patients and vena caval dilation and thrombosis or extension of tumors from the inferior vena cava to the right heart chambers have been diagnosed. The hepatic veins, their size, connection, and flow dynamics can be characterized with combined use of two-dimensional and Doppler echocardiography. Although visualization of all four pulmonary veins is not feasible in the majority of adult patients with use of the transthoracic approach, transesophageal echocardiography permits clear visualization of the pulmonary vein connections.

Indications for echocardiography

Class I
1. Acute aortic root dilation or clinical suspicion of aortic dissection
2. First-degree relatives of patients with genetically transmitted connective tissue disorders

Class II
1. Chronic aortic root dilation
2. Suspected connective tissue disorder in athletes
3. All other suspected disease of the great vessel

Class III
None

PULMONARY DISEASE

As a general rule, patients who have primary pulmonary disease are not ideal subjects for echocardiographic examinations because the hyperinflated lung is a poor conductor of ultrasound. Despite these technical limitations, transthoracic echocardiography can still be very informative in some patients with primary lung disease. The usual precordial or parasternal windows are frequently unavailable in patients with hyperinflated lungs. However, in these same patients the diaphragms are frequently lower than normal. Thus, the subcostal or subxyphoid transducer position can offer an ideal window for echocardiographic examinations.[105] For those few patients in whom transthoracic and subcostal echocardiographic windows are totally unavailable, there is now the transesophageal approach, which provides an unobstructed view of the heart in patients with lung disease. As a result, with use of one examining technique or another, almost all patients with primary lung disease can be studied echocardiographically.

If lung disease does not result in an anatomic or physiologic alteration of cardiac structure or function, the findings on the echocardiogram will be normal. Although a normal result on echocardiography does not indicate a diagnosis of lung disease, the differential diagnosis of cardiac versus pulmonary symptoms can often be made on the basis of the echocardiogram. Since a patient's shortness of breath can be due to either a lung or a heart condition, normal findings on the echocardiogram can be extremely helpful in such a differential diagnosis.

In those patients whose lung disease is affecting cardiac function, the echocardiogram can be of significant value. Pulmonary hypertension is one of the most common complications of primary lung disease, and echocardiography is helpful in evaluating the presence and severity of pulmonary hypertension. The right ventricle commonly dilates and can be detected on both the M-mode and two-dimensional echocardiogram. With marked systolic or diastolic overload of the right ventricle, the shape or motion, or both, of the interventricular septum is distorted, bulging abnormally toward the left ventricle. In patients with increased pulmonary vascular resistance, the M-mode recording of the pulmonary valve shows a distinctive early to mid-systolic notch. A somewhat similar pulmonary velocity flow pattern is seen on the Doppler recording in such patients.

Any valvular regurgitation resulting from pulmonary hypertension can be detected with Doppler techniques. If adequate tricuspid and pulmonary valve regurgitation signals are obtained, Doppler techniques can be used to accurately calculate right ventricular systolic and pulmonary artery diastolic pressure.[72] This type of determination can be made in a high percentage of patients with significant pulmonary hypertension. Doppler echocardiography can also be utilized to estimate pulmonary artery mean pressure (from the pulmonary acceleration time).

Indications for echocardiography

Class I

1. Unexplained pulmonary hypertension
2. Pulmonary emboli and suspected clots in the right atrium or ventricle

Class II

1. Lung disease with clinical suspicion of cardiac involvement
2. Pulmonary emboli

Class III

None

HYPERTENSION

In adults, hypertension is the most common cause of concentric left ventricular hypertrophy and congestive heart failure.[106] Data from the Framingham Study[106] have shown that both the risk of cardiac failure and mortality are increased in patients with electrocardiographic (ECG) criteria of left ventricular hypertrophy compared with patients who have hypertension and normal findings on electrocardiography. More recently, in the same population, an association of echocardiographic left ventricular mass with coronary heart disease events has been demonstrated that is independent of traditional coronary risk factors.[107]

Echocardiography must now be considered the noninvasive procedure of choice in evaluating the cardiac effects of systemic hypertension. M-mode and two-dimensional echocardiographic estimates of left ventricular mass are more sensitive and specific than either the ECG or chest roentgenogram in diagnosing the presence of left ventricular hypertrophy,[108] and these estimates have been shown to correlate accurately with left ventricular mass at necropsy.[109,110] These techniques have been used to evaluate the relation of left ventricular mass to rest and exercise blood pressure as well as to multiple other physiologic variables.[111] Echocardiography can also be used to evaluate systolic and diastolic properties of the left ventricle, such as speed and extent of contraction, end-systolic wall stress, and the rate of ventricular filling throughout diastole.[111]

A decrease in left ventricular mass in hypertensive patients through control of blood pressure or weight loss has been demonstrated in several studies.[112] The need for serial quantitation of left ventricular mass in assessing drug therapy for hypertension is underscored by the poor association of blood pressure control with regression of left ventricular hypertrophy.[111] However, although preliminary data are encouraging, more study will be required to prove that regression of left ventricular hypertrophy alters cardiac morbidity and mortality and that echocardiography is a cost-effective method for both the detection and follow-up evaluation of the large number of patients with hypertension.

Indications for echocardiography

Class I
1. Hypertension with clinical evidence of heart disease

Class II
1. Hypertension without signs or symptoms of heart disease

Class III
1. Borderline hypertension without signs or symptoms of heart disease

DYSPNEA

Dyspnea is a common cardiac symptom in patients with lung or cardiac disease. The role of echocardiography in patients with lung disease is addressed in the section on pulmonary disease. Impairment of left ventricular systolic function is the most common cause of heart failure. Recently, it has been recognized that up to one third of patients who have dyspnea of cardiac origin have abnormalities of left ventricular diastolic function as the cause of their symptoms.[113,114] Diastolic abnormalities severe enough to cause symptoms without systolic dysfunction are most commonly seen in elderly patients who have left ventricular hypertrophy and a history of hypertension. Evidence suggests that diastolic abnormalities precede detectable left ventricular systolic dysfunction and are associated with increased cardiovascular morbidity.[115] Since treatment to improve systolic cardiac performance may not benefit or may even be detrimental to diastolic function, a noninvasive method to help determine the cause of cardiac dyspnea should ideally be able to evaluate both systolic and diastolic cardiac performance.

With its ability to assess cardiac anatomy, chamber sizes, and myocardial and valvular function, echocardiography is a powerful noninvasive tool to investigate possible causes of dyspnea of cardiac origin. Echocardiography is a good method for detecting and quantitating left ventricular hypertrophy[111] and has been shown to be comparable to cardiac catheterization for assessing the severity of valvular and congenital heart disease. In most patients who have pulmonary and tricuspid valve regurgitation, estimates of pulmonary artery systolic and diastolic pressures can be made with use of the modified Bernoulli equation.[116] Abnormalities of left ventricular diastolic filling can be assessed by either M-mode or Doppler echocardiography; the results of both have been compared favorably with those of angiographic[117] and radionuclide[118] techniques. Therefore, echocardiography can be recommended for the evaluation of dyspnea in patients with clinical findings suggestive of significant coronary, valvular, or hypertensive heart disease. However, because dyspnea is a common symptom in patients without organic heart disease, echocardiography cannot be recommended as an initial diagnostic study in patients with normal blood pressure and physical examination.

Indications for echocardiography

Class I

None

Class II

1. Dyspnea with clinical evidence or suspicion of heart disease
2. Unexplained dyspnea

Class III

1. Dyspnea without clinical evidence of heart disease, pulmonary hypertension, or significant lung disease
2. Hyperventilation syndrome

CHEST PAIN

There are many cardiac causes of chest pain. The most common clinical entity that presents as chest pain is coronary artery disease (see section on ischemic heart disease). Hypertrophic cardiomyopathy, aortic stenosis, aortic dissection, mitral valve prolapse, and even acute pulmonary embolism can present with fairly distinctive and diagnostic findings on echocardiography.

The role of echocardiography in patients whose chest pain raises suspicion of coronary artery disease is being defined. In patients with ischemic heart disease, the role of echocardiography can be similar to that of electrocardiography. A person can have extensive coronary artery disease; however, if the coronary artery obstructions have not induced any malfunction of the ventricle, then the echocardiographic findings can be completely normal at rest. If the patient has had a previous known or unknown myocardial infarction, then the rest echocardiogram will help to confirm or evaluate that clinical event. Silent ischemia, even to the point of myocardial infarction, is not uncommon. A rest echocardiogram can detect a previously unknown myocardial infarction.

A patient may have coronary artery disease that is not producing angina but is interfering with blood flow so that myocardial function is impaired even in the resting state, as in hibernating myocardium. An echocardiogram can detect regional wall dysfunction and, theoretically, can be diagnostically useful in patients who are suspected of having coronary artery disease. The frequency with which a rest echocardiogram will be informative in such patients is still unknown.

The majority of patients with ischemic heart disease will have normal findings on rest echocardiography. If there is clinical evidence to suggest a prior myocardial infarction and confirmation or evaluation of the patient's global or regional ventricular function is desired, then the need for a rest echocardiogram can be more easily justified.

As with the ECG, a patient with coronary artery disease may exhibit an echocardiographic abnormality only when ischemia can be induced with some form of stress testing. Exercise is a commonly used form of stress to bring out ECG abnormalities, ventricular wall motion abnormalities, or perfusion defect abnormalities that are not present at rest. A similar strategy is possible with echocardiography. By inducing ischemia, either with exercise,[119-121] pharmacologic stress,[122,123] or pacing,[124] myocardial dysfunction can be produced that can be recognized on the echocardiogram as a wall motion abnormality. The feasibility of using echocardiography to detect ischemia-induced wall motion abnormalities has been well demonstrated.[73,125,126]

A major issue regarding the use of stress echocardiography is its practicality. However, with advances and improvements in echocardiographic techniques, echocardiographic equipment, and digital recording methods, the majority of patients can be successfully examined with stress echocardiography.[127-129]

Stress echocardiography is combined with routine exercise testing and offers supplemental information.[130] The sensitivity and specificity of the combined tests are improved, especially in certain subsets of patients.[131,132] The addition of echocardiography, however, substantially increases the cost of a routine stress test. For any patient whose physician believes that ECG stress testing with clinical evaluation alone needs to be supplemented with a test of ventricular function, stress echocardiography is a reasonable option.

Indications for echocardiography

Class I

1. Chest pain with clinical evidence of valvular, pericardial, or primary myocardial disease

Class II

1. Known or suspected coronary artery disease

Class III

1. Noncardiac chest pain

See previous section on chest pain for discussion of stress echocardiography.

MURMURS

Cardiac auscultation remains the most widely used method of screening for heart disease. In valvular and congenital forms of heart disease a murmur is usually the major evidence of the abnormality. Heart murmurs are produced by turbulent blood flow and are often signs of stenotic or regurgitant valve disease or of acquired or congenital defects. However, many murmurs are "innocent" and of no functional significance. When the characteristic findings of an individual murmur are considered together with other clinical data from the physical examination, the chest roentgenogram, and the ECG, the correct diagnosis can usually be established. However, echocardiography provides complementary information about cardiac structure and function as well as about blood flow. In some patients the echocardiogram is the only noninvasive method capable of identifying the cause of a heart murmur.

In the evaluation of heart murmurs the purposes of performing an echocardiogram are to:

- Define the primary lesion and judge its severity
- Detect coexisting abnormalities
- Detect lesions secondary to the primary lesion
- Evaluate cardiac function
- Establish a reference point for future observations
- Reevaluate the patient after an intervention

Echocardiography has replaced cardiac catheterization as the definitive study for many types of valvular and congenital heart disease and has become the method of choice for serial observation of patients with these conditions because it is accurate and painless. Furthermore, in many patients surgery can be performed without cardiac catheterization as long as the status of the coronary arteries is not a concern.

As valuable as echocardiography may be, the basic cardiovascular evaluation is still the most appropriate method to screen for cardiac disease and will establish many clinical diagnoses. Accordingly, echocardiography should not be used to replace the cardiovascular examination. Echocardiography can be helpful to determine the etiology and judge the severity of lesions.

Indications for echocardiography

Class I

1. An organic murmur in a patient with cardiorespiratory symptoms
2. A murmur in an asymptomatic patient if the clinical features indicate at least a moderate probability that the murmur is organic

Class II

1. A murmur in an asymptomatic patient in whom there is low probability of heart disease but in whom the diagnosis of heart disease cannot be reasonably excluded by the standard cardiovascular clinical evaluation

Class III

1. A typically innocent murmur in an asymptomatic patient without any other reason to suspect heart disease

NEUROLOGIC DISORDERS

Ischemic syndromes

By clinical criteria, cerebral embolism originating from the heart is believed to account for approximately 15% of all ischemic strokes.[133] Using aggregate clinical data, the main condi-

---

tions believed to be associated with the formation of intracardiac thrombus by percentage are nonrheumatic atrial fibrillation (45%), acute myocardial infarction or left ventricular aneurysm (15%), rheumatic mitral stenosis (10%), and prosthetic aortic or mitral valves (10%). Mitral valve prolapse, idiopathic dilated cardiomyopathy, valvular vegetations, calcific aortic stenosis, patent foramen ovale, and left atrial myxoma are other possible sources of cerebral emboli.

Two-dimensional echocardiography is recognized as a sensitive and specific noninvasive method for the diagnosis of intracardiac thrombi.[134] Although it can confirm the presence of abnormalities associated with cerebral emboli, an abnormal result cannot rule out the heart as an embolic source. Two-dimensional echocardiography has a sensitivity of 75% to 95% and a specificity of approximately 85% for detecting left ventricular thrombi that are >4 mm in diameter.[134] Two-dimensional echocardiography has a sensitivity and specificity of approximately 70% to 90% for identifying thrombi in the body of the left atrium,[134] but the sensitivity for clots located in the left atrial appendage is <15%. More recently, transesophageal echocardiography has been reported to have an increased sensitivity for diagnosing clots in the left atrium and left atrial appendage that approaches 95%.[135] This is notable since the appendage is the most frequent site for clot formation.

Previous studies have established that at least one third of patients with ischemic strokes have evidence of cardiac disease by history, physical examination, chest x-ray film, or ECG.[136] Because this incidence is higher than that estimated for cerebral embolism from a cardiac source, [133] a causal relation between the two cannot be assumed. Therefore, echocardiography appears warranted in patients with stroke who have clinical evidence for heart disease. Echocardiography is frequently performed in stroke patients <45 years of age, regardless of clinical findings, to rule out intraatrial communications or mitral valve prolapse as a possible source of embolism.[137] If Doppler echocardiography and color flow imaging do not detect a shunt, a two-dimensional contrast bubble study is frequently performed in these patients because it is the most sensitive method for detecting small intraatrial shunts. Routine echocardiography does not appear warranted as an initial diagnostic study in the majority of stroke patients >45 years old who do not have clinical evidence for cardiac disease because these patients rarely have echocardiographic findings associated with peripheral emboli.[138]

Indications for echocardiography

Class I
1. Patients with cerebral embolism and clinical evidence of heart disease
2. Patients <45 years of age with a cerebrovascular event

Class II
1. Patients >45 years of age with suspicion of cardiogenic brain embolism but without clinical evidence of heart disease

Class III
1. Patients with known noncardiac causes of the neurologic disorder

Syncope

Determination of the etiology of a syncopal episode can be a difficult clinical problem. Despite a careful history and physical examination, it is often not possible to distinguish syncope of cardiac origin from syncope due to other causes.[139-141] Furthermore, because numerous cardiac-related mechanisms can cause a sudden decrease in cerebral perfusion, a diagnostic approach for ordering cardiac studies that is cost-effective should be based both on the features of the individual case and on an awareness of the most common pathophysiologic mechanisms that cause syncope.[139,141]

Syncope of cardiac origin is most commonly related to vasodepressor reflexes or cardiac bradyarrhythmia or tachyarrhythmias.[140,142] Uncommon causes of cardiac syncope include severe aortic stenosis, hypertrophic obstructive cardiomyopathy, or atrial myxoma. Therefore, echocardiography should not be performed as an initial diagnostic step in patients with syncope unless the physical examination suggests the presence of a pathologic murmur or valvular heart disease. The decision on performing echocardiography in patients who still have unexplained syncope after evaluation for cardiac arrhythmias should be individualized with the knowledge that the yield of the test is expected to be low.

Indications for echocardiography

Class I
1. Patients with a murmur suggestive of significant valvular heart disease or obstructive cardiomyopathy

Class II
1. Patients without clinical evidence of heart disease and normal findings on evaluation for noncardiac causes of syncope

Class III
1. Patients with known noncardiac causes of syncope

PERIPHERAL EMBOLI

Patients with documented peripheral emboli involving major arteries should undergo echocardiographic study regardless of clinical findings because the heart is the only likely source for such large emboli. Transesophageal echocardiography improves the ability to detect left atrial thrombi, especially in the appendage, and to detect venous thrombi that have entered the central or peripheral circulation through a patent foramen ovale. Echocardiography should also be performed to look for evidence of endocarditis in patients with fever who have peripheral arterial emboli or embolic findings in the extremities or fundi. Transesophageal echocardiography improves the detection of ascending or descending aortic abnormalities, such as aneurysms, dissecting hematomas, or ulcerations.

Indications for echocardiography

Class I
None

Class II
1. Patients with peripheral emboli involving major arteries
2. Patients with evidence of infection and peripheral emboli

Class III
None

ARRHYTHMIAS AND PALPITATION

Echocardiography is useful in defining the cardiac milieu in which arrhythmias occur and therefore is a useful adjunct in the management of cardiac arrhythmias.

Arrhythmias associated with palpitation can be divided into several types. Minor arrhythmias, such as isolated premature contractions, can occur without structural heart disease and further evaluation is not required. Although an echocardiogram may reveal a minor abnormality such as mitral valve prolapse in such patients, the diagnostic yield is low and unlikely to change management.

Some arrhythmias are frequently associated with underlying organic heart disease or may predispose the patient to hemodynamic deterioration. Atrial fibrillation and flutter are examples of arrhythmias in which the echocardiogram frequently is appropriate to assess such an underlying disorder. A specific common use of the ultrasound examination is to quantitate left atrial size in patients with atrial fibrillation before considering cardioversion.

Certain arrhythmias are more prone to deteriorate into unstable or life-threatening forms. In these patients, there is an important relation between the underlying substrate to sustain the arrhythmia and the need for special treatment. Increasing degrees of cardiac abnormality or dysfunction are associated with greater need to treat specific arrhythmias. Echocardiography is an excellent tool for assessing the presence and degree of cardiac dysfunction and therefore provides essential information for the management of these patients. Furthermore, the assessment of ventricular function may also influence the choice of antiarrhythmic agent, as some have significant negative inotropic effects.

In patients with arrhythmias capable of hemodynamic compromise or life-threatening potential, an echocardiogram can serve as an integral part of the cardiac evaluation.

Indications for echocardiography

Class I
1. Arrhythmias with evidence of heart disease
2. Family history of genetic disorder associated with arrhythmias

Class II
1. Arrhythmias commonly associated with, but without evidence of, heart disease
2. Atrial fibrillation or flutter

Class III
1. Palpitation without evidence of arrhythmias
2. Minor arrhythmias without evidence of heart disease

EDEMA

The causes of peripheral edema are numerous and include both cardiogenic and noncardiogenic etiologies. Echocardiographic study could be recommended in any patient who has evidence for an elevated central venous pressure, significant valvular or coronary artery disease, cor pulmonale, or pulsus paradoxus. Uncommon cardiac disorders that might be detected by echocardiography in patients with abnormal findings on physical examination include constrictive pericarditis,[80] restrictive cardiomyopathy,[80] and amyloid heart disease.[143] Echocardiography cannot be routinely recommended in patients with mild peripheral edema who have no evidence for an increase in central venous pressure or clinical findings of heart disease because the diagnostic yield in such patients is expected to be low. In patients in whom central venous pressure cannot be estimated with certainty on physical examination, echocardiographic evaluation of respiratory collapse of the inferior vena cava diameter can determine if the central venous pressure is elevated.[144]

Indications for echocardiography

Class I
1. Edema with other evidence of cardiac disease

Class II
1. Edema without evidence of cardiac disease

Class III
1. Edema of noncardiac origin

EVALUATION OF VENTRICULAR FUNCTION

Global systolic function

Echocardiographic methods can be used to define several indexes of global left ventricular systolic function,[145] including M-mode measurements (fractional minor axis shortening, mitral-septal separation), two-dimensional measurements (fractional area change, ejection fraction), Doppler measurements (peak aortic flow velocity and acceleration), and combined indexes (cardiac output, stroke volume). The M-mode indexes are prone to significant errors in patients with inadequate acoustic access, abnormally shaped ventricles, extreme dilation, and segmental wall motion abnormalities. Two-dimensional data, including linear (fractional shortening), area-based (fractional area change), and volume-based (ejection fraction) measurements, correlate well with independent standards such as chest roentgenogram findings and radionuclide ventriculography and are, therefore, useful in patients in whom studies of adequate quality can be obtained. Doppler indexes may be useful in the serial evaluation of a given patient and less useful for comparisons among patients.

Global right ventricular systolic function in adults is difficult to quantitate by echocardiography because of the frequent difficulty in obtaining accurate geometric information concerning the unusually shaped right ventricular chamber. Useful qualitative assessment of right ventricular size and function may be obtained with echocardiography. In children, useful quantitative measures of right ventricular function may be made. Doppler-derived data may be of more use, particularly in serial studies of a patient or in the determination of pulmonary to systemic flow ratios in patients with shunt lesions.

Regional left ventricular function

Echocardiography is an excellent technique for determining regional contractile function of the left ventricle.[146] The attributes of high spatial and temporal resolution and the ability to define regional wall thickening, as well as endocardial excursion, make echocardiography extremely useful in defining regional dysfunction due to ischemic disease, cardiomyopathy, contusion, and other disorders. Considerable controversy still surrounds the optimal method of analyzing echocardiographic data to extract information on regional left ventricular function, but virtually all carefully tested methods have yielded data useful in the clinical examination of regional function.

Right ventricular regional function may also be assessed by echocardiography, but the difficulties mentioned, coupled with the different mechanisms of contraction of the right and left ventricles, combine to make echocardiographic data on regional right ventricular contraction abnormalities less quantitatively accurate than data for the left ventricle. Nonetheless, clinically useful evidence of regional right ventricular dysfunction, such as that due to infarction, can be garnered from echocardiograms.

Diastolic left ventricular function

Recent interest in the noninvasive evaluation of diastolic function has produced a large number of indexes based on information from M-mode, two-dimensional, or Doppler echocardiographic studies.[147,148] In addition, echocardiography has been used experimentally to obtain complex measures of regional diastolic stress-strain characteristics.[149] Unfortunately, virtually all clinically available indexes of diastolic function (including echocardiography) are of somewhat limited usefulness. This is due to several factors, including (1) the complex nature of diastolic function, which differs in its mechanism in early diastole (when active cellular relaxation occurs) from that in late diastole (when passive muscle material properties are important); (2) the load dependence of the commonly described echocardiographic variables; and (3) the lack of careful validation of most of the variables by comparison to appropriate independent standards. For these reasons, echocardiographic indexes of diastolic function find their greatest usefulness in the serial examination of a given patient but less usefulness in comparing patients or in identifying the degree of diastolic dysfunction.

Indications for echocardiography

Class I
1. To evaluate global left ventricular function
2. To evaluate regional left ventricular function
3. Qualitative right ventricular function

Class II
1. Diastolic left ventricular function

Class III
1. Quantitative right ventricular function (except in children)

SCREENING

Screening tests for cardiac disease can be valuable but may not be very cost-effective. The intent of screening tests is to find those persons who have a serious, potentially treatable abnormality but are unaware of the problem. Although waiting for the patient to have some sort of complaint before investigating the possibility of a treatable illness is common, significant abnormalities can occur in the asymptomatic patient that at times lead to severe organ damage.

The criteria for an ideal screening test include being accurate, harmless, rapid, painless, and inexpensive. Echocardiography meets some of these criteria. The examination is painless and accurate, and as best can be determined, it is harmless. The test is relatively rapid, depending on the information desired. Unfortunately, echocardiography is not inexpensive. The examination is less costly than some other sophisticated procedures, such as invasive testing, or other noninvasive tests, such as nuclear stress testing, computed tomography scanning, or nuclear magnetic resonance imaging. On the other hand, it is considerably more expensive than an ECG or a chest roentgenogram. There are certain groups of persons who might benefit from a routine echocardiogram because of a relatively high risk of cardiac disease; an example might be patients with a family history of inheritable cardiovascular disease.

In general, echocardiography is too costly to be considered as a routine screening test for the general population. There may be certain subgroups of persons for whom the cost of this procedure may be warranted, provided that there is a reasonable likelihood that the results of the test will influence an individual patient's management or prognosis.

Indications for echocardiography

Class I

1. Patients with a family history of cardiovascular disease that is clearly inheritable

Class II

1. Competitive athletes

Class III

1. General population

USE OF ECHOCARDIOGRAPHY IN THE PEDIATRIC PATIENT

Echocardiography has become the definitive diagnostic method for the recognition and assessment of congenital and acquired heart disease in children. Its use has eliminated the need for invasive or other noninvasive studies in some and decreased the frequency and improved the timing and performance of invasive studies in other patients.[150-155] Serial evaluations in some conditions improve medical or surgical management. Echocardiographic evaluation reduces trauma to the child with insignificant cardiac abnormality and provides reassurance to the family. The outcome is improved for those patients with significant cardiac abnormality by guiding management decisions and providing early education and support for the family.

Although congenital heart disease is the most common type of cardiovascular disease recognized in the pediatric population, the appearance of Kawasaki disease and human immunodeficiency virus–related myocarditis and the recrudescence of rheumatic heart disease have increased the prevalence of inflammatory diseases in this age group. Cardiomyopathy, whether familial, acquired, or idiopathic, is also commonly seen. Additionally, a variety of serious cardiopulmonary diseases occur in neonates.

Serial follow-up studies are frequently utilized to follow the late cardiovascular adaptation to surgical repair or palliation, to demonstrate the recurrence of abnormalities, and to provide new knowledge about the relative benefits of new surgical techniques, such as the arterial switch procedure for transposition of the great arteries.[156-171] Such information serves retrospectively to enlighten the clinician in the selection of the correct interventional approach and its timing. For these reasons, echocardiography provides improved outcome and lowered health care costs by the streamlined use of medical resources.

Congenital heart disease

Two-dimensional echocardiography provides essential structural information in all forms of cardiac and great vessel disease in pediatric patients. Doppler echocardiography provides important physiologic information that, when combined with anatomic data, is sufficient to guide therapeutic management in some diagnostic categories. Serial examinations allow tracking of hemodynamic changes such as those occurring during the transition phase from fetal to newborn and infancy periods.[172] Echocardiography provides clinical information for the initial evaluation, before medical or surgical intervention, during medical or surgical intervention, and in postoperative patients.

Perinatal physiologic changes often mask or obscure the presence of hemodynamically important cardiovascular lesions. Echocardiography allows early recognition of lesions in which either the pulmonary or the systemic circulation is dependent on the patency of the ductus arteriosus.[173-175] Definitive diagnosis in these lesions before ductal closure may prevent death or severe morbidity. Infants with a loud murmur, signs of congestive heart failure, cyanosis, or failure to thrive have a high probability of significant heart disease and should undergo echocardiographic evaluation.

Congenital heart disease in the child or adolescent commonly presents as an asymptomatic heart murmur; nevertheless, the cardiac murmurs of this age group are more commonly functional than pathologic. History and physical examination by a skilled observer are usually sufficient to distinguish functional from pathologic murmurs.[176] In the presence of ambiguous clinical findings, echocardiography can demonstrate the presence or absence of abnormalities such as bicuspid aortic valve, mildly obstructive subaortic stenosis, mitral valve prolapse, or cardiomyopathy. Such determination directs a need for further follow-up or endocarditis prophylaxis, or both. For patients with clinical findings of hemodynamically significant heart disease, anatomic and physiologic data provided by serial two-dimensional and Doppler echocardiography may provide a definitive diagnosis and allow the most efficient timing of invasive or interventional procedures.

Echocardiography may be employed in concert with cardiac catheterization to limit the quantity of radiographic contrast material and to direct interventional maneuvers.

Intraoperative echocardiography has been utilized to provide timely information about the success of septal defect closure and valve palliation.[177-180] In some lesions, the ability to scan the heart by direct transducer placement on the heart surface or by transesophageal echocardiography allows the patient to undergo surgical repair without prior cardiac catheterization.

Indications for echocardiography

Class I

1. Cyanosis, respiratory distress, abnormal arterial pulses, or cardiac murmur in a neonate

2. Loud or abnormal murmur or other abnormal cardiac finding in an infant or older child
3. Failure to thrive in the presence of an abnormal or unusual cardiac finding
4. Presence of a syndrome associated with cardiovascular disease and dominant inheritance or multiple affected family members
5. Presence of a syndrome associated with heart disease, with or without abnormal cardiac findings, for which an urgent management decision is needed
6. Cardiomegaly on chest radiograph
7. Dextrocardia, abnormal pulmonary, or visceral situs
8. Most ECG abnormalities
9. Postoperative congenital or acquired heart disease
10. Postcardiac or cardiopulmonary transplant

Class II
1. Murmur of uncertain etiology
2. Failure to thrive in the absence of definite abnormal clinical findings
3. Clinical findings of small ventricular septal defect after the neonatal period
4. Presence of a syndrome associated with a high incidence of congenital heart disease for which there are no abnormal cardiac findings and no urgency of management decisions

Class III
1. An asymptomatic heart murmur in a child or adolescent that is positively identified by an experienced observer as functional or innocent

The common categories of congenital heart disease are summarized as follows:

Diagnostic groups	Information provided
1. Left-to-right shunts	Presence, position, configuration, and size of defect, direction of flow and gradient across defect, pulmonary/systemic flow, ventricular compensation, associated lesions[181,182]
2. Obstructive lesions	Location, configuration, and severity of obstruction, ventricular compensation, associated lesions[8,175,183-185]
3. Regurgitant lesions	Valve configuration, assessment of severity, chamber dilation, ventricular compensation, associated lesions[160,186,187]
4. Venous connections	Location and connections of all systemic and pulmonary veins, assessment of left-to-right and right-to-left shunts, associated lesions[164,188]
5. Conotruncal abnormalities	Position of great arteries, location of ventricles and ventricular septal defect, nature of subarterial obstruction, great artery anatomy, associated lesions, ventricular compensation[189-192]

Diagnostic groups	Information provided
6. Coronary anomalies	Origin, size, and flow in coronary arteries, ventricular compensation
7. Complex lesions	Cardiac segmental analysis of situs and connections, size and location of all cardiac chambers, atrioventricular valve morphology, subarterial and arterial obstruction, interatrial and interventricular communications, venous and great artery anatomy, ventricular compensation

Inflammatory diseases

Kawasaki disease may result in abnormalities in the proximal or distal coronary circulation, myocarditis, myocardial infarction, and pericardial effusion. Baseline and serial evaluations by echocardiography are recommended in all patients with clinical stigmata of this disease because echocardiographic findings influence management decisions.[193,194] Since long-term abnormalities of the coronary arteries have been noted after resolution of initial aneurysms, these patients may require lifelong follow-up.

Children with human immunodeficiency virus infection acquired during the fetal or newborn period have an aggressive form of the disease with early and prominent myocardial involvement and therefore should have a baseline study and serial follow-up studies as indicated by the appearance of tachycardia, congestive heart failure, and respiratory distress.[195]

There is a resurgence of acute rheumatic fever in the United States. Newer diagnostic criteria include echocardiographic assessment of mitral valve function, ventricular function, and pericarditis. Echocardiography is an important component of the diagnostic evaluation of children with fever, new cardiac murmur, migratory polyarthritis, and chorea.

See previous sections for discussion of pericardial disease and infective endocarditis.

Indications for echocardiography

Class I

1. Baseline and follow-up studies on all pediatric patients with suspected or documented Kawasaki disease, human immunodeficiency virus infection, or rheumatic fever

Class II

1. Follow-up examinations after occurrence of acute rheumatic fever in patients with normal cardiac findings
2. Long-term follow-up studies in patients with Kawasaki disease who have no coronary abnormalities during the acute phase of the disease process

Class III

None

Myocardial disease

Echocardiography provides diagnostic information in patients with hypertrophic, congestive, and infiltrative cardiomyopathy, viral myocarditis, toxic cardiomyopathy, and idiopathic cardiomyopathy. Patients receiving anthracycline or other cardiotoxic agents should have baseline and serial follow-up studies. Echocardiographic assessment of patients with renal disease provides guidance in management of hemodialysis and hypertensive medications. Echocardiography is useful in detecting hypertrophic cardiomyopathy and in determining the presence of subaortic and subpulmonary obstruction, mitral insufficiency, and diastolic compliance abnormalities. Echocardiography is useful in screening family members in all types of cardiomyopathy associated with a dominant or recessive pattern of inheritance.

Indications for echocardiography

Class I

1. Patients with a family history of genetically transmitted myocardial disease, with or without abnormal cardiac findings
2. Patients with clinical evidence of myocardial disease
3. Baseline and serial examinations of patients receiving cardiotoxic therapeutic agents
4. Patients with severe renal disease and an abnormal cardiac finding
5. Recipients and donors undergoing evaluation for cardiac transplantation

Class II

None

Class III

None

Arrhythmia

Rhythm abnormalities in children may be associated with Ebstein anomaly of the tricuspid valve, cardiac tumor, cardiomyopathy, mitral valve prolapse, glycogen storage disease, or stimulation from migrated central catheters.

Echocardiography is an important component in evaluation of these patients. Mild rhythm disturbances, such as sinus arrhythmias and low-grade supraventricular ectopic beats, or brief and infrequent runs of supraventricular tachycardia, are rarely associated with cardiac pathology. In addition, atrial contraction can sometimes be characterized by echocardiography when findings are obscured on the surface ECG.

Indications for echocardiography

Class I

1. Arrhythmia requiring treatment
2. Arrhythmia in the presence of an abnormal cardiac finding
3. Arrhythmia in a patient with a family history of a genetically transmitted cardiac lesion associated with arrhythmia, such as tuberous sclerosis or rhabdomyoma
4. Appearance of arrhythmia in a patient with a central venous catheter

Class II

1. Recurring arrhythmia not requiring treatment in the presence of normal findings on cardiac examination

Class III

1. Sinus arrhythmia or isolated extrasystoles in a child with otherwise normal findings

---

on cardiac examination and no family history of a genetically transmitted abnormality associated with arrhythmia

Cardiopulmonary diseases

A variety of cardiopulmonary diseases are seen in the neonates. Premature infants may have respiratory failure based on a combination of processes: lung immaturity, hyaline membrane disease, persistence of the ductus arteriosus, inflammatory disease, or congenital heart disease. Echocardiography determines the patency of the ductus arteriosus, direction and degree of shunting at the ductal level, and ventricular compensation for left ventricular volume overload. An indirect assessment of pulmonary artery hypertension can also be made. Echocardiography study also rules out a ductal-dependent lesion when pharmacologic or surgical ductal closure is planned.

Term newborn infants with primary pulmonary hypertension of the newborn (persistent fetal circulation) may present with or without associated meconium staining or aspiration. Differentiation of this entity from cyanotic heart disease often requires echocardiography. In addition to excluding structural abnormalities, Doppler echocardiography provides additional information about atrial and ductal shunting, pulmonary artery pressure, and ventricular function. Serial studies are useful in monitoring the therapeutic response. In patients with severe disease progressing to extracorporeal membrane oxygenation, this information is useful in assessing the contribution of extracorporeal circulation to ventricular output, the appearance and course of "stunned myocardium," and flow across the ductus arteriosus. Children with upper airway disease, cystic fibrosis, human immunodeficiency virus infection, and other chronic immunologic disorders may have clinical or ECG evidence of pulmonary artery hypertension. As discussed in a previous section, echocardiography provides indirect documentation of pulmonary artery hypertension and estimation of severity. Follow-up studies reflect response to therapy and are useful in guiding management.

Indications for echocardiography

Class I
1. Respiratory distress or cyanosis in the newborn
2. Any patient with clinical findings of pulmonary artery hypertension

Class II
1. Baseline study of patients with cystic fibrosis and no findings of cor pulmonale
2. Newborn, premature, or term infants with respiratory distress who respond rapidly to initial pulmonary management

Class III
None

Thromboembolic disorders

Stroke and other manifestations of thromboembolism that occur in childhood may result from intracardiac thrombus, tumor, or vegetation. In some groups of patients, long-term indwelling catheters in the central veins or atria may predispose to thrombus formation or infection. Because children have a lower incidence of distal cardiovascular disease as a cause of stroke or loss of pulse, the yield of echocardiography to rule out an intracardiac cause may be somewhat higher than for adults.

Indications for echocardiography

Class I

1. Thromboembolic event in an infant, child, or adolescent

Class II

None

Class III

None

Fetal echocardiography

Widespread use of general fetal ultrasound examinations among women receiving prenatal care has resulted in increased referrals for specific cardiac analysis. Definition of fetal cardiac structures is currently possible at 10 to 12 weeks' gestation, with the use of vaginal probes with high-resolution transducers. By 16 to 18 weeks' gestation, accurate segmental analysis of cardiac structure is possible with a conventional transabdominal approach.[196,197] Doppler examination provides important information about blood flow across the cardiac valves, great arteries, ductus arteriosus, and umbilical arteries.[198] A general fetal ultrasound examination usually includes a four-chamber or inflow view of the fetal heart. This view is sensitive to abnormalities of the inflow portions of the heart but is insensitive to some septal defects, outflow lesions, and conotruncal abnormalities. Patients are referred for specific fetal echocardiographic examination because of an abnormality of structure or rhythm noted on ultrasound examination or because the patient is in a high-risk group for fetal heart disease. Early recognition of fetal heart disease allows the opportunity for transplacental therapy, as in the case of arrhythmias.[199] When a potentially life-threatening cardiac anomaly is found, the delivery can be planned at a tertiary care center where supportive measures can be instituted before severe hypoxia, shock, or acidosis ensues. Education of the parents can be initiated early so that complex therapeutic choices can be reviewed and informed consent obtained. When the fetal heart appears normal, the family may be reassured.

Diagnostic difficulties may arise because of modulation of the anatomic and physiologic presentation of certain lesions by the fetal circulation and dramatic changes in the heart and great vessels that may occur throughout gestation. As an example, the severity of pulmonary stenosis cannot be assessed by quantification of valve gradient because of the variability in right ventricular output and the condition of the ductus arteriosus. The outcome of fetal heart disease is often suggested only after serial studies to determine growth of cardiac chambers and vascular structures and changes in blood flow patterns. The spectrum of congenital cardiac lesions is broader than that seen in the neonates and infants because of the presence of nonviable subcategories of disease. The maternal history of a given congenital heart lesion recognized prenatally is not always the same as that of one diagnosed postnatally. A knowledge of prenatal maternal history is as necessary as good imaging in providing proper care for these patients. An additional degree of difficulty is imposed by the inability to see the fetus for orientation reference and the inability to examine the fetus for clinical findings that might guide the performance and interpretation of the echocardiogram.

In skilled hands, the diagnostic accuracy of fetal echocardiography may reach the high sensitivity and specificity of echocardiography in the neonate; however, not all pediatric cardiology centers have specially trained fetal echocardiographers. Such experts may be pediatric cardiologists, obstetricians, or radiologists with special training or experience in fetal ultrasound imaging and a comprehensive knowledge of congenital heart disease, fetal cardiac anatomy and physiology, and arrhythmias. Where specific expertise in fetal echocardiography does not exist, close collaboration between a pediatric cardiologist/echocardiographer and a fetal ultrasonographer may produce similar results once a learning curve has been completed. The collaboration of a multidisciplinary perinatal team provides support for diagnostic and therapeutic decisions.

Indications for echocardiography

Class I

1. Abnormal-appearing heart on general fetal ultrasound examination
2. Fetal tachycardia, bradycardia, or irregular rhythm on clinical or screening ultrasound examination
3. Maternal/family risk factors for cardiovascular disease, such as a parent, sibling, or first-degree relative with congenital heart disease
4. Maternal diabetes
5. Maternal systemic lupus erythematosus
6. Teratogen exposure during a vulnerable period
7. Other fetal system abnormalities (including chromosomal) if pregnancy management decisions are required
8. Performance of transplacental therapy or the presence of a history of significant, but intermittent, arrhythmia or a family history of left or right heart obstructive lesions. Serial examinations are required in these conditions.

Class II

1. Fetal distress or dysfunction of unclear etiology
2. Previous history of multiple fetal losses
3. Presence of other system abnormality and an unclear prognosis for fetal outcome

Class III

1. Multiple gestations
2. Low-risk pregnancies with normal anatomic findings on ultrasound examination
3. Occasional premature contractions without sustained tachycardia or signs of dysfunction or distress
4. Presence of a noncardiovascular system abnormality when evaluation of the cardiovascular system will not alter either management decisions or fetal outcome

REFERENCES

1. Pearlman AS, Gardin JM, Martin RP et al: Guidelines for optimal physician training in echocardiography: recommendations of the American Society of Echocardiography Committee for Physician Training in Echocardiography, *Am J Cardiol* 60:158-163, 1987.
2. Seventeenth Bethesda Conference: Adult cardiology training, November 1, 2, 1985, Bethesda, Maryland, *J Am Coll Cardiol* 7:1191-1218, 1986.
3. Meyer RA, Hagler D, Huhta J, Smallhorn J, Snider R, Williams R: Guidelines for physician training in pediatric echocardiography: recommendations of the Society of Pediatric Echocardiography Committee on Physician Training, *Am J Cardiol* 60:164-165, 1987.

4. Peller OG, Wallerson DC, Devereux RB: Role of Doppler and imaging echocardiography in selection of patients for cardiac valvular surgery, *Am Heart J* 114:1445-1461, 1987.
5. Adhar GC, Nanda NC: Doppler echocardiography. Part II. Adult valvular heart disease, *Echocardiography* 1:219-241, 1984.
6. Richards KL: Doppler echocardiography in the diagnosis and quantification of valvular disease, *Mod Concepts Cardiovasc Dis* 56:43-48, 1987.
7. Pérez JE, Ludbrook PA, Ahumada GG: Usefulness of Doppler echocardiography in detecting tricuspid valve stenosis, *Am J Cardiol* 55:601-603, 1985.
8. Lima CO, Sahn DJ, Valdes-Cruz LM et al: Noninvasive prediction of transvalvular pressure gradient in patients with pulmonary stenosis by quantitative two-dimensional echocardiographic Doppler studies, *Circulation* 67:866-871, 1983.
9. Suzuki Y, Kambara H, Kadota K et al: Detection and evaluation of tricuspid regurgitation using a real-time, two-dimensional, color-coded, Doppler flow imaging system: comparison with contrast two-dimensional echocardiography and right ventriculography, *Am J Cardiol* 57:811-815, 1986.
10. Levine RA, Stathogiannis E, Newell JB, Harrigan P, Weyman AE: Reconsideration of echocardiographic standards for mitral valve prolapse: lack of association between leaflet displacement isolated to the apical four chamber view and independent echocardiographic evidence of abnormality, *J Am Coll Cardiol* 11:1010-1119, 1988.
11. Krivokapich J, Child JS, Dadourian BJ, Perloff JK: Reassessment of echocardiographic criteria for diagnosis of mitral valve prolapse, *Am J Cardiol* 61:131-135, 1988.
12. Stamm RB, Martin RP: Quantification of pressure gradients across stenotic valves by Doppler ultrasound, *J Am Coll Cardiol* 2:707-718, 1983.
13. Currie PJ, Hagler DJ, Seward JB et al: Instantaneous pressure gradient: a simultaneous Doppler and dual catheter correlative study, *J Am Coll Cardiol* 7:800-806, 1986.
14. Otto CM, Pearlman AS: Doppler echocardiography in adults with symptomatic aortic stenosis: diagnostic utility and cost-effectiveness, *Arch Intern Med* 148:2553-2560, 1988.
15. Hatle L, Angelsen B, Tromsdal A: Noninvasive assessment of atrioventricular pressure half-time by Doppler ultrasound, *Circulation* 60:1096-1104, 1979.
16. Loyd D, Eng D, Ask P, Wranne B: Pressure half-time does not always predict mitral valve area correctly, *J Am Soc Echo* 1:313-321, 1988.
17. Thomas JD, Wilkins GT, Choong CYP et al: Inaccuracy of mitral pressure half-time immediately after percutaneous mitral valvotomy: dependence on transmitral gradient and left atrial and ventricular compliance, *Circulation* 78:980-993, 1988.
18. Thomas JD, Weyman AE: Doppler mitral pressure half-time: a clinical tool in search of theoretical justification, *J Am Coll Cardiol* 10:923-929, 1987.
19. Nakatani S, Masuyama T, Kodama K, Kitabatake A, Fujii K, Kamada T: Value and limitations of Doppler echocardiography in the quantification of stenotic mitral valve area: comparison of the pressure half-time and the continuity equation methods, *Circulation* 77:78-85, 1988.
20. Sahn DJ, Maciel BC: Physiological valvular regurgitation: Doppler echocardiography and the potential for iatrogenic heart disease, *Circulation* 78:1075-1077, 1988.
21. Yoshida K, Yoshikawa J, Shakudo M et al: Color Doppler evaluation of valvular regurgitation in normal subjects, *Circulation* 78:840-847, 1988.
22. Pearlman AS, Otto CM: The use of Doppler techniques for quantitative evaluation of valvular regurgitation, *Eur Heart J* 8(suppl C):35-43, 1987.
23. Smith MD, Grayburn PA, Spain MG, DeMaria AN, Kwan OL, Moffett CB: Observer variability in the quantitation of Doppler color flow jet areas for mitral and aortic regurgitation, *J Am Coll Cardiol* 11:579-584, 1988.
24. Yoshikawa J, Yoshida K, Akasaka T, Shakudo M, Kato H: Value and limitations of color Doppler flow mapping in the detection and semiquantification of valvular regurgitation, *Int J Card Imaging* 2:85-91, 1987.
25. Martin RP, Rakowski H, Kleiman JH, Beaver W, London E, Popp RL: Reliability and reproducibility of two dimensional echocardiographic measurement of the stenotic mitral valve orifice area, *Am J Cardiol* 43:560-568, 1979.
26. Mügge A, Daniel WG, Frank G, Lichtlen PR: Echocardiography in infective endocarditis: reassessment of prognostic implications of vegetation size determined by the transthoracic and the transesophageal approach, *J Am Coll Cardiol* 14:631-638, 1989.
27. Rubenson DS, Tucker CR, Stinson EB et al: The use of echocardiography in diagnosing culture-negative endocarditis, *Circulation* 64:641-646, 1981.

28. Sagar KB, Wann LS, Paulsen WHJ, Romhilt DW: Doppler echocardiographic evaluation of Hancock and Björk-Shiley prosthetic valves, *J Am Coll Cardiol* 7:681-687, 1986.
29. Burstow DJ, Nishimura RA, Bailey KR et al: Continuous wave Doppler echocardiographic measurement of prosthetic valve gradients: a simultaneous Doppler-catheter correlative study, *Circulation* 80:504-514, 1989.
30. Reisner SA, Meltzer RS: Normal values of prosthetic valve Doppler echocardiographic parameters: a review, *J Am Soc Echo* 1:201-210, 1988.
31. Wilkins GT, Gillam LD, Kritzer GL, Levine RA, Palacios IF, Weyman AE: Validation of continous-wave Doppler echocardiographic measurements of mitral and tricuspid prosthetic valve gradients: a simultaneous Doppler-catheter study, *Circulation* 74:786-795, 1986.
32. Maze SS, Kotler MN, Parry WR: Regurgitant signals in normally functioning valves: Doppler characteristics of the Medtronic-Hall valve, *Am J Noninvas Cardiol* 2:164-168, 1988.
33. Come PC: Pitfalls in the diagnosis of periprosthetic valvular regurgitation by pulsed Doppler echocardiography, *J Am Coll Cardiol* 9:1176-1179, 1987.
34. Alam M, Rosman HS, Lakier JB et al: Doppler and echocardiographic features of normal and dysfunctioning bioprosthetic valves, *J Am Coll Cardiol* 10:851-858, 1987.
35. Seward JB, Khandheria BK, Oh JK et al: Transesophageal echocardiography: technique, anatomic correlations, implementation, and clinical applications, *Mayo Clin Proc* 63:649-680, 1988.
36. Tennant R, Wiggers CJ: The effect of coronary occlusion on myocardial contraction, *Am J Physiol* 112:351-361, 1935.
37. Kerber RE, Abboud FM: Echocardiographic detection of regional myocardial infarction, *Circulation* 47:997-1005, 1973.
38. Horowitz RS, Morganroth J, Parrotto C, Chen CC, Soffer J, Pauletto FJ: Immediate diagnosis of acute myocardial infarction by two-dimensional echocardiography, *Circulation* 65:323-329, 1982.
39. Weiss JL, Bulkley BH, Hutchins GM, Mason SJ: Two-dimensional echocardiographic recognition of myocardial injury in man: comparison with postmortem studies, *Circulation* 63:401-408, 1981.
40. Nixon JV, Narahara KA, Smitherman TC: Estimation of myocardial involvement in patients with acute myocardial infarction by two-dimensional echocardiography, *Circulation* 62:1248-1255, 1980.
41. Gibson RS, Bishop HL, Stamm RB, Crampton RS, Beller GA, Martin RP: Value of early two dimensional echocardiography in patients with acute myocardial infarction, *Am J Cardiol* 49:1110-1119, 1982.
42. Heger JJ, Weyman AE, Wann LS, Rogers EW, Dillon JC, Feigenbaum H: Cross-sectional echocardiographic analysis of the extent of left ventricular asynergy in acute myocardial infarction, *Circulation* 61:1113-1118, 1980.
43. Distante A, Picano E, Moscarelli E, Palombo C, Benassi A, L'Abbate A: Echocardiographic versus hemodynamic monitoring during attacks of variant angina pectoris, *Am J Cardiol* 55:1319-1322, 1985.
44. Shibata J, Takahashi H, Itaya M et al: Cross-sectional echocardiographic visualization of the infarcted site in myocardial infarction: correlation with echocardiographic and coronary angiographic findings, *J Cardiogr* 12:885-894, 1982.
45. Shen WK, Khandheria BK, Oh JK et al: Quantitative correlation between echocardiographic wall-motion abnormalities and left ventricular infarct size determined by pathology, *Circulation* 74(suppl II):II-479, 1986.
46. O'Boyle JE, Parisi AF, Nieminen M, Kloner RA, Khuri S: Quantitative detection of regional left ventricular contraction abnormalities by 2-dimensional echocardiography, comparison of myocardial thickening and thinning and endocardial motion in a canine model, *Am J Cardiol* 51:1732-1738, 1983.
47. Parisi AF, Moynihan PF, Folland ED, Strauss WE, Sharma GVRK, Sasahara AA: Echocardiography in acute and remote myocardial infarction, *Am J Cardiol* 46:1205-1214, 1980.
48. Horowitz RS, Morganroth J: Immediate detection of early high-risk patients with acute myocardial infarction using two-dimensional echocardiographic evaluation of left ventricular regional wall motion abnormalities, *Am Heart J* 103:814-822, 1982.
49. Bhatnagar SK, Moussa MAA, Al-Yusuf AR: The role of prehospital discharge two-dimensional echocardiography in determining the prognosis of survivors of first myocardial infarction, *Am Heart J* 109:472-477, 1985.
50. Nelson GR, Cohn PF, Gorlin R: Prognosis in medically treated coronary artery disease: influence of ejection fraction compared to other parameters, *Circulation* 52:408-412, 1975.
51. Isner JM, Roberts WC: Right ventricular infarction complicating left ventricular infarction secondary to coronary heart disease: frequency, location, associated findings and significance from analysis of 236 necropsy patients with acute or healed myocardial infarction, *Am J Cardiol* 42:885-894, 1978.
52. D'Arcy B, Nanda NC: Two-dimensional echocardiographic features of right ventricular infarction, *Circulation* 65:167-173, 1982.
53. DeMaria AN, Bommer W, Neumann A et al: Left ventricular thrombi identified by cross-sectional echocardiography, *Ann Intern Med* 90:14-28, 1979.
54. Spirito P, Bellotti P, Chiarella F, Domenicucci S, Sementa A, Vecchio C: Prognostic significance and natural history of left ventricular thrombi in patients with acute anterior myocardial infarction: a two-dimensional echocardiographic study, *Circulation* 72:774-780, 1985.

55. Visser CA, Kan G, Meltzer RS, Dunning AJ, Roelandt J: Embolic potential of left ventricular thrombus after myocardial infarction: a two-dimensional echocardiographic study of 119 patients, *J Am Coll Cardiol* 5:1276-1280, 1985.

56. Gueret P, Dubourg O, Ferrier A, Farcot JC, Rigaud M, Bourdarias JP: Effects of full-dose heparin anticoagulation on the development of left ventricular thrombosis in acute transmural myocardial infarction, *J Am Coll Cardiol* 8:419-426, 1986.

57. Keating EC, Gross SA, Schlamowitz RA et al: Mural thrombi in myocardial infarctions: prospective evaluation by two-dimensional echocardiography, *Am J Med* 74:989-995, 1983.

58. Keren A, Goldberg S, Gottlieb S et al: Natural history of left ventricular thrombi: their appearance and resolution in the posthospitalization period of acute myocardial infarction, *J Am Coll Cardiol* 15:790-800, 1990.

59. Lehmann KG, Francis CK, Dodge HT: Mitral regurgitation in early myocardial infarction is the strongest predictor of mortality, *Circulation* 74(suppl II):II-304, 1986.

60. Nishimura RA, Schaff HV, Shub C, Gersh BJ, Edwards WD, Tajik AJ: Papillary muscle rupture complicating acute myocardial infarction: analysis of 17 patients, *Am J Cardiol* 51:373-377, 1983.

61. Godley RW, Wann LS, Rogers EW, Feigenbaum H, Weyman AE: Incomplete mitral leaflet closure in patients with papillary muscle dysfunction, *Circulation* 63:565-571, 1981.

62. Miyatake K, Izumi S, Okamoto M et al: Semiquantitative grading of severity of mitral regurgitation by real-time two-dimensional Doppler flow imaging technique, *J Am Coll Cardiol* 7:82-88, 1986.

63. Rogers EW, Glassman RD, Feigenbaum H, Weyman AE, Godley RW: Aneurysms of the posterior interventricular septum with postinfarction ventricular septal defect: echocardiographic identification, *Chest* 78:741-746, 1980.

64. Chandraratna PAN, Balachandran PK, Shah PM, Hodges M: Echocardiographic observations on ventricular septal rupture complicating acute myocardial infarction, *Circulation* 51:506-510, 1975.

65. Miyatake K, Okamoto M, Kinoshita N et al: Doppler echocardiographic features of ventricular septal rupture in myocardial infarction, *J Am Coll Cardiol* 5:182-187, 1985.

66. Eisenberg PR, Barzilai B, Perez JE: Noninvasive detection by Doppler echocardiography of combined ventricular septal rupture and mitral regurgitation in acute myocardial infarction, *J Am Coll Cardiolmain4:617-620, 1984.*

67. Gatewood RP Jr, Nanda NC: Differentiation of left ventricular pseudoaneurysm from true aneurysm with two dimensional echocardiography, *Am J Cardiol* 46:869-878, 1980.

68. Visser CA, Kan G, Meltzer RS et al: Incidence, timing and prognostic value of left ventricular aneurysm formation after myocardial infarction: a prospective, serial echocardiographic study of 158 patients, *Am J Cardiol* 57:729-732, 1986.

69. Erlebacher JA, Weiss JL, Weisfeldt ML, Bulkley BH: Early dilation of the infarcted segment in acute transmural myocardial infarction: role of infarct expansion in acute left ventricular enlargement, *J Am Coll Cardiol* 4:201-208, 1984.

70. Weyman AE, Peskoe SM, Williams ES, Dillon JC, Feigenbaum H: Detection of left ventricular aneurysms by cross-sectional echocardiography, *Circulation* 54:936-944, 1976.

71. Visser CA, Kan G, David GK, Lie KI, Durrer D: Echocardiographic-cineangiographic correlation in detecting left ventricular aneurysm: a prospective study of 422 patients, *Am J Cardiol* 50:337-341, 1982.

72. Currie PJ, Seward JB, Chan KL et al: Continuous wave Doppler determination of right ventricular pressure: a simultaneous Doppler-catheterization study in 127 patients, *J Am Coll Cardiol* 6:750-756, 1985.

73. Wann LS, Faris JV, Childress RH, Dillon JC, Weyman AE, Feigenbaum H: Exercise cross-sectional echocardiography in ischemic heart disease, *Circulation* 60:1300-1308, 1979.

74. Maurer G, Nanda NC: Two dimensional echocardiographic evaluation of exercise-induced left and right ventricular asynergy: correlation with thallium scanning, *Am J Cardiol* 48:720-727, 1981.

75. Visser CA, van der Wieken RL, Kan G et al: Comparison of two-dimensional echocardiography with radionuclide angiography during dynamic exercise for the detection of coronary artery disease, *Am Heart J* 106:528-534, 1983.

76. Brandenburg RO, Chazov E, Cherian G et al: Report of the WHO/ISFC Task Force on Definition and Classification of Cardiomyopathies, *Circulation* 64:437A-438A, 1981.

77. Shah PM: Echocardiography in congestive or dilated cardiomyopathy, *J Am Soc Echo* 1:20-30, 1988.

78. Rakowski H, Sasson Z, Wigle ED: Echocardiographic and Doppler assessment of hypertrophic cardiomyopathy, *J Am Soc Echo* 1:31-47, 1988.

79. Appleton CP, Hatle LK, Popp RL: Demonstration of restrictive ventricular physiology by Doppler echocardiography, *J Am Coll Cardiol* 11:757-768, 1988.

80. Hatle LK, Appleton CP, Popp RL: Differentiation of constrictive pericarditis and restrictive cardiomyopathy by Doppler echocardiography, *Circulation* 79:357-370, 1989.
81. Klein AL, Hatle LK, Burstow DJ et al: Doppler characterization of left ventricular diastolic function in cardiac amyloidosis, *J Am Coll Cardiol* 13:1017-1026, 1989.
82. Feigenbaum H: Echocardiographic diagnosis of pericardial effusion, *Am J Cardiol* 26:475-479, 1970.
83. Clark JG, Berberich SN, Zager JR: Echocardiographic findings of pericardial effusion mimicked by fibrocalcific pericardial disease, *Echocardiography* 2:475-480, 1985.
84. Callahan JA, Seward JB, Nishimura RA et al: Two-dimensional echocardiographically guided pericardiocentesis: experience in 117 consecutive patients, *Am J Cardiol* 55:476-479, 1985.
85. Armstrong WF, Schilt BF, Helper DJ, Dillon JC, Feigenbaum H: Diastolic collapse of the right ventricle with cardiac tamponade: an echocardiographic study, *Circulation* 65:1491-1496, 1982.
86. Gillam LD, Guyer DE, Gibson TC, King ME, Marshall JE, Weyman AE: Hydrodynamic compression of the right atrium: a new echocardiographic sign of cardiac tamponade, *Circulation* 68:294-301, 1983.
87. Singh S, Wann LS, Schuchard GH et al: Right ventricular and right atrial collapse in patients with cardiac tamponade—a combined echocardiographic and hemodynamic study, *Circulation* 70:966-971, 1984.
88. Himelman RB, Kircher B, Rockey DC, Schiller NB: Inferior vena cava plethora with blunted respiratory response: a sensitive echocardiographic sign of cardiac tamponade, *J Am Coll Cardiol* 12:1470-1477, 1988.
89. Appleton CP, Hatle LK, Popp RL: Cardiac tamponade and pericardial effusion: respiratory variation in transvalvular flow velocities studied by Doppler echocardiography, *J Am Coll Cardiol* 11:1020-1030, 1988.
90. Burstow DJ, Oh JK, Bailey KR, Seward JB, Tajik AJ: Cardiac tamponade: characteristic Doppler observations, *Mayo Clin Proc* 64:312-324, 1989.
91. Pandian NG, Skorton DJ, Kieso RA, Kerber RE: Diagnosis of constrictive pericarditis by two-dimensional echocardiography: studies in a new experimental model and in patients, *J Am Coll Cardiol* 4:1164-1173, 1984.
92. Thurber DL, Edwards JE, Achor RWP: Secondary malignant tumors of the pericardium, *Circulation* 26:228-241, 1962.
93. Hynes JK, Tajik AJ, Osborn MJ, Orszulak TA, Seward JB: Two-dimensional echocardiographic diagnosis of pericardial cyst, *Mayo Clin Proc* 58:60-63, 1983.
94. Pool PE, Seagren SC, Abbasi AS, Charuzi Y, Kraus R: Echocardiographic manifestations of constrictive pericarditis: abnormal septal motion, *Chest* 68:684-688, 1975.
95. Gibson TC, Grossman W, McLaurin LP, Moos S, Craige E: An echocardiographic study of the interventricular septum in constrictive pericarditis, *Br Heart J* 38:738-743, 1976.
96. Schnittger I, Bowden RE, Abrams J, Popp RL: Echocardiography: pericardial thickening and constrictive pericarditis, *Am J Cardiol* 42:388-395, 1978.
97. Tei C, Child JS, Tanaka H, Shah PM: Atrial systolic notch on the interventricular septal echogram: an echocardiographic sign of constrictive pericarditis, *J Am Coll Cardiol* 1:907-912, 1983.
98. Wann LS, Weyman AE, Dillon JC, Feigenbaum H: Premature pulmonary valve opening, *Circulation* 55:128-133, 1977.
99. Kansal S, Roitman D, Sheffield LT: Two-dimensional echocardiography of congenital absence of pericardium, *Am Heart J* 109:912-915, 1985.
100. Ruys F, Paulus W, Stevens C, Brutsaert D: Expansion of the left atrial appendage is a distinctive cross-sectional echocardiographic feature of congenital defect of the pericardium, *Eur Heart J* 4:738-741, 1983.
101. Fyke FE III, Seward JB, Edwards WD et al: Primary cardiac tumors: experience with 30 consecutive patients since the introduction of two-dimensional echocardiography, *J Am Coll Cardiol* 5:1465-1473, 1985.
102. Khandheria BK, Tajik AJ, Taylor CL et al: Aortic dissection: review of value and limitations of two-dimensional echocardiography in a six-year experience, *J Am Soc Echo* 2:17-24, 1989.
103. Erbel R, Daniel W, Visser C et al: Echocardiography in diagnosis of aortic dissection, *Lancet* 1:457-461, 1989.
104. Mohr-Kahaly S, Erbel R, Rennollet H et al: Ambulatory follow-up of aortic dissection by transesophageal two-dimensional and color-coded Doppler echocardiography, *Circulation* 80:24-33, 1989.
105. Rogers EW, Feigenbaum H, Weyman AE: Echocardiography for quantitation of cardiac chambers. In Yu PN, Goodwin JF, editors: *Progress in cardiology*, Philadelphia, 1979, Lea & Febiger, vol 8, pp 1-28.
106. Kannel WB, Gordon T, Offutt D: Left ventricular hypertrophy by electrocardiogram: prevalence, incidence, and mortality in the Framingham Study, *Ann Intern Med* 71:89-105, 1969.
107. Levy D, Garrison RJ, Savage DD, Kannel WB, Castelli WP: Left ventricular mass and incidence of coronary heart disease in an elderly cohort: the Framingham Heart Study, *Ann Intern Med* 110:101-107, 1989.
108. Devereux RB, Alonso DR, Lutas EM, Pickering TG, Harshfield GA, Laragh JH: Sensitivity of echocardiography for detection of left ventricular hypertrophy. In ter Keurs HEDJ, Schipperheyn JJ, editors: *Cardiac left ventricular hypertrophy*. Boston, 1983, Martinus Nijhoff Publishing, pp 16-37.
109. Devereux RB, Reichek N: Echocardiographic determination of left ventricular mass in man: anatomic validation of the method, *Circulation* 55:613-618, 1977.
110. Devereux RB, Alonso DR, Lutas EM et al: Echocardiographic assessment of left ventricular hypertrophy: comparison to necropsy findings, *Am J Cardiol* 57:450-458, 1986.

111. Liebson PR, Devereux RB, Horan MJ: Hypertension research: echocardiography in the measurement of left ventricular wall mass, *Hypertension* 9(suppl II):II-2-II-5, 1987.
112. Liebson PR, Savage DD: Echocardiography in hypertension: a review. II. Echocardiographic studies of the effects of antihypertensive agents on left ventricular wall mass and function, *Echocardiography* 4:215-249, 1987.
113. Soufer R, Wohlgelernter D, Vita NA et al: Intact systolic left ventricular function in clinical congestive heart failure, *Am J Cardiol* 55:1032-1036, 1985.
114. Dougherty AH et al: Congestive heart failure with normal systolic function, *Am J Cardiol* 54:778-782, 1984.
115. Harizi RC, Bianco JA, Alpert JS: Diastolic function of the heart in clinical cardiology, *Arch Intern Med* 148:99-109, 1988.
116. Yock PG, Popp RL: Noninvasive estimation of right ventricular systolic pressure by Doppler ultrasound in patients with tricuspid regurgitation, *Circulation* 70:657-662, 1984.
117. Rokey R, Kuo LC, Zoghbi WA, Limacher MC, Quinones MA: Determination of parameters of left ventricular diastolic filling with pulsed Doppler echocardiography: comparison with cineangiography, *Circulation* 71:543-550, 1985.
118. Spirito P, Maron BJ, Bonow RO: Noninvasive assessment of left ventricular diastolic function: comparative analysis of Doppler echocardiographic and radionuclide angiographic techniques, *J Am Coll Cardiol* 7:518-526, 1986.
119. Ginzton LE, Conant R, Brizendine M, Lee F, Mena I, Laks MM: Exercise subcostal two-dimensional echocardiography: a new method of segmental wall motion analysis, *Am J Cardiol* 53:805-811, 1984.
120. Heng MK, Simard M, Lake R, Udhoji VH: Exercise two-dimensional echocardiography for diagnosis of coronary artery disease, *Am J Cardiol* 54:502-507, 1984.
121. Ryan T, Vasey CG, Presti CF, O'Donnell JA, Feigenbaum H, Armstrong WF: Exercise echocardiography: detection of coronary artery disease in patients with normal left ventricular wall motion at rest, *J Am Coll Cardiol* 11:993-999, 1988.
122. Picano E, Lattanzi F, Masini M, Distante A, L'Abbate A: Usefulness of the dipyridamole-exercise echocardiography test for diagnosis of coronary artery disease, *Am J Cardiol* 62:67-70, 1988.
123. Berthe C, Pierard LA, Hiernaux M et al: Predicting the extent and location of coronary artery disease in acute myocardial infarction by echocardiography during dobutamine infusion, *Am J Cardiol* 58:1167-1172, 1986.
124. Chapman PD, Wann LS: Two-dimensional echocardiography during transesophageal pacing, *Practical Cardiol* 13:105-108, 1987.
125. Morganroth J, Chen CC, David D et al: Exercise cross-sectional echocardiographic diagnosis of coronary artery disease, *Am J Cardiol* 47:20-26, 1981.
126. Crawford MH, Amon KW, Vance WS: Exercise two-dimensional echocardiography: quantitation of left ventricular performance in patients with severe angina pectoris, *Am J Cardiol* 51:1-6, 1982.
127. Robertson WS, Feigenbaum H, Armstrong WF, Dillon JC, O'Donnell J, McHenry PW: Exercise echocardiography: a clinically practical addition in the evaluation of coronary artery disease, *J Am Coll Cardiol* 2:1085-1091, 1983.
128. Presti CF, Armstrong WF, Feigenbaum H: Comparison of echocardiography at peak exercise and after bicycle exercise in evaluation of patients with known or suspected coronary artery disease, *J Am Soc Echo* 1:119-126, 1988.
129. Jaarsma W, Visser CA, Kupper AJ, Res JCJ, van Eenige MJ, Roos JP: Usefulness of two-dimensional exercise echocardiography shortly after myocardial infarction, *Am J Cardiol* 57:86-90, 1986.
130. Armstrong WF, O'Donnell J, Dillon JC, McHenry PL, Morris SN, Feigenbaum H: Complementary value of two-dimensional exercise echocardiography to routine treadmill exercise testing, *Ann Intern Med* 105:829-835, 1986.
131. Applegate RJ, Dell'Italia LJ, Crawford MH: Usefulness of two-dimensional echocardiography during low-level exercise testing early after uncomplicated acute myocardial infarction, *Am J Cardiol* 60:10-14, 1987.
132. Ryan T, Armstrong WF, O'Donnell JA, Feigenbaum H: Risk stratification after acute myocardial infarction by means of exercise two-dimensional echocardiography, *Am Heart J* 114:1305-1316, 1987.
133. Cardiogenic brain embolism: cerebral Embolism Task Force, *Arch Neurol* 43:71-84, 1986.
134. Meltzer RS, Visser CA, Fuster V: Intracardiac thrombi and systemic embolization, *Ann Intern Med* 104:689-698, 1986.
135. Matsumura M, Shah P, Kyo S, Omoto R: Advantages of transesophageal echo for correct diagnosis on small left atrial thrombi in mitral stenosis, *Circulation* 80(suppl II):II-678, 1989.
136. Nishide M, Irino T, Gotoh M, Naka M, Tsuji K: Cardiac abnormalities in ischemic cerebrovascular disease studied by two-dimensional echocardiography, *Stroke* 14:541-545, 1983.

137. Harvey JR, Teague SM, Anderson JL, Voyles WF, Thadani U: Clinically silent atrial septal defects with evidence for cerebral embolization, *Ann Intern Med* 105:695-697, 1986.

138. Lovett JL, Sandok BA, Giuliani ER, Nasser FN: Two-dimensional echocardiography in patients with focal cerebral ischemia, *Ann Intern Med* 95:1-4, 1981.

139. Kapoor WN, Karpf M, Wieand S, Peterson JR, Levey GS: A prospective evaluation and follow-up of patients with syncope, *N Engl J Med* 309:197-204, 1983.

140. Wayne HH: Syncope: physiologic considerations and an analysis of the clinical characteristics in 510 patients, *Am J Med* 31:418-438, 1961.

141. Kapoor WN, Karpf M, Maher Y, Miller RA, Levey GS: Syncope of unknown origin: the need for a more cost-effective approach to its diagnostic evaluation, *JAMA* 247:2687-2691, 1982.

142. Day SC, Cook EF, Funkenstein H et al: Evaluation and outcome of emergency room patients with transient loss of consciousness, *Am J Med* 73:15-23, 1982.

143. Klein AL, Oh JK, Miller FA, Seward JB, Tajik AJ: Two-dimensional and Doppler echocardiographic assessment of infiltrative cardiomyopathy, *J Am Soc Echo* 1:48-59, 1988.

144. Simonson JS, Schiller NB: Sonospirometry: a new method for noninvasive estimation of mean right atrial pressure based on two-dimensional echographic measurements of the inferior vena cava during measured inspiration, *J Am Coll Cardiol* 11:557-564, 1988.

145. Force TL, Folland ED, Aebischer N, Sharma S, Parisi AF: Echocardiographic assessment of ventricular function. In Marcus ML, Skorton DJ, Schelbert HR, Wolf GL, Braunwald E, editors: *Cardiac imaging—principles and practice*, Philadelphia, WB Saunders (in press).

146. Collins SM, Kerber RE, Skorton DJ: Quantitative analysis of left ventricular regional function by imaging methods. In Miller DD, Burns RJ, Gill JB, Ruddy TD, editors: *Clinical cardiac imaging*, New York, 1988, McGraw-Hill, pp 233-259.

147. Danford DA, Huhta JC, Murphy DJ Jr: Doppler echocardiographic approaches to ventricular diastolic function, *Echocardiography* 3:33-40, 1986.

148. Colan SD, Sanders SP, MacPherson D, Borow KM: Left ventricular diastolic function in elite athletes with physiologic cardiac hypertrophy, *J Am Coll Cardiol* 6:545-549, 1985.

149. McPherson DD, Skorton DJ, Kodiyalam S et al: Finite element analysis of myocardial diastolic function using three-dimensional echocardiographic reconstructions: application of a new method for study of acute ischemia in dogs, *Circ Res* 60:674-682, 1987.

150. Huhta JC, Glasow P, Murphy DJ Jr et al: Surgery without catheterization for congenital heart defects: management of 100 patients, *J Am Coll Cardiol* 9:823-829, 1987.

151. Krabill KA, Ring WS, Foker JE et al: Echocardiographic versus cardiac catheterization diagnosis of infants with congenital heart disease requiring cardiac surgery, *Am J Cardiol* 60:351-354, 1987.

152. George B, DiSessa TG, Williams R et al: Coarctation repair without cardiac catheterization in infants, *Am Heart J* 114:1421-1425, 1987.

153. Alboliras ET, Seward JB, Hagler DJ, Danielson GK, Puga FJ, Tajik AJ: Impact of two-dimensional and Doppler echocardiography on care of children aged two years and younger, *Am J Cardiol* 61:166-169, 1988.

154. Leung MP, Mok CK, Lau KC, Lo R, Yeung CY: The role of cross sectional echocardiography and pulsed Doppler ultrasound in the management of neonates in whom congenital heart disease is suspected: a prospective study, *Br Heart J* 56:73-82, 1986.

155. Lipshultz SE, Sanders SP, Mayer JE, Colan SD, Lock JE: Are routine preoperative cardiac catheterization and angiography necessary before repair of ostium primum atrial septal defect? *J Am Coll Cardiol* 11:373-378, 1988.

156. Gewitz MH, Werner JC, Kleinman CS, Hellenbrand WE, Talner NS, Taunt KA: Role of echocardiography in aortic stenosis: pre- and postoperative studies, *Am J Cardiol* 43:67-73, 1979.

157. Smallhorn JF, Pauperio H, Benson L, Freedom RM, Rowe RD: Pulsed Doppler assessment of pulmonary vein obstruction, *Am Heart J* 110:483-486, 1985.

158. Vick GW III, Murphy DJ Jr, Ludomirsky A et al: Pulmonary venous and systemic ventricular inflow obstruction in patients with congenital heart disease: detection by combined two-dimensional and Doppler echocardiography, *J Am Coll Cardiol* 9:580-587, 1987.

159. Valdes-Cruz LM, Pieroni DR, Roland JMA, Shematek JP: Recognition of residual postoperative shunts by contrast echocardiographic techniques, *Circulation* 55:148-152, 1977.

160. Meijboom EJ, Ebels T, Anderson RH et al: Left atrioventricular valve after surgical repair in atrioventricular septal defect with separate valve orifices ("ostium primum atrial septal defect"): an echo-Doppler study, *Am J Cardiol* 57:433-436, 1986.

161. Meijboom EJ, Wyse RKH, Ebels T et al: Doppler mapping of postoperative left atrioventricular valve regurgitation, *Circulation* 77:311-315, 1988.

162. Chin AJ, Sanders SP, Willimas RG, Lang P, Norwood WI, Castaneda AR: Two-dimensional echocardiographic assessment of caval and pulmonary venous pathways after the Senning operation, *Am J Cardiol* 52:118-126, 1983.

163. Satomi G, Nakamura K, Takao A, Imai Y: Two-dimensional echocardiographic detection of pulmonary venous channel stenosis after Senning's operation, *Circulation* 68:545-549, 1983.

164. Smallhorn JF, Burrows P, Wilson G, Coles J, Gilday DL, Freedom RM: Two-dimensional and pulsed Doppler echocardiography in the postoperative evaluation of total anomalous pulmonary venous connection, *Circulation* 76:298-305, 1987.

165. Fyfe DA, Currie PJ, Seward JB et al: Continuous-wave Doppler determination of the pressure gradient across pulmonary artery bands: hemodynamic correlation in 20 patients, *Mayo Clin Proc* 59:744-750, 1984.

166. Stevenson JG, Kawabori I, Bailey WW: Noninvasive evaluation of Blalock-Taussig shunts: determination of patency and differentiation from patient ductus arteriosus by Doppler echocardiography, *Am Heart J* 106:1121-1132, 1983.

167. Marx GR, Allen HD, Goldberg SJ: Doppler echocardiographic estimation of systolic pulmonary artery pressure in patients with aortic-pulmonary shunts, *J Am Coll Cardiol* 7:880-885, 1986.

168. Hagler DJ, Seward JB, Tajik AJ, Ritter DG: Functional assessment of the Fontan operation: combined M-mode, two-dimensional and Doppler echocardiographic studies, *J Am Coll Cardiol* 4:756-764, 1984.

169. DiSessa TG, Child JS, Perloff JK et al: Systemic venous and pulmonary arterial flow patterns after Fontan's procedure for tricuspid atresia or single ventricle, *Circulation* 70:898-902, 1984.

170. Nakazawa M, Nojima K, Okuda H et al: Flow dynamics in the main pulmonary artery after the Fontan procedure in patients with tricuspid atresia or single ventricle, *Circulation* 75:1117-1123, 1987.

171. Borow KM, Colan SD, Neumann A: Altered left ventricular mechanics in patients with valvular aortic stenosis and coarction of the aorta: effects on systolic performance and late outcome, *Circulation* 72:515-522, 1985.

172. Musewe NN, Smallhorn JF, Benson LN, Burrows PE, Freedom RM: Validation of Doppler-derived pulmonary arterial pressure with ductus arteriosus under different hemodynamic states, *Circulation* 76:1081-1091, 1987.

173. Leung MP, Mok CK, Hui PW: Echocardiographic assessment of neonates with pulmonary atresia and intact ventricular septum, *J Am Coll Cardiol* 12:719-725, 1988.

174. Bash SE, Huhta JC, Vick GW III, Gutgesell HP, Ott DA: Hypoplastic left heart syndrome: is echocardiography accurate enough to guide surgical palliation? *J Am Coll Cardiol* 7:610-616, 1986.

175. Huhta JC, Gutgesell HP, Latson LA, Huffines FD: Two-dimensional echocardiographic assessment of the aorta in infants and children with congenital heart disease, *Circulation* 70:417-424, 1984.

176. Newburger JW, Rosenthal A, Williams RG, Fellows K, Miettinen OS: Noninvasive tests in the initial evaluation of heart murmurs in children, *N Engl J Med* 308:61-64, 1983.

177. Sahn DJ: Intraoperative applications of two-dimensional and contrast two-dimensional echocardiography for evaluation of congenital, acquired and coronary heart disease in open-chested humans during cardiac surgery. In Rijsterborgh H, editor: *Echocardiology*, The Hague, 1981, Martinus Nijhoff Publishing, pp 9-23.

178. Takamoto S, Kyo S, Adachi H et al: Intraoperative color flow mapping by real-time two-dimensional Doppler echocardiography for evaluation of valvular and congenital heart disease and vascular disease, *J Thorac Cardiovasc Surg* 90:802-812, 1985.

179. Gussenhoven EJ, van Herwerden LA, Roelandt J, Ligtvoet KM, Bos E, Witsenburg M: Intraoperative two-dimensional echocardiography in congenital heart disease, *J Am Coll Cardiol* 9:565-572, 1987.

180. Czer LSC, Maurer G, Bolger AF et al: Intraoperative evaluation of mitral regurgitation by Doppler color flow mapping, *Circulation* 76:108-116, 1987.

181. Bierman FZ, Williams RG: Subxiphoid two-dimensional imaging of the interatrial septum in infants and neonates with congenital heart disease, *Circulation* 60:80-90, 1979.

182. Bierman FZ, Fellows K, Williams RG: Prospective identification of ventricular septal defects in infancy using subxiphoid two-dimensional echocardiography, *Circulation* 62:807-817, 1980.

183. Simpson IA, Sahn DJ, Valdes-Cruz LM, Chung KJ, Sherman FS, Swensson RE: Color Doppler flow mapping in patients with coarctation of the aorta: new observations and improved evaluation with color flow diameter and proximal acceleration as predictors of severity, *Circulation* 77:736-744, 1988.

184. Murphy DJ Jr, Ludomirsky A, Huhta JC: Continuous-wave Doppler in children with ventricular septal defect: noninvasive estimation of interventricular pressure gradient, *Am J Cardiol* 57:428-432, 1986.

185. Huhta JC, Latson LA, Gutgesell HP, Cooley DA, Kearney DL: Echocardiography in the diagnosis and management of symptomatic aortic valve stenosis in infants, *Circulation* 70:438-444, 1984.

186. Silverman NH, Hudson S: Evaluation of right ventricular volume and ejection fraction in children by two-dimensional echocardiography, *Pediatr Cardiol* 4:197-203, 1983.

187. Colan SD, Borow KM, Neumann A: Left ventricular end-systolic wall stress-velocity of fiber shortening relation: a load-independent index of myocardial contractility, *J Am Coll Cardiol* 4:715-724, 1984.

188. Huhta JC, Gutgesell HP, Nihill MR: Cross-sectional echocardiographic diagnosis of total anomalous pulmonary venous connection, *Br Heart J* 53:525-534, 1985.

189. Sanders SP, Bierman FZ, Williams RG: Conotruncal malformations: diagnosis in infancy using subxiphoid 2-dimensional echocardiography, *Am J Cardiol* 50:1361-1367, 1982.

190. Trowitzsch E, Colan SD, Sanders SP: Global and regional right ventricular function in normal infants and infants with transposition of the great arteries after Senning operation, *Circulation* 72:1008-1014, 1985.

191. Borow KM, Keane JF, Castaneda AR, Freed MD: Systemic ventricular function in patients with tetralogy of Fallot, ventricular septal defect and transposition of the great arteries repaired during infancy, *Circulation* 64:878-885, 1981.

192. Van Doesburg NH, Bierman FZ, Williams RG: Left ventricular geometry in infants with d-transposition of the great arteries and intact interventricular septum, *Circulation* 68:733-739, 1983.

193. Satomi G, Nakamura K, Narai S, Takao A: Systematic visualization of coronary arteries by two-dimensional echocardiography in children and infants: evaluation in Kawasaki's disease and coronary arteriovenous fistulas, *Am Heart J* 107:497-505, 1984.

194. Anderson TM, Meyer RA, Kaplan S: Long-term echocardiographic evaluation of cardiac size and function in patients with Kawasaki disease, *Am Heart J* 110:107-115, 1985.

195. Lipshultz SE, Chanock S, Sanders SP, Colan SD, Perez-Atayde A, McIntosh K: Cardiovascular manifestations of human immunodeficiency virus infection in infants and children, *Am J Cardiol* 63:1489-1497, 1989.

196. Sahn DJ, Lange LW, Allen HD et al: Quantitative real-time cross-sectional echocardiography in the developing normal human fetus and newborn, *Circulation* 62:588-597, 1980.

197. Schmidt KG, de Araujo LMD, Silverman NH: Evaluation of structural and functional abnormalities of the fetal heart by echocardiography, *Am J Cardiac Imaging* 2:57-76, 1988.

198. Kenny JF, Plappert T, Doubilet P et al: Changes in intracardiac blood flow velocities and right and left ventricular stroke volumes with gestational age in the normal human fetus: a prospective Doppler echocardiographic study, *Circulation* 74:1208-1216, 1986.

199. Kleinman CS, Donnerstein RL, Jaffe CC et al: Fetal echocardiography: a tool for evaluation of in utero cardiac arrhythmias and monitoring of in utero therapy: analysis of 71 patients, *Am J Cardiol* 51:237-243, 1983.

Index

Page numbers in *italics* indicate illustrations.

539